D1481076

MOLECULAR AND CELLULAR PHYSIOLOGY OF NEURONS

Molecular and Cellular Physiology of Neurons

GORDON L. FAIN

HARVARD UNIVERSITY PRESS

Cambridge, Massachusetts
London, England   1999

Illustrations by Margery J. Fain

Library of Congress Cataloging-in-Publication Data
Fain, Gordon L.
    Molecular and cellular physiology of neurons / Gordon L. Fain.
      p. cm.
    Includes bibliographical references and index.
    ISBN 0-674-58155-5 (alk. paper)
    1. Neurons. 2. Neurophysiology.
   3. Molecular neurobiology. I. Title.
QP363.F35   1999
573.8'536—dc21   98-44886

To the memory of Susumu Hagiwara

Contents

Preface

Nullum esse librum tam malum ut non aliqua parte prodesset.
—PLINY

THIS BOOK emerged from a series of course notes I have used to teach advanced undergraduates and graduate students in the Neuroscience Program at UCLA. In both classes I describe what I believe to be a recent synthesis of neurophysiology at the level of the molecules and cells of the nervous system. The basic premise of the courses and of this book is that molecules and cells matter. This is not to say that the nervous system can be completely understood merely by studying events at the cellular level, but that it *cannot* be understood unless we know how single molecules and cells function. I make no effort in my courses or in this book to cover topics in higher-level integration, such as sensory or motor function, neural networks, or imaging. These topics are an essential part of any neuroscientist's formation, but they are covered in other courses taught at UCLA.

The level of this book reflects the needs of our students, who have in general had calculus and college physics, as well as an introductory course in biology including molecular biology. Since a few of our students are weak in these areas, I have included a review of resistance and capacitance in Chapter 2, and brief explanations of gene cloning, expression, and site-directed mutagenesis in Chapters 1, 6, and 9. Our students have not in general had physical chemistry, matrix algebra, or differential equations. I have therefore postponed topics such as current flow in finite cables, rate theory, and single-channel kinetics to later study.

My aim has been to provide as much cellular physiology as I believe to be necessary to any serious student of the nervous system, regardless of his or her particular orientation. In addition, we have provided up-to-date reviews of many of the subjects currently of interest to neuroscientists, including channel activation and diversity, mechanisms of transmitter release, neuromodulation (including long-term potentiation), and sensory transduction. I hope this book will be useful not only to beginning graduate students but to anyone interested in the role of molecules and cells in the central nervous system.

I am grateful to Michael Fisher, Kate Schmit, Kate Brick, and the staff of Harvard University Press for their interest in this project, their patience, and their helpful comments and revisions. I am also grateful to the many friends and colleagues who offered encouragement, provided useful suggestions, and helped with the immense literature. I have cited reviews and papers that I have found to be essential points of departure for students beginning to read original articles concerning the topics covered by the book. Some recent citations have been included in proof and are placed in a separate section at the end of the References. I regret the inevitable oversight of papers that have been left out, in some cases to keep the reference list to a manageable size but in other instances, I am sure, through inadvertence or the limitations of time and energy.

I am particularly grateful to the following people, who read one or more chapters in an earlier draft: Michael Barish, Francisco Bezanilla, Mariel Birnbaumer, Bruce Cohen, John Dowling, Peter Gillespie, Alan Grinnell, Shaul Hestrin, Sally Krasne, John Lisman, Hugh Matthews, Istvan Mody, Richard Olsen, Diane Papazian, Edwin Richard, A. P. Sampath, Kathy Sweadner, Roger Thomas, Julio Vergara, Robert Zucker, and Frank Zufall. I also wish to thank the neuroscience students at UCLA who have read and corrected previous drafts of the manuscript; and to the external reviewers of Harvard University Press, who made many useful suggestions. Finally, I express my deepest gratitude to my wife Margery, who did all the illustrations for the book, helped with the proofreading, and put up with my behavior, even more eccentric than usual, during the two years the writing of this book required.

1

Introduction

THE BASIC PREMISE of this book is that if we are to understand the brain, we must discover how the individual molecules and cells of the nervous system produce electrical activity. It may not be obvious why this should be so. After all, it is probably not necessary to understand how a diode or even a transistor works to understand processing in a computer. Why do we need to know about the molecules and cells of the nervous system?

For someone who has spent most of his scientific career studying the photoreceptors of the eye, the importance of molecules and cells is abundantly clear. Many essential features of our visual behavior are a direct consequence of events in the photoreceptors. The extraordinary sensitivity of the eye is the result of the ability of the photoreceptors to detect single photons of light (Baylor, Lamb, and Yau, 1979), a process that ultimately depends upon the way the molecules of the photoreceptors are organized to convert a sensory signal into an electrical response with very high gain (see Chapter 16). The ability of the visual system to adjust to varying light levels also begins in the photoreceptor (Baylor and Hodgkin, 1974; Fain, 1976), and this, too, is a direct consequence of the modulation of the molecules of transduction, mediated principally through the action of calcium ions (Koutalos and Yau, 1996; Fain, Matthews, and Cornwall, 1996). Even spatial contrast begins in the photoreceptors (Baylor, Fuortes, and O'Bryan, 1971). Similar statements could be made for the other senses, for which events in the receptor itself have profound implications for our ability to perceive sensory stimuli.

What about the brain? Are single molecules and cells equally important for the infinitely more complex processing that occurs in the middle of the central nervous system? Every neuron has many thousands of different proteins, and many of these are absolutely essential for receiving and processing neural signals. The brain contains many billions of such cells, each connected to other cells with thousands of junctions called *synapses*. Is it really sensible to suppose that events at the level of single molecules or cells make an important contribution to higher mental function?

The answer to this question, I believe, is an unqualified yes. My explanation of why this is so begins with the pyramidal cell of the cerebral cortex (Fig. 1.1). This cell, first described in detail by the great Spanish neuroanatomist Santiago Ramón y Cajal (1909), is a principal building block of integration in the cortex, the part of the brain thought to be responsible for our most complicated behavior. Pyramidal cells receive input from axons coming from other parts of the brain and from interneurons and other pyramidal cells, principally on terminal swellings of the dendrites called *spines* (Fig. 1.1C). The signals from these inputs converge upon the cell body and generate an output signal in the axon, which travels either from one region of cortex to another or out of the cortex to other brain structures or to the spinal cord. There is considerable evidence that these cells play an essential role in higher brain functions, such as sensory perception, learning, and consciousness.

Twenty years ago, many neuroscientists would have said that these cells were too complicated to be understood with any of the techniques then available, and only a few laboratories were attempting to study pyramidal cell biochemistry or electrophysiology. Now there are hundreds of laboratories around the world doing this. Dramatic progress has been made, and there is considerable hope that we may truly know much of importance about these cells within our lifetime.

What has happened to bring about this change? We have seen a revolution in our ability to study the molecules and cells of the nervous system. It began with the invention of the patch electrode by Neher and Sakmann (1976), which made possible direct recordings from the molecules responsible for electrical activity in the central nervous system (CNS) (Sakmann and Neher, 1995). A few years later, refinements in the techniques of molecular biology for cloning genes and expressing proteins led to the isolation and characterization of ion channels, receptors, and the other molecular building blocks of neural function. These discoveries have had many practi-

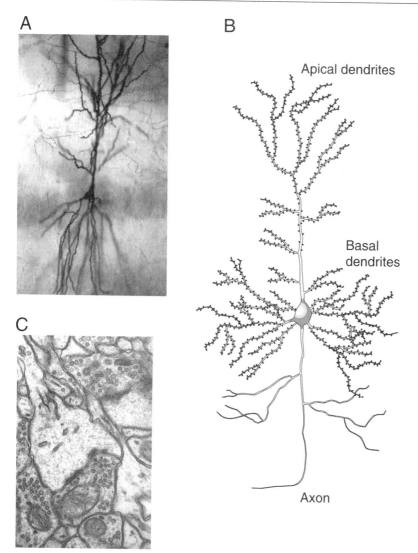

A

B

Apical dendrites

Basal dendrites

Axon

C

Fig. 1.1 Hippocampal pyramidal cell. **(A)** Micrograph of cell stained with the Golgi method by Kirsten M. Harris. **(B)** Schematic drawing of a typical pyramidal cell. Numerous spines cover the apical and basal dendrites. **(C)** High-power electron micrograph of portion of hippocampal cell dendrite. A spine is visible as the light gray area in the center of the micrograph. The synapse can be identified from the dark, electron-dense regions near the membrane of the spine, which are called "postsynaptic densities." Note the accumulation of synaptic vesicles in the cell synapsing onto the spine. The structure of synapses is described in more detail in Chapter 8 (see Figs. 8.8 and 8.9). (Photographs in **(A)** and **(C)** courtesy of Kirsten M. Harris.)

cal benefits, since they have provided a molecular basis for understanding neurological disorders and the effects of drugs on the nervous system. They have also completely altered the landscape of cellular neuroscience by demonstrating beyond any doubt that single molecules and cells can provide essential insight into mechanisms likely to be responsible for higher mental function.

Patch-Clamp Recording

Before the invention of the patch electrode by Neher and Sakmann, only a few methods were available for recording the electrical activity of cells in the brain. Some properties of pyramidal cells were deduced by registering the spiking output of axons with fine-tipped metal electrodes placed just outside the axon or soma of the cell. This method of *extracellular recording* proved to be especially useful in the visual cortex and provided the first information of the cellular events responsible for higher visual processing (Hubel and Wiesel, 1977). In the late 1940s, Ling and Gerard (1949) introduced the use of fine glass microelectrodes called *intracellular micropipettes*. These are made by pulling small tubes of glass over a heated coil or flame. The pipettes are filled with salt solution and are inserted through the plasma membrane of nerve and muscle cells to record membrane potentials and electrical activity. The discovery of newer and better mechanical devices for pulling these electrodes, and particularly the invention of the Flaming-Brown puller (Brown and Flaming, 1977), made possible the construction of very fine tipped pipettes, which could even be inserted into the small cell bodies of CNS neurons. Intracellular recording made possible many important discoveries, including the first information about the cellular basis of synaptic action in the nervous system (see for example Eccles, 1964). Furthermore, the combination of this technique with anatomical techniques such as electron microscopy provided a unified view of the nervous system as a cellular machine, driven by interactions between distinct cell types.

As useful as these techniques have been, they have now been largely superseded by the much more powerful methods made possible by the patch electrode. A patch electrode is made from fine glass tubing, much as an intracellular pipette, but the tip of the electrode must be fashioned so that it is very smooth, for example by polishing the end of the pipette with heat under a microscope. The pipette is then pressed against the cell body (or axon or dendrite) of a neuron or other cell type, and slight suction is applied, generally by mouth (Fig. 1.2). The cell membrane of the neuron then adheres to the rim of the pipette, forming a very high resistance seal. The strength of the seal greatly reduces the background

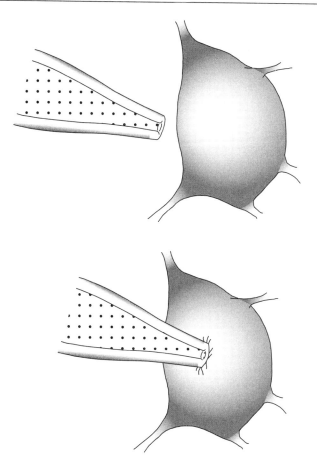

noise of the recording and makes it possible to visualize the electrical currents caused by ions flowing through single channels.

Before the invention of the patch electrode, we knew that electrical signals were produced by the flow of ions through protein channels in the membranes of nerve cells, and many inferences about the opening and closing of these protein "gates" had been made from voltage-clamp recordings (see Chapter 5) and from measurements of membrane noise (Katz and Miledi, 1972). To these deductions were suddenly added actual measurements of the current passing through the channels, giving an extraordinary view of the working of a single molecule. First acetylcholine receptors (Neher

A

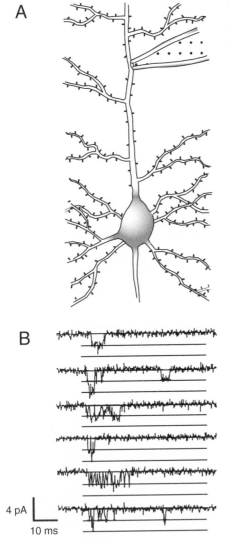

B

4 pA

10 ms

Fig. 1.3 Patch-clamp recording from primary apical dendrite of pyramidal cell. **(A)** Method of recording. **(B)** Single Na$^+$ channel openings recorded with cell-attached patch clamp from the apical dendrite of a CA1 pyramidal cell in a rat hippocampal slice. Openings were evoked as the membrane potential was raised from −70 mV to −40 mV. Figure presents consecutive recordings from a single patch. Horizontal lines indicate zero current level and incremental current levels of −1.7 picoamperes (pA), the size of the current produced by a single channel opening. Notice that in the second and sixth sweeps, two channels were open simultaneously for a brief period. Note also the scale bars at lower left, indicating the level of electrical activity by the vertical bar (in this case current), and time by the horizontal bar (in milliseconds). (Reprinted from Magee and Johnston, 1995, with permission of the authors and of the Physiological Society.)

and Sakmann, 1976) and then Na$^+$ channels (Sigworth and Neher, 1980) were studied by this technique, and in a very short time single-channel recordings were obtained from many of the principal channel molecules of the nervous system.

Figure 1.3 (from Magee and Johnston, 1995) illustrates some of the power of this method. In this case, a patch pipette has been pushed up against the principal apical dendrite of a cortical pyramidal cell, and depolarization of the membrane directly beneath the pipette produces brief openings of Na$^+$ channels on the dendrite membrane. These recordings, and those from other laboratories (Stuart and Sakmann, 1994), provided the first direct demonstration of the presence of Na$^+$ channels in pyramidal cell apical dendrites, and similar recordings from a variety of cell types have yielded important information about the molecular mechanisms of activation and inactivation for voltage-gated channels (see Chapter 6).

Excised-Patch and Whole-Cell Recording

Measurements of the kind shown in Figs. 1.2 and 1.3, which were the first kinds of recordings to be made with patch electrodes, are now called *on-cell* or *cell-attached* recordings. This sort of recording remains useful for certain kinds of experiments, but even more powerful are the techniques of *excised-patch* and *whole-cell* recording (see Hamill et al., 1981). As Fig. 1.4 shows, if a patch pipette sealed onto the membrane of a cell is gently lifted off, very often the membrane patch is carried along with it. This forms an *inside-out* patch: a piece of the membrane of the cell is spread over the orifice of the pipette, with the cytoplasmic surface of the membrane facing the outside of the pipette. This technique allows much better control of the voltage across the membrane and makes it possible directly to perfuse the inside surface of the membrane with substances like Ca^{2+}, cAMP, and protein kinases, to study the regulation of channel gating. Remarkably, many channels survive this treatment quite well, and inside-out recording has become an enormously powerful method for exploring channel function.

If the pipette remains in contact with the cell and the on-cell patch is subjected to additional suction (or to a sudden high-voltage pulse), the membrane beneath the cell often ruptures, al-

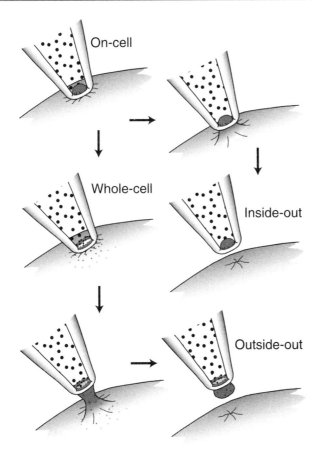

Fig. 1.4 Patch-clamp recording. Methods for making whole-cell and isolated patch recordings. (After Hamill et al., 1981.)

lowing a *whole-cell* recording. In this configuration, the inside of the pipette is in direct contact with the inside of the cell. This has several extraordinary implications. First, the solution inside the pipette exchanges with the solution inside the cell, so it is possible for the experimenter to alter the composition of ions inside the cell. Second messengers, enzymes, inhibitors, and Ca^{2+} indicator dyes can be introduced into the cell merely by placing them in the pipette. This is often a tremendous advantage for studying the effects of substances that are effective only when placed in the cytoplasm.

A second implication of the direct connection between the pipette and cell cytoplasm is that a patch pipette can be used much as an intracellular pipette to record the voltage difference across the cell membrane, but whole-cell recordings are more stable and can be made reliably even from small cells. Furthermore, since the resistance of a patch pipette is comparatively low, a whole-cell recording can be used to *voltage-clamp* the cell (Marty and Neher, 1995). Voltage-clamping was first implemented in the 1940s to study Na^+ and K^+ currents in squid axons, as I describe in detail in Chapter 5. With a voltage clamp, it is possible to measure membrane currents at constant membrane voltage. This is more useful than simply recording the membrane potential, since changes in current are a direct measure of the changes in conductance produced by channel opening and closing.

Before the development of whole-cell recording, voltage-clamping could be used only with relatively large cells, those which could be penetrated with two microelectrodes. Now even small cells can be clamped, routinely and with relatively little difficulty. It would not be too much of an exaggeration to say that whole-cell recording (with its near relation, the perforated patch—Horn and Marty, 1988) has entirely changed the way most scientists study single nerve cells. Recordings can be made not only from isolated cells but from cells in brain slices (see Edwards et al., 1989; Sakmann and Stuart, 1995). No cell in the nervous system is now beyond the reach of this method.

But this is not all. Having established a whole-cell recording, the experimenter can then gently lift the pipette off the cell. Then, in a way not clearly understood, the excised membrane of the cell will often flap around and reseal on the pipette, with its *outside* surface facing outward. This is called an *outside-out* recording (see Fig. 1.4) and is especially useful for investigating *ligand-gated* channels, like acetylcholine and glutamate receptors. Since these receptors are activated by the binding of synaptic transmitters on the extracellular surface of the receptor, they can be studied with outside-out recording simply by placing the transmitters in the bathing solution.

The Cloning of Membrane Proteins

At about the same time patch-clamp recording was invented, the first successful attempts were made to isolate the membrane proteins responsible for electrical activity. Henderson and Wang (1972) and Benzer and Raftery (1973) first showed that the Na^+ channels of nerves could be isolated using a specific toxin called tetrodotoxin (see Chapter 5), which binds with high affinity to the Na^+ channel protein. This binding was used as an assay to identify the protein in solubilized fractions of nerve membrane, a technique that ultimately led to the biochemical isolation of sodium channels (see Catterall, 1992). With similar methods, several other membrane proteins essential for nerve cell signaling were also purified.

At the time this work was being done, it was unclear to many scientists whether the isolation of these proteins would provide any useful information about their function. Signaling proteins like Na^+ channels are generally present in small amounts even in axons and are difficult to purify; moreover, the strong detergents that are required to pull these proteins out of the plasma membrane often produce large changes in protein conformation and activity. It is now quite clear, however, that these experiments have proved absolutely essential for the eventual characterization of membrane channels. Not only has study of the isolated proteins themselves provided much useful information about the subunit composition, stoichiometry, and structure of the molecules (see Chapters 6–10), it has also revealed partial amino acid sequences of the proteins; and from these sequences, it has been possible to make probes that have allowed the first channel protein genes to be cloned.

The first channel genes that were cloned were all cloned in the same way (Fig. 1.5). The channel was first separated from other proteins, generally with chromatography or electrophoresis, and identified by binding with a specific, high-affinity ligand like

Fig. 1.5 Method of cloning used for many of the first proteins whose genes were cloned from the nervous system. This method begins with the isolation and purification of the protein from tissue. The protein is then partially sequenced, and the peptide sequence is used to synthesize DNA or RNA complementary to the DNA coding for this sequence. These nucleotides are then used to probe a tissue library to determine clones containing the gene for the peptide. Alternatively, the purified protein can be used to produce antibodies, which can be used to screen an expression library. These methods were used for the first cloning of Na^+ channels, Ca^{2+} channels, GABA receptors, glycine receptors, and photoreceptor cyclic nucleotide-gated channels (see text for references). Other cloning methods were used for K^+ channels and glutamate receptors (see Chapters 6 and 9).

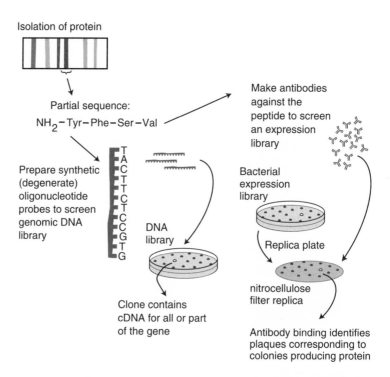

Cloning a gene from partial sequence of a protein

Isolation of protein

Partial sequence:

NH_2 – Tyr – Phe – Ser – Val

Make antibodies against the peptide to screen an expression library

Prepare synthetic (degenerate) oligonucleotide probes to screen genomic DNA library

DNA library

Bacterial expression library

Clone contains cDNA for all or part of the gene

Replica plate

nitrocellulose filter replica

Antibody binding identifies plaques corresponding to colonies producing protein

tetrodotoxin. The protein was then digested with a protease like trypsin, and a few small-molecular-weight peptides were isolated and sequenced. From the peptide sequence, synthetic nucleotide sequences were synthesized and used to screen a library of clones, made from RNA isolated from neural tissue. Alternatively, an antibody was made to the isolated channel protein, and the antibody was used to screen an expression library. The DNA of identified clones was then sequenced and examined for structures that might form ion channels (see Watson et al., 1992).

With this method, the first clones and sequences were obtained for the genes of: *Na+ channels* (Noda et al., 1984), *acetylcholine receptors* (Kubo et al., 1986), *Ca2+ channels* (Tanabe et al., 1987), *GABA receptors* (Schofield et al., 1987), *glycine receptors* (Grenningloh et al., 1987), and photoreceptor *cyclic nucleotide-gated channels* (Kaupp et al., 1989). Other methods described later (see Chapters 6 and 9) were used to clone and sequence the genes for K⁺ channels (Papazian et al., 1987; Tempel et al., 1987; Kamb, Iverson, and Tanouye, 1987; Pongs et al., 1988) and glutamate receptors (Hollman et al., 1989; Moriyoshi et al., 1991).

Ultimately, the identification of a DNA sequence as that of a channel-forming protein rests upon the demonstration that the DNA in question can direct the synthesis of a molecule with biological activity: if it looks like a channel, it must also walk and talk like a channel. This can be done by *expressing* the channel. The DNA of the identified clone can be used to make complementary RNA, or cRNA (Swanson and Folander, 1992), which is then

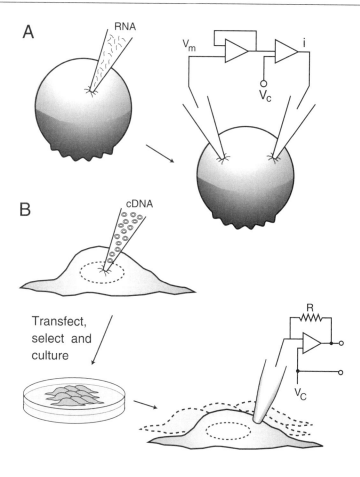

Fig. 1.6 Methods of expression. **(A)** RNA injected into a *Xenopus* oocyte directs the expression of protein, whose biological activity can be recorded by two-electrode voltage clamp or with patch electrodes (after removal of the oocyte's vitelline membrane). V_m, membrane potential; V_c, command potential; i, current. **(B)** Transfection. The DNA is incorporated into a plasmid or viral vector and introduced into the cell by one of several methods, including electroporation, Ca^{2+} shock, and direct injection into the nucleus. The DNA then becomes a part of the genome of the host cell, and the cells are cultured and selected for those expressing the clonal DNA. Once the cell has expressed the protein, its biological activity can be recorded with a patch electrode, either with whole-cell or excised-patch recording. V_c, command potential; R, feedback resistance of patch amplifier.

injected into an oocyte of the frog *Xenopus* (Fig. 1.6A—Goldin, 1992). In very many cases the cRNA is transcribed by the oocyte just as if it were native messenger RNA (mRNA), and channels are inserted into the oocyte's membrane. The oocyte can then be voltage-clamped and the biological activity of the channel recorded (Stühmer, 1992). Na$^+$ channel cRNA forms voltage-gated Na$^+$ currents, acetylcholine channel cRNA forms channels gated by acetylcholine, and so on. Remarkably, channels expressed from cloned genes often have properties quite similar to those of native channels. When differences exist, they have often been quite helpful in stimulating the search for new channel subunits.

An alternative method of expressing the protein is to incorporate DNA from the clone directly into the DNA of a cultured cell by a process called *transfection.* The DNA from the clone is placed in a *vector,* made from a virus or plasmid, which can be introduced into the cell by a variety of methods, including Ca^{2+} shock and direct injection into the nucleus (see Fig. 1.6B). The cloned DNA is directly incorporated into the DNA of the cell genome and, if properly linked to promoters or other regulatory elements, can be transcribed into RNA, which can be translated into protein. In some cases the transfection is transient, but in others a stable population of cells is produced expressing the protein. Transfection is often more convenient than RNA expression in oocytes, since cultured cell lines provide an excellent preparation for recording with patch-clamp electrodes, particularly for single-channel recording.

The identification of sequences for membrane channels has given us our first clues about the structure of these proteins. From the peptide sequence alone, reasonable guesses can be made about which amino acids lie within the hydrophobic interior of the membrane and which are more likely to face the cytoplasmic or extracellular solution: some amino acids (such as valine and isoleucine) are hydrophobic and much more likely to be surrounded by lipid or other protein, whereas others (such as aspartate and lysine) are hydrophilic or even charged and much more likely to be surrounded by water. By a process known as *hydropathy analysis,* the sequence of amino acids can be used to make inferences about how the protein folds and is integrated into the membrane.

Hydropathy analysis, though by no means free from uncertainty, has been remarkably helpful in producing hypothetical models of protein structure, which can then be subjected to experimentation. A variety of methods can be used to determine which parts of the protein face the intracellular or extracellular surface. For example, antibodies to specific sequences can be used to localize parts of the protein to one side of the membrane or the other. Sequences that can be identified as substrates for glycosylation (sugar addition) or protein phosphorylation (phosphate addition) are sometimes helpful in identifying regions that are extracellular or cytoplasmic. Even more helpful are sequences that can actually be shown to be glycosylated or phosphorylated. More recently, the techniques of molecular biology have been used to modify the protein sequence to test in a more rigorous way the location of particular parts of the protein.

Later in the book, many experiments will be described for which synthetic DNA was constructed with one or more altered nucleotides to produce *site-directed mutations* of single amino acids in predetermined positions. In other cases, the DNA was cleaved at designated sites to produce specific *deletions* of part of the protein sequence. Finally, regions of peptide sequence have been exchanged between related proteins to produce *chimeric* proteins, containing part of one protein and part of another. Experiments with these techniques have afforded remarkable insight into the relationship between the structure of channels and their physiology. These and other results have shown that ion channels are multimeric proteins with a central core providing the pathway for ion permeation (see Fig. 1.7), and they have helped to identify structures responsible for forming ion pores and for producing voltage-dependent gating and ligand binding. Ultimately, this information can be expected to give a detailed molecular description of channel function that will not only be fundamental to our understanding of how the nervous system works, but will also aid in drug design, genetic testing of hereditary neurological disorders, and eventually the treatment and cure of mental illness.

An Illustration: The NMDA Receptor

The development of the patch electrode and the cloning of many of the proteins important for nerve cell function have produced a

Fig. 1.7 Structure of ion channels viewed in cross-section and from the extracellular or intracellular space. **(A)** Voltage-gated channels, such as Na$^+$ and K$^+$ channels of axons. Only main (α) subunit is illustrated. Channel is either a multimer of four α subunits (K$^+$ channels) or is composed of a single α subunit with four distinct *repeat domains* (Na$^+$ and Ca^{2+} channels). See Chapter 6. **(B)** Ligand-gated channels, such as acetylcholine receptors. Channel is again a multimer but is composed of 5 subunits. See Chapter 9. For both voltage-gated and ligand-gated channels, the ion conductance pathway is thought to be formed by regions of the channel protein lining a pore in the middle of the multimeric structure (see Box 7.2).

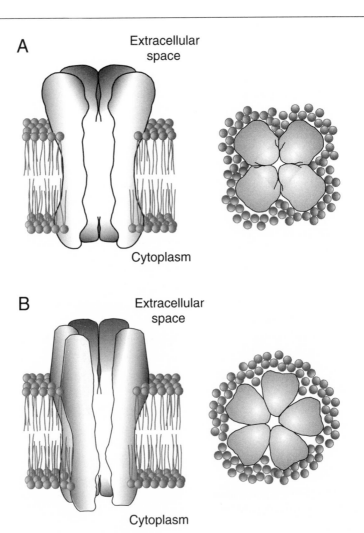

new synthesis of understanding of the physiology of the nervous system at the level of single molecules. One way of appreciating the importance of these new methods is to take a specific example. I have chosen the NMDA receptor, a synaptic receptor type found in pyramidal cells and in many (perhaps most) of the neurons of the CNS. NMDA receptors are activated by the amino acid glutamate, which is the most common chemical transmitter used at excitatory synapses in the brain. NMDA receptors can be distinguished from other glutamate receptors by their selective activation with the compound N-methyl-D-aspartate, and they are sites of action of many drugs, in particular the compound 1-(1-phenyl-cyclohexyl)piperidine, also known as PCP, phencyclidine, or *angel dust*. PCP was originally developed as a general anesthetic in the 1950s but was withdrawn from clinical use because of its dangerous side effects. It remains, unhappily, a popular drug of abuse. At the concentrations normally ingested, PCP is a selective blocker of NMDA receptors. A single dose can produce paranoia, hallucinations, and disturbances in attention and perception that can last days or even weeks. These symptoms in aggregate are clinically indistinguishable from those shown by patients with schizophrenia (see Javitt and Zukin, 1991). Furthermore, schizophrenics who ingest even a single low dose of PCP have aggravated symptoms that can last for many weeks.

Considerable insight into the function of NMDA receptors has been gained from studies of their molecular biology and physiology. The receptors are either tetramers or pentamers composed of four or five subunits of at least two different kinds, one called NR1 and the other NR2 (see Chapter 9). There seems to be only a single gene for NR1, but the RNA produced from this gene can be alternatively spliced to generate at least 8 different proteins, with dramatic effects on the pharmacology and physiology of the receptor (see McBain and Mayer, 1994; Zukin and Bennett, 1995). There are at least 4 genes for NR2, at least some of which also produce RNA that can be alternatively spliced. The different splice variants of NR1 and the different genes and splice variants for NR2 are produced in different parts of the brain and probably form receptors localized to different parts of the nervous system. This large diversity is typical of ion channels and other proteins important for CNS function and is interesting for two reasons. First, if different receptors are specific to different synapses, they are probably serving different functions. What these functions are is still unclear, but the differences probably exist for some good reason. Second, if the pharmacology of receptor subtypes is different, it may be possible to target different drugs to different subtypes. The pharmacology of the future may be just this: discovering drugs that act in particular locations rather than globally, to produce selective action with the fewest possible side effects.

NMDA Receptors are Coincidence Detectors

The physiology of NMDA receptors is unlike that of any other receptor we know and indicates that these molecules may have some special functions within the central nervous system. The NMDA receptor contains within itself an ion channel, opened by the binding of glutamate or the compound N-methyl-D-aspartate to sites on the extracellular surface of the receptor. In addition, the receptor contains binding sites for glycine, and these must also be occupied for channel opening to occur (Johnson and Ascher, 1987). Even with both glutamate and glycine bound to the channel, openings are rare and brief, since the channel is normally blocked at the resting membrane potential. This block can only be removed when strong excitation is produced by some other event at the synapse or elsewhere within the cell.

The block of the NMDA receptor is produced by extracellular Mg^{2+}, at its normal concentration in the extracellular spaces of the brain. This was discovered by two groups nearly simultaneously (Nowak et al., 1984; Mayer, Westbrook, and Guthrie, 1984). The recordings in Fig. 1.8 (from Ascher and Nowak, 1988) were made with patch electrodes from embryonic mouse neurons. They show representative openings of single NMDA channels from outside-out patches in the presence of glycine, NMDA at a concentration of

Fig. 1.8 Representative single-channel recordings from outside-out patches pulled from embryonic mouse neurons. Numbers above and to right of channel openings give Mg^{2+} concentration in μM. Openings were induced by perfusion with 10 μM NMDA in the presence of glycine. **(A)** Membrane potential, −60 mV. **(B)** Membrane potential, +40 mV. Note the increasing channel blocking (a flickering effect) with increasing Mg^{2+} concentration at −60 mV, but lack of blocking at +40 mV. (From Ascher and Nowak, 1988; reprinted with permission of the authors and of the Physiological Society.)

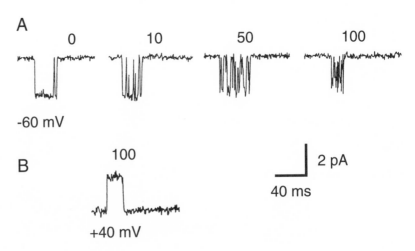

10 μM, and Mg^{2+} at concentrations from 0 to 100 μM. Remember that an outside-out patch has its extracellular surface facing the bath and its cytoplasmic surface facing the inside of the patch pipette (see Fig. 1.4). Outside-out patches are particularly useful for studying NMDA responses, since NMDA (and glycine and Mg^{2+}) can be perfused across the outside surface of the patch to activate and modulate the receptor.

The recordings in Fig. 1.8 were made at two different potentials: at −60 mV, near the normal resting potential of the cell (part A); and at a considerably more positive potential, +40 mV (part B). At −60 mV and in Mg^{2+}-free solution, the openings of the channel produce a trace with a characteristically simple shape when the outside-out patch is exposed to NMDA and glycine. The downward deflection of the recording at −60 mV is produced by an inward current, suddenly activated as the channel opens. After some period of time—of random duration, like the decay of a radioactive isotope—the NMDA (or glycine) falls off the receptor and the channel closes.

In the presence of Mg^{2+}, on the other hand, the channel opens and then rapidly flickers between open and closed. This produces a burst of brief openings. The length of the burst is again largely determined by the length of binding of NMDA and glycine to the receptor, but the openings within the burst are a function of Mg^{2+} concentration; the greater the concentration, the shorter the openings and the more rapid the flickering. This happens for the most part because Mg^{2+} enters the channel pore and blocks the channel, but the Mg^{2+} then comes rapidly off and back onto its binding site, producing rapid channel block and unblock. The block is facilitated by the negative membrane potential of the cell, since negativity inside the cell attracts the positively charged Mg^{2+} ion from the external solution into the channel pore. At physiological concentrations of Mg^{2+} (2.4 mM in the cerebrospinal fluid), the channel is almost entirely blocked at the resting membrane potential. As the membrane potential is made positive, the positivity inside the cell repels the Mg^{2+}, so that the probability of channel opening increases. At progressively more positive membrane potentials, the block by Mg^{2+} becomes less and less probable; and at very positive membrane potentials, the Mg^{2+} is almost without effect (Fig. 1.8B).

Fig. 1.9 Voltage-dependent block of NMDA channel by Mg^{2+}. *Left:* NMDA receptor shown as pentameric—but see Laube, Kuhse, and Betz (1998) and Chapter 9. With membrane potential *(Vm)* at −60 mV, neither glutamate nor glycine is bound to the receptor, and the channel is in closed conformation.

Middle: Glutamate and glycine are bound to the channel, which has assumed an open conformation; but at a membrane potential close to the resting membrane potential, the channel is blocked by external Mg^{2+}. Schema is not meant to indicate number or position of glutamate or glycine binding sites (see Chapter 9).

Right: Glutamate and glycine are bound to channel and channel is in open conformation. Membrane potential is now at a more positive value, as the result of excitation produced by some other input. The Mg^{2+} block is relieved and Ca^{2+} and other cations can now permeate the channel.

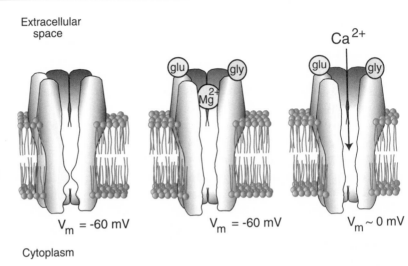

Extracellular space

Ca^{2+}

V_m = -60 mV V_m = -60 mV V_m ~ 0 mV

Cytoplasm

The voltage-dependent block of Mg^{2+} may be responsible for some of the most interesting properties of the NMDA receptor (Fig. 1.9). Since at negative membrane potentials the channel is blocked, the activation of the NMDA receptor by glutamate and glycine is not sufficient *by itself* to permit the receptor channel to open for a significant period of time. The cell containing the receptor must also be excited rather strongly by some other process, to make the membrane potential of the cell more positive and relieve some part of the Mg^{2+} block. Excitation may result from activation of other types of glutamate receptors in the vicinity of the NMDA receptors, or from more global influences, such as action potentials produced at the cell body and propagating back into the dendrites (Markram et al., 1997). The NMDA receptor is therefore a coincidence detector: only when both glutamate and glycine bind *and* the cell is strongly excited by some other mechanism will ions flow through the channel.

When the channel finally does open, it permits the flow of cations like Na^+ and K^+, but it also facilitates the influx of the important second messenger ion Ca^{2+} (see Fig. 1.9), which can produce changes in other second messengers, like cyclic AMP and nitric oxide, and directly activate protein kinases and phosphatases to modulate the activity of receptors and other molecules of importance in synaptic function (see Chapter 13). There is increasing evidence that NMDA receptor activation and Ca^{2+} influx at the spines of some kinds of pyramidal cells are responsible for a very long-lasting change in the efficacy of synaptic transmission, called *long-term potentiation (LTP)*. During LTP, the amplitude of the synaptic response can increase several-fold, and this effect can last for days or even weeks. LTP has been proposed to be an important mechanism of learning and memory (see Chapter 14), although this notion has not yet been firmly established. Regardless of the specific function of LTP, there can be little question that large changes in synaptic efficacy lasting for such long periods of time must have an important role in higher brain function.

Molecules and Cells

The example of the NMDA receptor demonstrates without doubt, I believe, that understanding the molecules and cells of the nervous system is absolutely essential to understanding the function of the brain. The unique properties of this multimeric protein have provided a surprising new perspective on the way certain circuits in the nervous system may be facilitated or depressed. The properties of this receptor are fundamental to many of the most interesting new models that attempt to explain the cellular basis of learning and memory.

This receptor has also taught us several other lessons of importance. Since the block of the NMDA receptors can be relieved when excitation spreads from one part of the pyramidal cell to another, it is clearly important to know how signals are conducted throughout the dendrites of a neuron. The Ca^{2+} permeability of NMDA receptors illustrates how important it is to understand the *ion selectivity* of a channel—that is, to know which ions can permeate the conductance pore. The Mg^{2+} block is voltage-dependent: we need to know about cell voltages, how they are produced and maintained, and how they are altered. To understand long-term changes in synaptic processing, it is essential to understand the basic mechanisms responsible for synaptic transmitter release and for the opening and closing of channels. Finally, we need to know about second messengers and signal modulation to understand processes such as LTP.

The philosopher Otto Neurath said that doing science was like building a ship in the open sea. Planks must be put in place sometimes provisionally, then new planks added to support or replace the old. To understand recent developments in molecular and cellular neurophysiology, we must begin with some of the oldest, most encrusted timbers, which still sit squarely among the floorboards. I therefore start by giving an introduction to the electrical properties of cell membranes. This serves two purposes: it provides a review of simple electrical circuits, essential for much of the rest of the book; and it conveys something of the power of recent techniques for understanding the shape of nerve cells. I then proceed to membrane potentials, ion permeability, and homeostasis. Whole-cell recording has made investigations of channel selectivity much easier and more accurate than previously, and these methods have been used in many more recent studies that probe the structure of channel pores.

Once the oldest beams of this ship have been inspected, I then proceed to the classic experiments of Hodgkin and Huxley, which are examined in detail in Chapter 5. These serve as prelude for more recent experiments on voltage-gated channels described in Chapters 6 and 7. In a similar way, the experiments of Katz, Miledi, and their colleagues on synaptic transmission in Chapter 8 are used to place in context newer revelations about the proteins responsible for transmitter release and the postsynaptic receptors responsible for excitatory and inhibitory transmission (Chapters 9 and 10).

The remainder of the book follows these established themes and describes, in Chapters 11–13, the receptors, G proteins, effector molecules, and second messengers responsible for metabotropic transmission. I describe many important new biochemical discoveries about these molecules, not to provide a comprehensive treatment of the chemistry of the nervous system, but to shed light on how these molecules regulate nerve cell behavior. This part of the book culminates in Chapter 14, with a discussion of long-term potentiation. The final two chapters describe the molecules and cellular events responsible for sensory transduction.

I hope to show not only what we know but how we know it. Each chapter provides details on individual experiments taken from the literature. Some of these (such as those of Hodgkin and Huxley) are well enough established to have entered the pantheon of the greats, and some are less well known but also illustrate the techniques and approaches that have formed our present view of nerve cell function. These experiments are described in enough detail so that the papers themselves can be consulted, and an extensive list of citations has been provided for this purpose, including many reviews of current literature.

My goal is to explain the responses of nerve cells in terms of their molecular components. Although it is not yet possible to do this as completely as one would like, much can be said about how channels, receptors, second messengers, and signaling enzymes alter the electrical potential across the nerve cell membrane. I hope to convey some of the excitement of these new discoveries, while at the same time providing a solid foundation in cellular neurophysiology, essential to any student of the brain.

PART ONE

Electrical Properties of Cells and Homeostasis

2

Passive Electrical Properties
of Neurons

A NERVE CELL integrates incoming signals by performing simple calculations. It adds and subtracts inputs from excitatory and inhibitory synapses, and the results of these calculations are reflected in the output signal that the cell transmits to other cells. For the pyramidal cell in Fig. 1.1, for example, there are many excitatory synapses onto spines (Fig. 1.1C). At these synapses, a presynaptic neuron releases a transmitter (glutamate) that activates receptors on the plasma membrane of the spine, and this produces a positive change (called a "depolarization") in the spine membrane potential. These depolarizations are summed and communicated to other parts of the pyramidal cell's dendritic tree and to the cell body and axon. The depolarization of the axon produces action potentials (see Chapter 5), which are propagated sometimes for very long distances to other parts of the nervous system.

The spread of signals throughout the dendritic tree allows inputs in different parts of the cell to interact with one another (Yuste and Tank, 1996). For pyramidal cells in the hippocampus, the spread of excitation from one dendrite to the next may have important implications for our behavior, since these cells are thought to participate in some forms of learning. Learning in many cases is *associative:* that is, learning occurs more easily if one event is paired with another. The summing of synaptic inputs within the dendritic tree may be in part responsible for this phenomenon (see Chapter 14).

Signal Spread

The principal means of signal spread in the dendritic tree of a neuron is *passive spread* or *electrotonic decay.* This is the spread of voltage (or current) that occurs purely as the result of the resistance

Fig. 2.1 Electrical equivalent of plasma membrane. *R,* resistance; *C,* capacitance.

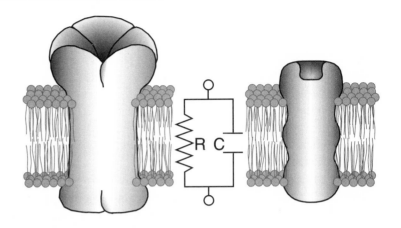

and capacitance of the cell membrane. The membrane of neurons, like the membrane of other cells in the body, is composed mostly of phospholipid and protein, and membrane of this composition behaves much like a resistance in parallel with a capacitance (Fig. 2.1). Dendrites are long cylinders of membrane that behave like electrical cables. This means that electrical signals can spread down the dendrite, though the signal progressively decreases in amplitude and speed the farther down the cable it proceeds.

In some cells, passive spread is the *only* means of signal propagation. Consider the cell in Fig. 2.2, which is called a *starburst amacrine cell.* This cell is found in the retina of the eye in probably every vertebrate species, including our own. It is nothing like a pyramidal cell: it has no axon and (in mature animals) does not produce action potentials (Zhou and Fain, 1996). Furthermore, it has a complex and nearly symmetric dendritic tree. Inputs to this cell are uniformly distributed throughout the dendrites, but outputs, *which also occur on the dendrites,* are restricted to the distal one-third of each dendritic branch (Famiglietti, 1991). It would therefore be possible, at least in theory, for each dendrite to act as a semi-independent unit, receiving input and sending output, perhaps unaffected by processing in other parts of the cell. Starburst cells are thought by many to play some role in sensing the direction of movement, and it is conceivable that each dendrite analyzes motion in a different direction.

To see if the dendrites of this cell *do* behave in this way, we would need some method of studying signal spread. We could imagine approaching the cell with a patch pipette and forming a seal on a dendrite, much as for the pyramidal cell's apical dendrite in Fig. 1.3. We could *imagine* doing such a thing, but unfortunately the dendrites of these cells are less than a micron in diameter, much smaller in diameter than the apical dendrite of a pyramidal cell and smaller even than the tip of a typical patch electrode (Sakmann and Neher, 1995). Other methods of recording, such as intracellular recording with a fine-tipped electrode, are equally impractical, at least with the techniques we presently have.

If electrical recording is not possible, what can we do to study this cell? One answer is this: we can use what we know about passive signal spread and the electrical properties of neurons to create a reasonable electrical model of the amacrine cell. From this model (and with the help of one of a number of readily available computer programs), we can *calculate* how signal spreads from one dendrite to another. Although a model of this sort is less satisfactory than an actual experimental measurement, it is probably accurate enough to teach us a great deal about how postsynaptic responses spread throughout the dendritic tree. Furthermore, at least for the amacrine cell in Fig. 2.2, a model of this sort may at present

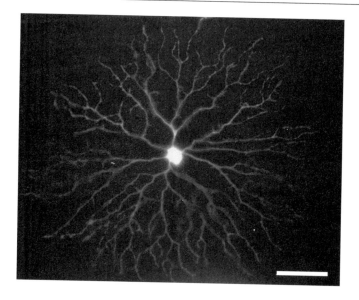

Fig. 2.2 Starburst amacrine cell. Cell stained in rabbit retina during whole-cell recording with pipette filled with dye Lucifer Yellow™. Scale bar, 50 μm. (Photograph courtesy of Z. J. Zhou.)

be the only way we can learn anything about the details of signal processing in a cell of this sort.

In this chapter, I describe how to make an electrical model of a cell, beginning with simple geometries, such as spheres and infinite cables, and then proceeding to more complex configurations. Along the way, I review some elementary principles of electrical circuits; and at the end of the chapter, I will return to the starburst amacrine cell and present the calculations that model signal spread from one main dendrite down to the soma and out to other dendrites.

Principles of Electrical Circuits

Resistance

The resistance of a circuit element is defined by Ohm's law:

$$V = iR \tag{1}$$

In this equation V is the voltage (in *volts*, V), R is the resistance (in *ohms*, Ω), and i is the current (in *amperes*, A). By convention, current is carried by positive charge. Thus, current always flows from a more positive voltage to a less positive voltage (see Fig. 2.3A). In a wire, current is actually carried by electrons, which are negatively charged, and the direction of current flow is opposite to the direction of motion of the electrons. In a cell, current across the cell membrane is often carried by cations (Na^+, K^+, Ca^{2+}), which move in the same direction as the current; but sometimes it is carried by anions (Cl^-, HCO_3^-), which move in an opposite direction, as electrons do.

If two resistive elements (called *resistors*) are placed end to end *(in series)*, as in Fig. 2.3B, their resistances simply add. Since the same current flows through both resistors, the voltage is

$$V = V_1 + V_2 = iR_1 + iR_2 = i(R_1 + R_2) \tag{2}$$

and the total resistance equals $R_1 + R_2$. In most cases, we need to combine the resistances of adjacent patches of membrane, and in so doing the resistors are placed not in series but in parallel (Fig.

2.3C). In this configuration, different currents flow through each resistor. Notice, however, that the *voltage* across each resistor must be the same. The reason for this is perhaps obvious: the ends of each of the resistors placed in parallel are connected to one another by wires that are assumed to have negligible resistance, so the voltage across one resistor must be the same as that across any other. The current that flows across each resistor is given by

$$i_1 = \frac{V}{R_1}, \quad i_2 = \frac{V}{R_2}, \quad i_3 = \frac{V}{R_3}, \quad \dots, \quad i_n = \frac{V}{R_n} \tag{3}$$

so the total current flow is given by

$$i = \frac{V}{R_T} = V(\frac{1}{R_1} + \frac{1}{R_2} + \frac{1}{R_3} + \dots + \frac{1}{R_n}) = V\sum_j^n (\frac{1}{R_j}) \tag{4}$$

and the total resistance is given by

$$\frac{1}{R_T} = \sum_j^n \frac{1}{R_j} \tag{5}$$

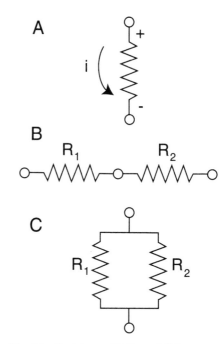

Fig. 2.3 Resistance. **(A)** Current *(i)* flows through a resistor from positive (+) to negative (−) voltage. **(B)** Resistances in series. **(C)** Resistances in parallel.

In many cases it will be simpler to think not of the resistance of a patch of membrane but rather of its conductance. The conductance *g* is equal to the inverse of the resistance,

$$g = \frac{1}{R} \tag{6}$$

From Eqns. (5) and (6) it is easy to see that conductances in parallel simply add,

$$g_T = g_1 + g_2 + g_3 + \dots g_n = \sum_j^n g_j \tag{7}$$

The unit of conductance is the *siemens (S)*, sometimes given as the *mho* in older literature.

Since the conductance of a lipid bilayer is very low, the conductance of the cell membrane of a typical neuron is mostly de-termined by proteins spanning the membrane, particularly by ion channels. I will say much more about ion channels later in the book. For now, assume that channels have been evenly distributed throughout the membrane, and ignore small differences in conduc-tance from one membrane patch to another. That is, always select a patch of membrane large enough to contain a sufficiently large number of channels, so that regional differences in the distribution of the channels can be ignored.

Capacitance

Capacitance is the ability of a circuit element to store charge and is defined by

$$C = \frac{q}{V} \tag{8}$$

where V is again the voltage in *volts*, q is the charge in *coulombs*, and C is the capacitance in *farads (F)*. Circuit elements called *capacitors* are typically made from two parallel conductive plates, separated by an insulator (such as glass or a plastic like polystyrene or Teflon™). For the cell membrane, the insulator is the lipid of the bilayer, and the two conductive plates are the ion-containing solu-tions on either side of the membrane (Fig. 2.4A).

As for the resistance, we ignore regional differences in the lipid composition of the cell membrane and assume that the capacitance is everywhere the same. This is true to a fairly good approximation. For capacitors in parallel (Fig. 2.4B), the voltage across each capac-itor will be assumed to be the same. Each capacitor stores charge, and the total charge stored by all of the capacitors is given by

$$q_T = q_1 + q_2 + q_3 + \ldots + q_n$$
$$= C_1 V + C_2 V + C_3 V + \ldots + C_n V = V \sum_{i}^{n} C_i \tag{9}$$

The total capacitance of several capacitors in parallel is the sum of their capacitances. For capacitors in series, the inverse of the total

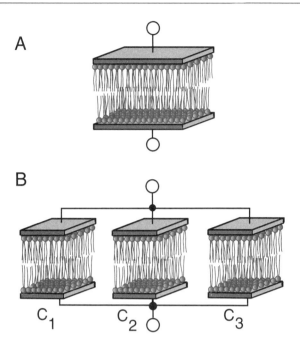

A

B

C_1 C_2 C_3

Fig. 2.4 Membranes as capacitors. **(A)** Membrane, made of 2 layers of phospholipid, can be thought of as a nonconducting insulator (the lipid, shown here in gray at top and bottom of bilayer) that separates two conducting media, the intracellular and extracellular solutions (above and below the bilayer). **(B)** Capacitances in parallel.

capacitance is the sum of the inverses of each of the capacitances, just as for resistances in parallel.

The Small, Spherical Cell

It is helpful to think of the cell body of a neuron as a small sphere. To calculate the total resistance of the membrane of a sphere, we connect the resistances of many small patches of membrane in parallel. A simpler way to do this is to sum conductances, since conductances in parallel simply add. If the conductance of each small patch of membrane is a function of the density and conductances of the ion channels in that membrane, then *adding more membrane* will add more channels and more pathways for ion flow. This is another way of saying that the conductance of a spherical cell can be obtained by summing the conductances of the patches of membrane that compose the cell, and the bigger the cell, the greater its conductance.

If we assume that the cell membrane conductance is uniform, then we can characterize the cell by its surface area and its *specific conductance*—that is, the conductance per unit area (always expressed per *cm²* of membrane). The specific conductance of the membrane of a neuron (g_m) is typically of the order of 10^{-4}–10^{-5} S cm^{-2}. For a sphere 20 μm in diameter (with radius, *a*, equal to 10 μm, or 10^{-3} cm), the surface area is given by $4\pi a^2$ (about 10^{-5} cm²), and the total conductance can be obtained by multiplying the specific conductance by the surface area, giving 10^{-9}–10^{-10} S. The total resistance can be calculated by taking the inverse of the total conductance, or 1–10 gigaohm (GΩ) or 10^9–10^{10} Ω.

Physiologists are more accustomed to giving the specific *resistance* of a cell membrane rather than the specific conductance. If the specific conductance is 10^{-4}–10^{-5} S cm^{-2}, then the specific resistance (R_m) is 10^4–10^5 Ω cm² (note the units). The total resistance of a spherical cell can then be calculated by *dividing* the specific resistance by the surface area. The result for a cell 20 μm in diameter is again about 1–10 GΩ. The total capacitance is obtained by multiplying the membrane's *specific capacitance (C_m)*, which is typically of the order of 0.7–1.0 $\times$ 10^{-6} F cm^{-2}, by the surface area. For a cell 20 μm in diameter, the total capacitance is of the order of 10^{-11} farad or 10 picofarad (pF).

Notice that in calculating both total capacitance and total resistance, we assumed that adjacent patches of membrane were connected in parallel, and that *the voltage across each patch of membrane is the same.* That is, we have assumed that the ends of the resistances and capacitances in each membrane patch are connected to those in the adjacent membrane patch by a path of negligible resistance, like the wires in Figs. 2.3 and 2.4. We are obliged to make this assumption in order to use Eqns. (4), (7), and (9). The connecting links for adjacent membrane patches are of course not wires but rather the ion-containing solutions which bathe the inside and outside surface of the cell. We are in effect assuming that the voltage inside the cell is everywhere the same, and that there are no regional differences in voltage in the solution bathing the cell.

The assumption that the voltage within the cell is everywhere the same is called the assumption of *isopotentiality,* and it is never strictly true. Cytoplasm, like any solution, has resistance, though the resistance is small; and currents that flow across this resistance produce a voltage given by Ohm's law. Making an assumption of isopotentiality is equivalent to ignoring the resistance of the cell cytoplasm or of the external solution. We can get away with this for a small cell, because the resistance through the cytoplasm or external

Box 2.1

SAMPLE PROBLEM I

A. Suppose a spherical cell 20 μm in diameter is penetrated with a fine glass micropipette containing salt solution, which is used to pass positive current into the cell. If the specific resistance of the cell membrane is 10^4 Ω cm^2, calculate the change in voltage produced by a current of 100 pA (10^{-10} A) at steady state.

Answer. First calculate the surface area of the cell. It is $4\pi(10^{-3}$ cm)^2, or 1.26×10^{-5} cm^2. Now calculate the total resistance of the cell: $(10^4$ Ω cm$^2)/(1.26 \times 10^{-5}$ cm$^2) = 7.96 \times 10^8$ Ω. The change in voltage is given by $V = iR = (7.96 \times 10^8$ $\Omega)(10^{-10}$ A) $= 7.96 \times 10^{-2}$ V (about 80 mV).

B. Suppose the pipette used to penetrate the cell in A contains a high concentration (3 M) of a potassium salt, such as potassium acetate. Assume that when positive current is injected into the cell, all of this current is carried by K^+. Calculate the number of K^+ ions injected into the cell if a 100 pA current is injected for 10 seconds. How much would this increase the K^+ concentration inside the cell (in mM)?

Answer. To calculate the number of K^+ ions injected into the cell, we must first calculate the number of coulombs of charge we have injected. This is (100 pA)(10 s) = $(10^{-10}$ A)(10 s) = 10^{-9} coulomb. The value of a single electronic charge is 1.60×10^{-19} coulomb. So the number of charges injected is $(10^{-9}$ coulomb)/$(1.60 \times 10^{-19}$ coulomb/charge) = 6.25×10^9 charges (K^+ ions), or 1.04×10^{-14} mole. The volume of a sphere is $4\pi a^3/3$, and so the volume of the cell is just $4\pi(10^{-3}$ cm)$^3/3 = 4.19 \times 10^{-9}$ cm$^3 = 4.19 \times 10^{-12}$ liter. The change in K^+ concentration is $(1.04 \times 10^{-14}$ mole/4.19×10^{-12} liter) = 2.48×10^{-3} mole per liter, or about 2.5 mM. Since the normal K^+ concentration inside the cell is about 100 mM, the change in K^+ concentration is about 2.5 percent.

solution is proportional to the distance the current flows, which is not very large if the cell is small. We will not be able to make the same assumption for more extended cell geometries: when we derive the cable equation for axons and dendrites, we will have to take the resistance of the cytoplasm explicitly into account.

Time Constants for Membranes

A physiologist does not normally *calculate* a cell's resistance and capacitance, he measures them. A fine glass microelectrode is inserted into a cell (or a whole-cell recording is made with a patch-clamp electrode—see Fig. 1.4), and current is passed from inside the cell to the outside across the cell membrane. A circuit diagram illustrating how this experiment is done is given in Fig. 2.5. The interlocking circles to the right of the diagram represent an ideal current generator. When the switch is closed at $t = 0$, current is injected into the cell, and the current flows outward through the parallel combination of the cell's resistance *(R)* and its capacitance *(C)*.

The current flowing through the resistance is given by Ohm's law, $i = V/R$, and if current flows outward across the cell membrane, then the inside of the cell becomes more positive, and the cell is said to *depolarize* (see Fig. 2.3A). What about the current

Fig. 2.5 Electrical equivalent of current injection into a small spherical cell. The plasma membrane of the neuron has been represented as a parallel combination of a capacitance (symbolized by two parallel lines) and a resistance. The double circles to the right are the symbol for an ideal current generator, which is connected in series with a switch. When the switch is thrown to complete the circuit, a current is injected into the inside of the neuron (the total current, i_T), which then passes across the membrane to the outside of the cell, partially across the resistance (i_R) and partially (as displacement current) across the capacitance (i_C).

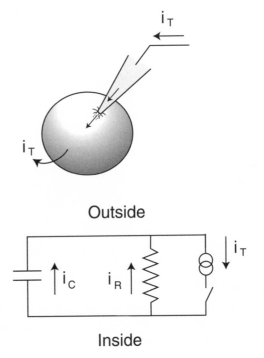

that flows through the capacitance? How can ions flow through an insulator like the lipid of the bilayer? The answer to this question is that ions do not actually flow *through* the lipid bilayer, not at least at a very high density, since the lipid bilayer is so highly resistive. However, the charge on the two sides of the capacitance must be changed for the voltage across the capacitance to be changed, and this change occurs only if charge is added or removed from the two sides of the membrane. A change in charge behaves as a current, often called a *displacement* current. If $C = q/V$, then

$$q = CV \quad \text{and} \quad \frac{dq}{dt} = i = C\frac{dV}{dt} \tag{10}$$

The total current (i_T) across the parallel combination of the resistance and the capacitance in Fig. 2.5 is equal to the sum of the current through the resistance (i_R) and the displacement current across the capacitance (i_C). From Eqns. (1) and (10), we have

$$i_R = \frac{V}{R}, \quad i_C = C\frac{dV}{dt}; \quad \text{so} \quad i_T = \frac{V}{R} + C\frac{dV}{dt} \tag{11}$$

When the switch is first closed, the voltage begins to change. Initially, most of the current will be capacitive or displacement current, which will alter the charge across the membrane capacitance and therefore alter the voltage across the capacitance. As the voltage across the capacitance changes, the voltage across the resistance also changes (since R and C are in parallel, and the voltage across each must be the same). As the voltage across the resistance changes, current begins to flow through the resistance. At later times, the current through the capacitance will diminish and the resistive current will dominate. At steady state, dV/dt is equal to zero, there is no capacitive current, and all of the current flows through the resistance.

The voltage at any time t can be calculated as follows. Rearranging the equation for i_T given above, we have

$$(V - i_T R) = -RC\frac{dV}{dt} \tag{12}$$

So

$$\frac{dV}{(V - i_T R)} = -\frac{dt}{RC} \tag{13}$$

If this expression is integrated from $t = 0$ to $t = t$ and from $V = 0$ to $V = V$, remembering that

$$\int \frac{dx}{x + c} = ln(x + c)$$

we obtain

$$\ln(V - i_T R) - \ln(-i_T R) = -\frac{t}{RC} \tag{14}$$

Rearranging and taking antilogs of both sides of the equation, we have

$$V = i_T R(1 - e^{-t/\tau}), \quad \text{with} \quad \tau = RC \tag{15}$$

The rise in voltage is exponential (see Fig. 2.6A), with a time constant τ equal to the product of the resistance and the capacitance. If, after waiting a sufficiently long time for the voltage to stabilize, we now reopen the switch, the voltage declines according to

$$V = V_0 (e^{-t/\tau}) \tag{16}$$

where V_0 is the voltage at steady state, given by $i_T R$ (Fig. 2.6B).

The time constant τ can be measured by recording the membrane potential of a cell with a microelectrode while injecting a square-wave pulse of current. During the rise of voltage, the time after the beginning of the pulse is equal to the time constant ($t = \tau$) when the voltage is equal to $i_T R(1 - e^{-1})$, or $0.63 V_0$ (see Fig. 2.6A). During the falling phase, $t = \tau$ when V is equal to $V_0 e^{-1}$ or $0.37 V_0$ (see Fig. 2.6B). These values can be obtained directly from the record of voltage as a function of time. Alternatively, a plot of the $\log_{10}$ of

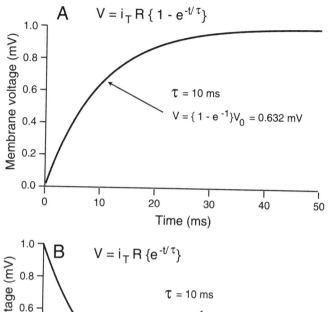

A

$$V = i_T R \{ 1 - e^{-t/\tau} \}$$

$\tau = 10$ ms

$V = \{ 1 - e^{-1} \} V_0 = 0.632$ mV

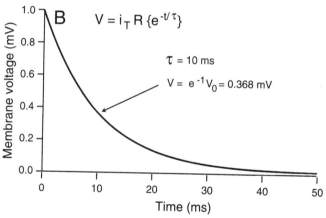

B

$$V = i_T R \{ e^{-t/\tau} \}$$

$\tau = 10$ ms

$V = e^{-1} V_0 = 0.368$ mV

Fig. 2.6 Voltage as a function of time for circuit as in Fig. 2.5. **(A)** Response of a small spherical cell to the onset of current injection. Curve is the solution of Eqn. (15) for a cell with a time constant of 10 ms and a voltage response at steady state ($V_0 = i_T R$) of 1 mV. **(B)** Response after turning off the stimulation pulse. Curve is solution of Eqn. (16) for same assumptions as in **(A)**.

voltage versus time will give a straight line for the decline of voltage after the current pulse is turned off. If we take the $\log_{10}$ of both sides of Eqn. (16), we have

$$\log_{10} V = \log_{10} V_0 + \log_{10}(e^{-t/\tau}) \tag{17}$$

Remembering that

$$\log_{10}(x) = \frac{\ln x}{\ln 10} = \frac{1}{2.303} \ln x \tag{18}$$

we can convert Eqn. (17) into,

$$\log_{10} V = \log_{10} V_0 - \frac{t}{2.303\tau} \tag{19}$$

The slope of the line during the decline of voltage ($\Delta\log_{10} V/\Delta t$) is equal to $-1/(2.303\tau)$, from which the time constant can be easily calculated. Actual time constants for neurons are typically of the order of 10–50 milliseconds (see for example Spruston and Johnston, 1992; Major et al., 1994).

Once we have measured the time constant of a spherical cell, we can calculate individual values for the total membrane resistance and capacitance. We do this by observing the value of the voltage produced by current injection at steady state. Since at steady state the capacitive current is zero, the voltage is just $i_T R$, from which we can determine the resistance. The capacitance can then be calculated from the relation $\tau = RC$.

The Cable Equation

Most cells are poorly represented by small spheres. Cells have axons and often quite complicated dendritic trees (think of the pyramidal cell of Fig. 1.1). Axons and dendrites are cables: thin cylinders whose cytoplasm represents a significant resistance to current flow. As a consequence, axons and dendrites cannot be assumed to be isopotential, and both voltage and current decay along their length. To take this into consideration, we must introduce the cable equation, which describes how voltage declines down a cylinder composed of patches of parallel combinations of resistances and capacitances.

As for the spherical cell, we assume that a cable is composed only of passive circuit elements (like resistors and capacitors). This is nearly true for most real axons and dendrites in the region of membrane potential near the resting potential. For the small spherical cell, we neglected the resistance of the cytoplasm, on the excuse that, for a small cell, the resistance between any two points within the cytoplasm is small, and the cell for all practical purposes is

---

Box 2.2

SAMPLE PROBLEM 2

A step of current of amplitude 1 pA (10^{-12} A) is injected into a small, spherical cell whose resistance is 2×10^9 Ω and whose capacitance is 0.5 pF. What is the value of the voltage after 1 millisecond? After 5 milliseconds?

Answer. First calculate $\tau = RC = (2 \times 10^9$ Ω$)(0.5 \times 10^{-12}$ F$) = 10^{-3}$ s, or 1 ms. Use Eqn. (15): $V = i_T R(1 - e^{-t/\tau})$. When $t = 1$ ms, $e^{-t/\tau} = e^{-1}$, so $V = (10^{-12}$ A$)(2 \times 10^9$ Ω$)(1 - e^{-1}) = (2 \times 10^{-3})$ $(0.63) = 1.26 \times 10^{-3}$ V $= 1.26$ mV. When $t = 5$ ms, $e^{-t/\tau} = e^{-5}$, so $V = (10^{-12}$ A$)(2 \times 10^9$ Ω$) \times (1 - e^{-5}) = (2 \times 10^{-3})(0.993) = 1.99 \times 10^{-3}$ V $= 1.99$ mV. At steady state, the voltage would be $V = (10^{-12}$ A$)(2 \times 10^9$ Ω$) = 2$ mV, so after just 5 milliseconds (or 5τ), the voltage of the cell is within 0.5 percent of its steady-state value.

---

isopotential. For a cable we must include the internal resistance (r_a) in our calculations, since distances from one point in the cable to another can be quite large (think of the motoneurons from the spinal cord that innervate the muscles in your toes). We shall assume that the cable is bathed in a chamber of large volume and shall therefore neglect the *external* resistance, but later I will show how the external resistance can be taken into account, should this be necessary for an actual neuron.

Figure 2.7A represents a cable as a series of small segments of plasma membrane, each composed of a resistance and capacitance in parallel. We use little r_m and c_m to represent the resistance and capacitance *of a unit length* (cm) of cable. They are related to the specific resistance and capacitance of the cell membrane (R_m and C_m) by the circumference of the cable, $2\pi a$, where a is the cable radius:

$$r_m = \frac{R_m}{2\pi a}, \quad c_m = C_m 2\pi a \tag{20}$$

Fig. 2.7 **(A)** Equivalent circuit of a cable: r_a, resistance of a unit length (cm) of cytoplasm; r_m, resistance of a unit length (cm) of membrane; c_m, capacitance of a unit length (cm) of membrane. **(B)** Electrical equivalent of current injection into a cable. Total current i_T is injected inside the cable and passes down the cable length across the intracellular resistance. Current also moves outward across patches of membrane, composed of parallel combinations of resistance and capacitance. The value of the current across the membrane (i_m) is equal to the change (a decrease) in current moving along the inside of the cable (Δi_a).

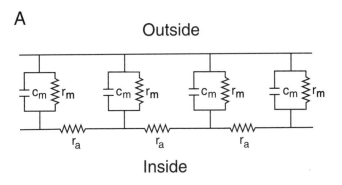

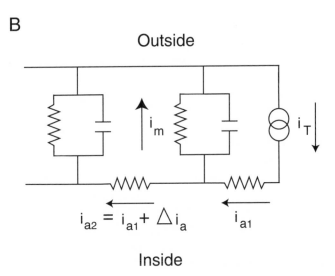

Let r_a be the resistance per unit length of the cytoplasm of a cable. This can be calculated from the specific resistance of the cytoplasm, R_a, by the equation $r_a = R_a/A$, where A is the cross-sectional area of the cable (πa^2). Note that we divide by the cross-sectional area, since the greater the cross-sectional area, the greater the number of pathways for current flow through the cytoplasm, the greater the conductance, and the *less* the resistance.

Derivation of Cable Equation

Suppose we penetrate the cable with a fine, glass microelectrode at some arbitrary point in the middle, which we call $x = 0$. Now we apply a current. If the cable were loss free (if no current were lost across the plasma membrane), a constant current would move down the middle of the cable, and the change in voltage within the cytoplasm as the current moved down the cable would be given by Ohm's law:

$$\Delta V = -i_a r_a \Delta x \qquad (21)$$

Here i_a is the current traveling down the cable through the cytoplasm, r_a is the internal (cytoplasmic) resistance per unit length of cable, and Δx is the distance the current travels. Total resistance is equal, then, to $r_a \Delta x$. In the limit, as Δx goes to zero,

$$\frac{\partial V}{\partial x} = -i_a r_a \qquad (22)$$

Of course, no cable transmits current without loss—certainly axons and dendrites do not. Transmission without loss would occur only if the resistance of the membrane of the axon or dendrite were infinite. Since the resistance of the plasma membrane is finite, some of the current traveling down the cytoplasm passes across the plasma membrane into the external medium. The passage of current across the plasma membrane produces a decrease in the value of the current moving down the cytoplasm and a decrease in the voltage across the cable membrane, much as volume and pressure decrease as fluid passes down a leaky pipe (see Fig. 2.8).

The amount of this decrease is easy to calculate. Consider a part of the cable very near the electrode. It should be clear from Fig. 2.7B that the decrease in the value of the cytoplasmic current *per unit length of cable* is equal to i_m, the membrane current *per unit length* (called the *membrane current density*). For a distance Δx

Fig. 2.8 Pressure applied at the pipe head would be maintained down the length of the pipe if no fluid escaped *(top)*, but the leakage of fluid across the surface of the pipe produces a decrease in both the volume of the fluid flowing from the outlet and the pressure of the fluid along the entire length of the pipe *(bottom)*. In the same way, the leakage of ions across the membrane of an axon or dendrite decreases both the current flowing down the cytoplasm and the voltage across the cable membrane.

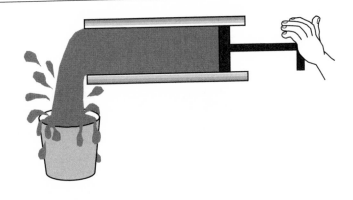

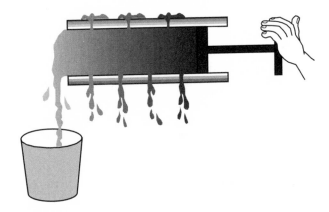

from the origin, the total decrease in cytoplasmic current, Δi_a, is given by

$$\Delta i_a = -i_m \Delta x \tag{23}$$

We must multiply i_m, the membrane current per unit length, by the length Δx to give the total current. In the limit, as Δx goes to zero,

$$\frac{\partial i_a}{\partial x} = -i_m \tag{24}$$

Combining Eqns. (22) and (24), we have

$$\left(\frac{1}{r_a}\right)\left(\frac{\partial^2 V}{\partial x^2}\right) = i_m \tag{25}$$

This gives a single equation for i_m as a function of voltage and distance.

We can obtain a second equation for i_m from the passive properties of the membrane. For any infinitesimal part of the cable containing resistance and capacitance, the membrane current is given by the same equation that we used for i_T for the small spherical cell (see Eqn. 11):

$$i_m = c_m \frac{\partial V}{\partial t} + \frac{V}{r_m} \tag{26}$$

In this equation, i_m is the membrane current per unit length (cm) of cable, and c_m and r_m are the capacitance and resistance of a unit length. Combining equations (25) and (26) gives the cable equation:

$$\lambda^2 \frac{\partial^2 V}{\partial x^2} - \tau_m \frac{\partial V}{\partial t} - V = 0 \tag{27}$$

where

$$\lambda = \sqrt{\frac{r_m}{r_a}} \quad \text{and} \quad \tau_m = r_m c_m \tag{28}$$

We refer to λ as the length constant for reasons that will become apparent shortly. The value τ_m is, of course, the time constant. Note that in cases for which the extracellular resistance is appreciable, the form of the cable equation is identical, but λ is now given by

$$\lambda = \sqrt{\frac{r_m}{(r_a + r_o)}} \tag{29}$$

where r_o is the external resistance per unit length of extracellular solution.

Solving the Cable Equation

Eqn. (28) is a partial differential equation in two variables and is in general quite difficult or even impossible to solve analytically (that is, in the form of an equation). A solution has been obtained in several special cases (Jack, Noble, and Tsien, 1975), of which the most useful may be that for a "step" input of current beginning at $t = 0$. Imagine that we have penetrated the cable (the axon or dendrite) at $x = 0$ with a microelectrode and then flipped a switch to turn on a current. If a current step of amplitude I_0 is applied by intracellular injection at the point $x = 0$ and at time $t = 0$, the solution to the cable equation is

$$V = \frac{r_a I_o \lambda}{4} [\exp(-X)\mathrm{erfc}(\frac{X}{2\sqrt{T}} - \sqrt{T})$$
$$- \exp(X)\mathrm{erfc}(\frac{X}{2\sqrt{T}} + \sqrt{T})] \tag{30}$$

where the normalized variables X and T are given by

$$X = \frac{x}{\lambda} \quad \text{and} \quad T = \frac{t}{\tau} \tag{31}$$

The function $erfc$ is the complement of the error function, that is, $1 - erf$. The error function is defined as

$$erf(x) = \frac{2}{\sqrt{\pi}} \int_o^x \exp(-y^2)dy \tag{32}$$

and values of the error function can be obtained from tables. Although Eqn. (30) seems impossibly complicated, it is actually rather easy to obtain graphical solutions for this equation in one of a number of readily available software packages, such as Mathcad© (see Box 2.3).

Equation (30) was first obtained by Hodgkin and Rushton (1946). It is the solution for an *infinite* cable—that is, a cable so long that we do not have to consider how the cable is terminated. It describes in a quantitative fashion how the distribution of voltage down the cable changes with time after the beginning of a current step. In order to develop some notion of what the voltage distribution looks like, we must first consider two special cases of this solution.

Voltage at Steady State

If the current pulse is sufficiently long, after a time the voltage distribution of the cable will converge to steady state. We can obtain the solution for the steady-state distribution from the general solution since, when T goes to infinity, $erfc(T)$ goes to zero and $erfc(-T)$ goes to 2. The solution to Eqn. (30) then becomes

$$V = \frac{r_a I_o \lambda}{2}(e^{-x/\lambda})$$ (33)

Voltage drops exponentially from either side of $x = 0$, falling e^{-1} of its steady-state value in a distance λ. Now it is clear why λ is referred to as the length constant.

The value of the steady-state voltage at $x = 0$ (at the point of current injection) can also be obtained from Eqn. (33), since if $x = 0$, $e^{-x/\lambda} = 1$, and $V = r_a I_0 \lambda/2$. From this relation we can calculate the *input resistance* of the cable. The input resistance (R_{in}) is the resistance measured for a cell or cable (or, for that matter, a piece of hamburger) *at the position of current injection*. For a small spherical cell, the input resistance is just R, the total resistance of the cell membrane. For a cable, the input resistance can be obtained from the ratio of the voltage to the current (that is, from V/I_0) at the position of current injection. It is $r_a\lambda/2$. From our previous definitions of r_a and λ, the input resistance can be shown to be

$$R_{in} = \frac{\sqrt{R_m R_a / 2}}{2\pi\sqrt{a^3}} \quad \text{or} \quad \frac{(R_m R_a / 2)^{1/2}}{2\pi(a^{3/2})}$$ (34)

Eqn. (34) contains the important result that the input resistance of a cable (or an axon or dendrite) varies inversely as the 3/2 power of *a*, the fiber radius.

Time Course of Voltage Change

We now consider the solution of the cable equation as a function of time at a single point, the point of current injection ($X = 0$). If $X = 0$, then Eqn. (30) becomes

$$V = \frac{r_a I_o \lambda}{4} [erfc(-\sqrt{T}) - erfc(\sqrt{T})] \tag{35}$$

Since $erfc(x) = 1 - erf(x)$ and $erf(-x) = -erf(x)$, Eqn. (35) can be simplified to

$$V = \frac{r_a I_o \lambda}{4} [2erf(\sqrt{T})] = \frac{r_a I_o \lambda}{2} [erf(\sqrt{T})] \tag{36}$$

This can be further simplified if we remember that $r_a I_o \lambda / 2$ is equal to V_0, the steady-state value of the voltage at $x = 0$ (see Eqn. (33)). Eqn. (36) is then equivalent to

$$V = V_o [erf(\sqrt{T})] \tag{37}$$

and $erf(\sqrt{T})$ determines the rise of V.

Fig. 2.9 compares the time dependence of the rise of voltage for a cable at the point of current application with that for a small cell (from Jack, Noble, and Tsien, 1975). Since $erf(1) = 0.84$, V rises to 84 percent of its steady-state value in a cable within one time constant—considerably faster than the exponential rise of voltage for a spherical cell. It may seem paradoxical that voltage rises faster for an axon than for a spherical cell for the same values of R_m and C_m. The reason for this is that the change in voltage is limited by the rate at which the capacitance of the membrane can be charged. For a small spherical cell, the whole of the plasma membrane must be charged uniformly. For the axon or dendrite, charging of the mem-

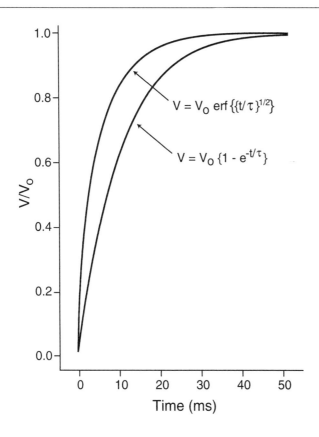

Fig. 2.9 Comparison of voltage change during current injection for small, spherical cell and a cable. The voltage change for the charging of a spherical cell is given by Eqn. (15), $V = V_0 (1 - e^{-t/\tau})$, while that for an infinite cable (recorded at the point of current injection) is given by Eqn. (37), $V = V_0\ erf(\sqrt{T})$. (Remember that $T = t/\tau$.) Curves plot V/V_0 (which is 1.0 at steady state) versus time in milliseconds. For both curves, the time constant τ was assumed to be 10 ms.

brane occurs nonuniformly and is quickest in the direct vicinity of the point of application of the current (i.e., at $x = 0$). As we shall see, for more remote regions, the charging of the membrane capacitance occurs much more slowly.

More General Solutions of the Cable Equation

To investigate the rate of charging of the membrane at locations other than $x = 0$, we use a computer program (as in Box 2.3) and show the results in the form of graphs. The first (Fig. 2.10A) shows the rate of charging of the membrane as a function of time at various distances from the point of application of the current. Note that x and t have been replaced by the dimensionless variables X and T from Eqn. (31). For $X = 0$, the time dependence of voltage

---

Box 2.3

A SOLUTION FOR EQN. (30)

Although solving the cable equation may seem a formidable task, it is actually fairly easy with the right software. One way to obtain a solution is to use the program Mathcad©, from Mathsoft in Cambridge, Massachusetts. Here is a program in Mathcad© that gives the voltage as a function of time at a specified position down the length of the cable. The program first defines the index j and gives it a range from 1 to 1000. Then 1000 time points are defined (in milliseconds) from 1/20 ms to $1000/20 = 50$ ms, and the variable T is obtained by dividing each of these time points by the cable time constant, assumed to be 10 ms. Finally a position is specified, in this case $X = 0$, and a value is assumed for $r_a I_0 \lambda / 4$ (I have set this equal to 5 mV). Mathcad© then solves the cable equation (introducing the appropriate values of the error function automatically) for each of these time points. If we then use Mathcad© to define a graph to plot V_j (in mV) against T_j, we obtain a function of the same form as the one for the cable in Fig. 2.9.

---

increase is determined by $erf(\sqrt{T})$, as previously explained, and is rather rapid. For distances away from the point of current application, the steady-state responses become smaller, and the membrane charges more slowly and with a progressively greater delay.

The delay can be appreciated more clearly in the second graph (Fig. 2.10B), which shows the potential as a function of distance at various times after the beginning of a pulse. Just after the beginning of the pulse (say at $T = 0.1$), only the part of the cable adjacent to the point of current application shows any significant change in voltage. The change in voltage spreads outward with increasing T, and at large T voltage reaches the steady-state distribution, as described at Eqn. (33) (V declines exponentially with a length constant λ).

Passive Spread of Synaptic Potentials

To appreciate the implications of passive spread down a cable for signal processing in an actual cell, imagine that current is injected

Calculations for Cable Equation

$$j := 1\ldots1000 \qquad t_j := \frac{j}{20} \qquad T_j := \frac{t_j}{10} \qquad X := 0$$

$$V_j := 5 \cdot \left[\exp(-X) \cdot \left[1 - \text{erf}\left[\frac{X}{2 \cdot (T_j)^{1/2}} - (T_j)^{1/2} \right] \right] \right.$$
$$\left. - \exp(X) \cdot \left[1 - \text{erf}\left[\left[\frac{X}{2 \cdot (T_j)^{1/2}} \right] + (T_j)^{1/2} \right] \right] \right]$$

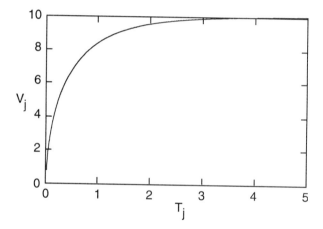

A similar graph for voltage versus distance at constant time (like the graphs in Fig. 2.10B) can be constructed by altering the beginning of the program to define the variables x_j as $j/20$ and X_j as x_j/λ, and by setting a value for T. The same equation can be used, and a graph would have to be defined to plot V_j against X_j.

into a dendrite by the opening of ion channels at a synapse remote from the cell body. What will the synaptic potential—the change in voltage produced by synapse activation—look like as a function of distance from the site of the synapse? The answer to this question depends very much on the geometry of the cell. Consider the simplest case. Suppose we inject a brief pulse of current (of duration $0.1\,T$) into our cable and solve the cable equation as a function of T

Fig. 2.10 Solutions of the cable equation (Eqn. 30) for an infinite cable. The voltage responses to a current step are calculated on the assumption that voltage at steady state at the point of current injection is V_0. **(A)** Voltage as a function of time ($T = t/\tau$). Calculated responses are graphed for voltage measured at the point of current injection ($X = 0$) and at various distances from the site of current injection, as indicated at right. Distances are given relative to the length constant of the cable ($X = x/\lambda$). **(B)** Voltage as a function of distance ($X = x/\lambda$). Calculated responses are graphed for voltage measured at the times given in the figure, relative to the time constant of the cable ($T = t/\tau$).

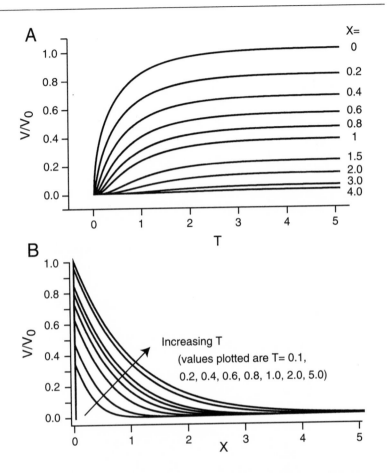

for various values of X. Solutions of this kind (Jack, Noble, and Tsien, 1975), showing the waveform of the voltage produced by a current pulse as a function of distance away from the site of current injection, are given in Fig. 2.11A. Note that the synaptic potential becomes smaller the further away it is measured, and that the waveform changes in shape. Electrotonic conduction causes the signal to become progressively smaller and progressively slower in time course.

Fig. 2.11B gives actual measurements by Fatt and Katz (1951) of the amplitude of the postsynaptic (endplate) potential of a muscle as a function of distance from the motor synapse. A striated muscle fiber is long enough and of small enough diameter to be satisfactorily described over much of its length by the equation for an infinite cable. The line fitted to the measurements (from Jack, Noble, and Tsien, 1975) gives the predicted amplitude of the postsynaptic potential following a rectangular current pulse of duration $0.1T$, for a length constant of 2.4 mm.

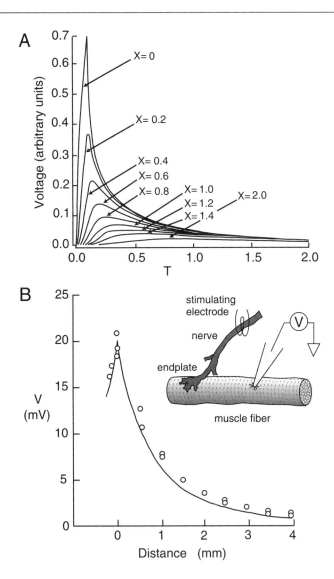

Fig. 2.11 Passive spread of synaptic potentials. **(A)** Waveform of voltage change produced by brief injection of current into an infinite cable. Distances are given relative to the length constant of the cable ($X = x/\lambda$), and time relative to the time constant of the cable ($T = t/\tau$). Voltage is plotted on the ordinate in arbitrary units. Waveforms are calculated responses to the injection of a square pulse of current of duration $0.1T$. Calculations show voltage change as a function of time at the point of current injection ($X = 0$) and at increasing distance from current injection. (From Jack, Noble, and Tsien, 1975, reprinted with permission of the authors and of Oxford University Press.) **(B)** Amplitude of voltage response as a function of distance from the synapse of the endplate for frog skeletal muscle. The neuromuscular junction in vertebrates is called an *endplate,* and the *endplate potential* is the name given to the synaptic response in a muscle cell. (Data points are actual voltages and distances, taken from Fatt and Katz, 1951. Curve is a calculation of cable equation for a square wave of input current of duration $0.1T$, taken from Jack, Noble, and Tsien, 1975; reprinted with permission of the authors and of Oxford University Press.)

Box 2.4

SAMPLE PROBLEM 3

A. What is the length constant of a cable whose specific resistance of the membrane (R_m) is 1000 Ω cm², whose radius (a) is 10 μm, and whose specific resistance of the cytoplasm (R_a) is 100 Ω cm? The resistance of the extracellular fluid may be neglected.

Answer. First calculate $r_m = R_m/2\pi a = (10^3 \ \Omega \ \text{cm}^2)/(2 \times 3.14159 \times 10^{-3} \ \text{cm}) = 1.59 \times 10^5 \ \Omega \ \text{cm}$. Now $r_a = R_a/\pi a^2 = (10^2 \ \Omega \ \text{cm})/(3.14159) (10^{-3} \ \text{cm})^2 = 3.18 \times 10^7 \ \Omega \ \text{cm}^{-1}$. Hence $\lambda = (r_m/r_a)^{1/2} = [(1.59 \times 10^5 \ \Omega \ \text{cm})/(3.18 \times 10^7 \ \Omega \ \text{cm}^{-1})]^{1/2} = 7.07 \times 10^{-2}$ cm, or about 0.71 mm.

B. For the same cable as in A, what is the input resistance?
Answer. You could do this calculation from the equation

$$\frac{(R_m R_a/2)^{1/2}}{2\pi(a^{3/2})}$$

but why bother? R_{in} is also just $r_a\lambda/2$ (from Eqn. 33), which in this case is $(3.18 \times 10^7 \ \Omega \ \text{cm}^{-1}) (7.07 \times 10^{-2} \ \text{cm})/2 = 1.12 \times 10^6 \ \Omega$, or 1.12 megohm (M$\Omega$).

C. For the same cable, let us assume that the specific capacitance of the membrane (C_m) is 10^{-6} F cm^{-2}. A step of current 10 nA $(= 10^{-8}$ A) in amplitude is injected into the axon. Calculate the value of the voltage *at the point of current injection* after 1 ms and after 5 ms.

Answer. In this case $X = 0$, the appropriate equation (from Eqn. 36) is

$$V = \frac{r_a I_0 \lambda}{2} \, erf[(t/\tau_m)^{1/2}]$$

We have $r_a = 3.18 \times 10^7 \ \Omega \ \text{cm}^{-1}$, $I_0 = 10^{-8}$ A, $\lambda = 7.07 \times 10^{-2}$ cm, and $\tau_m = r_m c_m = R_m C_m = 10^{-3}$ s = 1 ms. After 1 ms, $erf[(t/\tau_m)^{1/2}]$ is just $erf(1)$ or 0.843. Hence $V = [(3.18 \times 10^7 \ \Omega \ \text{cm}^{-1}) (10^{-8} \ \text{A}) (7.07 \times 10^{-2} \ \text{cm}) / 2](0.843) = (11.2 \times 10^{-3} \ \text{V})(0.843) = 9.48$ mV. After 5 ms, $erf[(t/\tau_m)^{1/2}] = erf[(5/1)^{1/2}] = erf(2.24) = 0.998$ (this comes from a table or from Mathcad©), so the voltage has now reached $(11.2 \times 10^{-3} \ \text{V})(0.998) = 11.18$ mV, almost its maximum value of 11.2 mV.

Electrical Models of Real Neurons

Real neurons are not small spheres or infinite cables; they have cell bodies, or somas, of irregular shape, with axons and often quite elaborate dendritic trees. Many methods now exist for modeling passive spread in a complicated neuronal structure. These methods generally begin with the assumption that the cell body of the neuron is uniform and can be described entirely by its passive electrical properties (by its specific resistance R_m and capacitance C_m). Dendrites are also generally assumed to be uniform in their electrical properties, though this is not strictly necessary. For example, it is possible to assume that some dendrites have greater resistance than others, or that the membrane resistance of the soma is different from that of the dendrites. Usually the intracellular (cytoplasmic) resistance is assumed to be uniform, though again this is not strictly necessary.

Methods for modeling nerve cells were all greatly influenced by the work of Wilfrid Rall (Segev, Rinzel, and Shepherd, 1995). Rall (1959, 1960) first described a mathematical treatment for combining an electrical model of the soma with electrical (cable) models of dendrites and axons to produce a model of a whole cell (see also Rall, 1977, 1989; Jack, Noble, and Tsien, 1975, chap. 7). In general, the dendrites are broken into segments, each of which represents a separate "compartment" of the cell. The compartments are then connected according to the branching configuration of the dendritic tree. A cable equation (Eqn. 27) is written for each compartment, with values for τ and λ given by the diameter of each dendritic segment, the cytoplasmic resistivity, the specific membrane resistance, and the specific membrane capacitance (as in Eqn. 28). Since dendritic compartments will in general be too short to be modeled as *infinite* cables, it is also necessary to determine the length of each dendritic compartment and to assume *boundary* conditions for each compartment—that is, whether the ends of the dendrites are sealed (as would occur at the very tips of the dendritic tree) or open (as would occur for dendrites connected to other dendrites or to the soma).

The result of such a model is a series of simultaneous partial differential equations similar to the cable equation for each of the compartments of the cell. The solution of these equations is fairly straightforward in certain special cases (for example, at steady state—see Rall, 1959) and for cells with very simple geometries (Rall, 1969) but can be enormously complicated for cells with complicated geometries (Koch and Poggio, 1985; Major, Evans, and Jack, 1993). Furthermore, a solution is in general possible only if the dendrites and the soma of the cell are assumed to behave passively, as combinations of resistances and capacitances that are constant and not functions of voltage. Dendrites often do not behave passively but have voltage-dependent conductances and even generate action potentials (Segev and Rall, 1998).

Two methods have been proposed for simplifying the modeling of cells with complicated dendritic morphologies, both first suggested by Rall. The first of these is called the *equivalent-cylinder* model and the second the *compartmental* model.

Equivalent-Cylinder Model

Rall demonstrated that a complicated branching structure could be reduced to an "equivalent cylinder" if the electrical properties of the dendrites are uniform and if the branching structure of the dendritic tree satisfies two requirements. First, at each branching point the dendritic tree must obey the "three-halves rule":

$$D^{3/2} = \sum_{j}^{n} d_j^{\,3/2} \tag{38}$$

where D is the diameter of the process coming into the branch and d_j is the diameter of each of the n processes coming out of the branch. This is equivalent to assuming the input resistance of the process coming into the branch is equal to the sum of the input resistances of the processes coming out of the branch, since the resistance of a cable varies as the 3/2 power of the diameter (or radius—see Eqn. 34).

If the three-halves rule is satisfied at a branch point, then the dendritic compartments on the two sides of the branch behave electrically as if the branch were not present, since there is no change in input resistance. The compartments on either side of the branch can then be replaced by a single compartment. If the three-halves rule is satisfied at *all* of the branch points of a main dendrite of a neuron, then the whole main dendrite can be represented by an equivalent cylinder. A further transformation can be made if each of the equivalent cylinders of the main dendrites satisfies a second requirement: if the main dendrites all have the same *electrotonic length*—that is, if the value of X (or of x/λ) measured from the soma to the end of each main dendrite is the same. In this case, all of the primary dendrites can be lumped together into a *single* cylinder (Fig. 2.12). We now have converted a complicated dendritic morphology into a soma connected to a single cable.

Equivalent-cylinder models are important historically, since solutions of simplified models of this kind were readily obtainable even before powerful computers became commonly available and relatively inexpensive. Even a simple model of this sort can be useful for studying the response of the cell to currents injected uniformly into all of the processes simultaneously, or for currents injected into the soma.

Compartmental Models

A much more powerful approach is to divide the dendritic tree into a series of compartments and to make these compartments sufficiently short so that each compartment can be assumed to be isopotential (Rall, 1964; Segev, Fleshman, and Burke, 1989). Each compartment can be modeled as a resistance in parallel with a capacitance, connected to adjacent compartments by resistances whose values are determined by the resistance of the cytoplasm (Fig. 2.13).

There are several advantages to using compartmental models. First, many cells seem not to satisfy the three-halves rule (for example, pyramidal cells—see Major et al., 1994) and so cannot be reduced to equivalent cylinders. Second, it is possible with numerical methods and a personal computer to solve the equations of a compartmental model in a reasonable time, even for models with several hundred compartments. Several computer programs are available (NEURON, GENESIS, NODUS) for these calculations, and they are easy to use and inexpensive (or free). Third, the dendritic tree does not have to be uniform in its properties. The dendrite does not even need to be passive. It is possible to add, for each

Fig. 2.12 Modeling dendrites by the equivalent-cylinder method. Dendritic tree of neuron
(in this case, retinal starburst amacrine cell) is
reduced to a simplified model, by the assumption that each of the major dendrites can be replaced with an equivalent cylinder, if at all of the
branch points the three-halves rule can be assumed to be satisfied (see Eqn. 38). A further
simplification can be made if each of the main
dendrites can be assumed to have the same
electrotonic length—a reasonable assumption
for this cell. In this case, all of the main dendrites can be replaced with a single cylinder.
(Modified from Rall, 1962, with starburst
amacrine from Wong and Collin, 1989, reprinted with permission of the authors and of
John Wiley and Sons, Inc.)

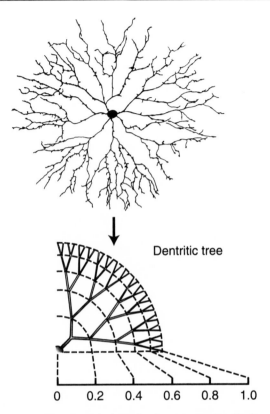

Dentritic tree

Electrotonic length of equivalent cylinder

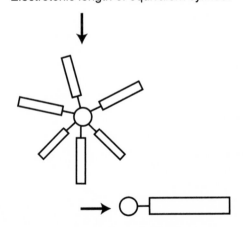

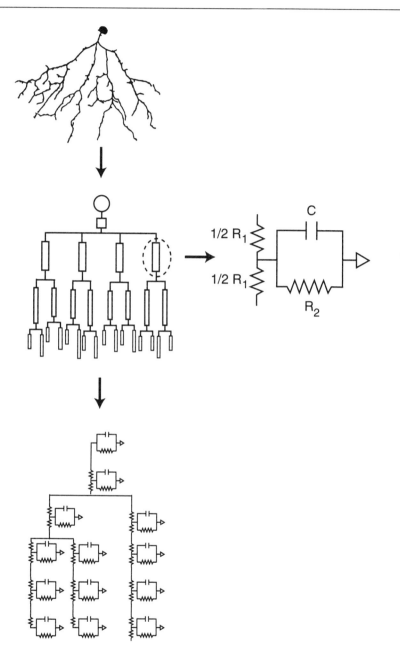

Fig. 2.13 Compartmental modeling. A single main dendritic branch of a starburst amacrine cell has been divided into a number of compartments, which were chosen to be small enough so that we may assume isopotentiality. Each compartment is modeled by the parallel combination of a resistance and a capacitance and is joined to the other compartments by resistances whose values are determined by the resistance of the cytoplasm. R_1, total resistance of cytoplasm of compartment; R_2, resistance of membrane of compartment; C, capacitance of compartment. (After Segev, Fleshman, and Burke, 1989, with starburst amacrine from Wong and Collin, 1989; reprinted with permission of the authors and of John Wiley and Sons, Inc.)

compartment, resistances that are voltage-dependent and in parallel with the passive membrane resistance, in order to model voltage-gated channels (see Chapter 5). Synaptic conductances can also be added to the model. Voltage-gated and synaptic channels can be distributed nonuniformly. Clearly, it is possible with compartmental models to investigate in much more detail the physiology of a nerve cell and the dependence of its responses on the morphology of the dendritic tree.

In order to illustrate the usefulness of compartmental models, I return now to the starburst amacrine cell (Fig. 2.14A). Begin by dividing the dendritic tree into small compartments, each of which is less than 0.01λ in length. Since the compartments are so small, it is possible to assume without too much error that each compartment is effectively isopotential. The diameters of the dendrites and the shape of the cell can be taken from published articles (Famiglietti, 1991; Wong and Collin, 1989). Fig. 2.14B is an enlargement of part of a cell, with only two of the main dendritic branches shown. The compartments for these two branches are illustrated in Fig. 2.14C in a diagram known as a *dendrogram,* which makes explicit the connections of each of the compartments of the dendrites.

As in many calculations of this sort, the cytoplasmic resistivity is not known but can be assumed to be the same as that measured in other neurons, of the order of 70–100 Ω cm (see for example Hodgkin and Rushton, 1946). The specific membrane capacitance, C_m, has been measured for many different cell types and is typically of the order of 10^{-6} F/cm². The specific membrane resistance, R_m, can be obtained directly from experiment, as for a spherical cell, by injecting a pulse of constant current. For a real neuron with a complex dendritic tree, however, the decay of voltage to a current pulse is not given by a single exponential, as for a spherical cell (Eqn. 16), but rather by the sum of a series of exponentials (Rall, 1969),

$$V = C_o e^{-t/\tau_o} + C_1 e^{-t/\tau_1} + C_2 e^{-t/\tau_2} + \ldots + C_n e^{-t/\tau_n}$$
$$= \sum_{j=0}^{n} C_j e^{-t/\tau_j} \tag{39}$$

where $\tau_0 = R_m C_m$, and the other time constants τ_1–τ_n (called *equalizing time constants*) are caused by the spread of current between

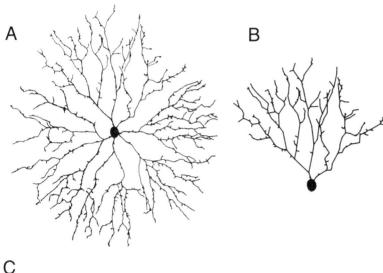

A

B

Fig. 2.14 Partial compartmental model of starburst amacrine. **(A)** Drawing of a complete starburst amacrine cell. (From Wong and Collin, 1989, reprinted with permission of the authors and of John Wiley and Sons, Inc.) **(B)** The portion of the cell in **(A)** for which compartmental model calculations were performed. Only two main dendritic branches are shown, both emerging from the soma. **(C)** Dendrogram showing each of the compartments used to model the two main dendrites for the portion of the cell shown in **(B).** Two squares (labeled *Distal 1* and *Distal 2*) indicate positions at the tips of the two dendrites that are used as points of reference in Fig. 2.15.

C

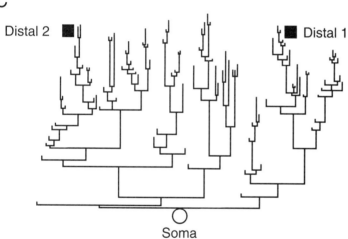

Distal 2   Distal 1

Soma

different parts of the cell, which are polarized to different degrees by the current pulse. Fortunately, τ_0 is the slowest time constant and is often sufficiently separated in time from τ_1–τ_n so that $R_m C_m$ can be obtained from the voltage waveform. Alternatively, different values of R_m can be inserted into the model, and Eqn. (39) solved and fitted to responses to current pulses actually recorded from the cell. The time constant τ_0 for a starburst amacrine cell is typically 10–15 milliseconds (ms).

The results of some calculations performed for this cell with the program NODUS (De Schutter, 1989, 1992) are shown in Fig. 2.15 (Zhou, Cheney, and Fain, 1996). Fig. 2.15A simulates the injection of a current pulse into the soma, with voltage calculated at the soma and at two points near the distal ends of the two branches, at positions indicated by the squares in Fig. 2.14B. Voltage spreads quite readily from the soma to the ends of the dendritic tree. Fig. 2.15B simulates the reverse experiment: a current is injected into a distal dendrite, and the voltage is calculated at the point of current injection, at the soma, and at a distal branch of the other main dendrite. Now voltage spreads less efficiently. This is of some interest, since it suggests that voltages in this cell communicate more efficiently within a single main dendritic branch than from one main dendritic branch to another.

Fig. 2.15 Results of calculations for model in Fig. 2.14, performed with the program NODUS. **(A)** Current pulse injected into the soma. Delay in rise and decay of voltage is result of passive properties of cell. Peak amplitude of voltage change is nearly identical in soma and at the distal ends of the two dendrites. **(B)** Current pulse injected into distal site 1 (see Fig. 2.14C). Now amplitude of voltage change is much reduced at soma and at the other distal compartment, because of *impedance mismatching*. Reduction would have been even larger if all of the dendritic branches of the cell had been included in the model and not just the two shown in Fig. 2.14B. (Calculations made with the assistance of Z. J. Zhou and M. Cheney.)

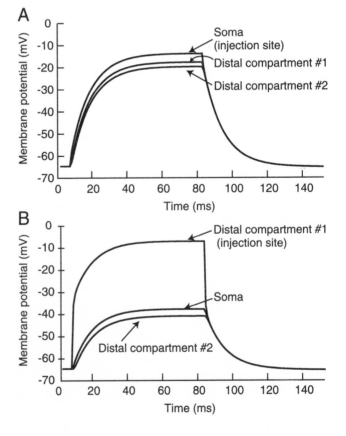

The reason for the poorer spread of current from dendrites to soma in a starburst amacrine cell is called *impedance mismatching*. Because the diameter of the soma is relatively large, its input resistance is relatively small (remember, the bigger a cell, the bigger its conductance and smaller its resistance). To change the voltage of the soma, Ohm's law says that a fairly large current would have to be injected (Fig. 2.15A), and the current would spread throughout the cell and cause a large voltage change even in remote dendrites. The dendrites, on the other hand, are tiny. Since the input resistance of a dendrite (or of any cable) varies inversely as the 3/2 power of the dendritic radius, the small dendrites of starburst amacrine cells have a relatively high input resistance, and only a small current needs be injected to change their voltage. Some of the current injected into the dendrite spreads into the soma but produces a smaller voltage change there, because of the lower resistance of the soma. The voltage further diminishes (though by a smaller proportion) as current spreads from the soma into the other main dendritic branches. A similar effect has also been demonstrated for this cell with an equivalent-cylinder model (Miller and Bloomfield, 1983).

These calculations lead to some interesting conclusions that would have been difficult to obtain in any other way. Synaptic input coming into a starburst amacrine cell dendrite can spread to other parts of the dendrite and also to the soma, but the spread of the voltage into the soma or into the other main dendritic branches is not very efficient. The principal dendrites *do* seem to function somewhat independently of one another (see Velte and Miller, 1997). It is quite striking how small the dendrites of this cell are, and how abruptly the diameter of the cell changes from the soma to the principal dendrites. It is also interesting that each of the principal dendrites terminates in the soma: the radial symmetry of the cell seems almost to have been designed to isolate signals in different parts of the cell. This is unlike the pyramidal cell, where the apical dendrites all converge into a single large process that terminates in the cell body, as if to funnel synaptic input into the soma.

The lesson is that the shape of a cell can tell us something about what the cell does. Different cells have different shapes, and there are probably very good reasons that they are. Studying the electrical properties of cells is a powerful tool for investigating the relationship between morphology and function for the many hundreds or thousands of different cell types in the central nervous system.

Summary

The passive electrical properties of neurons may be modeled according to the principles of electrical circuits. Simple rules for combining passive circuit elements can be used to model voltage changes in small spherical cells and in cables. For example, the spread of voltage down a cable is, in general, *decremental:* the voltage decreases in amplitude and slows in waveform.

Membranes, too, may be understood as electrical circuits, the properties of which can be used to construct models of whole neurons, by either the equivalent-cylinder approach or compartmental models. Models of this sort are necessarily approximate, since accurate values for the cytoplasmic resistance and membrane capacitance are not available for very many cell types. Nevertheless, even these rudimentary calculations can provide interesting insight about the way signals generated in the dendrites are communicated to the rest of the cell.

The passive or decremental conduction described in this chapter was once thought to be the only mode of signal spread down dendrites, but we now know that this is not true (Llinás, 1988; Yuste and Tank, 1996; Johnston et al., 1996). Dendrites also contain a second mechanism for the spread of voltage, which is mediated by voltage-gated Na^+ and Ca^{2+} channels. Na^+ and Ca^{2+} channels are membrane proteins that are opened and closed by changes in membrane voltage. Although we usually associate Na^+ channels with axons, where they produce regenerative events called *action potentials,* Na^+ channels (and Ca^{2+} channels) can also occur in dendrites and may provide a form of signal boosting that increases both the amplitude and rapidity of synaptic events (Deisz, Fortin, and Zieglgänsberger, 1991; Stuart and Sakmann, 1995). Perhaps more important, dendritic Na^+ channels may allow action potentials produced by the soma and axon of the cell to propagate back up into the dendrites, to depolarize the dendritic membrane and modulate synaptic input (Stuart and Sakmann, 1994). Signal spread boosted by voltage-gated Na^+ and Ca^{2+} channels is known as *active conduction* and will be the subject of Chapters 5–7.

3

Ion Permeability and Membrane Potentials

EVEN THE MOST complicated forms of processing in the brain—including sensory detection, higher mental function, and consciousness—all have their basis in electrical signals, produced by changes in voltage across the plasma membrane of particular collections of nerve cells. These changes in voltage are produced when the resting membrane potential, typically -70 mV, is altered by the opening or closing of ion channels, triggered by the voltage change itself or by the binding of extracellular neurotransmitters or intracellular second messengers. The channels act as gates for the entry of ions, such as Na^+ or K^+. For neurons, as for other cells in the body, all of the ions of physiological importance are asymmetrically distributed across the plasma membrane (Fig. 3.1). Differences in concentration occur because the membranes of animal cells contain metabolically fueled pumps and transporters, which move ions selectively between the inside and outside of the cell (see Chapter 4). This movement produces a gradient of concentration for each ion, so when the channels open, ions flow in one direction or another across the membrane.

Imagine the neuron in Fig. 3.1 with all of its channels closed and with the membrane potential initially at zero. Suppose a large number of K^+ channels were now opened. What effect would this have on the voltage across the cell membrane? Since there is more K^+ inside the cell than outside, K^+ would initially be more likely to leave the cell than to enter. As K^+ leaves the cell, the inside of the cell becomes negative: the departure of K^+ leaves a deficit of charge inside the cell. The asymmetry of charge across the cell membrane capacitance will produce a voltage, given by $V_m = \Delta q/C_T$, where V_m is the membrane potential, Δq is the charge deficit inside the cell, and C_T is the total cell capacitance (Chapter 2, Eqn. 8). As more K^+

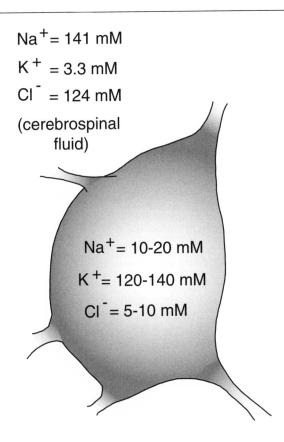

Fig. 3.1   Typical concentrations of Na^+, K^+, and Cl^- inside and outside a neuron in the central nervous system.

$Na^+ = 141$ mM

$K^+ = 3.3$ mM

$Cl^- = 124$ mM

(cerebrospinal fluid)

$Na^+ = 10\text{-}20$ mM

$K^+ = 120\text{-}140$ mM

$Cl^- = 5\text{-}10$ mM

leaves, the voltage across the cell becomes increasingly negative. This makes it increasingly difficult for additional K^+ ions to leave, since to do so they must move across an increasingly larger electric field, and the negativity inside the cell prevents additional positive charge from leaving. Eventually the voltage across the membrane becomes large enough to oppose the diffusion of K^+ outward, and the cell reaches electrochemical equilibrium with a resting membrane potential determined by the K^+ concentrations on the two sides of the membrane.

The asymmetry of charge across membrane that is responsible for the resting potential is actually quite small. For a typical neuron 20 µm in diameter, the total capacitance is of the order of 10^{-11} F (see Chapter 2). For a membrane potential of -100 mV, or -10^{-1} V (with the inside of the cell negative relative to the outside), the charge deficit $\Delta q = C_T V_m = (10^{-11}$ F$)(10^{-1}$ V$) =$ about 10^{-12} coulombs (more positive charges outside than inside). There are approximately 10^5 coulombs per mole for a univalent ion like K^+, so 10^{-12} coulombs is 10^{-17} moles of K^+, in a cell volume of about 4×10^{-12} liter. Thus the deficit of charge amounts to a difference in K^+ concentration of only about $(10^{-17}$ mol$)/(4 \times 10^{-12}$ l$) = 0.25 \times 10^{-5}$ mol l$^{-1} = 2.5$ µM—negligible by comparison to the total concentration of K^+ in the cytosol.

In this chapter I describe the relationship between ion concentration and membrane potential, and I explain how the resting membrane potential can be calculated if the resting permeabilities and concentration gradients are known for each ion. The pumps and transporters that establish the concentration gradients will be the subject of the following chapter.

Membrane Potential at Equilibrium: The Nernst Equation

For a cell at equilibrium, the laws of physical chemistry allow us to calculate how large the membrane potential will be. Consider the simplest case, that of two solutions (labeled 1 and 2), separated by a semipermeable membrane, each containing the same ion at concentrations $c(1)$ or $c(2)$ (Fig. 3.2A). At equilibrium, the *chemical potential* for the solute on both sides of the membrane is the same. The chemical potential (μ) is the Gibbs free energy *(G)* per mole *(n)*,

$$\mu = \frac{\partial G}{\partial n} \tag{1}$$

and equilibrium occurs when

$$\mu(1) = \mu(2) \tag{2}$$

Fig. 3.2 Model cell consisting of solutions separated by a semipermeable membrane (dotted line). **(A)** Solutions 1 and 2 each contain a single solute at concentrations $c(1)$ and $c(2)$. **(B)** Solutions 1 and 2 each contain concentrations $c_1(1)$, $c_2(1)$, and $c_3(1)$ for solution 1 and $c_1(2)$, $c_2(2)$, and $c_3(2)$ for solution 2.

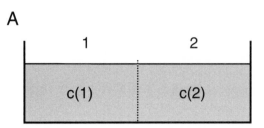

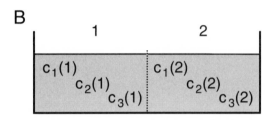

where $\mu(1)$ and $\mu(2)$ represent the chemical potentials in solutions 1 and 2.

At constant temperature, pressure, and volume, for dilute solutions, it can be shown that the chemical potential is given by

$$\mu = \mu^0 + RT \ln(c) + zF\psi \tag{3}$$

The quantity μ^0 is called the *standard chemical potential* (the chemical potential under "standard conditions"), R is the gas constant (8.31 joule per degree per mole), T is the absolute temperature, z is the valence, F is the faraday (96,487 coulomb per mole), and ψ is the electrical potential of the solution. The concentration is of course c, which should be replaced with activities unless the concentrations are dilute.

At equilibrium, since $\mu(1) = \mu(2)$,

$$\mu^0 + RT \ln(c(1)) + zF\psi(1) = \mu^0 + RT \ln(c(2)) + zF\psi(2) \tag{4}$$

Box 3.1

SAMPLE PROBLEM I

Calculate the Nernst potential for a cell at 25°C whose membrane is permeable only to Cl$^-$ if [Cl$^-$]$_i$ = 2 mM and [Cl$^-$]$_o$ = 100 mM.

Answer. Since z_{Cl} is −1, the Nernst equation for Cl$^-$ is V_m = RT/F ln([Cl$^-$]$_i$/[Cl$^-$]$_o$). At 25°C, RT/F is 25.7 mV. So we have (25.7 mV)[ln (2/100)] = −101 mV.

Subtracting one side of the equation from the other gives

$$\psi(2) - \psi(1) = \Delta\psi = \frac{RT}{zF} \ln \frac{c(1)}{c(2)} = 2.303 \frac{RT}{zF} \log_{10} \frac{c(1)}{c(2)} \qquad (5)$$

since $2.303\log_{10}(x) = \ln(x)$ (see Eqn. 18 of Chapter 2).

Eqn. (5) is called the *Nernst equation.* The difference in electrical potential across the membrane at equilibrium is called the *equilibrium potential* (E_j for the jth ion species) and is given by the product of a series of constants (equal for $z = 1$ to 25.7 mV at 25°C or 26.7 mV at 37°C) times the natural logarithm of the ratio of the concentrations; equivalently, the equilibrium potential may be calculated as 59.2 mV (at 25°C) or 61.5 mV (at 37°C) times the logarithm to the base 10 of the ratio of the concentrations.

The Nernst-Planck Equation

The Nernst equation gives the value of the resting membrane potential at equilibrium, and this would be the value of the resting membrane potential for the cell in Fig. 3.1 if the membrane were permeable only to a single ion species, such as K$^+$. Unfortunately, life is not so simple: no living cell is so selectively permeable or is in electrochemical equilibrium. To calculate the membrane potential for a cell permeable to more than one ion species, we must understand the movement of ions across cell membranes under *non-*

equilibrium conditions; and to do this, we need to consider the forces acting on ions in solution.

We begin with the same simple system consisting of two solutions separated by a membrane at constant pressure and at thermal equilibrium. Now we imagine that the solution contains more than one ion species to which the membrane is permeable (Fig. 3.2B). What determines the flux of the *j*th ion (Φ_j) from one solution to the other?

Two forces act on the ion. One is called *electrophoresis:* ions move as charged particles in response to a difference of potential across the membrane. The other force is *diffusion:* ions move from a region of high concentration to one of low concentration. If a membrane is placed between two solutions containing ions at different concentrations, the total flux—that is, the rate at which ions will move from one solution to the other across the membrane—is determined by the sum of the fluxes due to electrophoresis and to diffusion.

To calculate this flux, let us begin with the component (Φ_j^e) due to electrophoresis. First consider the *mobility (u_j),* which is the ratio of the velocity of the ion to the amplitude of the electric field; u_j quantifies the ease with which the ion moves across the membrane in response to a voltage gradient. With this definition, the electrophoretic component of the flux is equal to the product of the concentration of the ion, its valence, its mobility through the membrane, and the electric field, which provides the driving force for charge movement. The electric field *(E)* in turn is equal to the negative of the gradient of the voltage, or $E = -d\psi/dx$ for a single dimension across the membrane. This means that the electrophoretic component Φ_j^e of the flux of the *j*th ion across the membrane, in units of moles per second per square centimeter of membrane, is given by

$$\Phi_j^e = -c_j z_j u_j \frac{d\psi}{dx} \qquad (6)$$

The second component of flux, Φ_j^d, is produced by diffusion. It is given by Fick's first law, which states that the flux is proportional to the amplitude of the concentration gradient. For a single dimension across the membrane, Fick's first law is

$$\Phi_j^d = -D_j \frac{dc_j}{dx} \tag{7}$$

where D_j is the diffusion constant for the jth ion. The sign is negative, since diffusion always occurs in a direction opposite in sign to the concentration gradient, that is, from high concentration to low.

It will be convenient in many cases to express the diffusion constant in terms of the mobility. The mobility is related to the diffusion constant by the Einstein relation, $u = De/kT$, where e is the elementary charge and k is Boltzmann's constant. Fick's law is then

$$\Phi_j^d = -\frac{u_j kT}{e} \frac{dc_j}{dx} \tag{8}$$

Multiplying both the numerator and the denominator of Eqn. (8) by Avogadro's number, N_A (and remembering that $R = kN_A$ and $F = eN_A$), we have

$$\Phi_j^d = -\frac{u_j RT}{F} \frac{dc_j}{dx} \tag{9}$$

Summing the diffusional and electrophoretic components (Eqns. 6 and 9) gives

$$\Phi_j = -u_j c_j \left(\frac{RT}{Fc_j} \frac{dc_j}{dx} + z_j \frac{d\psi}{dx} \right) \tag{10}$$

This expression is known as the *Nernst-Planck equation.*

It will be helpful in many cases to convert this equation from an equation for flux into an equation for current flow. We can do this by multiplying the flux by $z_j F$, where z_j is the valence or charge per ion and F (the faraday) is 96,487 coulombs per mole. We then have the Nernst-Planck equation for the current density (I_j, expressed in amperes per square centimeter):

$$I_j = -z_j u_j (RT \frac{dc_j}{dx} + c_j z_j F \frac{d\psi}{dx}) \qquad (11)$$

Nernst-Planck Equation for a Simple Salt

It is instructive to begin by solving the Nernst-Planck equation for the simplest case, that of a membrane permeable only to K^+. From Eqn. (11), remembering that z_K is equal to 1, we have for K^+:

$$I_K = -u_K RT \frac{d[K^+]}{dx} - u_K [K^+] F \frac{d\psi}{dx} \qquad (12)$$

If the system is at steady state, then the net flow of K^+ across the membrane is zero, and I_K is zero. So

$$0 = -u_K RT \frac{d[K^+]}{dx} - u_K [K^+] F \frac{d\psi}{dx} \qquad (13)$$

Combining terms and multiplying through by dx, we have

$$d\psi = -\frac{RT}{F} \frac{d[K^+]}{[K^+]} \qquad (14)$$

Recalling that $dx/x = d(\ln x)$, we can integrate both sides of this equation across the membrane from solution 1 to solution 2:

$$\psi_2 - \psi_1 = -\frac{RT}{F} \ln \frac{[K^+]_2}{[K^+]_1} \qquad (15)$$

We now adopt the convention that solution 1 is "inside" and solution 2 is "outside" and that the membrane potential is defined as *inside* minus *outside*. This means that $V_m = \psi_1 - \psi_2$ and

$$V_m = \frac{RT}{F} \ln \frac{[K^+]_o}{[K^+]_i} = 2.303 \frac{RT}{F} \log_{10} \frac{[K^+]_o}{[K^+]_i} \qquad (16)$$

Eqn. (16) is identical in form to the Nernst equation. This is a comforting result. If a cell is permeable only to a single species of ion, the cell is at equilibrium *and* at steady state, and it should not matter whether we calculate the membrane potential with the Nernst equation or the Nernst-Planck equation. This means that for a membrane permeable only to K^+, V_m is equal to the equilibrium potential for potassium, E_K.

Using the Nernst Equation to Calculate Membrane Potential

To use the Nernst equation to calculate membrane potentials for a nerve cell permeable only to a single ion species, we might take the values of ion concentrations given in Fig. 3.1. For simplicity of notation, we let K_o and K_i stand for $[K^+]_o$ and $[K^+]_i$. If at rest the membrane were exclusively permeable to K^+, we would expect the membrane potential (at 37°C) to be (26.7 mV)$\ln(K_o/K_i)$, or between (26.7 mV)$\ln(3.3/120) = -96$ mV and (26.7 mV)$\ln(3.3/140)$ $= -100$ mV. This is more negative than the normal resting membrane potential of a typical neuron (-70 to -80 mV), suggesting that most nerve cells at rest are not exclusively permeable to K^+. More evidence for this will be given later in this chapter.

If the membrane were suddenly to become exclusively permeable to Na^+ (as nearly occurs at the peak of the action potential), the membrane potential would go to (26.7 mV)$\ln(Na_o/Na_i)$, or between 52 and 71 mV. An increase in Na^+ permeability should cause the membrane potential to become more positive. On the other hand, the equilibrium potential for Cl^- (since $z_{Cl} = -1$) is $-(26.7$ mV)$\ln(Cl_o/Cl_i)$ or (26.7 mV)$\ln(Cl_i/Cl_o)$, between -67 and -86 mV for a typical neuron. This is near to the resting membrane potential, which means that a large increase in conductance to Cl^- (produced, for example, by inhibitory input) might be expected to leave the resting membrane potential nearly unchanged. This is likely to be an oversimplification. In some cells, or in some regions of cells, inhibitory input causes the membrane potential to become more negative (to *hyperpolarize*), probably because there is active transport of Cl⁻ out of the cell interior. In other cells or regions of cells, inhibition causes the membrane potential to become more positive (to *depolarize*), because there is active transport of Cl⁻ *into* the cell (Chapter 4).

The Goldman-Hodgkin-Katz (GHK) Current Equation

A general expression for calculating the membrane potential at steady state when the membrane is permeable to more than one ion species was first derived by Goldman (1943). This derivation uses the Nernst-Planck equation and, in many respects, is quite similar to the one just given for a membrane permeable to a single ion (Eqn. 5). Goldman, however, added a further assumption about the form of the electric field across the membrane. Goldman made the simplest possible assumption, that the electric field *(E)* is constant with distance through the thickness of the membrane. Recall that for a single dimension (i.e., perpendicular to the membrane), $E = -d\psi/dx$. Suppose we integrate E across the membrane (from $x = 0$ to $x = \delta$) for a membrane of thickness δ. If E is a constant (we shall call the value of this constant E), then

$$\Delta\psi = \int_0^\delta Edx \quad \text{and} \quad \Delta\psi = E\delta \tag{17}$$

The drop of potential across the membrane is illustrated in Fig. 3.3.

With this assumption, called the *constant-field* assumption, it is possible to derive an expression for the current of a particular ion across the membrane as a function of the voltage and ion concentration. This expression is called the *Goldman* or *GHK current equation,* and its derivation is given in Box 3.2. For Na⁺, the GHK current equation can be obtained by substituting the Na⁺ concentrations into Eqn. (30) in Box 3.2, giving

$$I_{Na} = P_{Na}V_m \frac{F^2}{RT} \frac{[Na^+]_o - [Na^+]_i e^{FV_m/RT}}{1 - e^{FV_m/RT}} \tag{18}$$

The expression for K⁺ is similar and is given below as Eqn. (31).

For Cl⁻, the negative valence introduces negative exponentials

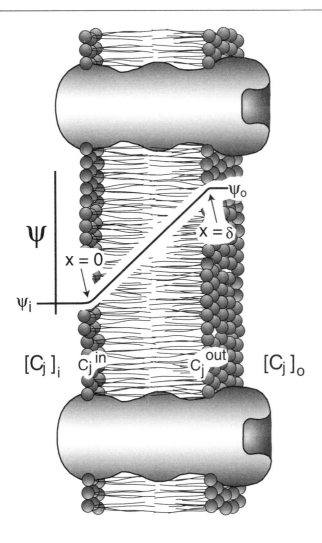

Fig. 3.3 Assumptions of the Goldman-Hodgkin-Katz equation. Lipid membrane (including two membrane proteins) separates two solutions, each containing ions of species j at a concentration of $[C_j]_i$ (on the intracellular side of the membrane) and $[C_j]_o$ (on the extracellular side of the membrane). The concentrations of the ions just inside the membrane, at the membrane-solution border, are assumed to be proportional to their concentrations in solution (see Box 3.2, Eqn. 29) and are given by c_j^{in} and c_j^{out}. The assumption of a constant electric field within the membrane is equivalent to assuming that the potential changes linearly from ψ_i at the intracellular surface of the membrane (at $x = 0$) to ψ_o at the extracellular surface (at $x = \delta$).

in both the numerator and denominator of Eqn. (30). That is, $e^{z_j FV_m/RT}$ becomes $e^{-FV_m/RT}$. We can substitute these negative exponentials with $1/e^{FV_m/RT}$, multiply both the numerator and denominator within the brackets of Eqn. (30) by $-e^{FV_m/RT}$, and obtain

$$I_{Cl} = P_{Cl}V_m \frac{F^2}{RT} \frac{[Cl^-]_i - [Cl^-]_o e^{FV_m/RT}}{1 - e^{FV_m/RT}} \qquad (19)$$

Box 3.2

DERIVATION OF GHK CURRENT EQUATION

In order to derive the Goldman (or GHK) current equation, we give the transmembrane potential ($\Delta\psi$) as V_m, so that Eqn. (17) becomes $V_m = E\delta$. Therefore,

$$E = -\frac{d\psi}{dx} = \frac{V_m}{\delta} \tag{20}$$

and we can substitute $-V_m/\delta$ for $d\psi/dx$ in the Nernst-Planck equation, which greatly simplifies this equation and allows us to solve it. With the further assistance of the Einstein relation ($u_j = D_j F/RT$), we can transform Eqn. (11) into

$$I_j = -D_j F z_j \frac{dc_j}{dx} + \frac{D_j F^2 z_j^2 V_m}{RT\delta} c_j \tag{21}$$

(Remember that $d\psi/dx = -V_m/\delta$). Eqn. (21) can be rewritten as

$$\frac{dc_j}{dx} - \frac{F z_j V_m}{RT\delta} c_j = -\frac{I_j}{D_j F z_j} \tag{22}$$

which is of the form

$$\frac{dc_j}{dx} + ac_j = b, \text{ with } a = -\frac{F z_j V_m}{RT\delta}, b = -\frac{I_j}{D_j F z_j} \tag{23}$$

This is a first-order, linear differential equation, whose solution can be obtained (e.g., by the method of integrating factors) as

$$c_j = \frac{b}{a} + c_j' e^{-ax} \tag{24}$$

where c_j' is a constant. This solution can be inserted back into Eqn. (23) to verify that it is correct.

   The next step is to evaluate c_j'. To do this, we assign a value to the concentration of the jth ion at the position $x = 0$, just inside the membrane adjacent to the internal solution (see Fig. 3.3). We call this concentration c_j^{in}, so at $x = 0$, $c_j = c_j^{in}$. Substituting this into Eqn. (24), we have $c_j^{in} = b/a + c_j'$ (since $e^0 = 1$), so that $c_j' = c_j^{in} - b/a$. Eqn. (24) now becomes

$$c_j = \frac{b}{a} + (c_j^{in} - \frac{b}{a})e^{-ax} \qquad (25)$$

At the other side of the membrane, $x = \delta$, and we let $c_j = c_j^{out}$. So

$$c_j^{out} = \frac{b}{a} + (c_j^{in} - \frac{b}{a})e^{-a\delta} \qquad (26)$$

After expanding and rearranging, we have

$$\frac{b}{a} = \frac{c_j^{out} - c_j^{in} e^{-a\delta}}{1 - e^{-a\delta}} \qquad (27)$$

Reintroducing a and b, we have an expression for the current:

$$I_j = \frac{D_j F^2 z_j^2 V_m}{RT\delta} \left[\frac{c_j^{out} - c_j^{in} e^{z_j FV_m/RT}}{1 - e^{z_j FV_m/RT}} \right] \qquad (28)$$

The final step is to make some assumptions about the concentrations of the ions just at the border of the membrane (at $x = 0$ and $x = \delta$). Following Hodgkin and Katz (1949), we assume that c_j^{in} and c_j^{out} are proportional to the concentrations of c_j in the bulk solution (in Fig. 3.3, $[C_j]_i$ and $[C_j]_o$) with a proportionality constant called the partition coefficient (β_j), such that

$$c_j^{in} = \beta_j [C_j]_i \text{ and } c_j^{out} = \beta_j [C_j]_o \qquad (29)$$

We then define the permeability constant for the jth ion (P_j) as $P_j = D_j\beta_j/\delta$. This relationship and Eqn. (29) are then inserted into Eqn. (28) to give

$$I_j = P_j V_m z_j^2 \frac{F^2}{RT} \left[\frac{[C_j]_o - [C_j]_i e^{z_j FV_m/RT}}{1 - e^{z_j FV_m/RT}} \right] \qquad (30)$$

Equation (30) is called the Goldman (or GHK) *current* equation. It gives the current of a particular ion species across the membrane as a function of voltage, permeability, and concentration.

Current-Voltage Curves

Since the GHK current equation gives the current density as a function of voltage, we can use it to construct a graph of current *versus* voltage, known as an "*i–V* curve." We must keep in mind the assumptions made in deriving the GHK equation: that the membrane is homogeneous, that the electric field is constant through the membrane, that ions move in the membrane as in free solution, that ions behave independently (do not interact), and that the concentrations of the ions at the edges of the membrane are proportional to their concentrations in bulk solution. These assumptions are likely to be only approximately true for biological membranes under physiological conditions. Nevertheless, calculating the current-voltage curve from the GHK current equation gives important insights into the voltage and concentration dependence of permeation.

In the following example, we calculate the K^+ current as a function of concentration and voltage. First, we set $[K^+]_i$ equal to 100 mM and vary $[K^+]_o$, using values of 2, 10, 20, 40, 60, 70, and 100 mM (Fig. 3.4A). We use a permeability constant for K^+ *(P_K)* of 2 x 10^{-6} cm s^{-1} (similar to the one given by Hodgkin and Katz, 1949, for the squid giant axon), and we assume that the permeability of K^+ does not depend upon the membrane potential. The ordinate gives current density in units of amps per square centimeter of membrane. Outward currents (produced by K^+ flowing out of the cell) are positive, and inward currents are negative. Notice that for $[K^+]_i = [K^+]_o = 100$ mM, the current-voltage curve passes through the origin and is linear. The curve passes through the origin since at the equilibrium potential for K^+, there is no net K^+ current through the membrane; and the equilibrium potential for K^+ is given by the Nernst equation,

$$E_K = \frac{RT}{F} \ln \frac{[K^+]_o}{[K^+]_i}$$

which is zero, since $\ln(1) = 0$.

The curve for $[K^+]_i = [K^+]_o$ is linear since the Goldman current equation for K^+ is

$$I_K = P_K V_m \frac{F^2}{RT} \frac{[K^+]_o - [K^+]_i e^{FV_m/RT}}{1 - e^{FV_m/RT}} \qquad (31)$$

If $[K^+]_i = [K^+]_o$, then the concentration terms in the numerator of Eqn. (31) become $[K^+]_i(1 - e^{FV_m/RT})$, and the exponential terms in the numerator and denominator cancel. The current then becomes a constant function of voltage:

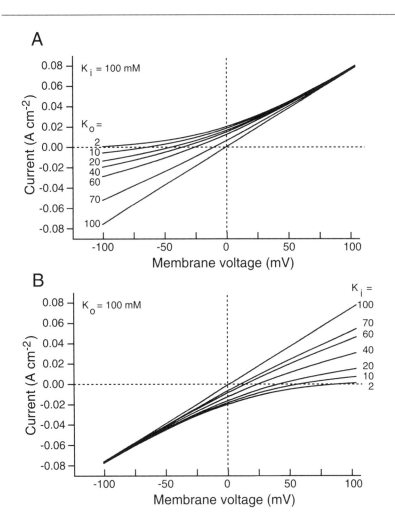

Fig. 3.4 Solutions of Goldman-Hodgkin-Katz current equation for K^+ (Eqn. 31). Current plotted as a function of voltage, with permeability constant for K^+ (P_K) assumed to be 2×10^{-6} cm s^{-1}. **(A)** $[K^+]_i$ set to 100 mM, and $[K^+]_o$ varied as shown. **(B)** $[K^+]_o$ set to 100 mM, and $[K^+]_i$ varied as shown.

$$I_K = P_K \frac{F^2}{RT} [K^+]_i V_m \qquad (32)$$

For $[K^+]_i > [K^+]_o$, the curves pass through the current axis at progressively more negative values, since the equilibrium potential becomes progressively more negative at lower external K^+ concentrations. The curves also decline in slope ("flatten out") at negative voltages. This is called *outward rectification* and is a form of *Goldman rectification* or *constant-field rectification*. The term *rectification* indicates that the current is a nonlinear function of voltage, which means that current passes more easily in one direction than in the other. For the curves in Fig. 3.4A, positive currents are larger than negative currents, so current passes more easily outward (thus *outward* rectification). The reason rectification occurs for $[K^+]_i > [K^+]_o$ in Fig. 3.4A is quite simple. As the extracellular K^+ concentration is made smaller, there are fewer ions to carry inward current, and the inward current decreases. In the limit of $[K^+]_o = 0$, the GHK current equation becomes

$$I_K = P_K V_m \frac{F^2}{RT} [K^+]_i \frac{-e^{FV_m/RT}}{1 - e^{FV_m/RT}} \qquad (33)$$

At large negative V_m, the term in the numerator goes to zero, and the current goes to zero. At large positive V_m, the exponential terms in numerator and denominator nearly cancel, and the current approaches the value given in Eqn. (32) for $[K^+]_i = [K^+]_o$.

In Fig. 3.4B, $[K^+]_o$ is equal to 100 mM, and $[K^+]_i$ varies over the values of 2, 10, 20, 40, 60, 70, and 100 mM. For $[K^+]_o > [K^+]_i$, the equilibrium potentials are positive and the curves decrease in slope at positive voltages. This is called *inward rectification*, since current passes more easily in an inward direction than in an outward direction. Goldman rectification is an important consequence of an asymmetry in the concentrations of permeant ions across membranes and occurs in many cases of physiological interest.

Box 3.3

SAMPLE PROBLEM 2

For a neuron whose internal and external solutions both consist of 100 mM NaCl and whose membrane is impermeable to Cl⁻, a current of 1 nA was recorded at a membrane potential of 100 mV and at 25°C. If the surface area of the cell is 100 μm², use the GHK current equation to estimate the Na⁺ permeability.

Answer. Since $[Na^+]_o = [Na^+]_i$, we can write the GHK current equation as in Eqn. (32): $I_{Na} = P_{Na}F^2[Na^+]_iV_m/RT$. So $P_{Na} = I_{Na}RT/F^2[Na^+]_iV_m$. Remember that I_{Na} in this equation is the current *density* (A cm⁻²). $I_{Na} = (10^{-9}$ A$)/(10^{-6}$ cm²$) = 10^{-3}$ A cm⁻² or 10^{-3} coulombs per second per square centimeter (C s⁻¹ cm⁻²). We can now calculate P_{Na} as $(10^{-3}$ C s⁻¹ cm⁻²$)(8.31$ J °K⁻¹ mol⁻¹$)(298$ °K$)/(96,487$ J V⁻¹ mol⁻¹$)(96,487$ C mol⁻¹$)(10^{-4}$ mol cm⁻³$)(0.1$ V$) = 2.66 \times 10^{-5}$ cm s⁻¹. Notice that we expressed the Na⁺ concentration in units of moles per cubic centimeter, so that 100 mM became 10^{-4} mol cm⁻³. We also expressed the Faraday two different ways, once as joules per volt per mole and once as coulombs per mole. That a joule per volt is equal to a coulomb is clear if you remember that, for an electrical circuit, the power expenditure P (in watts, or joules per second) is given by $P = iV$. That is, (J s⁻¹) = (C s⁻¹)(V), so C = J V⁻¹.

Rectification of Receptor Currents

Throughout this book there are many examples of rectification, both inward and outward. As Fig. 3.4 shows, rectification can be produced merely by a difference in the concentrations of ions on the two sides of the membrane, but this is not the only cause of rectification. Fig. 3.5 gives the current-voltage curve for the current evoked by glycine in a neuron dissociated from the spinal cord and recorded with a patch-clamp electrode in the whole-cell recording mode (from Bormann, Hamill, and Sakmann, 1987). This curve shows a pronounced outward rectification, much like that in Fig. 3.4A. Could it be the result of Goldman rectification?

We can answer this question quite definitely, since we know (in part as the result of the data in this same paper) that glycine

Fig. 3.5 Rectification of current through a glycine channel. **(A)** Net change in membrane current induced by glycine for dissociated embryonic neuron from mouse spinal cord. Current recordings were made under voltage clamp with whole-cell patch recording. **(B)** Chord conductance calculated from currents in **(A)** and the equation $\Delta i_m = \Delta g (V_m - E_{rev})$. **(C)** Definition of chord conductance as $\Delta g = \Delta i_m / (V_m - E_{rev})$. The value of the chord conductance can be obtained by drawing a chord *(dotted lines)* between the point at which $i = 0$ (where the curve crosses the voltage axis at the reversal potential) and the value of the current at voltage V_m. The slope of the chord will be equal to the ratio of Δi_m (the rise of the chord) and $V_m - E_{rev}$ (the run of the chord). Two chords are shown here, one for $V_m = -100$ mV and one for $V_m = 100$ mV. The greater slope of the second chord illustrates the point made in the text that the conductance change, $\Delta g = \Delta i_m / (V_m - E_{rev})$, increases as the membrane is depolarized. (Parts **(A)** and **(B)** taken, with minor modifications, from Bormann, Hamill, and Sakmann, 1987, and reprinted with permission of the authors and the Physiological Society.)

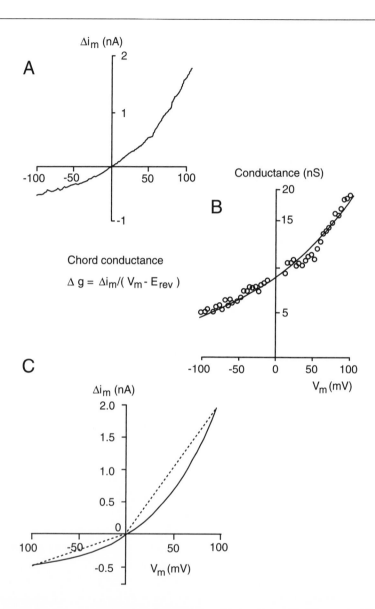

channels are very selective for anions. Since the experiment in Fig. 3.5 was done with whole-cell recording, Bormann and colleagues could control both the intracellular and extracellular ion concentrations. The only anion present in either solution was Cl⁻, at a concentration of 148 mM outside and 146 mM inside. Cl⁻ would have had a slightly greater tendency to flow inward, which would have produced a small *outward* rectification, since Cl$^-$ is negatively charged, and an inward movement of Cl$^-$ produces an outward current. However, a calculation much like that performed for Fig. 3.4 will show that this concentration difference is much too small to account for the rectification observed for the glycine current in Fig. 3.5. If Goldman rectification is not responsible, some other process must produce the nonlinearity of the $i-V$ curve.

For glycine receptors, the most probable explanation is that the channel has an intrinsic voltage dependence: even with glycine bound, the channel is more likely to open and let ions enter when the membrane potential is positive than when it is negative. Fig. 3.5B is a plot of the change in membrane conductance produced by glycine, estimated from the following equation:

$$\Delta i_m = \Delta g(V_m - E_{rev})\qquad(34)$$

where Δi_m is the change in membrane current produced by ions flowing through glycine-gated channels, Δg is the change in conductance produced by the opening of the channels, V_m is the membrane potential, and E_{rev} is the reversal potential. The reversal potential is defined as the membrane voltage for which glycine produces no change in current. Eqn. (34) says that when V_m is equal to E_{rev}, Δi_m is zero regardless of the size of the conductance change. E_{rev} is called the reversal potential because the sign of the current reverses for voltages positive and negative of E_{rev}. The quantity $(V_m - E_{rev})$ is often called the *driving force*.

The conductance calculated from Eqn. (34) is usually referred to as the *chord conductance,* because it is equivalent to the slope of the line drawn as a chord on the $i-V$ curve between the points at which voltage equals V_m and E_{rev} (see Fig. 3.5C). It is also possible to define conductance from Ohm's law as di/dV, and this is usually referred to as the *slope conductance.* The slope conductance is obtained from the instantaneous slope of the current-voltage curve at any voltage V_m. The slope of the current-voltage curve will have units of conductance, since the slope is given by the instantaneous change in current divided by the instantaneous change in voltage. Note that the slope and chord conductances have the same

Box 3.4

SAMPLE PROBLEM 3

After considerable effort, you have succeeded in extracting a biologically active peptide from the poison gland of the toad, *Bufo marinus*. You prefuse this peptide, which you have decided to call "Z peptide," onto a neuron that you have dissociated from the nucleus obscurus, and then you voltage-clamp with the whole-cell recording method. You see an inward current at the resting membrane potential, which your patient investigations show to be due to a change in Cl^- conductance. You then record the complete current-voltage curve under voltage clamp for the net current response to Z peptide, with 100 mM Cl^- in the external solution and 20 mM Cl^- in your pipette (i.e., in the cell), at 25°C:

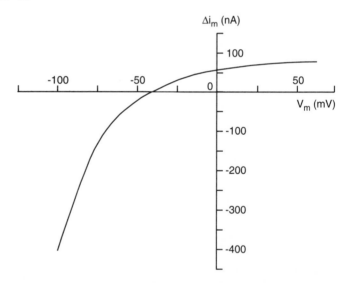

A. Does Z peptide open channels or close them? How do you know?

Answer. If the channels are permeable only to Cl^-, then the reversal potential can be calculated from the Nernst equation (Eqn. 5). Since RT/F is 25.7 mV at 25°C, we have (25.7 mV)[ln(20/100)], or about −41 mV (see Box 3.1). Notice that the current-voltage curve passes through the x-axis at about this voltage. To find out if channels open or close, we calculate the chord conductance. That is, we insert values for currents and voltages into the equation

$$\Delta i_m = \Delta g(V_m - E_{rev})$$

Take $V_m = -100$ mV. We have from the graph $\Delta i_m = -400$ nA $= \Delta g[-100 - (-41)$ mV$] = \Delta g(-59$ mV$)$. Since both Δi_m and $(V_m - E_{rev})$ are negative, Δg must be positive. Alternatively, at $V_m = +50$ mV, $\Delta i_m = +75$ nA $= \Delta g[50 - (-41)$ mV$] = \Delta g(91$ mV$)$, and again Δg is positive. That Δg is positive can also be inferred from the shape of the curve, which is monotonically rising with positive slope, with the chord and slope conductances everywhere positive. Since Δg is positive—that is, since conductance is increasing—Z peptide must be opening channels.

B. Is the rectification of the current-voltage curve inward or outward? Can it be due to Goldman rectification? Why (or why not)?

Answer. The rectification is inward: currents pass more easily in an inward (negative) direction than in an outward direction. This can be seen from the graph, since for voltages equidistant from the reversal potential, inward currents are much larger than outward currents. Since the ion carrying the current in this case is Cl^-, the movement of the ion is opposite in direction to the movement of the current, and Cl^- moves more easily outward. This is opposite to the expected direction, since there is more Cl^- outside the cell than inside. Cl^- would therefore be expected to move more easily inward, and the Goldman equation would predict outward rectification. Thus the rectification for the channels opened by Z peptide cannot be due to Goldman rectification.

value only if the current-voltage curve is a straight line. By either measure, the conductance increase produced by glycine becomes larger as the membrane is depolarized, and this is evidence that the glycine channel has an intrinsic sensitivity to membrane voltage similar to (though much smaller than) the voltage dependence of voltage-gated Na^+ and K^+ channels (Chapters 5–7).

The Goldman (GHK) Voltage Equation

Although the GHK current equation is often helpful in understanding the electrical behavior of single cells, a much more widely used expression is the GHK voltage equation. This equation can be used to calculate the membrane potential at steady state when the membrane is permeable to more than one species of ion. The GHK voltage equation can be derived from the current equation if we assume that there is no net current across the membrane, that is,

$$\sum_j I_j = 0 \tag{35}$$

Let us suppose that the only ions of physiological interest are Na^+, K^+, and Cl^-. At steady state, Eqn. (35) requires that $I_{Na} + I_K + I_{Cl} = 0$. From Eqns. (18), (19), and (31), we have

$$P_{Na}[Na^+]_o - P_{Na}[Na^+]_i e^{FV_m/RT} + P_K[K^+]_o - P_K[K^+]_i e^{FV_m/RT} \tag{36}$$
$$+ P_{Cl}[Cl^-]_i - P_{Cl}[Cl^-]_o e^{FV_m/RT} = 0$$

Combining terms and taking the logarithm, we have

$$V_m = \frac{RT}{F} \ln \frac{P_{Na}[Na^+]_o + P_K[K^+]_o + P_{Cl}[Cl^-]_i}{P_{Na}[Na^+]_i + P_K[K^+]_i + P_{Cl}[Cl^-]_o} \tag{37}$$

Note that for Cl^-, the inside concentration is in the numerator, because the valence of chloride is negative (see Eqns. 19 and 36). This is the most common form of the Goldman (GHK) voltage equation, often just called the Goldman equation.

The Goldman voltage equation is of more general applicability than the current equation. Although it was necessary to assume a constant field within the membrane to derive the current equation, and although (following Hodgkin and Katz, 1949) we have derived the voltage equation *from* the current equation, it can be shown that the voltage equation can actually be derived directly from the Nernst-Planck equation for any voltage profile through the membrane (Hille, 1975). It isn't even necessary that the diffusion coefficients *(D_i)* be constant, provided that everywhere within the membrane the D_j's for the different ions remain in fixed proportion. The voltage equation is also unaffected by channel block or saturation of the current through the membrane at high concentrations of the permeant ion. This makes the GHK voltage equation particularly useful to the cellular neurophysiologist, and I use it extensively in the remainder of the book.

Calculating the Resting Membrane Potential

To illustrate how this equation can be used to calculate the resting membrane potential, I have chosen one famous example. Nerve and muscle cells at rest (and animal cells in general) are primarily permeable to K^+, as noted earlier. When, however, the external $[K^+]_o$ is varied, the resting potential typically deviates from the Nernst potential, particularly at low values of $[K^+]_o$. Figure 3.6, from the paper of Hodgkin and Horowicz (1959), gives the membrane potential for a muscle fiber as a function of $[K^+]_o$. The muscle fiber in this experiment was perfused with zero $[Cl^-]_o$ medium for a fairly long time before the experiments were begun, so it is probably safe to assume that all the Cl^- would have come out of the cell, and that both $[Cl^-]_o$ and $[Cl^-]_i$ were zero. The Goldman equation is then

$$V_m = \frac{RT}{F} \ln \frac{P_{Na}[\text{Na}^+]_o + P_K[\text{K}^+]_o}{P_{Na}[\text{Na}^+]_i + P_K[\text{K}^+]_i} \tag{38}$$

If we let α equal P_{Na}/P_K, then this equation simplifies to

$$V_m = \frac{RT}{F} \ln \frac{\alpha[\text{Na}^+]_o + [\text{K}^+]_o}{\alpha[\text{Na}^+]_i + [\text{K}^+]_i} \tag{39}$$

The data in Fig. 3.6 have been fitted with Eqn. (39) for $\alpha = 0$ and for $\alpha = 0.01$. For $\alpha = 0$, Eqn. (39) becomes the Nernst equation. The Nernst equation gives a poor fit, especially at low $[K^+]_o$. A much better fit is obtained if some Na^+ permeability is assumed. Using similar methods, Hodgkin and Katz (1949) showed that the

Fig. 3.6 Resting membrane potential of a frog skeletal muscle fiber as a function of $[K^+]_o$. Muscle fibers were equilibrated for one hour in Cl^--free solution (chloride was replaced with sulphate), and the Cl^- concentration after equilibration was assumed to be zero both inside and outside the muscle fiber. Membrane potential was recorded with a fine intracellular micropipette connected to a voltage preamplifier. Filled circles are measurements made after 10–60 min in the indicated extracellular K^+ concentration, and open circles are measurements made only 20–60 s after a concentration change. Data have been fitted with the Nernst equation and with the Goldman-Hodgkin-Katz voltage equation, with 2.303 $RT/F = 58$ mV (see Eqn. 5). Intracellular K^+ concentration was assumed to have remained constant during the experiments and equal to 140 mM. The value of $\alpha[Na]_i$ was assumed to be negligible in comparison to $[K]_i$. The fit to the GHK equation assumes a ratio of Na^+ to K^+ permeability (P_{Na}/P_K) of 0.01. (Redrawn from Hodgkin and Horowicz, 1959.)

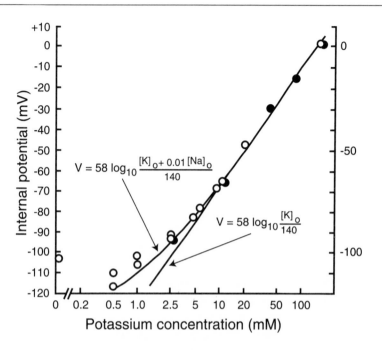

resting membrane of the squid axon is primarily permeable to K^+ but also shows significant permeability to Na^+ and even to Cl^-.

Estimating Ion Selectivity

The Goldman or GHK voltage equation is also useful for estimating ion selectivity—that is, the relative permeabilities of a channel to different ions. One of the most interesting and important properties of an ion channel is its ability to admit certain ions and exclude others. The selectivity of the resting membrane of a nerve to K^+ is, for example, responsible for the negative resting membrane potential, and the opening of channels selective for Na^+ produces the large positive upswing of the action potential. Ion channels, however, are not exclusively permeable to just one ion type: Na^+ channels, for example, are permeable not only to Na^+ but also to Li^+, NH_4^+, and even sparingly to K^+. From measurements of ion selectivity we may learn about the structure of the channel pore and about differences in the structure and function of different types of channels.

Box 3.5

SAMPLE PROBLEM 4

What is the resting membrane potential of a cell whose internal (cytoplasmic) solution is 100 mM KCl and whose external solution is 10 mM KCl (with sucrose added to preserve osmotic balance), if $P_{Cl}/P_K = 0.2$? If $P_{Cl}/P_K = 0.1$? Assume a temperature of 25°C.

Answer. We use the Goldman voltage equation. Let $\alpha = P_{Cl}/P_K$ and $RT/F = 25.7$ mV. Since no Na^+ is present, the Goldman equation reduces to

$$V_m = \frac{RT}{F} \ln \frac{[K^+]_o + \alpha[Cl^-]_i}{[K^+]_i + \alpha[Cl^-]_o}$$

For $\alpha = 0.2$,

$$V_m = (25.7\,\text{mV})\left[\ln \frac{10\,\text{mM} + (0.2)(100\,\text{mM})}{100\,\text{mM} + (0.2)(10\,\text{mM})}\right]$$

$$= (25.7\,\text{mV})\left[\ln \frac{30}{102}\right] = -31.5\,\text{mV}$$

For $\alpha = 0.1$, $V_m = (25.7\,\text{mV})[\ln(20/101)] = -41.6$ mV.

SAMPLE PROBLEM 5

Suppose you record a resting potential from a neuron of -70 mV at 25°C, and the resting ion concentrations are as follows: $[Na^+]_o = 150$ mM, $[Na^+]_i = 20$ mM, $[K^+]_o = 2.5$ mM, $[K^+]_i = 120$ mM, $[Cl^-]_o = 150$ mM, and $[Cl^-]_i = 5$ mM.

A. What is P_{Na}/P_K if $P_{Cl} = 0$?

Answer. We again use the GHK equation, but because $P_{Cl} = 0$, now

$$V_m = \frac{RT}{F} \ln \frac{[K^+]_o + \alpha[Na^+]_o}{[K^+]_i + \alpha[Na^+]_i}$$

where α is P_{Na}/P_K. Plugging in the numbers and using 25.7 mV for RT/F, we have:

continued

−70 mV = (25.7 mV) ln [(2.5 + 150α)/(120 + 20α)], so −2.72 = ln [(2.5 + 150α)/(120 + 20α)]. Taking natural antilogs of both sides, we have 0.066 = (2.5 + 150α)/(120 + 20α), and 7.875 + 1.313α = 2.5 + 150α. Simplifying, we have 5.375 = 148.7α, and α = 0.036.

B. What is P_{Na}/P_{Cl} if $P_K = 0$?
   Answer. Now the equation becomes

$$V_m = \frac{RT}{F} \ln \frac{\alpha[Na^+]_o + [Cl^-]_i}{\alpha[Na^+]_i + [Cl^-]_o}$$

where α is P_{Na}/P_{Cl}. We have −70 mV = (25.7 mV) ln [(150α + 5)/(20α + 150)]. Now 0.066 is equal to (150α + 5)/(20α + 150), and using the same procedure as in A we calculate that α is 0.033. As expected from the negative resting potential, the membrane is much more permeable to Cl^- under these circumstances than to Na^+.

To demonstrate how the Goldman equation can be used in this way, I begin with some experimental results. The recordings in Fig. 3.7 are again from the study by Bormann, Hamill, and Sakmann (1987) of the glycine and GABA responses of neurons dissociated from the spinal cord. The upper trace (Fig. 3.7A) graphs currents recorded after a brief application of glycine, under conditions identical to those in Fig. 3.6; i.e., with $[Cl^-]_o = 148$ mM and $[Cl^-]_i = 146$ mM. The traces in Fig. 3.7B are recordings for which most of the Cl^- in the intracellular (pipette) solution was substituted with Br^-, I^-, or SCN^- (thiocyanate).

For each ion in the internal and external medium, we can write an equation for the current through the glycine channels using the GHK current equation,

$$I_j = P_j V_m z_j^2 \frac{F^2}{RT} \left[\frac{[C_j]_o - [C_j]_i e^{z_j F V_m / RT}}{1 - e^{z_j F V_m / RT}} \right] \tag{30}$$

At the reversal potential, there is no net flow of current through the GABA channels, so

$$\sum_j I_j = 0 \tag{35}$$

This means that, just as for the resting membrane potential, the value of the reversal potential is given by the GHK voltage equation,

$$E_{rev} = \frac{RT}{F} \ln \frac{P_{Na}[\text{Na}^+]_o + P_K[\text{K}^+]_o + P_{Cl}[\text{Cl}^-]_i}{P_{Na}[\text{Na}^+]_i + P_K[\text{K}^+]_i + P_{Cl}[\text{Cl}^-]_o} \tag{37}$$

which again can be used in a wide variety of circumstances for virtually any profile of the electric field through the membrane, provided the diffusion constants for the various ions either remain constant or in fixed proportion to one another (Hille, 1975).

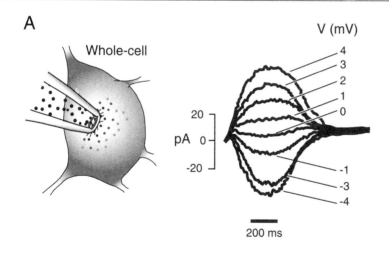

A

Whole-cell

V (mV)

20

pA 0

-20

200 ms

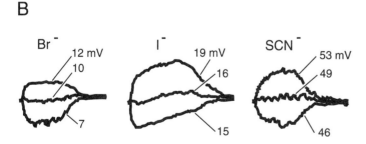

B

Br⁻

I⁻

SCN⁻

Fig. 3.7 Measurement of the reversal potential of the change in membrane current elicited by glycine, recorded with whole-cell voltage clamp from dissociated embryonic neurons of mouse spinal cord. Traces show the change in membrane current induced by a brief application of 10 μM glycine at the membrane potential indicated for each response. **(A)** Extracellular solution contained 148 mM Cl⁻ and intracellular solution 146 mM Cl⁻. Reversal potential (the voltage at which current does not change) is near 0 mV. **(B)** Intracellular solution now contains 140 mM of Br⁻, I⁻, or SCN⁻ plus 4 mM Cl⁻. Note changes in reversal potential. (Reprinted from Bormann, Hamill, and Sakmann, 1987, with permission of the authors and of the Physiological Society.)

We can use the GHK voltage equation to calculate the reversal potentials for each of the anions in Fig. 3.7. In Fig. 3.7A, the reversal potential is very close to zero, since the Cl^- concentrations on the two sides of the membrane were nearly the same:

$$E_{rev} = \frac{RT}{F} \ln \frac{P_{Cl}[Cl^-]_i}{P_{Cl}[Cl^-]_o} \tag{40}$$

(remember $z = -1$), and this can be calculated to be -0.3 mV, with RT/F equal to 25.4 mV (the temperature in these experiments was about 22°C).

For the experiments in Fig. 3.7B, the external anion was always Cl^- at a concentration of 148 mM, and the internal anions were Cl^- at a concentration of 4 mM and X^- (i.e., Br^-, I^-, or SCN^-) at a concentration of 140 mM. From Eqn. (43), we have

$$E_{rev} = \frac{RT}{F} \ln \frac{P_{Cl}[Cl^-]_i + P_X[X^-]_i}{P_{Cl}[Cl^-]_o} \tag{41}$$

Strictly speaking, activities should be used in this equation rather than concentrations: instead of $[X^-]$ and $[Cl^-]$, we should use $\gamma_X[X^-]$ and $\gamma_{Cl}[Cl^-]$, where the γ's are the activity coefficients. The activity coefficients can in this case be ignored, since for all of the anions used in these experiments the activity coefficients were nearly equal and canceled out. The permeability ratios P_X/P_{Cl} can then be calculated for the various anions from Eqn. (41); by inserting ion concentrations, taking the natural antilog of both sides of the equation (i.e., raising both to the power of e), and rearranging:

$$\frac{P_X}{P_{Cl}} = \frac{148e^{E_{rev}/25.4} - 4}{140} \tag{42}$$

The reversal potentials were found to be 9, 15, and 49 mV for Br^-, I^-, and SCN^- (see Fig. 3.7B); with these numbers substituted for E_{rev} above, the permeability ratios are approximately 1.5, 2, and 7. Note that all of these ions are significantly more permeable than Cl^- through the glycine channel.

Box 3.6

SAMPLE PROBLEM 6

Suppose a recording is made with the whole-cell patch-clamp method from a small spherical neuron having ligand-gated channels for the neurotransmitter glutamate. Suppose the interior of the cell is dialyzed (from the patch pipette) with 100 mM KCl, and the exterior solution contains 100 mM NaCl. If the reversal potential of the response of the cell to glutamate is +5 mV, and if the glutamate channels can be assumed to be impermeable to Cl^-, what is the relative permeability of the glutamate channels to Na^+ and K^+ (P_{Na}/P_K)? Assume the activity coefficients of Na^+ and K^+ at these concentrations are nearly the same, and use RT/F = 25 mV.

Answer. Since at the reversal potential the net current produced by the opening of the glutamate channels is zero, we can use the GHK voltage equation:

$$E_{rev} = \frac{RT}{F} \ln \frac{P_{Na}[Na^+]_o + P_K[K^+]_o + P_{Cl}[Cl^-]_i}{P_{Na}[Na^+]_i + P_K[K^+]_i + P_{Cl}[Cl^-]_o}$$

Since the only cation in the external solution is Na^+ and the only cation in the internal solution is K^+, we have (with $z = 1$)

$$+5 \text{ mV} = \frac{RT}{F} \ln \frac{P_{Na}[Na^+]_o}{P_K[K^+]_i}$$

where we have used concentrations instead of activities since the activity coefficients were assumed to be nearly the same for Na^+ and K^+ (and will therefore cancel). Since $[Na^+]_o = [K^+]_i$ and RT/F = 25 mV,

$$\frac{5 \text{ mV}}{25 \text{ mV}} = \ln \frac{P_{Na}}{P_K} = 0.2$$

so P_{Na}/P_K is equal to 1.2.

SAMPLE PROBLEM 7

The graph below shows hypothetical *i–V* curves (recorded from a dissociated cell with whole-cell voltage clamp) for the net

continued

change in membrane current produced by application of the neurotransmitter histamine at 25°C.

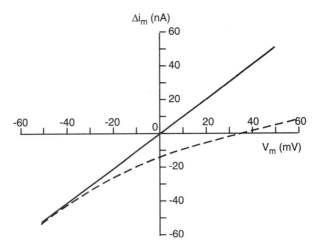

The pipette (intracellular) solution was the same for both curves
and contained 120 mM KCl. The extracellular solutions differed: the solid-line curve was recorded in 120 mM NaCl, and
the dashed-line curve in 30 mM NaCl (an uncharged solute like
sucrose was added to keep the osmolarity of the extracellular solution constant).

A. To which ion or ions are the histamine-gated channels permeable? Why?

Answer. Consider first the solid-line curve. With NaCl outside
and KCl inside at the same concentration, the reversal potential
is zero. This means that the channels cannot be selective for either Na^+ or K^+ but could be equally selective for both (i.e., *cation*-selective). If the channels were equally selective to both Na^+
and K^+, the GHK equation would reduce to $E_{rev} = RT/F[\ln (120/
120)]$, and since the log of 1 is zero, E_{rev} would be zero. Alterna-
tively, the channels could be selective for Cl^-, since for this curve
the Cl^- concentration on the two sides of the membrane is the
same. A third possibility is that the channels are not selective, so
that both cations and anions freely permeate.

These hypotheses can be tested with the results of the other
curve *(dashed line)*. If the channels were equally selective for
both Na^+ and K^+ but not permeant to Cl^-, the reversal potential

for this curve should be $E_{rev} = RT/F[\ln (30/120)]$, or about -36 mV ($RT/F = 25.7$ mV). If the channels were Cl$^-$-selective, $E_{rev} = RT/F[\ln (120/30)]$, or about $+36$ mV—remember that for anions, the *inside* concentration is in the numerator. If the channels are not selective, the ion permeabilities are all equal and cancel. The reversal potential is then $(RT/F) \ln [(120 + 30)/(30 + 120)]$, and this is zero just as for the solid-line curve. Since the dashed curve crosses the voltage axis very near to $+36$ mV, the channels must be primarily permeable to Cl$^-$.

B. What process might be responsible for the rectification of the dashed curve?

Answer. This is probably just Goldman rectification, since when the Cl$^-$ concentration on the two sides of the membrane is the same (as for the solid curve), the *i–V* relation is linear. For the dotted curve, inward (negative) currents are larger than outward currents, and this is the expected direction for Cl$^-$ since there is more Cl$^-$ inside the cell than out.

Summary

A complete representation of the electrical properties of cell membranes requires batteries as well as the resistances and capacitances introduced in Chapter 2. These batteries represent differences in electrical potential, produced by differences in ion concentration between the cytosol and the extracellular solution. An understanding of how these electrical potentials are generated may be gained from deriving the Nernst equation, which gives the potential difference created by the concentration gradient of a single ion species (for example, K$^+$) at equilibrium. This equation is useful for calculating approximate values of membrane potentials. It can also be used to estimate reversal potentials for channels (such as the Na$^+$ channels of nerve cells) that, under physiological conditions, are primarily permeable to only one ion species.

The Nernst equation is limited in its usefulness, since living cells are not at equilibrium and many channel types have significant permeability to more than one kind of ion. The next step, then, is to take into consideration the electrophoretic and diffusive forces on ions to derive the Nernst-Planck equation. From this equation and the simplifying *constant field assumption* the GHK current equation is derived, giving the current for a particular species of ion as a function of ion concentration, permeability, and voltage. This leads to the concept of rectification: in many situations of physiological importance, current flow is not symmetric across the plasma membrane; rather, ions move more easily in one direction than the other. As the GHK current equation demonstrates, rectification for a particular ion species can occur merely as a result of a difference in the concentration of this ion on the two sides of the membrane. Rectification can also be caused by channel block and by a voltage dependence of channel opening; we shall encounter many examples of rectification in the remainder of the book.

One of the most fundamental properties of ion channels is their ability to admit certain ions and exclude others. The selective permeability of channels is responsible for the negativity of the resting membrane potential, as well as the sudden positive change that produces the action potential (see Chapter 5). The GHK voltage equation, derived from the Nernst-Planck equation, can be used to calculate the resting membrane potential of a cell permeable to more than one ion type. It can also be used to provide detailed measurements of the ion selectivity of channels of physiological interest. As I shall describe later in the book, measurements of selective permeability are being used in conjunction with the powerful techniques of X-ray crystallography and molecular biology to study the structure of ion channels and to alter their amino acid sequence almost at will. These methods may eventually tell us how channel structure is responsible for the highly specific selectivity of channel proteins for different ions (see Box 7.2).

4

Ion Pumps and Homeostasis

THE ASYMMETRIC ion concentrations that produce the electrochemical driving forces for ion movement are created by pumps
and transporters, which move ions into or out of the cell. Membrane proteins—such as the Na$^+$/K$^+$ ATPase—use the high-energy
bond of the terminal phosphate of ATP to move Na$^+$ and K$^+$ across
the plasma membrane, creating the unequal distributions of these
ions that drive Na$^+$ and K$^+$ currents during action potentials and
excitatory synaptic stimulation. Other transporters establish gradients for Ca^{2+}, Cl$^-$, and H$^+$ (i.e., for pH). This chapter reviews the
structure and function of these proteins and the physiological consequences of ion transport. It focuses on how transporters produce
the resting (steady-state) concentrations of ions, and how these
concentrations are restored after ion influx or efflux.

I: SODIUM AND POTASSIUM

In an unstimulated neuron at steady state, the Na$^+$ and K$^+$ concentration gradients across the plasma membrane are very far from
equilibrium. A typical vertebrate neuron has an intracellular Na$^+$
concentration of 10–20 mM and an extracellular concentration of
141 mM (see Fig. 3.1). Typical K$^+$ concentrations are 120–140 mM
inside and 3.3 mM outside the cell. From the Nernst equation (see
Eqn. 5 in Chapter 3) we can calculate the equilibrium potentials
for Na$^+$ and K$^+$ to be: E_{Na} between 52 and 71 mV, and E_K in the
neighborhood of -96 mV to -100 mV. Since the resting membrane
potential of a typical neuron (V_m) is between -70 and -80 mV,
there is a large driving force for inward Na$^+$ movement ($V_m - E_{Na}$
$= -120$ to -150 mV). Although the driving force for outward K$^+$

movement is smaller ($+20$ to $+30$ mV), the resting permeability of a typical neuron for K^+ is sufficiently large, so that the outward movement of K^+ would quickly dissipate the resting membrane potential of the cell in the absence of active K^+ transport.

Na$^+$/K$^+$ ATPase: The "Sodium Pump"

The mechanism by which Na^+ and K^+ gradients are maintained across the neuronal cell membrane is now well known. Na^+ is transported outward and K^+ inward by an enzyme, the Na^+/K^+ ATPase, which couples the hydrolysis of ATP to the movement of ions (Sweadner, 1991, 1995; Horisberger et al., 1991; Lingrel, 1992; Glynn, 1993; Mercer, 1993; Lingrel and Kuntzweiler, 1994). The Na^+/K^+ ATPase consists of two subunits (see Fig. 4.1), an α subunit (with molecular weight about 110 kDa) and a β subunit (35–55 kDa, depending on the extent of glycosylation). The α subunit contains the binding sites for Na^+, K^+, and ATP, and it is this part of the Na^+/K^+ ATPase that is actually responsible for ion transport. The β subunit does not appear to contribute to ion pumping directly but is essential for the stability and proper assembly and targeting of the α subunit to the membrane (see for example Kawamura and Noguchi, 1991). The protein may exist in the membrane as a multimer of both subunits, perhaps with the stoichiometry $\alpha_2\beta_2$.

There are at least three different α subunits, called $\alpha 1$–$\alpha 3$, which are coded by different genes and which are widely distributed throughout the body (Sweadner, 1991). All three are found in the CNS, but the distribution is not the same for the different subunits. This distribution has been explored by Sweadner and her colleagues using antibodies specifically targeted to the different isoforms of the enzyme. For hippocampal pyramidal cells, for example (McGrail, Phillips, and Sweadner, 1991), the cell bodies are intensely stained for antibodies directed against $\alpha 3$, and the somata are also stained (though less heavily) by antibodies against $\alpha 2$. Antibodies against $\alpha 1$ produce only a peculiar punctate staining of the cell body, but they also appear to stain pyramidal cell dendrites. For photoreceptors and bipolar cells in the retina, on the other hand, only $\alpha 3$ staining was observed (McGrail and Sweadner, 1989). The different α isoforms have somewhat different properties (reviewed by Sweadner, 1991; Lingrel, 1992; Glynn, 1993). For example, all of the Na$^+$/K$^+$ ATPases are blocked by the cardiac glycoside *ouabain*, but in rodents the α1 has a much lower affinity for ouabain than the α2 or α3. There are also differences in the Na$^+$ affinities of the different isoforms. It is still uncertain why different cells or different parts of the same cell would have different forms of the enzyme.

All the α subunit isoforms are similar in sequence, and proteins of the same isoform are remarkably similar from one organism to another. The α subunit is an integral membrane protein whose amino acid sequence makes several passes through the membrane, but the details of the structure remain a subject of intense controversy (reviewed by Lingrel and Kuntzweiler, 1994; see Fig. 4.1). Both the amino and carboxyl termini of the α subunit are on the cytoplasmic side of the membrane, so the protein must have an even number of membrane-spanning regions. There is general agreement that there are four membrane-spanning regions near the amino terminus (left-hand side of Fig. 4.1) and that there is a large cytoplasmic region between the fourth and fifth membrane-

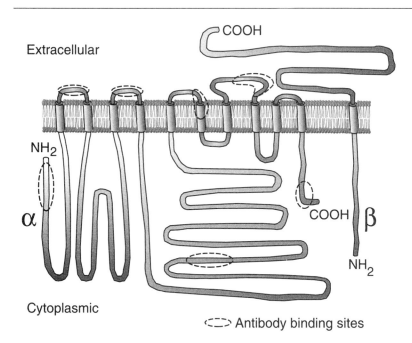

Fig. 4.1 Structure of α and β subunits of Na$^+$/K$^+$ ATPase. Amino and carboxyl termini are indicated by NH$_2$ and COOH labels at ends of protein sequences. Dotted lines show approximate locations of antibody-binding sites that have been used in studies of the membrane conformation of the α subunit. (After Fig. 2 of Lingrel and Kuntzweiler, 1994.)

spanning regions. There is, however, no general agreement about the number of membrane-spanning regions near the carboxyl terminus, though most investigators believe there are either 8 or 10 in the α subunit as a whole, since a considerable part of the protein seems to lie within the membrane (Maunsbach, Skriver, and Hebert, 1991). These questions are being approached with a variety of techniques and are an active area of investigation (see for example Mohraz, Arystarkhova, and Sweadner, 1994). The β subunit is also a transmembrane protein, though it appears to span the membrane only once (Fig. 4.1). It is highly glycosylated, and most of the protein is extracellular.

Mechanism of Pumping

The stoichiometry of the pumping reaction was first determined for erythrocytes by Post and Jolly (1957), who showed that 3 Na^+ ions are transported outward for 2 K^+ ions inward. The pump is therefore electrogenic—i.e., it produces a net flow of current. Similar experiments have also been done on squid axons and snail neurons with similar results. The electrogenicity of the pump (the ratio of Na^+ pumped outward to K^+ pumped inward) is 1.5. There is no evidence that the electrogenicity varies from species to species (as used to be thought) or depends (say) on the concentration of Ca^{2+} or other internal messengers. The electrogenicity seems also not to depend upon membrane voltage (Rakowski, 1991). Under certain rather extreme conditions (such as very low cytoplasmic Na^+ and low pH), changes in the ratio of pumping of Na^+ to K^+ can take place (Blostein and Polvani, 1991), but these are unlikely to occur under physiological conditions. The transport of 3 Na^+ outward for 2 K^+ inward is accompanied by the hydrolysis of one ATP molecule to ADP and an inorganic phosphate (P_i) (Garrahan and Glynn, 1967).

The mechanism of Na^+ and K^+ pumping (called the Post-Albers or "ping-pong" mechanism) seems to be as follows (see Fig. 4.2 and Läuger, 1991; Sachs, 1991; Glynn, 1993). The Na^+/K^+ ATPase can assume two basic conformations, called E_1 and E_2. Each of these conformations can be either unphosphorylated (E_1, E_2) or phosphorylated ($E_1 \cdot P$ or $E_2 \cdot P$). Three Na^+ ions bind to E_1 on the intracellular side of the pump, forming $E_1 3Na \cdot ATP$. The protein then undergoes a change in conformation so that the Na^+ ions are

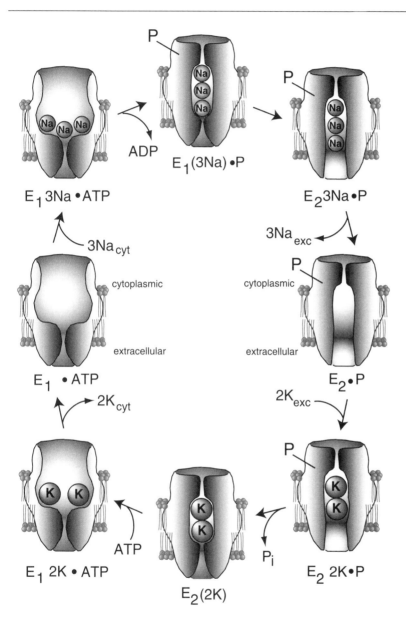

P

$E_1(3Na) \cdot P$

P

ADP

$E_1 3Na \cdot ATP$

P

$E_2 3Na \cdot P$

$3Na_{cyt}$

$3Na_{exc}$

cytoplasmic

P

cytoplasmic

extracellular

extracellular

$E_1 \cdot ATP$

$E_2 \cdot P$

$2K_{cyt}$

$2K_{exc}$

P

K   K

K

K

K

K

ATP

P_i

$E_1 2K \cdot ATP$

$E_2(2K)$

$E_2 2K \cdot P$

Fig. 4.2 Ping-pong scheme for pumping cycle of Na^+/K^+ ATPase. Cycle begins at top left, with the enzyme in the form $E_1 3Na \cdot ATP$. (Note that in this rendering the extracellular side is below each enzyme molecule and the cytoplasmic side above.) After a series of reactions as described in the text, the enzyme is in the form $E_1 \cdot ATP$ (at middle, left). Three Na^+ ions from inside the cell enter the pump, and the cycle begins again. (Redrawn from Läuger, 1991).

"occluded" and can no longer exchange with Na^+ ions in the cytoplasm, and ATP phosphorylates an aspartate residue on the cytoplasmic side of the α subunit within the large intracellular loop. This form of the enzyme is referred to as $E_1(3Na) \bullet P$. The enzyme then spontaneously converts to $E_23Na \bullet P$ and then to $E_2 \bullet P$, delivering the 3 Na^+ ions to the extracellular space and exposing binding sites for K^+. The binding of two K^+ ions leads to the formation of $E_22K \bullet P$, which triggers the occlusion of the K^+ ions and the dephosphorylation of the enzyme (to produce the $E_2(2K)$ form). The spontaneous reversion to E_12K and binding of ATP releases the K^+ ions into the cell, forming $E_1 \bullet ATP$ and completing the cycle. This mechanism is called "ping-pong" because the transport of Na^+ and K^+ is accomplished by independent half-reactions that occur sequentially.

Contribution of Na^+/K^+ Pump to Resting Membrane Potential

Since the Na^+/K^+ pump is electrogenic, transporting 3 Na^+ outward for every 2 K^+ inward, it acts as a current source moving charge directly out of the cell. This asymmetric removal of charge from the inside of the cell can (and often does) contribute directly to the resting membrane potential of a neuron. We calculate the amplitude of this contribution by first assuming that the cell is at steady state, and we ignore Cl^- by supposing either that membrane permeability for Cl^- is small or that Cl^- is not actively transported and is passively distributed across the membrane. Most neurons have only a small resting permeability to Cl^-, though the assumption that Cl^- is passively distributed is likely to be wrong for many neurons (see section III of this chapter). Still, the error produced by an active transport of Cl^- is likely to be modest in the derivation that follows.

If the cell is at steady state at its resting membrane potential, then the passive currents through the resting permeabilities must equal the active currents generated by the pump. Call the passive currents i_K and i_{Na} and the pump currents $i\rho_K$ and $i\rho_{Na}$. For both the K^+ and Na^+ currents at steady state,

$$i_K + i\rho_K = 0 \quad \text{and} \quad i_{Na} + i\rho_{Na} = 0 \tag{1}$$

since at steady state the resting currents carried by Na^+ and K^+ must be exactly countered by active pump currents for the two ions, equal in amplitude but opposite in sign. Let the electrogenicity of the pump be r (see Thomas, 1972). The value of r is given by the absolute value of the ratio of $i\rho_{Na}$ and $i\rho_K$, so

$$r = \left| \frac{i\rho_{Na}}{i\rho_K} \right| \quad \text{and} \quad ri\rho_K + i\rho_{Na} = 0 \tag{2}$$

From the work of Post and Jolly (1957), we know that r is 1.5. Eqn. (2) therefore says that if the potassium pump current is multiplied by 1.5 and *added* to the sodium pump current (which is opposite in sign), the two sum to zero. This follows simply from the definition of r. Furthermore, since from Eqn. (1) $i\rho_K = -i_K$ and $i\rho_{Na} = -i_{Na}$,

$$ri_K + i_{Na} = 0 \tag{3}$$

From the GHK current equations, we now write expressions for the K^+ and Na^+ currents (see Chapter 3). These are

$$I_K = P_K V_m \frac{F^2}{RT} \frac{[K^+]_o - [K^+]_i e^{FV_m/RT}}{1 - e^{FV_m/RT}} \tag{4}$$

and

$$I_{Na} = P_{Na} V_m \frac{F^2}{RT} \frac{[Na^+]_o - [Na^+]_i e^{FV_m/RT}}{1 - e^{FV_m/RT}} \tag{5}$$

If we insert Eqns. (4) and (5) into Eqn. (3) and simplify, we have

$$rP_K([K^+]_o - [K^+]_i e^{FV_m/RT}) + P_{Na}([Na^+]_o \\ - [Na^+]_i e^{FV_m/RT}) = 0 \tag{6}$$

Now we let P_{Na}/P_K be given by α. Then from Eqn. (6),

$$r([K^+]_o - [K^+]_i e^{FV_m/RT}) + \alpha([Na^+])_o - [Na^+]_i e^{FV_m/RT}) = 0 \quad (7)$$

and so

$$\frac{r[K^+]_o + \alpha[Na^+]_o}{r[K^+]_i + \alpha[Na^+]_i} = e^{FV_m/RT} \quad (8)$$

This means that the resting membrane potential at steady state in the presence of active Na^+ and K^+ pumping is not given by the Goldman equation, but rather by

$$V_m = \frac{RT}{F} \ln \frac{r[K^+]_o + \alpha[Na^+]_o}{r[K^+]_i + \alpha[Na^+]_i} \quad (9)$$

The contribution of the pump to the resting membrane potential (V_p) can be calculated as the difference between Eqn. (9) and the Goldman voltage equation (Thomas, 1972):

$$V_p = \frac{RT}{F} \ln \frac{r[K^+]_o + \alpha[Na^+]_o}{r[K^+]_i + \alpha[Na^+]_i} - \frac{RT}{F} \ln \frac{[K^+]_o + \alpha[Na^+]_o}{[K^+]_i + \alpha[Na^+]_i} \quad (10)$$

For $r = 1.5$, $\alpha = 0.01$, and the K^+ and Na^+ concentrations given in Fig. 3.1, V_p is about 3 mV at 37°C. The value of V_p increases as α increases, and for $\alpha = 1$ (which is nearly the case for a vertebrate photoreceptor), the contribution of the pump to the resting membrane potential is approximately 9.7 mV. The maximum value of V_p at steady state was shown by Philippe Ascher to be $(RT/F)\ln(1/r)$, which is about 11 mV for $r = 1.5$ at 37°C (see Thomas, 1972).

Experimental Confirmation of the Contribution of the Na^+/K^+ Pump

The first convincing demonstration that the Na^+/K^+ pump contributes directly to the resting membrane potential of a neuron was that of Gorman and Marmor (1970). They showed that the rest-

Box 4.1

SAMPLE PROBLEM I

Suppose a nerve cell at rest has an intracellular ion composition of 100 mM KCl and 10 mM NaCl and is bathed in a solution of 100 mM NaCl and 10 mM KCl. If the ratio of Na^+ to K^+ permeability for the resting membrane is 0.05 (i.e., $\alpha = P_{Na}/P_K = 0.05$), what is the resting membrane potential in the presence of electrogenic Na^+/K^+ pump activity? Suppose the pump is now blocked with ouabain. What initial change in membrane potential would you expect as the result of blocking the activity of the pump? Assume that the internal and external ion concentrations are not altered (at least initially) by ouabain, and use $RT/F = 25$ mV.

   Answer. To calculate the membrane potential with pump activity, we use

$$V_m = \frac{RT}{F} \ln \frac{r[K^+]_o + \alpha[Na^+]_o}{r[K^+]_i + \alpha[Na^+]_i}$$

with $\alpha = 0.05$ and $r = 1.5$. This gives

$$V_m = (25 \text{ mV}) \ln \frac{1.5(10) + 0.05(100)}{1.5(100) + 0.05(10)} = -50.5 \text{ mV}$$

Now calculate the membrane potential without pump activity:

$$V_m = \frac{RT}{F} \ln \frac{[K^+]_o + \alpha[Na^+]_o}{[K^+]_i + \alpha[Na^+]_i}$$

With $\alpha = 0.05$,

$$V_m = (25 \text{ mV}) \ln \frac{10 + 0.05(100)}{100 + 0.05(10)} = -47.6 \text{ mV}$$

Thus treatment with ouabain, which blocks the pump, should depolarize the cell about 3 mV.

ing potential of a molluscan neuron could be described by the Goldman equation only at low temperature (4°C), when the metabolism (ATP production) of the cell would be expected to be slower; or in the presence of ouabain, which blocks the Na$^+$/K$^+$ ATPase. At higher temperatures in the absence of ouabain, the membrane potential was consistently more hyperpolarized than predicted by the GHK voltage equation. This is demonstrated in Fig. 4.3, where the membrane potential is plotted as a function of [K$^+$]$_o$ at two different temperatures. At 4°C, the fit of the Goldman equation to the membrane potential is quite good. At higher temperatures, there are significant deviations, which can be abolished by treatment of the cell with ouabain.

Activation of Na$^+$/K$^+$ Pump by Increases in [Na$^+$]$_i$

Although the stoichiometry of the pump appears to be fixed at a transport ratio of 3 Na$^+$ to 2 K$^+$ and to be unaffected (for example)

Fig. 4.3   Effect of Na$^+$/K$^+$ ATPase on resting membrane potential of neuron from the marine mollusc *Anisodoris nobilis.* Membrane potential, measured with an intracellular microelectrode, is graphed as a function of extracellular K$^+$ concentration at two different temperatures. Data are given as means of five experiments, and error bars are standard errors. At 4°C, the metabolic rate of the neuron should have been sufficiently slowed that the Na$^+$/K$^+$ ATPase would be expected to contribute minimally to the resting membrane potential, and the measurements of V_m can be satisfactorily fit with the GHK voltage equation (P_{Na}/P_K was assumed to be 0.028 and [K$^+$]$_i$ was assumed to be 235 mM). At 17°C, the Na$^+$/K$^+$ ATPase would be expected to make some contribution to the resting potential, and the membrane potential is consistently more hyperpolarized than predicted by the GHK equation for the same assumptions as for the 4°C recordings. Note that the voltage scale plots increasing negativity upward. (Modified from Gorman and Marmor, 1970.)

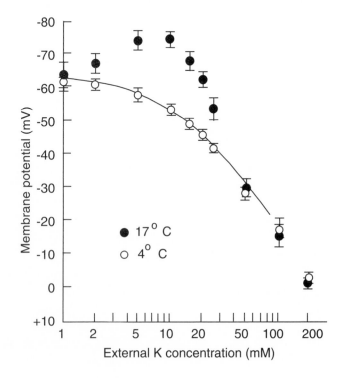

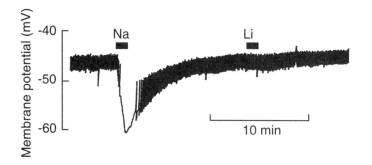

Fig. 4.4 Activation of Na$^+$/K$^+$ ATPase by intracellular Na$^+$ but not by Li$^+$. Membrane potential of a neuron of the common land snail, *Helix aspersa*, was measured with an intracellular micropipette; two additional microelectrodes were inserted into the cell to inject Na$^+$ and Li$^+$, by the method of "interbarrel iontophoresis." A current stimulator well isolated from the rest of the recording electronics was used to pass current between an electrode containing NaAc (sodium acetate) and another electrode containing LiAc (lithium acetate). Positive current injected from the NaAc electrode to the LiAc electrode caused positively charged sodium to move out of the NaAc pipette and negatively charged acetate to move out of the LiAc pipette, in such a way that NaAc accumulated inside the cell but no net current passed across the cell membrane. In this way, the Na$^+$ could be injected without altering the membrane potential. When the current direction was reversed and positive current was injected from the LiAc electrode, LiAc accumulated inside the cell. Note that an increase in intracellular Na$^+$ caused a transient hyperpolarization of the membrane potential, whereas Li$^+$ injection had little effect. Rapid depolarizations of membrane potential during the experiment (briefly eliminated by Na$^+$-induced hyperpolarization) are action potentials, but these are not visible in detail because of the limited frequency response of the pen recorder used to record the data. (Reprinted from Thomas, 1969, with permission of the author and the Physiological Society.)

by second messengers or membrane voltage, the *rate* of pumping is altered by the intracellular Na$^+$ concentration ([Na$^+$]$_i$) and can be modulated in many tissues by hormones, including insulin and vasopressin. Other hormones (like aldosterone) have been demonstrated to alter the *number* of active pump molecules in the membrane of nonneuronal tissues—for example, in kidney and large intestine.

The modulation of pump rate by sodium concentration is likely to have important consequences for the physiology of neurons. In a resting cell, the Na$^+$/K$^+$ ATPase pumps at a fraction of its maximal rate, which can be increased by increasing [Na$^+$]$_i$. This was shown directly by Roger Thomas (1969, 1982), who recorded intracellularly from a snail neuron while injecting Na$^+$ into the cell. The neurons he recorded from were so large that it was possible to place up to four electrodes inside the cell at the same time. Different electrodes were used to inject Na$^+$ and to record the membrane potential of the cell or the membrane current under voltage clamp.

A typical result from these experiments is given in Fig. 4.4. The bars above the record indicate the duration of the injections. When Na$^+$ was injected, the resting membrane potential became more negative (hyperpolarized). Injection of Li$^+$ as a control produced little or no effect.

The evidence that this hyperpolarization was produced by the Na$^+$/K$^+$ ATPase is as follows. First, when the pump was poisoned with 10 μM ouabain, the membrane potential depolarized and the effect of the Na$^+$ injection was greatly diminished (see Fig. 4.5A) or nearly eliminated, if the ouabain exposure was prolonged (Thomas, 1982). Second, when K$^+$ was removed from the external solution, the effect of the Na$^+$ injection also disappeared (Fig. 4.5B). If there is no K$^+$ in the external solution, the Na$^+$/K$^+$ ATPase is able to cycle through its "ping-pong" sequence to the form identified as E$_2 \bullet$P in Fig. 4.2 but can go no further, since there is no K$^+$ available to bind to the pump and allow it to cycle back to form E$_1$. Notice that as soon as the K$^+$ is restored, the membrane potential immediately hyperpolarized (Fig. 4.5B), since the Na$^+$ accumulated during the injection could then be pumped outward.

The change in membrane potential produced by the Na$^+$ injection could be quite large, nearly 15 mV in Figs. 4.4 and 4.5 and up to 25 mV for larger injections (Thomas, 1982). These are much larger hyperpolarizations than would be expected from our calculations of V_ρ, the contribution of the pump to the resting membrane potential. Recall that V_ρ is typically 3 mV or so and cannot exceed $10-11$ mV. However, V_ρ is the pump contribution *for the resting membrane potential,* calculated under the assumption that the neuron is at steady state. Clearly, much larger changes in membrane potential can be observed transiently, when the Na$^+$ concentration in the cell increases as a result of a large Na$^+$ influx.

Fig. 4.5 Effect of ouabain and K$^+$-free solution on Na$^+$ injections. Methods and preparation as in Fig. 4.4. **(A)** Hyperpolarization produced by Na$^+$ injection (indicated by black bar) is substantially reduced after addition of ouabain *(arrow).* **(B)** Hyperpolarization produced by Na$^+$ injection is nearly abolished by superfusion with extracellular solution lacking K$^+$ *(arrows).* Note that reintroduction of K$^+$ *(second arrow)* produces a large hyperpolarization, due to the pumping out of Na$^+$ accumulated within the cell during the Na$^+$ injection. (Reprinted from Thomas, 1969, with permission of the author and the Physiological Society.)

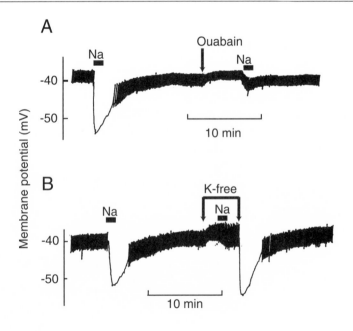

Physiological Significance of Na+/K+ Pump Modulation

If it is possible to increase the rate of the Na$^+$/K$^+$ pump by injecting Na$^+$ into the cell body, the pump should also be activated under physiological conditions, when stimulation leads to an increase in cytoplasmic Na$^+$ concentration. In a cell with a small surface-to-volume ratio, such as a squid axon, the amount of Na$^+$ entering the cell during an action potential, or even a train of several hundred action potentials, is too small to cause a significant increase in the intracellular Na$^+$ concentration. The Na$^+$ entry for a single impulse in squid axon has been estimated to be of the order of 4×10^{-12} moles (4 picomoles) per square centimeter of membrane (Hodgkin, 1964). This means that for an axon whose diameter is 500 μM, a single action potential would change the internal Na$^+$ concentration by less than 0.5 μM. Over 10,000 action potentials would be required to change the Na$^+$ concentration by 5 mM. For a small cell with a comparable density of Na$^+$ channels, much larger

---

Box 4.2

Na$^+$ CHANNEL ACTIVITY AND CHANGES IN INTRACELLULAR Na$^+$ CONCENTRATION

Consider a small spherical cell of radius a and surface area $4\pi a^2$. If the density of Na$^+$ channels is the same for this cell as for the squid axon, then the number of moles of Na$^+$ ions entering the cell per impulse would be 4×10^{-12} moles times $4\pi a^2$, or about $(5 \times 10^{-11})\ a^2$ moles per impulse (with a given in cm). The volume of such a cell is $4/3\pi a^3$, expressed in cubic centimeters. Since there are 10^3 cm^3 per liter, the volume is about $(4.2 \times 10^{-3})\ a^3$ liters. Thus the change in the intracellular concentration of Na$^+$ per impulse in moles per liter is $[(5 \times 10^{-11})\ (a^2)]/[(4.2 \times 10^{-3})\ (a^3)]$ moles per liter, or $(1.2 \times 10^{-8})/a$ moles per liter, with a given in cm. So for a cell 5 μm in radius (10 μm in diameter), the change in Na$^+$ concentration per impulse is 24 μM, and 100 impulses change the Na$^+$ concentration by 2.4 mM. This is of the order of 10–20 percent of the normal Na$^+$ concentration (see Fig. 3.1).

Fig. 4.6 After-hyperpolarization in leech sensory neurons. Intracellular recordings of membrane potential from leech mechanoreceptors during and after mechanical stimulation to the skin. Mechanical stimulation was delivered by poking with a fine needle connected to a mechanical transducer (a piezo-electric element). **(A)** Response to touches delivered for 10 seconds at 20 per second. The resting potential of the cell before stimulation was −42 mV. Stimulation produced action potentials, which were clipped by the pen recorder (as in Figs. 4.4 and 4.5). Stimulation is followed by a long-lasting hyperpolarization. **(B)** After-hyperpolarization blocked by strophanthidin. Skin stimulated at 40 per second for 6 seconds: *a*, control response; *b*, 2 min after perfusion with 130 μM strophanthidin; *c*, recovery of response 15 min after return to normal bathing medium. (From Baylor and Nicholls, 1969, reprinted with permission of the authors and the Physiological Society.)

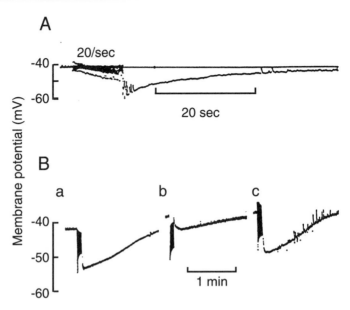

changes in sodium concentration can occur (see Box 4.2). These changes would be expected to increase the rate of the Na^+/K^+ pump and hyperpolarize the membrane potential by an amount that depends upon the product of the pump current and the resting membrane resistance.

There are two well-documented cases for which the entry of Na^+ under physiological conditions produces a large hyperpolarization of membrane potential mediated by the Na^+/K^+ ATPase. Baylor and Nicholls (1969) showed that stimulation of mechanoreceptors in the leech often produces a large hyperpolarization following a train of action potentials. The after-hyperpolarization seems to be produced by the entry of Na^+ during the action potentials and stimulation of the Na^+/K^+ ATPase, and it can occur under physiological conditions. Thus, direct stimulation of the receptors by delivering touches to the skin produces a train of action potentials, followed by a large hyperpolarization (Fig. 4.6A). The amplitude of the hyperpolarization can be as large as 30 mV after several hundred action potentials. Baylor and Nicholls showed that this hyperpolarization was reduced by cooling and blocked by ouabain or by strophanthidin, a cardiac glycoside similar to ouabain (Fig. 4.6B).

Prominent after-hyperpolarizations produced by the Na^+/K^+

ATPase can also occur for many invertebrate photoreceptors—for example, in the barnacle (Koike, Brown, and Hagiwara, 1971) and in the horseshoe crab, *Limulus* (Brown and Lisman, 1972). In these cells, stimulation with light opens a channel in the cell membrane that is permeable to Na^+. This causes Na^+ to flow into the cell, and the maintained increase in Na^+ conductance is large enough in bright light to cause a significant increase in intracellular Na^+. When the light is turned off there is a large after-hyperpolarization, which is not accompanied by a conductance change and which can be reduced or blocked with zero-K^+ Ringer solution or cardiac glycosides.

II: CALCIUM

The concentration of Ca^{2+} in the cerebrospinal fluid bathing the cells of the central nervous system is 2.5 mM, but the concentration of Ca^{2+} in the cytosol is much lower. A freshly dissected squid axon contains a total calcium concentration of the order of 100 μmoles per kilogram of axoplasm, and this value may be typical of neurons in the brain. This is the total Ca^{2+} concentration, but the physiological effects of Ca^{2+} depend not upon its total concentration but rather upon its *free* concentration, or its *activity*. The free Ca^{2+} concentration in a typical neuron is in the range 50–200 *nano*molar (50–200 $\times$ 10^{-9} M), over 4 orders of magnitude smaller than the concentration in the cerebrospinal fluid. There is therefore a very large gradient for the inward movement of Ca^{2+}—a gradient that must be established and maintained by active transport. Because of the importance of changes in Ca^{2+} concentration for transmitter release and intracellular signaling (see Chapters 8 and 13), neurons have a variety of mechanisms for regulating the intracellular Ca^{2+} concentration.

When Ca^{2+} enters a nerve cell—for example, as the result of the opening of Ca^{2+} channels during transmitter release—most of the Ca^{2+} is rapidly bound to proteins or other metabolites or sequestered into intracellular compartments. If we define the *buffering power* (or *buffering capacity*) as the ratio of Ca^{2+} entering to the change in free Ca^{2+} concentration, the buffering power for Ca^{2+} has been estimated to be of the order of 10^2–10^3 (*e.g.* Brindley,

1978; Requena et al., 1991; Neher and Augustine, 1992; Tse, Tse, and Hille, 1994). Thus for every 100–1,000 Ca^{2+} ions entering the cell, one (on average) remains free. Buffering power is a rather inexact concept, since Ca^{2+} buffering is a steep function of time: the Ca^{2+} ions that enter the cell do so as unbound Ca^{2+}, and all Ca^{2+} ions remain unbound for a short time. This has the consequence that high concentrations of Ca^{2+} (called *microdomains*) can occur in the vicinity of the plasma membrane (see Chapter 8). With a time constant of the order of 10–100 μs (Allbritton, Meyer, and Stryer, 1992), most of this Ca^{2+} appears to bind to proteins or other intracellular components and is then sequestered within the endoplasmic reticulum (ER) or mitochondria, or transported out of the cell across the plasma membrane.

This high buffering power has several important consequences. In the first place, the diffusion of Ca^{2+} in the cytoplasm is much slower than it is in free solution. The diffusion constant of Ca^{2+} in the cytoplasm is less than that in free solution by at least a factor of ten (Hodgkin and Keynes, 1957; Allbritton, Meyer, and Stryer, 1992). The high buffering capacity also means that, in the absence of a specific mechanism for propagation, increases in Ca^{2+} can occur only very locally. This is likely to be of considerable importance in the mechanism of synaptic transmitter release (Chapter 8).

The mechanisms responsible for Ca^{2+} homeostasis in neurons are summarized in Fig. 4.7 (Blaustein, 1988; Petersen, Petersen, and Kasai, 1994; Pozzan et al., 1994). They can be divided into three basic categories: Ca^{2+} *binding* to cytoplasmic proteins *(CaBPr)*, Ca^{2+} *sequestration* into cytoplasmic organelles (smooth ER and mitochondria), and Ca^{2+} *extrusion* across the plasma membrane.

Ca^{2+} Binding

The cytoplasm and membranes of neurons contain a variety of specific Ca^{2+}-binding proteins, such as calmodulin, parvalbumin, calbindin D–28K, calreticulin, calcineurin, and calretinin (Heizmann and Hunziker, 1990). Calmodulin is found in most of the cells of body. It is present in squid axon at a concentration of 10 μM and is also abundant in mammalian brain. Parvalbumin, which was originally described as a Ca^{2+}-binding protein in skeletal mus-

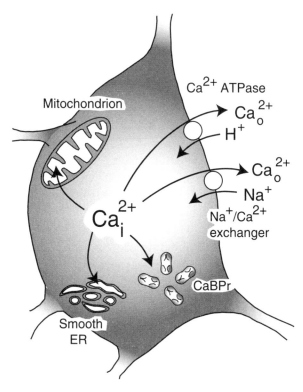

Fig. 4.7 Mechanisms of Ca^{2+} homeostasis in neurons. ER, endoplasmic reticulum; CaBPr, Ca binding proteins. (Modified from Blaustein, 1988.)

cle, is present in many neurons and may be preferentially contained in cells that use GABA as a transmitter. In addition to Ca^{2+}-binding proteins, Ca^{2+} can bind with low affinity to the negatively charged head groups of phospholipids.

Ca^{2+} Sequestration

Ca^{2+} is sequestered principally by two groups of intracellular organelles: smooth endoplasmic reticulum, or calcisomes, and mitochondria. Most cells in the body, including neurons, contain a specialized group of membranous inclusions that are thought by some to be part of the smooth endoplasmic reticulum and by others to be separate organelles (these have been called calcisomes—see Pozzan et al., 1994). These organelles contain a calmodulin-insensitive ATP-dependent Ca^{2+} pump that pumps Ca^{2+} from the cytosol into the organelle. This pump, called the sarco/endoplasmic reticulum

Ca^{2+} ATPase (or SERCA), is an approximately 110 kDa protein with a structure and mechanism of action similar to the α subunit of the Na^+/K^+ ATPase (Kirtley, Sumbilla, and Inesi, 1990; Inesi and Kirtley, 1992; Pozzan et al., 1994). The mechanism of Ca^{2+} pumping is probably also "ping-pong": Ca^{2+} binds to an intracellular binding site, and ATP hydrolysis causes the Ca^{2+} to be occluded. The protein then changes conformation to one in which the occluded Ca^{2+} is now exposed to the inside of the vesicle, and the affinity of Ca^{2+} binding is lowered so that Ca^{2+} can be released. Finally, dephosphorylation of the enzyme causes it to change conformation again, perhaps in conjunction with the binding of H^+. This re-exposes the binding site to the cytosol, so that Ca^{2+} can bind and the cycle can begin anew.

Most of the Ca^{2+} pumped into the smooth ER or calcisome is bound to specialized Ca^{2+}-binding proteins, such as calsequestrin and calreticulin. These organelles act as fairly effective Ca^{2+} storage devices. The Ca^{2+} pump has a high affinity and can pump Ca^{2+} into the organelle even at low cytosolic Ca^{2+} concentrations. Because of this property, Ca^{2+} pumping into ER or calcisomes is thought to be the most important mechanism for Ca^{2+} sequestration under resting (unstimulated) conditions. The ER or calcisomes have another important function: they appear to be the organelles that mediate inositol trisphosphate (IP_3)-dependent and Ca^{2+}-dependent Ca^{2+} release, which will be described in more detail when the role of Ca^{2+} as a second messenger is discussed (see Chapter 13).

Mitochondria also accumulate Ca^{2+} as the result of a large (~180 mV) potential across the mitochondrial inner membrane, inside negative, which results from the H^+ concentration gradient generated by oxidative phosphorylation. The Ca^{2+} is actually carried across the inner membrane by a transporter or channel. Ca^{2+} efflux can occur by at least two different mechanisms: a Na^+-dependent mechanism, perhaps some form of Na^+/Ca^{2+} exchange (see below); and a Na^+-independent mechanism, about which little is known (see Gunter and Pfeiffer, 1990).

Under physiological conditions, Ca^{2+} is cycled into and out of the mitochondria at a rather low rate, because the affinity of the Ca^{2+} transporter (or conductance of the channel) is low. As a result, the mitochondria accumulate little Ca^{2+}. The rate of Ca^{2+} entry via the transporter or channel increases dramatically with increasing

Ca²⁺ concentration, and when the free Ca²⁺ concentration in the cytosol exceeds 1 μM, significant Ca²⁺ can accumulate within the mitochondria. Such high cytosolic Ca²⁺ concentrations were once thought to occur only under pathological conditions, but we now know that this is not the case. The Ca²⁺ entry responsible for synaptic transmitter release can produce an increase in concentration—exceeding several tens of micromolar—though only very locally, in the vicinity of the plasma membrane (see Chapter 8). The capacity of the mitochondria in most cells greatly exceeds that of the ER or calcisome fraction, which means that under conditions of greatly elevated Ca²⁺, most of the cytosolic Ca²⁺ is sequestered into mitochondria. One of the reasons the capacity is so high is that when large amounts of Ca²⁺ enter the mitochondrion, much of the Ca²⁺ does not remain free but precipitates as calcium phosphate.

In summary, the picture that emerges, then, is of two major Ca²⁺-sequestering systems in cells: one of high affinity but relatively low capacity (ER or calcisomes), which is of greater importance under resting conditions; and the other of low affinity but high capacity (the mitochondrion), which is much more important when the cell is stimulated or injured.

Ca²⁺ Extrusion

Although mechanisms of binding and sequestration are of considerable importance in the response of the cell to Ca²⁺ loads, ultimately all of the Ca²⁺ that enters a cell must be expelled. Furthermore, at steady state the leakage of Ca²⁺ into the cell must be exactly balanced by the transport of Ca²⁺ out of the cell. The difference in free energy for Ca²⁺ inside and outside the cell can be calculated from the difference in the electrochemical gradient:

$$\Delta\mu_{Ca} = RT \ln \frac{Ca_i}{Ca_o} + zFV_m \qquad (11)$$

where $\Delta\mu_{Ca}$ is the change in free energy per mole of Ca²⁺, R is the gas constant (8.31 joules per degree per mole), Ca_i and Ca_o are the internal and external Ca²⁺ activities ($\sim 10^{-7}$ M and $\sim 10^{-3}$ M, respectively), z is the valence (+2), F is the faraday (96,487 coulombs per mole = 96,487 joules per volt per mole—see Box 3.3), and V_m

is the membrane voltage (about -70 mV). The difference in free energy at 37°C is about 37 kilojoules per mole. By comparison, the free energy of hydrolysis of ATP in a cell is 42–50 kilojoules per mole. There is thus a substantial electrochemical gradient favoring Ca^{2+} entry that, at steady state, must be countered by mechanisms for Ca^{2+} extrusion.

Two different transport systems are presently known to be used by neurons to expel Ca^{2+}: a plasma membrane Ca^{2+} ATPase (PMCA) and a Na^+/Ca^{2+} countertransporter. The plasma membrane Ca^{2+} ATPase is found in the membranes of most cells in the body, including most (if not all) neurons (Wuytack and Raeymaekers, 1992). It is a 135 kDa protein with many similarities in sequence to both the α subunit of the Na^+/K^+ ATPase and the SERCA Ca^{2+} ATPase. There is, however, one striking difference: a region, 27 amino acids long, near the carboxyl terminus that binds calmodulin. This is a regulatory site: the binding of Ca^{2+}-calmodulin appears to increase the rate of Ca^{2+} pumping. The plasma membrane Ca^{2+} ATPase pumps one Ca^{2+} per ATP hydrolyzed, probably in exchange for H^+ (see for example Schwiening, Kennedy, and Thomas, 1993). As our calculation of free energies shows, there is more than enough energy gain from the hydrolysis of a single ATP to pump one Ca^{2+} out of the cell against the energy difference at physiological free-Ca^{2+} concentrations.

Na^+–Ca^{2+} Exchange

In addition to the Ca^{2+} ATPase, the plasma membrane of most neurons contains a protein called the Na^+–Ca^{2+} exchange protein (also sometimes called the Na^+–Ca^{2+} *countertransporter* or the Na^+–Ca^{2+} *antiport*). This protein exchanges external Na^+ for internal Ca^{2+} or internal Na^+ for external Ca^{2+}, but in a neuron at rest it usually moves Ca^{2+} outward and Na^+ inward. It therefore functions as an important mechanism of Ca^{2+} homeostasis (Baker et al., 1969; for reviews, see Allen, Noble, and Reuter, 1989; Blaustein, DiPolo, and Reeves, 1991; Philipson and Nicoll, 1993; Reeves et al., 1994).

The Na^+/Ca^{2+} exchanger, first cloned and sequenced from cardiac muscle cells, is a protein of about 1,000 amino acids (Nicoll, Longoni, and Philipson, 1990). It appears to contain eleven α-helical membrane-spanning regions, a region of glycosylation near the amino terminus (which is therefore presumed to be extracellular), and a large intracellular region between membrane-spanning regions 5 and 6 (see Fig. 4.8). This large intracellular region is not essential for the operation of the exchanger but contains regulatory sites that modify its mode of action. Proteins similar to the one in cardiac muscle have now been cloned from several other tissues, including brain. Different isoforms of the Na^+/Ca^{2+} exchanger have been described, though little is known at present of their distribution in different tissues in the body. These isoforms are formed at least in part as the result of mRNA splicing.

The Na^+/Ca^{2+} exchanger uses the energy of the Na^+ gradient to expel Ca^{2+} from the cell. The mechanism of action may again be sequential or "ping-pong" in nature (see Hilgemann, Nicoll, and Philipson, 1991). One Ca^{2+} ion binds with high affinity to a binding site located on the cytoplasmic surface of the protein, and the protein then changes conformation, moving Ca^{2+} to the external surface of the cell. The Ca^{2+} is released from the binding site, and 3 Na^+ bind. The protein changes conformation again, delivering the Na^+ into the cell.

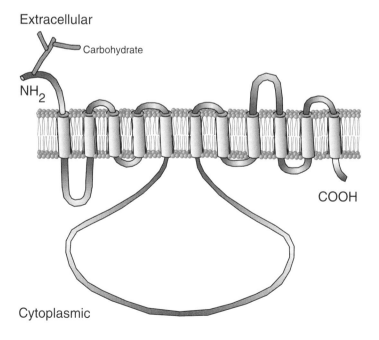

Fig. 4.8 Model of the membrane topology of Na^+/Ca^{2+} exchange protein. (After Philipson and Nicoll, 1993.)

One of the interesting things about this exchanger is that it is electrogenic: it transports 3 Na$^+$ inward for each Ca^{2+} outward, so that one extra positive charge moves into the cell for each Ca^{2+} ion removed. We can gain some insight into the reason for the electrogenicity of Na$^+$/Ca^{2+} transport by calculating the concentrations of Na$^+$ and Ca^{2+} at equilibrium as the result of the operation of the exchanger. Eqn. (11) gave the expression for the free-energy change for the movement of one mole of Ca^{2+} across the plasma membrane. We can write a similar equation for Na$^+$:

$$\Delta\mu_{Na} = RT \ln \frac{Na_i}{Na_o} + zFV_m \qquad (12)$$

If the exchange is electroneutral, then two Na$^+$ move for every one Ca^{2+}. The exchange of Na$^+$ for Ca^{2+} will reach equilibrium when $2\Delta\mu_{Na} = \Delta\mu_{Ca}$. Remembering that z is 2 for Ca^{2+} and 1 for Na$^+$, we can combine these equations to give

$$\frac{Ca_i}{Ca_o} = \frac{Na_i^2}{Na_o^2} \qquad (13)$$

For $Na_i = 11$ mM, $Na_o = 110$ mM, and $Ca_o = 1$ mM, Ca_i can be calculated to be 10 μM. This is too high to be of much use to the cell, since internal Ca^{2+} rarely rises above 1 μM, except very locally and for a very short time.

Suppose, however, that instead of being electroneutral, the pump is electrogenic and pumps 3 Na$^+$ ions for every Ca^{2+}. Then at equilibrium $3\Delta\mu_{Na} = \Delta\mu_{Ca}$. From the equations for the free energies, we have

$$RT \ln \frac{Ca_i}{Ca_o} + 2FV_m = 3RT \ln \frac{Na_i}{Na_o} + 3FV_m \qquad (14)$$

(remember that $z = 2$ for Ca^{2+}). So

$$\frac{Ca_i}{Ca_o} = \frac{Na_i^3}{Na_o^3} e^{FV_m/RT} \qquad (15)$$

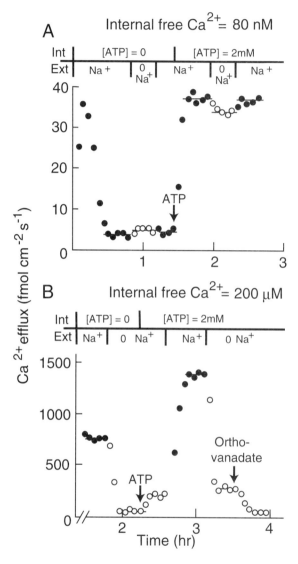

Fig. 4.9 Mechanisms of Ca²⁺ extrusion in squid giant axon. Ca²⁺ efflux measured by dialyzing axon with internal solution containing radioactive ⁴⁵Ca²⁺ and sampling at regular intervals the radioactivity accumulated in the external solution. *fmol,* femtomole (10⁻¹⁵ mole); *Int,* internal (dialysis) solution, replacing squid axoplasm; *Ext,* external (bathing) solution; open circles, efflux with Na⁺ removal; solid circles, efflux without Na⁺ removal. Dialysis media containing ATP also contained 5 mM phospho-arginine. **(A)** Ca²⁺ efflux for internal free-Ca²⁺ concentration of 80 nM. Ca²⁺ buffered with EGTA (see Chapter 13). At beginning of experiment, internal solution was changed to remove ATP. Note the fall in efflux. Efflux in zero-ATP solution is nearly insensitive to extracellular Na⁺ removal. Restoration of ATP produced an increase in Ca²⁺ efflux, which again was nearly insensitive to removal of extracellular Na⁺. **(B)** As in **(A)** but internal free-Ca²⁺ concentration of 200 μM. Note much larger scale on ordinate. Now removal of extracellular Na⁺ has a large effect, due to blocking of Na⁺/Ca²⁺ exchange. Residual efflux in zero Na⁺ was blocked by orthovanadate (which blocks the Na⁺/K⁺ ATPase). (Redrawn from Baker and DiPolo, 1984.)

Using the same values for F, R, T (37°C) and the same sodium concentrations as previously, we have for $V_m = -70$ mV that $Ca_i/Ca_o = 7.3 \times 10^{-5}$. For $Ca_o = 1$ mM, Ca_i can be as low as 73 nM. This would enable the exchanger to bring the Ca²⁺ concentration inside the cell to much lower levels.

There is now abundant evidence that the exchanger *is* electro-

genic. The stoichiometry in every system where it has been measured (except one; see Chapter 16) is 3 Na^+:1 Ca^{2+}. This stoichiometry is sufficient in theory to make the exchanger useful under
physiological conditions. In practice, the *rate* of transport is probably insufficient at resting Ca^{2+} concentrations for Na^+/Ca^{2+} exchange to contribute much to homeostasis. It seems likely that in
most neurons, the Ca^{2+} ATPase is the most important mechanism
for expelling Ca^{2+} at resting Ca^{2+} concentrations or under conditions of small Ca^{2+} increases. When increases in free-Ca^{2+} concentration become large, the Na^+/Ca^{2+} exchanger takes over.

A demonstration of the different roles of these two mechanisms for Ca^{2+} efflux is shown in Fig. 4.9. In this experiment, a
squid axon was loaded with radioactive $^{45}Ca^{2+}$, and the rate of
$^{45}Ca^{2+}$ efflux was measured as a function of extracellular Na^+,
intracellular Ca^{2+}, and internal ATP. Note that in part A of Fig. 4.9,
the intracellular Ca^{2+} concentration was 80 nM, close to the physiological concentration; whereas in part B it was much greater (200
μM). Also, note the different scales along the ordinates in two parts
of this figure. The results indicate that removing external Na^+
in the absence of ATP has little effect on Ca^{2+} efflux in low intracellular Ca^{2+} but a huge effect when the intracellular Ca^{2+} concentration is high. They also show that removing ATP in the absence
of Na^+ has a much greater effect as a percentage of total efflux
when intracellular Ca^{2+} concentration is low. These results strongly
suggest that the ATPase is the predominant source of Ca^{2+} efflux at
resting Ca^{2+} levels in squid axon, and this may also be true of neurons in the CNS.

III: ANIONS

The most abundant anions in cerebrospinal fluid are Cl^-, at a concentration of 124 mM, and HCO_3^-, at 21 mM. These are also the
principal small-molecular-weight anions in the cytosol, though the
cytoplasm also contains many anions of higher molecular weight,
including metabolites (like citric acid) and proteins. The concentration of Cl^- is typically much smaller inside a cell than outside (see
Fig. 3.1). The resting permeability of a neuron to Cl^- is usually

rather small but can increase dramatically during the activation of inhibitory synapses and the opening of GABA and glycine channels. Bicarbonate can also permeate GABA and glycine channels. I shall describe bicarbonate permeability in more detail later in this chapter, when I discuss pH regulation in neurons.

The Distribution of Cl⁻ across the Plasma Membrane of Nerve Cells

Imagine a cell whose resting membrane potential is largely determined by a resting permeability to K^+ and for which Cl^- is not pumped either into or out of the cell but is passively distributed across the membrane. If the external Cl^- concentration is 124 mM, as in cerebrospinal fluid, what will be the internal Cl^- concentration? A common response is to say that the Cl^- concentration inside the cell should be the same as that outside, if Cl^- isn't actively transported across the membrane; but this response ignores the resting membrane potential. If the inside of the cell is more negative than the outside, Cl^- will be driven out of the cell and will be at a lower concentration than outside, even in the absence of active transport.

The value of the intracellular Cl^- concentration is easy to calculate, since if V_m is set by the K^+ concentration gradient and Cl^- is passively distributed,

$$V_m = \frac{RT}{F} \ln \frac{[K^+]_o}{[K^+]_i} = \frac{RT}{F} \ln \frac{[Cl^-]_i}{[Cl^-]_o} \tag{16}$$

The membrane potential must be the same for both K^+ and Cl^-, since there is only one membrane whose potential is everywhere the same. The hypothetical situation just described is in fact nearly the case for vertebrate skeletal muscle fibers (Hodgkin and Horowicz, 1959), for which the Cl^- concentration inside the muscle is passively set by the membrane potential, which means that the Cl^- concentration gradient at steady state is nearly the same as the K^+ concentration gradient (though opposite in direction).

In some nerve cells, Cl^- may also be passively distributed. This means that for a cell whose membrane potential is -70 mV, the intracellular Cl^- concentration is approximately given by

$$\frac{-70\text{mV}}{25\text{mV}} = \ln \frac{[Cl^-]_i}{[Cl^-]_o} \qquad (17)$$

where we have assumed a value of 25 mV for RT/F. If the cell is bathed in a medium with a Cl^- concentration of 124 mM, $[Cl^-]_i$ is about 7.5 mM. In such a cell, the opening of Cl^- channels during inhibitory synaptic activity would produce no change in membrane potential.

As will be described in more detail in the section on GABA and glycine synaptic transmission (see Chapter 10), for most neurons the opening of Cl^- channels *does* produce a change in membrane potential, in some cases a hyperpolarization and in others a depolarization. If the opening of Cl^- channels produces a change in membrane potential, Cl^- cannot be passively distributed across the cell membrane but must be transported. If the opening of Cl^- channels causes a hyperpolarization, $[Cl^-]_i$ must be *lower* than it would be if it were passively distributed, and so Cl^- must be transported *out of* the cell. If the opening of Cl^- channels causes a depolarization, $[Cl^-]_i$ must be *higher* and so must be transported *into* the cell.

With the exception of an important H^+ transporter described in section IV of this chapter, little is known about mechanisms of Cl^- transport in nerve cells, though quite a lot is known about them in epithelia (see for example Reuss, Russell, and Jennings, 1993; Harvey and Nelson, 1994). Many epithelia contain a co-transporter, similar in molecular conformation to the Na^+/Ca^{2+} exchange protein, that simultaneously transports inward Na^+, K^+, and Cl^-, with a stoichiometry of 1 Na^+:1 K^+:2 Cl^-. This transporter generally works to transport Cl^- into the cell, using as an energy source the inwardly directed Na^+ gradient. It also transports K^+ inward *against* its concentration gradient, but a simple calculation—similar to those made above for Na^+/Ca^{2+} exchange—shows that the inward movement of Na^+ and Cl^- is energetically favorable in spite of the inward movement of K^+ against its gradient. The $Na^+/K^+/Cl^-$ cotransporter may be responsible for the transport of Cl^- into neurons, in the case where Cl^- is found at a higher concentration than would be expected from passive distribution. In the squid axon, for example, the internal Cl^- predicted from a membrane potential of -70 mV and an external Cl^- concentration (in sea water) of 540 mM can be calculated from Eqn. (17) to be about 33 mM, but actual measurement has shown the axoplasm to have considerably more Cl^- than this, with $[Cl^-]_i$ probably exceeding 100 mM (Keynes, 1963). There is evidence that this additional Cl^- is the result of inward transport via a $Na^+/K^+/Cl^-$ cotransporter (Russell, 1984; Russell and Boron, 1990). Similar observations of high internal Cl^- due to Na^+- and K^+-dependent transport have also been made for dorsal root ganglion cells (Alvarez-Leefmans et al., 1988).

Other transporters exist that could conceivably transport Cl^- out of cells. Some epithelial cells appear to have a K^+/Cl^- cotransporter (see for example Zeuthen, 1994). A K^+/Cl^- cotransporter has been suggested to transport Cl^- out of some neurons (see Alvarez-Leefmans, 1990), and this notion is supported by recent experiments (Riviera et al., 1999).

IV: H^+ AND THE REGULATION OF pH

It is relatively easy to show that H^+ cannot be passively distributed across the membrane of a nerve cell. If it were, the intracellular pH would be given by

$$V_m = \frac{RT}{F} \ln \frac{[H^+]_o}{[H^+]_i} = \frac{2.303RT}{F} (\text{pH}_i - \text{pH}_o) \qquad (18)$$

since $\text{pH} = -\log_{10}[H^+]$ and $\ln(x) = 2.303\log_{10}(x)$. This means that at a typical neuronal resting membrane potential of -70 mV at 25°C, the intracellular pH should be approximately 1.2 pH units smaller (more acidic) than the extracellular pH; since the pH of cerebrospinal fluid is 7.3 (Wright, 1978), the pH of the cytoplasm of a neuron would be 6.1 if H^+ were passively distributed. This is considerably more acidic than the values actually measured: 7.3 for squid axon (Boron, 1984), 7.1 for crayfish neurons (Moody, 1981), 7.4 for leech neurons (Schlue and Thomas, 1985), 7.1 for

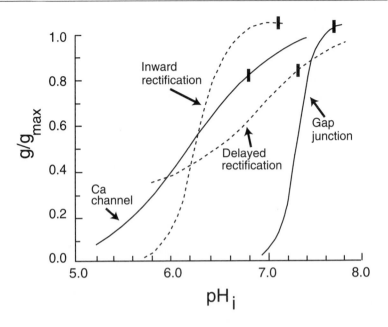

Fig. 4.10 Dependence of channel conductance on intracellular pH. Each curve is intersected by a vertical bar indicating the approximate resting pH_i of the cell from which the data were taken. (For original references, see Moody, 1984, from which this figure was reprinted with permission of the author and of Annual Reviews, Inc.)

Purkinje cells (Gaillard and Dupont, 1990), and 6.8 for pyramidal cells (Schwiening and Boron, 1994). Thus neurons must have mechanisms for removing H^+.

The control of the pH of the cytoplasm is crucially important for the physiology of a nerve cell, since ion channels are in general blocked at low pH_i. Figure 4.10 illustrates the effects of changes in pH_i on the relative conductance of several channel types, taken from the review of Moody (1984). The changes in conductance in this figure probably reflect changes in the probability of opening of the channel. If the pH of a cell were as low as 6.1, all of the channel types illustrated in this figure would be greatly affected. Decreases in pH can also produce changes in cytosolic Ca^{2+}, since H^+ and Ca^{2+} compete for binding sites on many Ca^{2+}-binding proteins.

Regulation of Intracellular pH

In order to prevent large changes in pH and keep the cytoplasm near neutrality, cells use two mechanisms. In the first place, the cytoplasm buffers pH rather effectively. The buffering capacity of a cell is defined as the amount of H$^+$ (in mM) needed to produce a 1-unit change in pH at the resting pH of the cell. This unit (mM per pH unit) is sometimes referred to as the *slyke*. In nerve cells, the buffering capacity is typically between 20 and 50 slykes (e.g., Purkinje cells, 37 slykes; see Gaillard and Dupont, 1990). A buffering capacity of 40 slykes is equivalent to 70 mM of the commonly used pH buffer HEPES at its pK$_a$: 40,000 H$^+$ ions have to be injected for each H$^+$ appearing as free in solution (Moody, 1984). This is quite a bit higher than the buffering capacity of the cytoplasm for Ca^{2+}. Much of the buffering is the result of the CO$_2$/HCO$_3^-$ equilibrium within the cell, which is facilitated by the enzyme carbonic anhydrase. Additional buffering is produced by proteins and small molecules that act as weak acids or bases.

In addition to buffering, cells also transport H$^+$ across their plasma membrane. It is the outward transport of H$^+$ that makes the pH of the cytoplasm so much less acidic than would be expected from passive distribution. There is considerable evidence that the most important system responsible for transporting H$^+$ in neurons is a protein that catalyzes the simultaneous exchange of both Na$^+$ and Cl$^-$ with H$^+$ and HCO$_3^-$. This protein has so far not been identified with molecular techniques, and we know nothing about its sequence or molecular structure; however, there is evidence from a wide variety of preparations that such a transporter exists and plays an active role in pH regulation (snail neurons: Thomas, 1977; crayfish neurons: Moody, 1981; squid axon: Boron, 1984; leech neurons: Schlue and Thomas, 1985; rat hippocampal pyramidal cells: Schwiening and Boron, 1994). The exchange of Na$^+$, Cl$^-$, and HCO$_3^-$ is so tightly coupled that it is most likely that all are transported by one protein.

In addition, at least two other transporters commonly found in animal cells may play a role in pH regulation: the band-3 protein and the Na$^+$/H$^+$ exchange protein. The band-3 or AE1 *(anion exchanger)* protein (Alper, 1991) exchanges Cl$^-$ for HCO$_3^-$. Cells effectively transport H$^+$ outward by transporting HCO$_3^-$ inward, since the transported HCO$_3^-$ reacts with intracellular H$^+$ to produce H$_2$O and CO$_2$,

$$HCO_3^- + H^+ = H_2O + CO_2 \qquad (19)$$

The H_2O and CO_2 then diffuse out of the cell. Many cells have been shown to express band-3 protein, and there is some evidence that this protein may actually function in nerve cells to regulate pH (Gaillard and Dupont, 1990).

Na^+/H^+ exchange proteins are integral membrane proteins that catalyze the electroneutral exchange of one Na^+ for one H^+ and thus use the energy of the Na^+ gradient to pump H^+ out of the cell. These proteins have been cloned and appear to be somewhat similar in molecular structure to the Na^+/Ca^{2+} exchanger (see Tse et al., 1993; Bianchini and Pouysségur, 1994), with 10–12 putative transmembrane sequences and a large intracellular C-terminal tail. Evidence for a role of the Na^+/H^+ exchanger in epithelia is quite strong (see for example Weinman and Shenolikar, 1993), and there is some evidence that nerve cells also use this family of proteins in pH regulation (Moody, 1981; Gaillard and Dupont, 1990; Schwiening and Boron, 1994).

Role of pH Regulation in the Physiology of Nerve Cells

Although changes in H^+ could in theory have large effects on the physiology of a neuron, it is fair to ask whether such changes actually occur during the normal life of a cell in the CNS. The answer to this question seems likely to be yes, because most CNS neurons receive inhibitory input from GABA and glycine synapses. Although we are accustomed to thinking of GABA and glycine channels as selective for Cl^- (see Chapter 10), these channels are in fact permeable to a wide variety of small-molecular-weight anions, as we have seen (see Chapter 3). This includes HCO_3^-: $P(HCO_3^-)/P(Cl^-)$ measured for spinal cord neurons is 0.18 for GABA channels and 0.11 for glycine (Bormann, Hamill, and Sakmann, 1987). Thus considerable movement of HCO_3^- would occur during the activation of GABA and glycine receptors unless HCO_3^- were passively distributed across the nerve cell membrane.

But HCO_3^- is *not* passively distributed. From Eqn. (19) and some freshman chemistry, we can derive what is usually referred to as the Henderson-Hasselbach equation,

$$pH = pK_a + \log \frac{[HCO_3^-]}{[CO_2]} \tag{20}$$

where pK_a is 6.1, and $[CO_2]$ can be calculated from the partial pressure and solubility coefficient for CO_2. An equation of this kind can be written for both the inside and outside of the cell. CO_2 is freely diffusible across the cell membrane, so $[CO_2]$ is likely to be nearly constant inside and outside. Since the pH is nearly the same on the two sides of the membrane, it follows from Eqn. (20) that HCO_3^- is also nearly the same inside and outside the cell. But if HCO_3^- were passively distributed, its concentration would be given by

$$V_m = \frac{RT}{F} \ln \frac{[HCO_3^-]_i}{[HCO_3^-]_o} \qquad (21)$$

and would be much lower inside the cell than outside. For a $[HCO_3^-]_o$ in the cerebrospinal fluid of 21 mM, $[HCO_3^-]_i$ would be expected to be 1.3 mM (with $V_m = -70$ mV and $RT/F = 25$ mV). The cytosolic bicarbonate concentration is therefore much larger than if bicarbonate were passively distributed, and there is a large driving force for HCO_3^- to exit the cell at a resting membrane potential of -70 mV, as the result of the difference between the membrane potential and the equilibrium potential for bicarbonate (which is near zero mV).

Imagine now what happens when GABA or glycine binds to its receptor. The channel of the receptor will open and there will be a net movement of Cl^- either inward or outward (or not at all), depending upon whether Cl^- is pumped outward or inward (or is passively distributed). Regardless of what Cl^- does, HCO_3^- will move outward, producing a small *inward* current (since bicarbonate is negatively charged) and a depolarization. Furthermore, as HCO_3^- leaves the cell, the pH of the cell will become more acidic (see Eqn. 19).

This effect can be rather large. Fig. 4.11 (from Kaila, Saarikoski, and Voipio, 1990) shows the effect of GABA on membrane potential and pH for a crayfish muscle. Even rather low concentrations of GABA can change the pH by 0.3–0.4 of a pH unit. At synapses in the central nervous system, the GABA concentration appears to rise as high as 0.5–1.0 mM (see Chapter 10), and it seems possible that local changes in pH could be large enough to have significant effects on the probability of opening of channels in the vicinity of the synapse.

Fig. 4.11 Effect of GABA receptor stimulation on membrane potential and pH_i of crayfish muscle fiber. Membrane potential was measured with an intracellular pipette, and pH_i was measured with an H^+-selective microelectrode also placed inside the muscle fiber. At the beginning of the record, the extracellular solution contained 1% CO_2 in air and 6 mM HCO_3^-. At the point indicated at the top of the figure, the solution was changed to one containing 5% CO_2 in air and 30 mM HCO_3^-. The increase in extracellular CO_2 produced an acidification of the cytoplasm, due to rapid entry of CO_2 into the cell and reaction of CO_2 with intracellular H_2O to produce H^+ and HCO_3^-. The pH_i was gradually restored to its resting value, presumably by H^+ extrusion. The cell was then exposed to solutions containing 20 and 80 μM GABA, which produced a graded acidification due to opening of anion-selective GABA channels and exit of HCO_3^- from the muscle fiber. Membrane potential (V_m) depolarized. (Reprinted from Kaila et al., 1990, with permission of the authors and of the Physiological Society.)

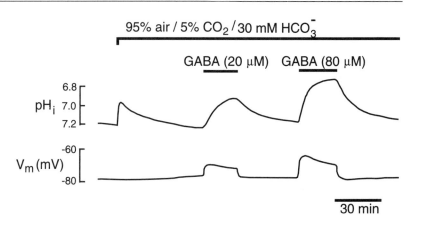

Summary

The electrical activity of neurons is caused by the movement of ions through channels in response to their electrochemical gradients. These gradients are produced by asymmetries in concentrations, which are the result of the transport of ions across the plasma membrane via specific membrane proteins. One of the most important molecules responsible for ion transport in the nervous system (and elsewhere in the body) is the Na^+/K^+ ATPase, an enzyme that uses the high-energy terminal phosphate bond of ATP to pump 3 Na^+ ions outward and 2 K^+ ions inward. This enzyme is responsible for establishing the gradients for K^+ and Na^+ across the cell membrane. Since 3 sodium ions are moved outward in exchange for only 2 potassium ions, there is a net transport of both particles and charge out of the cell. This interesting feature of the Na^+/K^+ ATPase has two important implications. First, the net export of particles from the cell helps maintain osmotic equilibrium, since the activity of this enzyme can produce a net change in the number of osmotically active particles in the cell. Second, the net transport of charge from the cell contributes to the membrane potential. This contribution is generally small for the cell at rest, but stimulation of the cell leading to an accumulation of intracellular Na^+ can in some cases produce large changes in V_m.

In addition to Na^+ and K^+ transporters, there are also important mechanisms for regulating cell Ca^{2+}. As Chapters 8 and 13 will show, Ca^{2+} plays an essential role in cell signaling, and the free concentration of Ca^{2+} is commonly several orders of magnitude lower in the cytoplasm than in the extracellular fluid. Neurons (in common with most cells in the body) have mechanisms for the cytoplasmic buffering of Ca^{2+}, including Ca^{2+}-binding proteins and sequestration within the endoplasmic reticulum (or calcisomes) and the mitochondria. There are also proteins in the plasma membrane specialized for extruding Ca^{2+}: an ATPase similar in structure and function to the Na^+/K^+ ATPase, and a Na^+/Ca^{2+} exchange protein. The Ca^{2+} ATPase is probably most important for regulating the Ca^{2+} concentration at rest, but when the Ca^{2+} level rises after stimulation or injury, the Na^+/Ca^{2+} countertransporter appears to play a more significant role.

Since Cl^- plays an important role in neuronal inhibition, cells in the CNS also have mechanisms for establishing and maintaining the Cl^- concentration. In some cells, cytoplasmic Cl^- is thought to be maintained at a concentration near its equilibrium value, without any active transport. Many neurons, however, are thought to have transporters either for importing or exporting Cl^-. There is evidence that inward transport may be mediated in some cells by $Na^+-K^+-Cl^-$ cotransport and outward transport by K^+-Cl^- cotransport, but much remains to be learned about neuronal mechanisms for Cl^- homeostasis.

Finally, nerve cells regulate cytoplasmic pH. The internal pH of a neuron is generally one pH unit or more higher (less acidic) than would be expected if H^+ were distributed across the plasma membrane at equilibrium. The mechanisms responsible for H^+ transport are still unclear but may include $Na^+-Cl^-/H^+-HCO_3^-$ transport, Cl^-/HCO_3^- exchange (via the so-called band-3 protein), and Na^+/H^+ countertransport. Since many if not all channel proteins are greatly affected by changes in intracellular pH, and since activation, for example, of GABA and glycine channels is likely to produce significant changes in pH in the vicinity of membrane channels, the regulation of cytoplasmic pH is likely to have important implications for nerve cell function.

PART TWO

Active Propagation of Neural Signals

5

Action Potentials:
The Hodgkin-Huxley Experiments

THE PASSIVE SPREAD of electrical signals down the axons and dendrites of nerve cells described in Chapter 2 is one way messages are communicated from one part of the nervous system to another. Passive spread is essential for the conveyance of synaptic potentials within the dendritic tree, and some cells (like the starburst amacrine cell of Fig. 2.2) appear to transmit electrical signals only by decremental conduction. These cells are probably exceptional. Many of the cells in the CNS are too large to be able to rely solely on passive spread. Pyramidal cells, for example, often convey signals over quite long distances within the brain or from the brain to the spinal cord. Some other mechanism must exist for the reliable transmission of electrical signals over these distances.

This mechanism is *active propagation* and is mediated by *action potentials,* also called *spikes.* An action potential is a large, regenerative depolarization produced by voltage-gated channels. In an axon, spikes are initiated by a depolarization of the membrane, for example from excitatory synaptic input. This depolarization facilitates a change in conformation of membrane proteins called *Na*$^+$ *channels,* leading to the opening of a pore selective for Na$^+$ (Fig. 5.1A). As Na$^+$ channels open, Na$^+$ flows into the cell. The entry of Na$^+$ causes a further depolarization of the membrane potential, by depositing additional positive charge in the cell (remember, $\Delta V = \Delta q/C$). When enough Na$^+$ channels have opened, the entry of Na$^+$ becomes large enough and the axon membrane sufficiently depolarized so that the membrane potential reaches threshold. At this point, it is no longer necessary to supply current from synaptic input to depolarize the cell, since the entry of Na$^+$ through the Na$^+$ channels is sufficient all by itself to continue the depolarization and initiate a *regenerative* cascade of positive feedback: the

Fig. 5.1 Action potentials. **(A)** Most of the Na⁺ channels are closed at the resting potential of a typical neuron, but depolarization—for example, by excitatory synaptic input—causes some of the channels to undergo a change in conformation. The opening of the channels permits Na⁺ ions to flow into the cell, and this depolarizes the cell further. The further depolarization of the cell causes even more Na⁺ channels to open, and a regenerative process results in the opening of a substantial fraction of the Na⁺ channels, producing an *all-or-none* event called an *action potential* or *spike*. **(B)** An early recording of the change in membrane potential during an action potential, from the giant axon of the squid *Loligo forbesi*. (After Hodgkin and Huxley, 1939, 1945.)

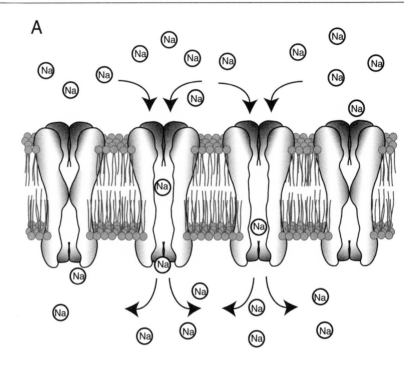

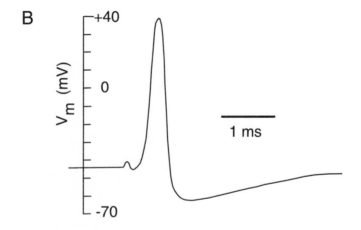

opening of channels produces more depolarization, which opens additional channels and produces further depolarization, until open Na+ channels constitute the major pathway for current flow through the cell membrane, and the membrane potential of the cell approaches E_{Na}.

Figure 5.1B is an early recording of an action potential from the squid *Loligo forbesi,* made by Hodgkin and Huxley (1939, 1945). The very rapid rising phase of the spike is produced by the rapid opening of Na+ channels, which produces a net change in membrane potential of about 100 mV. The falling phase of the spike is produced by the closing of the Na+ channels (by a process called *inactivation*), as well as by the opening of voltage-gated K+ channels. The K+ channels are also responsible for the rapid after-hyperpolarization of membrane potential, just following the falling phase of the spike.

Action potentials are much more useful than passive spread for communicating signals over long distances, since spikes can be propagated without any loss of signal amplitude. This happens in the following way. Spikes are initiated at a part of the axon called the *axon hillock,* often close to the point of the axon's attachment to the soma. They produce an entry of Na+ (as in Fig. 5.1A) that not only depolarizes the area in the immediate vicinity of the axon hillock but can also produce a decrementally spreading voltage change in nearby regions of axon. As nearby regions become depolarized, their Na+ channels begin to open. Eventually, the nearby regions also reach threshold and produce an action potential, which then depolarizes the next bit of axon membrane, and so on. In this way spikes can be communicated over long distances with no change in waveform at speeds of many tens of meters per second.

In this section of the book, I describe the voltage-gated channels responsible for producing action potentials and for directing the release of synaptic transmitter. I shall begin with the classic experiments of Hodgkin and Huxley on the squid giant axon. These experiments are important because they provided the first convincing description of the mechanism of the action potential. Furthermore, the methods used are of general applicability and are still being employed by many neuroscientists throughout the world to understand the physiology of ion channels.

The Squid Giant Axon

All of the experiments of Hodgkin and Huxley were performed on an extraordinary preparation, the very large, unmyelinated giant axon of the squid, first described by J. Z. Young (1936). The giant axon, as much as 1 mm in diameter, is dissected from the squid and placed in isolation in a recording chamber, after careful removal of the axon sheath and other adhering tissue. The axon is so large that it is possible to record the membrane potential merely by inserting a glass capillary down the length of the cell. It is even possible to squeeze all of the cytoplasm out of the axon and replace it with artificial medium (see Fig. 4.9 and Chapter 6). This makes this cell unusually favorable for studying the membrane properties of nerve cells.

Chemical analysis of the axoplasm of squid from the genus *Loligo* (used by Hodgkin and Huxley) shows that the ion concentrations inside the axon are $[Na^+]_i = 50$ mM, $[K^+]_i = 400$ mM, and $[Cl^-]_i = \sim 100$ mM (Keynes, 1963; Hodgkin, 1964). Electrical neutrality inside the cell is preserved by large concentrations of organic anions, such as isethionate. Hodgkin and Huxley usually used sea water as the bathing solution, since it is similar in composition to squid internal fluid. The ion concentrations in sea water are much higher than in mammalian blood or cerebrospinal fluid: $[Na^+]_o = 460$ mM, $[K^+]_o = 10$ mM, and $[Cl^-]_o = 540$ mM. Sea water also contains 10 mM Ca^{2+} and 53 mM Mg^{2+}, as well as several minor constituents in smaller concentration.

From the Nernst equation, the equilibrium potential for K^+ is found to be about -90 mV, the exact value depending upon the ambient temperature. When measurements were first made of the resting potential of squid giant axon (Hodgkin and Huxley, 1939; Curtis and Cole, 1942), less negative values were observed, in the neighborhood of -50 to -70 mV (see Fig. 5.1B). The reason for the difference is that the membrane at rest is permeable to Na^+ and Cl^- as well as to K^+ (see Chapter 3). These early experiments also showed that when the membrane of the axon is depolarized, an action potential is produced, during which V_m overshoots zero and reaches $+40$ to $+55$ mV at the peak of the spike (Fig. 5.1B).

The recording of an overshoot of the action potential in these early experiments was unexpected, since the German physiologist

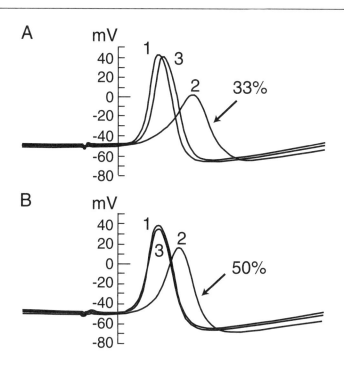

Fig. 5.2 Effect of reduced Na$^+$ on amplitude and waveform of action potential of squid giant axon. Membrane potential measured by inserting electrode down the length of axon under visual control (as in Fig. 5.3B but for voltage recording only). Concentration of Na$^+$ was reduced by diluting sea water with isotonic dextrose solution. **(A)** Exposure to 33% sea water, 67% isotonic dextrose. *1*, Response in sea water; *2*, after 16 min in 33% sea water; *3*, 13 min after reapplication of sea water. **(B)** Exposure to 50% sea water, 50% isotonic dextrose. *1*, Response in sea water; *2*, after 15 min in 50% sea water; *3*, 6 min after reapplication of sea water. (Reprinted from Hodgkin and Katz, 1949, with permission of the authors and the Physiological Society.)

Bernstein (1902, 1912) had predicted that the membrane potential ought only to go to zero, as a result of a general increase in conductance or nonselective "breakdown" of the membrane at the point of action potential generation. The overshoot was first explained by Hodgkin and Katz (1949), in the paper cited in Chapter 3 for the derivation of the GHK equations. Building on the demonstration by Overton (1902) that action potentials disappear in zero-Na$^+$ solution, Hodgkin and Katz varied the external Na$^+$ concentration and showed that the rate of rise and peak amplitude of the spike varied with [Na$^+$]$_o$ (see Fig. 5.2), as would be expected if the spike were initiated by a selective increase in the permeability of the axon membrane to Na$^+$.

Voltage-Clamping

The experiments in Fig. 5.2 were done simply by recording the membrane potential of the axon, but this approach is of rather limited utility for studying the Na$^+$ current responsible for the generation of an action potential. The Na⁺ conductance of the axon changes rapidly with both voltage and time, and the change in conductance produces a change in voltage as Na⁺ enters the axon. The change in voltage then produces a further change in conductance, to produce the regenerative activity that generates the spike. Since the conductance of the axon changes as the membrane potential changes, it is difficult if not impossible to understand how the change in Na⁺ conductance produces the rising phase of the spike by simple voltage recording.

To overcome this difficulty, Cole (1949), Marmont (1949), and Hodgkin, Huxley, and Katz (1952) introduced a new technique, *voltage-clamping*. This technique permits the investigator to hold the membrane voltage of the cell at a fixed value and to keep it at that value for a specified period of time, even when the conductance of the membrane is changing. To voltage-clamp the squid axon, Hodgkin, Huxley, and Katz (1952) introduced two wires into the middle of an isolated axon, one for recording voltage and the other for recording current, both wrapped around a fine glass tube. Over a part of their length the wires were insulated with shellac as indicated in Fig. 5.3A, and only the exposed parts of the wire could actually be used for recording voltage or applying current. Notice that the exposed portion of the current wire is longer than that of the voltage wire.

The axon voltage can then be clamped in the following way. The voltage wire is connected to the input of an amplifier, whose output (V'_m) is approximately equal to the membrane potential. The output of this amplifier is also connected to the negative input of a feedback amplifier (labeled *FBA*). The positive input to the feedback amplifier receives a voltage set by the experimenter, the *command potential* (V_c—the reason for this name will be revealed shortly). A feedback amplifier compares the difference in the voltages at its two inputs and sends a current proportional to this difference to the current wire (see Fig. 5.3B). Feedback amplifiers can now be purchased as integrated circuits and are exceedingly quiet and stable, but this was not the case in the late 1940s: Hodgkin, Huxley, and Katz used a circuit whose prototype was built from scratch with vacuum tubes, by their assistant R. H. Cook (Hodgkin, 1976).

The effect of the current from the feedback amplifier is to bring the measured value of the membrane potential (V'_m) nearly to the

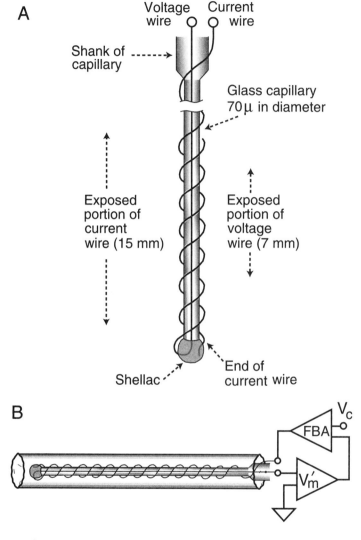

A

Voltage wire Current wire

Shank of capillary

Glass capillary 70µ in diameter

Exposed portion of current wire (15 mm)

Exposed portion of voltage wire (7 mm)

Shellac

End of current wire

B

V_c

FBA

V'_m

Fig. 5.3 Method used by Hodgkin and Huxley to voltage-clamp squid giant axon. **(A)** Construction of electrode. (Redrawn from Hodgkin, Huxley, and Katz, 1952.) **(B)** Insertion of electrode into axon (not drawn to scale), and connection with amplifiers used to measure voltage and apply current. *FBA*, feedback amplifier; V_c, command potential; V'_m, amplifier for measuring membrane voltage. The unlabeled triangle below V'_m is ground or earth and is connected to the solution bathing the axon.

same value as the command potential *(V_c)* and *keep it at that value.* A properly designed feedback amplifier will do this in a very short time (a few microseconds in the experiments of Hodgkin, Huxley, and Katz), so that a change in V_c will cause V'_m also to change, and V'_m rapidly becomes almost identical to V_c. Since it is the difference between the voltages at the inputs of the feedback amplifier that is responsible for the current at its output, V'_m and V_c cannot be exactly equal unless i_m is zero. The difference, however, can be small if the feedback amplifier is designed to have large gain, so that a small difference in the voltages at its inputs produces a large current output. Any propensity for V'_m to change from the value of the command potential set by the experimenter will cause the feedback amplifier rapidly to inject additional current to bring V'_m back nearly to V_c. Fluctuations in V'_m are therefore automatically minimized by the feedback circuitry, and the measured value of i_m is the current required to bring V'_m as close to V_c as the gain of the feedback amplifier will allow. This makes it possible for the experimenter to measure the membrane current *at almost constant membrane potential*. With the membrane potential clamped to the command potential, changes in membrane current are a direct reflection of changes in membrane conductance.

To understand how the voltage clamp measures membrane current, it is helpful to consider a simplified version of the circuit. In Fig. 5.4, *FBA* is again the feedback amplifier, and the triangle labelled V'_m is the amplifier that senses the membrane voltage. The box labeled *Mem* is the membrane of the axon. For the moment, the composition of the membrane will be left unspecified and treated as a "black box." The resistor labeled R_s is any resistance *in series* with the membrane—in the experiments of Hodgkin, Huxley, and Katz (1952) probably in part the resistance of the connective tissue and glia surrounding the axon. R_s is usually referred to as the *series resistance*. The current i_m is the current coming out of the feedback amplifier.

Since the input resistance of the voltage-measuring amplifier (labeled V'_m) is very high, very little of i_m enters its inputs. We can therefore disconnect this amplifier from the circuit and just assume that V'_m is measured and is led to one of the inputs of the feedback amplifier. We also assume that the feedback amplifier is of sufficiently high gain that it is able to keep the measured value of the membrane potential almost identical to V_c, and to do this so rapidly that (for practical purposes) we do not need to concern ourselves with how it does this. This means we can simplify the circuit to the one shown in the middle of Fig. 5.4. A voltage V_c is applied to the top of the circuit, and a current i_m flows through the membrane and series resistance to ground. If the active area of the current electrode is made larger than that of the voltage electrode (Fig.

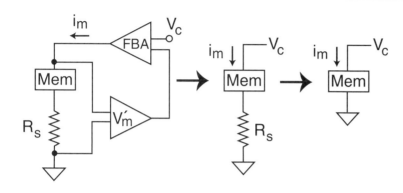

Fig. 5.4 A schematic drawing of the voltage clamp. *Mem*, axon membrane; R_s, series resistance; i_m, membrane current; *FBA*, feedback amplifier; V'_m, amplifier for measuring membrane voltage; V_c, command potential. The unlabeled triangles at bottom are grounds and are connected to the solution bathing the axon.

5.3A), the voltage change produced by the injection of current into the axon will be spatially uniform over the part of the axon containing the voltage electrode, since the nonuniform change in voltage produced at the regions of the axon near the *ends* of the current electrode can be ignored. In the experiments of Hodgkin and Huxley, membrane current was also measured only over the part of the axon containing the exposed voltage electrode. Thus the entire area of the axon from which the membrane potential and current were determined was clamped to the same value V'_m, and this part of the axon was therefore *isopotential* and is said to have been *space-clamped*.

Notice that the flow of current across the series resistance will produce a voltage (= $i_m R_s$) in series with the voltage across the membrane. This means that the potential actually measured by the voltage amplifier (which the feedback amplifier rapidly sets to V_c) is the sum of the membrane potential of the axon and an additional term, the voltage drop due to current flow through the series resistance:

$$V'_m = V_m + i_m R_s \qquad (1)$$

Thus V'_m differs from V_m by an amount equal to $i_m R_s$, which is often referred to as the *series resistance error*: the voltage-clamp circuit does not bring the membrane potential of the axon to V_c but rather to $V_c - i_m R_s$. It is possible to correct for the series resistance, for example by adding an additional voltage to V_c proportional to the membrane current, but this method has one serious limitation. As V_c is made larger, i_m also becomes larger, producing positive feedback that may cause the feedback amplifier to inject a massive current into the axon and destroy the preparation. In practice, only a portion of the series resistance can be compensated in this way.

For simplicity, we shall assume that R_s is zero (or that it has been perfectly compensated), as shown in the drawing to the right in Fig. 5.4. A voltage V_c (or V_m) is imposed across the axon by a current i_m that flows out of the feedback amplifier. This current *is the same current and is of the same sign as the current flowing across the membrane of the cell.* It is important to realize that there is, in principle, no difference between injecting a current into a cell and measuring the voltage, or imposing a constant voltage and measuring the current. If, for example, it were possible to inject current into a cell and vary its amplitude (say, by turning a knob) fast enough to keep the voltage of the cell constant, the current injected would be identical to the one injected by the voltage-clamp circuit. The advantage of the voltage clamp is that, in effect, the setup turns this knob automatically and rapidly enough to keep the voltage of the axon constant, even during the rapid opening and closing of Na$^+$ and K$^+$ channels.

Currents in Response to Voltage Steps

Suppose we begin by setting the command voltage equal to the resting membrane potential of the axon. What is the value of the membrane current? The answer is probably obvious: the membrane current is zero. It is nevertheless useful to solve the equivalent circuit of the membrane to see why this is so (see Fig. 5.5A).

At rest, and for a fairly wide range of potentials negative to rest, the membrane may be represented by a capacitance in parallel with the series combination of a resting conductance (called the leakage conductance—g_l) and its battery (E_l). In Fig. 5.5 the battery's negative pole (the smaller bar) points toward the inside (i.e., the cytoplasm), since the resting membrane potential of the axon is negative (about -65 mV).

Recall that the current through the capacitance is equal to $C_m(dV_m/dt)$. At rest $dV_m/dt = 0$, so there is no capacitive current. Since at rest the cell is at steady state, there can be no current

Box 5.1

VOLTAGE-CLAMPING SMALL CELLS

A small cell can be voltage-clamped, much as a squid axon. Two intracellular microelectrodes are introduced into the cell, one to measure voltage and the other to apply current. The voltage-clamp circuitry used for such experiments is usually quite similar to the one Hodgkin, Huxley, and Katz used, except that special care is often needed to prevent electrical interference between the two electrodes.

Although voltage-clamping can be done with two separate microelectrodes, in practice this method is limited in usefulness, since it is often quite difficult to get two intracellular pipettes into a cell without killing it, unless the cell is exceptionally hardy or rather large (as for snail neurons, see Fig. 4.4; or for *Xenopus* oocytes, see Fig. 1.6). A much more commonly used method is the whole-cell variant of patch-clamp recording. In this case, a single microelectrode is used both to measure voltage and to apply current (see Fig. 6.11 A).

How is this possible? Wouldn't the current of the voltage-clamp circuit pass across the resistance of the patch pipette and produce a voltage drop that would distort the measurement of membrane potential? The answer to this question is certainly yes. Any current passed down the patch pipette into the cell will produce a voltage drop at the pipette tip, and this voltage drop will be *in series with the membrane potential of the cell*. Thus the resistance of the pipette (and of the cell cytoplasm in the vicinity of the pipette tip) produces a *series resistance* like that of the axon sheath in the experiments of Hodgkin, Huxley, and Katz. The measured value of the cell membrane potential will therefore differ from the actual membrane potential.

Fortunately, this error is often fairly small. If the resistance of the patch pipette measured in Ringer solution is 2.5 MΩ (a typical value for whole-cell recording), the *series resistance* produced by the pipette and the cytoplasm of the cell in the vicinity of the pipette will be typically about double this or 5 MΩ. A current of 200 pA will produce a voltage error of $(5 \times 10^6 \ \Omega)(2 \times 10^{-10} \ \text{A})$ = 10×10^{-4} V, or 1 mV. This is not an excessively large error, and it is probably a manageable error in most experimental situations. Notice, however, that a larger current would produce a

continued

larger error: for a current of 2 nA, the error is 10 mV. Peak currents as large as 2 nA are often recorded from small cells for voltage-gated Na⁺ or K⁺ currents, and the voltage error in series with the membrane potential in such cases can be a sizeable fraction of the value of the voltage step. It is essential when voltage clamping with whole-cell patch-clamp recording to keep the series-resistance error as low as possible. This can be achieved by using small cells that have small currents or by proper compensation (some patch-clamp amplifiers allow over 90 percent of the series error to be compensated).

through g_l either. We ignore currents produced by metabolic pumps, since these are small by comparison to the other currents I shall be describing. So the total current across the membrane is zero. The voltage drop across the membrane, which from Ohm's law is the sum of i_l/g_l and E_l, is just E_l since there is no current through g_l. Thus E_l is the resting potential of the axon.

Suppose now the membrane potential is suddenly decreased from the resting potential to a new potential negative of rest (Fig. 5.5B). The feedback amplifier will impose across the membrane a potential V_m substantially equal to V_c (provided the series resistance is small or well enough compensated to be ignored). The current can again be analyzed as the sum of capacitive and resistive

Fig. 5.5   Equivalent circuit of resting axon membrane. **(A)** In absence of voltage clamp. **(B)** With voltage clamp at command potential V_c. C_m, membrane capacitance; g_l, resting or leakage conductance; E_l, resting or leakage battery (resting membrane potential); i_c, capacitive or displacement current; i_l, leakage current; i_m, total membrane current; *In*, intracellular side of circuit; *Out*, extracellular side.

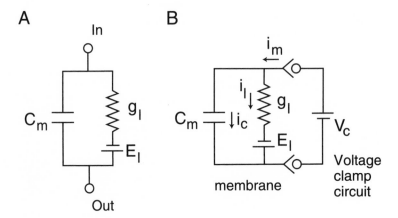

components. The capacitive current i_C is $C_m(dV_c/dt)$. What is the resistive component?

Since the three branches of the circuit in Fig. 5.5B are in parallel, the voltage across each of them must be the same and must be equal to V_c. This means that

$$V_c = E_l + \frac{i_l}{g_l} \qquad (2)$$

where i_l is the current through the leakage conductance, and i_l/g_l is the voltage drop across this conductance (from Ohm's law). If V_c can be assumed to be equal to V_m,

$$i_l = g_l(V_m - E_l) \qquad (3)$$

Eqn. (3) has already been introduced as the equation defining the chord conductance (Chapter 3, Eqn. 34). If we now add together the resistive and capacitive components of the current, the total membrane current is

$$i_m = C_m \frac{dV_m}{dt} + g_l(V_m - E_l) \qquad (4)$$

Fig. 5.6A, a recording from Hodgkin, Huxley, and Katz (1952), is the response of a squid giant axon to a voltage step from the resting potential (which Hodgkin et al. did not measure but which we shall assume from other measurements to be −65 mV) to a voltage 65 mV more negative (i.e., to −130 mV). The capacitive component of the current is virtually over in 50 microseconds (μs) and cannot be detected on the time scale of the figure. All that can be seen is the small negative deflection produced by the leakage current, which remains approximately constant for the duration of the voltage step. Why is the current negative? From Eqn. (3), with the value of the leakage battery (−65 mV) and the new membrane potential (−130 mV), we know that $i_l = (-65 \text{ mV})g_l$. Since g_l is the passive resistance of the membrane, it *must* be positive. So i_l must be negative. Since the voltage drop across g_l is negative, the current across g_l must be in an inward direction (see Chapter 2, Fig. 2.3A).

Fig. 5.6 Membrane currents of voltage-clamped squid axon in response to positive and negative voltage steps. **(A)** Negative voltage step of −65 mV, from resting membrane potential (assumed to be −65 mV) to −130 mV. Note small negative-going (inward) current response due to leakage conductance. **(B)** Positive voltage step of +65 mV from the resting membrane potential to 0 mV. Small initial positive-going current response due to leakage conductance is followed by large inward and then outward current. (Redrawn from Fig. 11 of Hodgkin, Huxley, and Katz, 1952, with polarity of current traces reversed; see also Hille, 1992.)

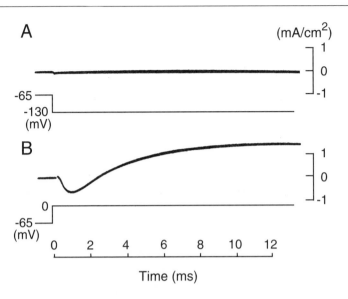

Parallel Conductance Model of Membrane

A much more interesting result is produced if instead of a hyperpolarizing voltage step, a depolarizing step to 0 mV is given (Fig. 5.6B). A small positive deflection can be detected just at the beginning of the trace, due to current through the leakage conductance (which is now outward, since the polarity of the voltage step has been reversed). This is followed by a much larger transient negative inward current, after which a maintained positive outward current occurs. Again, the capacitive component of the current cannot be resolved on this time scale.

There is now overwhelming evidence that the large inward current in Fig. 5.6B is caused by the inflow primarily of Na^+ through voltage-gated Na^+ channels. It is this inflow of Na^+ that is responsible for the upswing of the spike. The outward current is due to the efflux of K^+ through voltage-gated K^+ channels, and the outward flow of K^+ (together with the closing of the Na^+ channels) is responsible for the rapid decay of the action potential.

I shall describe some of the evidence for the ion selectivity of the inward and outward currents later in this chapter. For the moment, if we assume that the inward current is Na^+ and the outward current K$^+$, we can redraw the equivalent circuit of the membrane by adding appropriate conductance pathways, as in Fig. 5.7. Arrows have been drawn through g_{Na} and g_K to indicate that these conductances are variable with time and voltage.

The analysis of this circuit is as follows. Through each branch of the circuit a current flows, and the total membrane current i_m is the sum of each of these currents,

$$i_m = i_c + i_l + i_{Na} + i_K \tag{5}$$

The capacitive current is again given by $C_m(dV_c/dt)$. Since the voltage drop across each branch of the circuit must be the same and equal to V_c, we can write an equation like Eqn. (3) for i_l, i_{Na}, and i_K. The equation for the total membrane current is then

$$i_m = C_m \frac{dV_m}{dt} + g_l(V_m - E_l) + g_{Na}(V_m - E_{Na}) \tag{6}$$
$$+ g_K(V_m - E_K)$$

At rest, g_{Na} and g_K are small in comparison to g_l, and Eqn. (6) reduces to Eqn. (4). As sodium channels open during a depolarizing voltage step, g_{Na} initially becomes very large. As we shall see, both the Na$^+$ and K$^+$ channels are voltage-dependent and open with in-

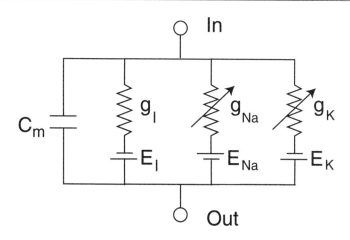

Fig. 5.7 Parallel conductance model of squid axon membrane. C_m, membrane capacitance; g_l, resting or leakage conductance; E_l, resting or leakage battery (resting membrane potential); g_{Na}, sodium conductance; E_{Na}, sodium battery; g_K, potassium conductance; E_K, potassium battery; *In*, intracellular side of circuit; *Out*, extracellular side. (Modified from Hodgkin and Huxley, 1952d.)

creasing depolarization. Since E_{Na} is about 55 mV, $(V_m - E_{Na})$ at V_m = 0 would be −55 mV, and the current produced by the increase in g_{Na} would be negative or inward. A similar calculation shows that the current produced by the delayed increase in g_K will be positive or outward.

At this point, it may be useful to emphasize that the only thing the voltage-clamp circuit is doing in Fig. 5.6B is rapidly moving the membrane potential from −65 mV to a new potential of 0 mV and *keeping it there*. What happens next is entirely the result of changes in the values of the conductances. The Na⁺ and K⁺ conductances change because they are functions of both time and voltage, as described in much more detail below. As these conductances change, the currents through the Na⁺ and K⁺ branches of the circuit in Fig. 5.7 also change. Since the conductances in Eqn. (6) are always positive, the sign of the current is entirely a function of the sign of the driving forces, $(V_m - E_{Na})$ or $(V_m - E_K)$. Since the driving force for Na⁺ is negative at $V_m = 0$, i_{Na} is inward; since that for K⁺ is positive, i_K is outward.

The circuit diagram in Fig. 5.7 representing the membrane as a series of separate conductance pathways for leakage, Na⁺, and K⁺ is often referred to as the *parallel conductance model*. The basic premise of this model is that Na⁺ and K⁺ flow through the membrane through separate and independent pathways. When Hodgkin and Huxley first published their experiments, this premise was quite controversial and widely debated. Now there is no longer any argument: Hodgkin and Huxley were correct. Evidence for separate conductance pathways is presented later in this chapter and in succeeding chapters.

Ion Selectivity of Currents

Inward Currents Carried by Na⁺

When most of the Na⁺ in the sea water bathing the axon was replaced with the larger organic cation choline⁺, the inward current disappeared with only a small reduction in the amplitude of the outward current (Hodgkin and Huxley, 1952a). Hodgkin and Huxley interpreted this experiment to mean that Na⁺ influx is mostly responsible for the rapid inward current and that choline⁺ doesn't permeate the Na⁺ channel. They then showed that if the

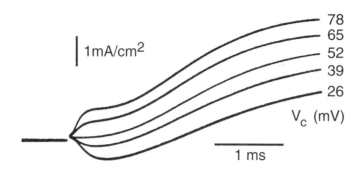

Fig. 5.8 Time course of currents recorded from voltage-clamped squid axon in response to large depolarizations. Resting membrane potential of axon was assumed to be −65 mV. Numbers to right of traces give values of the depolarizing command potentials used to evoke each of the recorded currents. (Redrawn from Fig. 14 of Hodgkin, Huxley, and Katz, 1952, with polarity of current traces reversed. See also Hodgkin, 1964.)

command potential was systematically changed in normal sea water, the inward current could be shown to reverse. In Fig. 5.8, the lowermost current record is the response to a voltage step from the resting potential, assumed to be −65 mV, to a membrane potential of +26 mV. It is similar in waveform to the trace in Fig. 5.6B: a transient inward current is followed by a more slowly developing outward current. As the value of the voltage step was increased further, the amplitude of the inward current became smaller, even though g_{Na} remained very large. Recall that if the inward current is produced by Na$^+$ influx, then $i_{Na} = g_{Na}(V_m - E_{rev})$. The current becomes smaller as V_m increases and approaches E_{rev}, even if g_{Na} remains large. When the voltage in Fig. 5.6B was stepped to 52 mV, there was no initial component of inward current but only a slowly rising outward current, since at a membrane potential of 52 mV, $V_m = E_{rev}$. For voltage steps more positive than 52 mV, the sign of the initial component of current reversed and the current became outward, since $V_m > E_{rev}$. The value of the reversal potential for the initial component of the current was of the order of +50 mV, near the estimated value of the equilibrium potential for Na$^+$.

Hodgkin and Huxley (1952a) then decreased the external Na$^+$ concentration, and the reversal potential of the inward current shifted to less positive values. To understand why this would be so, consider the measurement of the reversal potentials (ψ_1 and ψ_2) at two external Na$^+$ concentrations ([Na$^+$]$_1$ and [Na$^+$]$_2$). From the Nernst equation,

$$\psi_1 = \frac{RT}{F} \ln \frac{[Na^+]_1}{[Na^+]_i}, \quad \psi_2 = \frac{RT}{F} \ln \frac{[Na^+]_2}{[Na^+]_i} \tag{7}$$

where $[Na^+]_i$ is the Na^+ concentration in the axoplasm. If we assume that when we change the external Na^+ concentration, we do not change the *internal* concentration (probably a safe assumption, since the volume of the squid giant axon is so large in comparison to its membrane surface),

$$\psi_2 - \psi_1 = \frac{RT}{F} \ln \frac{[Na^+]_2}{[Na^+]_1} \tag{8}$$

Hodgkin and Huxley (1952a) showed that the change in the reversal potential corresponded very closely with the predictions of Eqn. (8) and concluded that the inward current was carried almost exclusively by Na^+.

More recent measurements indicate that Na^+ channels in axons, though selective for Na^+, can also be permeated by other ions. Although measurements of ion selectivity for the inward current could in principle be obtained as in Fig. 5.8, the measurements are easier and more accurate if the outward (K^+) currents are eliminated—for example, by replacing K^+ in the intracellular solution with Cs^+, which in most cases does not permeate K^+ channels, or by blocking the channels with quaternary ammonium ions, such as tetraethylammonium (TEA^+). (See Fig. 5.9A and Hille, 1967; Armstrong and Binstock, 1965; Armstrong, 1975.) The selectivity of the channels for ions other than Na^+ can then be measured by a method similar to the one described for glycine and GABA receptors. First, substitute all of the Na^+ in the external medium with another ion, say X^+. Then, from the GHK voltage equation, the difference between the reversal potentials in Na^+ (ψ_1) and in X^+ (ψ_2) is

$$\psi_2 - \psi_1 = \frac{RT}{F} \ln \frac{P_X[X^+]_o}{P_{Na}[Na^+]_o}, \tag{9}$$

provided there is no change in the concentrations of the ions inside the cell. Such measurements show that for vertebrate Na^+ channels P_X/P_{Na} is about 0.9 for Li^+, between 0.1 and 0.2 for organic cations such as NH_4^+ and guanidinium$^+$, about 0.1 for K^+, and less than

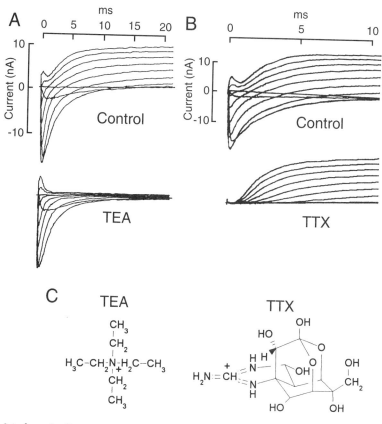

Fig. 5.9 Pharmacological isolation of Na^+ and K^+ currents. Voltage-clamp currents from frog myelinated nerve with a holding potential of −75 mV, in response to a series of depolarizing potentials at 15 mV intervals (first step was from −75 mV to −60 mV, second from −75 mV to −45 mV, and so on). **(A)** Currents in control solution (above) and in solution containing 6 mM tetraethylammonium (TEA). **(B)** Currents in control solution and in solution containing 300 nM tetrodotoxin (TTX). (Current records taken from figures 3a, 3b, 6a, and 6b of Hille, 1970, and reprinted with permission of the author and of Elsevier Science.) **(C)** Chemical structures of TEA and TTX.

0.01 for choline$^+$ (see Hille, 1975). Similar values have been obtained for squid axons (Chandler and Meeves, 1965).

Outward Currents Carried by K^+

Hodgkin and Huxley (1952a) observed that the delayed outward current was not much affected by the removal of Na_o and argued, mostly on the basis of evidence obtained by methods other than voltage-clamping, that the outward current was carried by K^+. More recently, the selectivity of the outward current has been investigated in great detail, largely in preparations for which the Na^+ current has been blocked by toxins, such as tetrodotoxin and saxitoxin. Tetrodotoxin (TTX), a poison from the puffer fish, and saxitoxin (STX), the poison contained in dinoflagellates responsible for "red tides," are both highly specific blockers of Na$^+$ channels (see Fig. 5.9B). After the Na$^+$ current is blocked, the K$^+$ current can be studied in isolation. Selectivity measurements like those for the Na$^+$ current have been made on K$^+$ channels in many different organisms (Latorre and Miller, 1983), with the conclusion that K$^+$ channels are quite selective for K$^+$. Of other monovalent cations only Tl$^+$, NH$_4^+$, and Rb$^+$ show significant permeability, and P_{Na}/P_K is often as low as 0.01.

Voltage and Time Dependence of Na$^+$ and K$^+$ Currents

If the peak amplitudes of inward and outward currents are plotted as a function of voltage, both are seen to be activated at membrane potentials above -50 mV (Fig. 5.10). Both then increase monotonically with increasing voltage. This steep increase in current reflects an increase in conductance, which is an important feature of the Na$^+$ and K$^+$ currents responsible for the action potential. As Fig. 5.1A illustrates, the currents are produced by proteins whose conformation is changed by voltage. Voltage-gated channels are proteins with charged amino acids, which respond to the change in membrane voltage by actually moving either toward or away from the inside of the cell (see Chapter 6). As these amino acids move, they change the conformation of the channel and open a conductance pore through which ions pass.

Gating of the channels could occur in two ways. The channel proteins might have a pore of fixed conductance, closed at negative potentials and opened as the membrane potential is depolarized. This would occur if, for example, the channel pore were occluded by an obstruction (perhaps a part of the protein) that swung open as a result of depolarization. The swinging open of this "gate" would reveal a pore of fixed conductance through which ions would flow. With increasing depolarization, more and more channels might open, each of the same unitary conductance. The voltage dependence of the current would then depend upon the voltage dependence of the gating of the channel, and the conductance of the pore would itself be independent of voltage.

On the other hand, it is possible to imagine that the pore of the channel is a more complicated structure, and that channel activa-

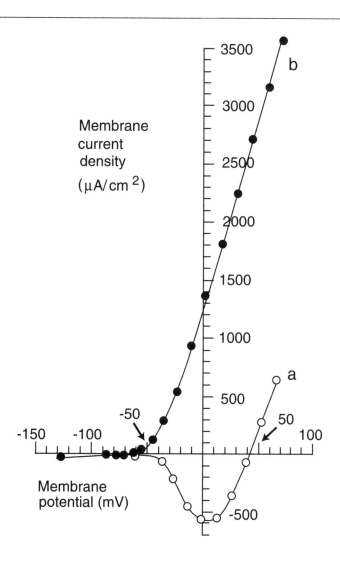

Fig. 5.10 Current-voltage curves of inward and outward currents from squid giant axon in normal solution (sea water). Open circles and curve labeled *a* give amplitude of inward current 0.63 ms after the beginning of the voltage step; solid circles and curve labeled *b* give outward current amplitude at "steady state," that is when the current appeared to have reached a steady value. (Data from fig. 13 of Hodgkin, Huxley, and Katz, 1952, with current and voltage polarities reversed and resting membrane potential assumed to be −65 mV.)

tion is inadequately described by the simple motion of a gate. The channel could, for example, undergo a series of conformational changes with increasing depolarization, and as a result channel pores of different conductance would be formed at different voltages. In this case the conductance of the channel would itself be a function of voltage.

Instantaneous i–V Curves

Hodgkin and Huxley (1952b) attempted to distinguish between these two possibilities by examining the conductance of the open channels with a novel measurement called the *instantaneous current-voltage curve*. The membrane potential of the axon was first stepped to a fixed depolarized value, called the *prepulse voltage* (V_1). The value of the prepulse voltage was selected to produce a large activation of current and was kept always the same, so that each prepulse opened the same *number* of channels in each experimental run. Then, near the peak of the current activated by the prepulse, the voltage was suddenly changed to a new value (V_2), which was varied. The current was measured just after the change from V_1 to V_2 (that is, "instantaneously" after the voltage change), before any change in the number of the channels could occur. In this way, Hodgkin and Huxley attempted to measure the i–V curve of the channels once they had been opened and before any alteration occurred in their gating.

The results Hodgkin and Huxley obtained for Na^+ channels are shown in Fig. 5.11A. The schema labeled at the top as *a* (to the left) shows the measurement of the peak Na^+ current, and the current-voltage curve for these measurements is given as the X's in the graph below. This is much like the curve for the Na^+ current shown in Fig. 5.10. The schema labeled *b* shows the measurement of the instantaneous i–V curve: the prepulse V_1 activated the Na^+ current, and the voltage was suddenly changed to a new value V_2. The current measured "instantaneously" just after the switch to V_2 is shown as i_2 and is plotted as the solid circles. The instantaneous i–V curve was linear. Similar results for the K^+ current are shown in Fig. 5.11B, obtained in Na^+-free sea water.

Since for both Na^+ and K^+ currents, the instantaneous current-voltage curves were linear (i.e., of constant slope) within the physiological range of voltages, Hodgkin and Huxley reasoned that the conductance of the channels was not a function of voltage—at least for the region of membrane potentials they investigated. If the conductance of the open channels is not a function of voltage, then the voltage dependence of the current measured from the whole axon must be the result of the voltage dependence of channel opening,

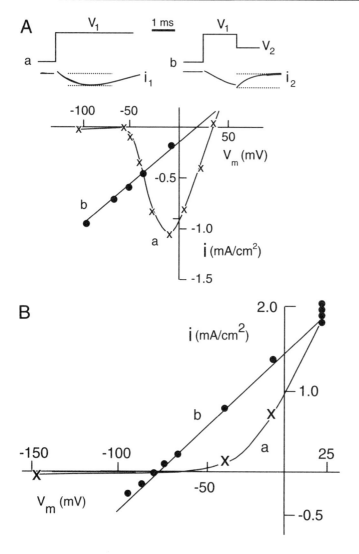

Fig. 5.11 Instantaneous current-voltage curve measured from voltage-clamped giant axon of squid. **(A)** Inward (Na⁺) current. Protocol for experiment shown above. For a, a single step was given to a variable voltage V_1, and the peak amplitude of the current was measured (i_1). For b, a prepulse was first given to voltage V_1. The value of this voltage was selected to evoke a large inward current, and the value of the prepulse voltage was kept constant throughout the experiment. Near the peak of the inward current, the voltage was changed to a second voltage, V_2, which was varied. The resulting current i_2 was measured just after the change from V_1 to V_2, that is, "instantaneously" after the voltage change. The values of the currents are plotted below. For curve a, i_1 has been plotted as a function of V_1; and for curve b, i_2 has been plotted as a function of V_2. (Data from fig. 6 of Hodgkin and Huxley, 1952b, with current and voltage polarities reversed and resting membrane potential assumed to be −65 mV.) **(B)** Outward (K⁺) current. Method similar to that in **(A)** except experiments were done in a solution for which the Na⁺ was replaced with the impermeant ion choline⁺. Instantaneous current-voltage curve is labeled b, and curve for single pulse is labeled a. (Data from fig. 12 of Hodgkin and Huxley, 1952b, with current and voltage polarities reversed and resting membrane potential assumed to be −65 mV.)

not the result of a voltage dependence of the conductance of the open channel pore.

This inference has been largely sustained by single-channel recordings (Chapters 6 and 7). Although the conductance of ion channels is not always completely independent of voltage (see for example MacKinnon and Yellen, 1990), for squid axon the conductance of Na⁺ and K⁺ channels is sufficiently constant within the physiological range of membrane potentials to justify the inferences Hodgkin and Huxley made. The notion that the voltage dependence of Na^+ and K^+ currents mostly reflects the voltage dependence of gating rather than that of the conductance of the pore was a remarkable insight—one of the most important intellectual achievements (among many) in the Hodgkin-Huxley papers.

Time Dependence of Gating

To study the time dependence of the sodium and potassium conductances, Hodgkin and Huxley realized that it would be necessary to separate the two currents so they could be studied independently. This can now be done rather easily with toxins like TTX and TEA^+ (see Fig. 5.9), though care must be taken to ensure that the block is complete and not a function of time or membrane voltage. Since Hodgkin and Huxley did not know about TTX or TEA^+, they used the following approach. They recorded currents in normal sea water and in sea water containing a reduced concentration of Na^+. On the assumption that the very beginning of the current trace was produced only by Na^+ currents, and that reducing the Na^+ reduced the Na^+ currents but did not change their time course or the time course of the K^+ currents, it was possible to compare the currents in normal and reduced-Na^+ sea water to estimate the form of the Na^+ currents; and to subtract these currents from the total ionic current in normal sea water to provide a measure of the waveform of K^+ currents.

These curves were then used to plot the time course of the conductance change for the Na^+ and K^+ currents. Conductances were calculated for each pathway from

$$g_{Na} = i_{Na} / (V_m - E_{Na}), \quad g_K = i_K / (V_m - E_K) \tag{10}$$

The results of these calculations (Fig. 5.12) indicate that even when the axon is voltage-clamped so that membrane potential is held at a constant value, the conductance change (and therefore the gating of the channels) is a complex function both of voltage and of time.

Inactivation of the Sodium Current

The curves in Fig. 5.12 show one remarkable feature: even in the presence of a maintained depolarization, the Na^+ conductance declines. The Na^+ channels, once they have opened, close again by a process that Hodgkin and Huxley (1952c) termed *inactivation*.

The inactivation of the Na^+ current depends upon both time and voltage. The time dependence is illustrated in Fig. 5.13. An 8 mV prepulse from $V_m = -65$ to $V_m = -57$ (called V_1) of variable length was given before a 44 mV depolarizing test pulse (to $V_m = -21$ mV—see Fig. 5.13). As the duration of the prepulse increased, i_{Na} produced by the test pulse declined. A summary of results for prepulses of different durations at several different membrane potentials is given in Fig. 5.14. The ordinate gives the current evoked by the test pulse after a prepulse $(i_{Na})_{V_1}$, divided by the current evoked by the test pulse in the absence of a prepulse $(i_{Na})_o$. The abscissa gives the duration of the prepulse. The current actually gets larger after hyperpolarizing prepulses, indicating that at the normal

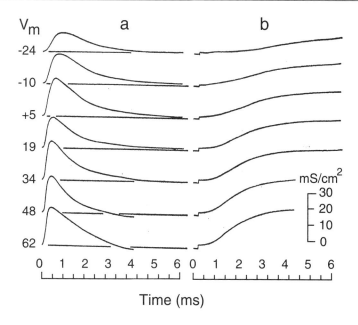

Time (ms)

Fig. 5.12 Curves of inward (Na^+) and outward (K^+) conductances (*a* and *b* respectively) as functions of time and voltage. Conductances were calculated as described in text. Waveforms are for voltage steps from rest to the voltages indicated to the left (in mV). (Data from fig. 8 of Hodgkin and Huxley, 1952a, with voltage polarities reversed and resting membrane potential assumed to be −65 mV.)

Fig. 5.13 Time dependence of Na$^+$ current inactivation for voltage-clamped axon of giant
squid. At left is the command potential pulse
protocol. Voltage was stepped initially 8 mV depolarized from resting potential of −65 mV to a
prepulse voltage of −57 mV. Voltage was then
left at the prepulse voltage for a variable length
of time. At the end of the prepulse, the voltage
was stepped to −21 mV and the amplitude of
the current measured. To the right of each protocol is the membrane current in response to
step to −21 mV. Vertical bars show amplitude of
Na$^+$ current in the absence of the prepulse.
(Data from fig. 1 of Hodgkin and Huxley, 1952c,
with current and voltage polarities reversed
and resting membrane potential assumed to
be −65 mV.)

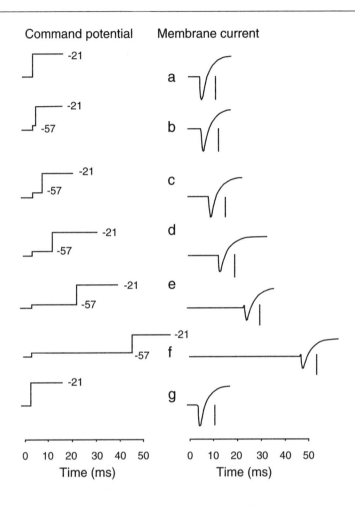

resting membrane potential the current is already partially inactivated. For depolarizing prepulses, the currents in response to the
test pulse become smaller.

To determine the voltage dependence of inactivation at steady
state, Hodgkin and Huxley (1952c) gave prepulses long enough
so that a steady state was reached regardless of the membrane potential. Fig. 5.14 shows that this occurs within 20–25 ms. The current in response to the test pulse declined continuously as the
value of the prepulse was made more depolarized (Fig. 5.15A).
These results are summarized in Fig. 5.15B. Once again the ordi-

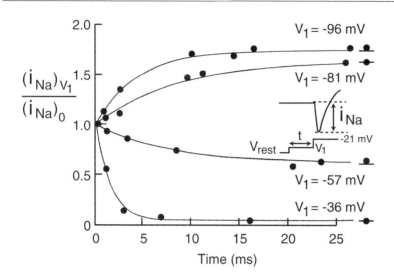

Fig. 5.14 Time dependence of inactivation. Ordinate gives the amplitude of the Na$^+$ current for a voltage step to -21 mV after presentation of a prepulse, normalized to the amplitude of the Na$^+$ current for the same voltage step in the absence of a prepulse. Prepulse amplitude was variable and is given as V_1 next to each of the curves. Abscissa gives duration of prepulse. Diagram at middle right presents the protocol for current measurements. (Data from fig. 3 of Hodgkin and Huxley, 1952c, with current and voltage polarities reversed and resting membrane potential assumed to be -65 mV.)

nate is the ratio of two currents: $(i_{Na})_V$, the peak Na$^+$ current following the prepulse; and $(i_{Na})_o$, the peak Na$^+$ current in the absence of a prepulse. This figure gives the steady-state inactivation of the sodium conductance as a function of potential and is called the h_∞ curve.

The inactivation of the Na$^+$ current has several important functional consequences. Since a fraction of the Na$^+$ channels is inactivated at the resting membrane potential, a brief hyperpolarization that removes inactivation can actually increase the excitability of the cell. A neuron in the CNS has Na$^+$ channels much like those in squid, and brief inhibitory synaptic input that hyperpolarizes the neuron and momentarily blocks the spiking of the cell also removes inactivation, actually making the neuron more likely to fire an action potential once the inhibitory input ceases.

When one action potential has occurred, another spike cannot be produced until the inactivation of the Na$^+$ channels is removed and the K$^+$ channels have reclosed. As a consequence, each spike is followed by a brief period of time, called the *refractory period*, before the axon or nerve cell can fire an additional spike. The time course of removal of inactivation is therefore one of the important determinants of the maximum frequency of spike firing of a neuron.

Fig. 5.15 Voltage dependence of inactivation at steady state. **(A)** Protocol similar to that in Fig. 5.13 except that prepulse duration was kept constant and voltage was varied. Voltage protocols at left, with amplitude of prepulse voltage given above each prepulse; second voltage pulse was always to −21 mV. Membrane currents traced at right. Vertical bar shows amplitude of Na$^+$ current in the absence of the prepulse. (Data from fig. 4 of Hodgkin and Huxley, 1952c, with current and voltage polarities reversed and resting membrane potential assumed to be −65 mV.) **(B)** Membrane-potential dependence of inactivation at steady state. Ordinate gives amplitude of current in presence of prepulse divided by amplitude of current in absence of prepulse, for currents evoked by steps to −21 mV. Abscissa is membrane potential of prepulse. (Data from fig. 5 of Hodgkin and Huxley, 1952c, with current and voltage polarities reversed and resting membrane potential assumed to be −65 mV.)

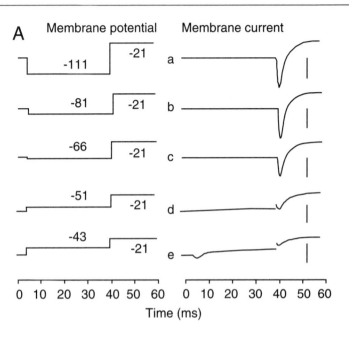

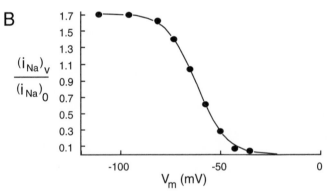

The Hodgkin-Huxley Model

Having described the basic features of the inward and outward currents, Hodgkin and Huxley (1952d) produced a mathematical model to reconstruct the time course and voltage dependence of the conductances and to calculate the form of the action potential. This model, which I shall refer to as the *Hodgkin-Huxley model,* was intended primarily as an empirical description of the currents. In this respect, their model succeeded admirably and still remains quite useful. Many studies have used and still use Hodgkin-Huxley-like models to represent ion channel currents—for example, to understand the contribution that particular channel types make to changes in spike threshold or firing frequency. Hodgkin-Huxley models are also quite useful for understanding the contribution of voltage-gated conductances to signal spread, as in dendrites with voltage-gated channels (see Fig. 1.3).

The basic assumption of the Hodgkin-Huxley model is that Na^+ and K^+ travel across the membrane through separate (parallel conductance) pathways, so that the total ionic current (i_m) can be written as a sum of currents, $i_m = i_l + i_{Na} + i_K$, with each of these currents given in turn by

$$i_l = g_l(V_m - E_l), \quad i_{Na} = g_{Na}(V_m - E_{Na}),$$
$$i_K = g_K(V_m - E_K) \tag{11}$$

Hodgkin and Huxley assumed that E_l, E_{Na}, and E_K are constants that do not change during voltage-clamp experiments or during the generation of an action potential. This is equivalent to saying that the concentrations, and hence the equilibrium potentials of the ions are not altered by the flow of Na^+ and K^+, which is likely to be true for a cell as large as a squid axon (see Box 4.2). Hodgkin and Huxley further assumed that g_l was not a function of either membrane potential or time. Thus to describe their results, they needed only to describe the time and voltage dependence of g_{Na} and g_K.

K^+ Conductance

Hodgkin and Huxley began with g_K, which seemed simpler since it did not show inactivation (at least during the short-duration voltage pulses used in their experiments). The time course of activation of g_K, obtained from conductance plots like those shown in Fig. 5.12, had a peculiar shape. The rise in current was sigmoidal and was poorly fit by a simple exponential function, $1 - \exp(-t/\tau)$, but could be fit by an exponential raised to a power, $[1 - \exp(-t/\tau)]^j$. Raising the exponential function to a power mimicked the delay in the rate of rise, with $j = 4$ giving the best fit. The *decay* of the K+ conductance was measured in experiments not yet described here (Hodgkin and Huxley, 1952b) by first activating g_K with a depolarizing voltage pulse and then repolarizing to a more negative potential, to measure the time course of current decline. In contrast to activation, the decline of current could be well fit by a simple exponential, $\exp(-t/\tau)$.

What physical model could explain this behavior? Hodgkin and Huxley argued (mostly for the sake of illustration) that there might be four gates in the membrane (or four protein subunits, or four regions of the K+ channel protein) that must change position so that the channel can open. Think of these gates as particles that move when the voltage is changed, perhaps because the particles are charged. Let us call n the probability of a particle moving across the membrane to an "open" position. If the channel opens only when *all four* of the particles have moved to the "open" position, then the rate of channel opening will go as n^4 (think of the probability of four coins all coming up heads).

Let us now suppose that the rate of movement of the particles (or subunits or protein regions) is first-order, linearly proportional to the concentration of the particles. The time course of particle movement would then be exponential (I shall show why this is so shortly). The time course of *channel opening,* however, would go as the *fourth power* of this exponential, or $[1 - \exp(-t/\tau)]^4$. When the channel closes, only one of the particles need move back for complete closing, so the rate of channel closing would just be exponential, as Hodgkin and Huxley observed.

The formal assumption Hodgkin and Huxley made was that

$$g_K = \overline{g_K} n^4 \tag{12}$$

where n varies between 0 and 1 and represents the proportion of particles in the proper position to cause channel opening, and "g_K-bar" is a constant equal to the maximum value of g_K. The proportion of channels in the "open" position is equal to the probability of the channels occupying the "open" position, provided the number of channels is large.

A first-order kinetic equation describing the movement of the particles is

$$\frac{dn}{dt} = \alpha_n(1-n) - \beta_n n \tag{13}$$

This equation says that the rate at which n increases is equal to the rate at which particles move from the closed to the open position minus the rate at which they move from the open to the closed position. The rate for particle motion from closed to open is the product of a rate constant (α_n) and the proportion of particles in the closed position ($1 - n$). Similarly, the rate from open to closed is equal to the rate constant for closing (β_n) times the proportion in the open position (n).

To solve this equation, we rearrange to get

$$\int dt = \int \frac{dn}{\alpha_n - (\alpha_n + \beta_n)n} \tag{14}$$

Since

$$\int \frac{dx}{ax+b} = \frac{1}{a}\ln(ax+b) \tag{15}$$

Eqn. (14) can be solved (from $t = 0$, $n = n_0$ to $t = t$, $n = n$) to obtain

$$\frac{\alpha_n - (\alpha_n + \beta_n)n}{\alpha_n - (\alpha_n + \beta_n)n_0} = \exp\left(-\frac{t}{\tau_n}\right) \tag{16}$$

where $\tau_n = 1/(\alpha_n + \beta_n)$. This equation can be usefully rearranged by multiplying both sides by $[\alpha_n - (\alpha_n + \beta_n)n_0]$ to give

$$\alpha_n - (\alpha_n + \beta_n)n = [\alpha_n - (\alpha_n + \beta_n)n_0]\exp\left(-\frac{t}{\tau_n}\right) \tag{17}$$

Hodgkin and Huxley next observed that as t goes to infinity, the exponential term on the right side of Eqn. (17) goes to zero. Thus the left side of the equation must also go to zero at $t = t_\infty$. If n_∞ is defined as the value of n at $t = t_\infty$, then $\alpha_n - (\alpha_n + \beta_n)n_\infty = 0$ and $n_\infty = \alpha_n/(\alpha_n + \beta_n)$. Now divide both sides of Eqn. (17) by $(\alpha_n + \beta_n)$ and introduce the definition of n_∞, to give the equation for n in the form Hodgkin and Huxley gave it:

$$n = n_\infty - (n_\infty - n_0)e^{-t/\tau_n} \tag{18}$$

Let us see what this equation says. At the beginning of the voltage step, $t = 0$, the exponential is equal to one, and $n = n_0$. If the voltage is changed to some new value, n changes. The reason for this is that the steady-state value of n is a function of voltage, so n rises (or falls) from n_0 to n_∞ along an exponential time course, with a time constant equal to τ_n, or $1/(\alpha_n + \beta_n)$. The conductance also changes as voltage changes but with a time course that goes as n^4. It is perhaps useful to keep in mind that n_0 and n_∞ both represent essentially the same variable, the steady-state value of n. The only difference is that n_0 is the steady-state value of n at the beginning of the pulse, and n_∞ its value at the end.

Hodgkin and Huxley fitted their measurements of conductance with Eqn. (12), using values for n obtained from Eqn. (18) by varying n_∞ and τ_n to obtain the best fit. The results of these calculations are shown in Fig. 5.16. The waveforms of the conductance are given in Fig. 5.16A, with circles showing the actual measurements and lines the results of the calculations. A graph of n_∞ as a function of voltage is given in Fig. 5.16B. It is of some interest that n_∞ is a rather steep function of membrane potential—it approaches zero only at rather negative potentials.

Na+ Conductance

To fit the data for Na+ conductance, Hodgkin and Huxley used a similar strategy, but for g_{Na} some alteration in the equations had to be made to accommodate inactivation. Largely to simplify the mathematics, they assumed that activation and inactivation of the Na+ channel occur independently, each governed by its own equation. As for the K+ conductance, they argued that activation might be thought of as regulated by the movement of particles through

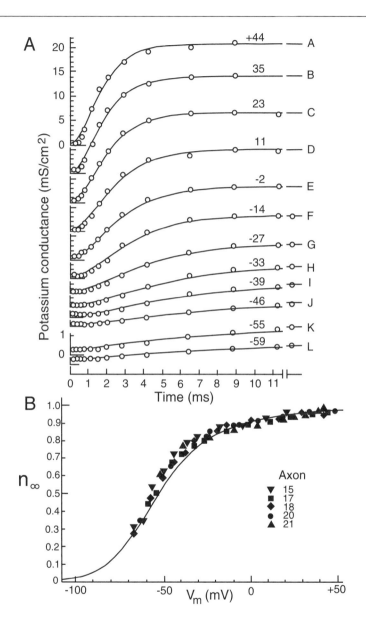

Fig. 5.16 Hodgkin-Huxley model of potassium conductance. **(A)** Fit of Eqns. (12) and (18) to measured values *(circles)* of potassium conductance as functions of time and voltage. Numbers above each curve give the membrane potential of the depolarizing voltage step (in mV). Scale of ordinate is the same for all traces except the two lowest (labeled *K* and *L*), for which a different scale is given. (Data from fig. 3 of Hodgkin and Huxley, 1952d, with voltage polarities reversed and resting membrane potential assumed to be −65 mV.)

(B) Voltage dependence of n_∞. Data points are values calculated from the potassium conductance at steady state (i.e., 10–15 ms after the beginning of the voltage step) and Eqn. (12). Each symbol gives measurements from a different axon. Curve is calculated from model. (Data and curve from fig. 5 of Hodgkin and Huxley, 1952d, with voltage polarities reversed and resting membrane potential assumed to be −65 mV.)

Fig. 5.17 Hodgkin and Huxley model of sodium conductance. **(A)** Fit of Eqns. (19) and (21) to measured values (circles) of sodium conductance as functions of time and voltage. Numbers above each curve give the membrane potential of the depolarizing voltage step (in mV). Conductance scales are different for different traces and are indicated to right of the curves in three groups, separated by dotted lines. (Data from fig. 6 of Hodgkin and Huxley, 1952d, with voltage polarities reversed and resting membrane potential assumed to be −65 mV.) **(B)** Voltage dependence of m_∞ (solid symbols) and of h_∞ (open symbols). Each symbol represents measurements from a different experiment. Lines are fitted from equations of model. (From figs. 8 and 10 of Hodgkin and Huxley, 1952d, with voltage polarities reversed and resting membrane potential assumed to be −65 mV.)

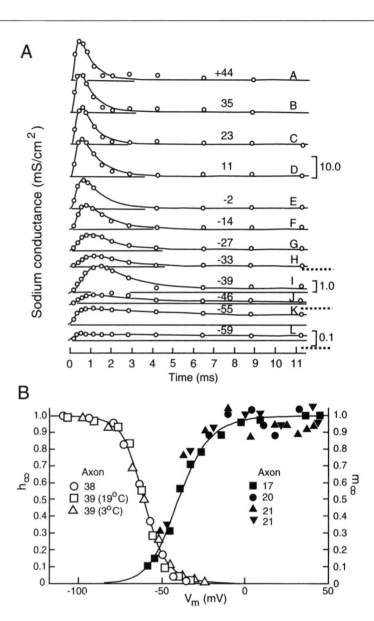

the membrane, which for g_{Na} they called m. Inactivation was governed by the independent movement of a different particle, called h. As for n, both m and h vary from 0 to 1, and g_{Na} is given by

$$g_{Na} = m^3 h \overline{g_{Na}} \qquad (19)$$

Notice that m is raised only to a power of 3, and h occurs without an exponent.

Following the treatment used for g_K, Hodgkin and Huxley assumed that both m and h follow first-order kinetic equations,

$$\frac{dm}{dt} = \alpha_m(1-m) - \beta_m m, \quad \frac{dh}{dt} = \alpha_h(1-h) - \beta_h h \qquad (20)$$

The solutions to these equations can be obtained just as for g_K, resulting in separate equations for m and h:

$$m = m_\infty - (m_\infty - m_0)e^{-t/\tau_m}, \quad h = h_\infty - (h_\infty - h_0)e^{-t/\tau_h} \qquad (21)$$

The τ's and m_∞ and h_∞ are defined just as for τ_n and n_∞. A comparison of the observed and calculated values of g_{Na} is given in Fig. 5.17A. From these calculations, best-fitting values of τ_m, τ_h, m_∞, and h_∞ were obtained (for graphs for m_∞ and h_∞, see Fig. 5.17B). The graph for h_∞ is of course identical to the steady-state inactivation curve for the Na^+ current, given in Fig. 5.15B.

The Mechanism of the Action Potential

An important feature of any theory is its predictive power. Having described the voltage and time dependence of both the Na^+ and K^+ currents, Hodgkin and Huxley attempted to use their descriptions to calculate the waveform of an action potential. From a theoretical point of view, the simplest situation occurs when an axon is stimulated not with a point source (such as a microelectrode) but rather with a current electrode, like the one Hodgkin and Huxley used for their voltage-clamp apparatus (see Fig. 5.3A). In this way, current is injected uniformly along the entire length of the axon,

Fig. 5.18 Membrane action potentials of squid giant axon. The axon was stimulated by applying current from an electrode over the greater part of the length of the axon, so that the axon's membrane potential changed nearly uniformly throughout its length. **(A)** Recorded voltages for four different strengths of electrical shock. Numbers near each trace give the strength of the shock in nanocoulombs per square centimeter. **(B)** Calculations of Hodgkin-Huxley model for initial depolarizations of 6, 7, 15, and 90 mV. (Traces for **(A)** and **(B)** from fig. 12 of Hodgkin and Huxley, 1952d, with voltage polarity reversed and resting membrane potential assumed to be −65 mV.)

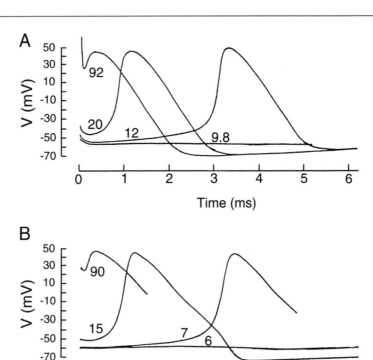

and an action potential is evoked everywhere at once. Hodgkin and Huxley called such action potentials *membrane action potentials.*

Examples of membrane action potentials are given in Fig. 5.18A. The changes in membrane potential are shown for a series of brief current injections, whose amplitude is labeled in the diagram in units of injected charge (nanocoulombs per square centimeter of membrane). As the strength of the injection was increased, the depolarization of the axon increased until the membrane potential exceeded a threshold voltage of about 8 mV positive of rest. For voltages above threshold, the current inward through the Na^+ channels exceeded the current through the leakage conductance, so that a net inward current entered the axon. The net increase in charge entering the cell produced a further depolarization, and the Na^+ current became regenerative. The axon gave an action potential whose amplitude did not change as the current was increased further, though the *latency* or time of onset of the action potential did change, since larger stimuli produced a more rapid initial depolarization and a faster activation of g_{Na}.

If the Na$^+$ and K$^+$ conductances Hodgkin and Huxley described in their voltage-clamp experiments are responsible for producing the action potentials, it should be possible to use the equations of the model to reconstruct this regenerative behavior. The membrane current of the axon is given by the sum of the currents through each of the conductances,

$$i_l = g_l(V_m - E_l), \quad i_{Na} = \overline{g_{Na}}\, m^3 h(V_m - E_{Na}),$$
$$i_K = \overline{g_K}\, n^4 (V_m - E_K) \tag{22}$$

and the total membrane current is:

$$i_m = C_m \frac{dV_m}{dt} + g_l(V_m - E_l) + \overline{g_{Na}}\, m^3 h(V_m - E_{Na})$$
$$+ \overline{g_K}\, n^4 (V_m - E_K) \tag{23}$$

Since all of the terms in this equation are either constants or known functions of time and voltage, it should be possible to solve this equation iteratively with the expressions for *n*, *m*, and *h*, and we can do this now on a computer of even moderate performance, such as a PC. Of course, Hodgkin and Huxley did not have a PC but would nevertheless not have had tremendous difficulty had not Cambridge University closed down its computing facility for modification just as Hodgkin and Huxley set to work. In the event, Huxley did the computations on a hand calculator. The results are shown in Fig. 5.18B for a brief current pulse injected at $t = 0$ into an axon at the resting membrane potential, with resting values of the τ's and n_∞, m_∞, and h_∞. The threshold is a bit lower than for the actual axon (6 mV positive of rest), but the agreement is otherwise rather good.

Action Potentials Propagate

In addition to being regenerative and all-or-none, action potentials move down the axon with no loss in amplitude at speeds of several tens of meters a second. They do so because the charge entering the axon through Na⁺ channels depolarizes not only the membrane directly adjacent to the open channels but also spreads down the axon to depolarize adjacent patches of membrane. In Chapter 2 I derived the equations that describe the spread of voltage down a cable, and these same equations can also be used to describe the propagation of the action potential. This is done by substituting Eqn. (25) of Chapter 2,

$$i_m = \frac{1}{r_a} \frac{\partial^2 V_m}{\partial x^2}$$

in Eqn. (23) of the present chapter, to give

$$\frac{1}{r_a} \frac{\partial^2 V_m}{\partial x^2} = C_m \frac{dV_m}{dt} + g_l(V_m - E_l) + \overline{g_{Na}} m^3 h(V_m - E_{Na})$$
$$+ \overline{g_K} n^4 (V_m - E_K) \tag{24}$$

Eqn. (24) is a second-order differential equation in two variables, which cannot be solved easily even on a fairly powerful computer. Hodgkin and Huxley simplified this equation by assuming that for an action potential propagating at constant velocity down the axon, the curve giving voltage as a function of time at any particular distance should have the same shape as the curve giving voltage as a function of distance at any particular time. The two curves should be linearly related to one another with a proportionality constant equal to the velocity of conduction. The derivative with respect to distance on the left side of Eqn. (24) can then be substituted with a derivative with respect to time, giving a second-order differential equation in only a single variable. This equation is still somewhat tedious to solve, since the conduction velocity is unknown, and wrong guesses cause V_m to explode to $\pm\infty$. It took Huxley (who actually manned the hand calculator) three weeks of work to get the solution (Hodgkin, 1976).

The solution, once obtained, again agrees very well with the form of the propagated action potential recorded experimentally. Figure 5.19 shows the voltage waveform as a function of time at

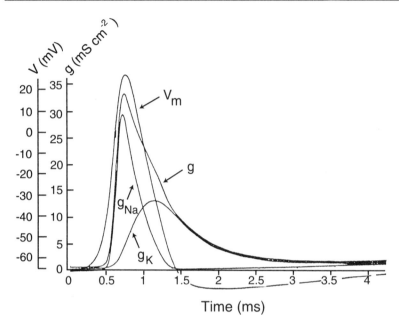

Fig. 5.19 Numerical solution of Hodgkin-Huxley equations for propagated action potential. Traces show separately the predictions for membrane potential V_m, total conductance g, sodium conductance g_{Na}, and potassium conductance g_K. (From fig. 17 of Hodgkin and Huxley, 1952d, with voltage polarity reversed and resting membrane potential assumed to be -65 mV.)

Time (ms)

one position along the axon, but this is also the mirror image of the waveform as a function of distance at any particular time. The calculated action potential (labeled V_m) should be compared with the recorded action potential in Fig. 5.1B.

The time dependence of the total membrane conductance (g) as well as of g_{Na} and g_K are also given in Fig. 5.19. Notice that g_{Na} begins to decay even before the voltage begins to decline from its maximum value, at the peak of the spike. The reason for this is the Na$^+$ channels begin to inactivate but are still open in sufficient number to bring V_m near to E_{Na}. During the decline of g_{Na}, there is a substantial activation of K$^+$ channels. The exit of K$^+$ from the axon produces a hyperpolarization of membrane potential, which actually causes V_m to dip below the resting membrane potential, producing the after-hyperpolarization.

Summary

The experiments of Hodgkin and Huxley, in which crucial discoveries of cellular neuroscience were made, represent one of the most impressive intellectual achievements of the twentieth century.

Hodgkin and Huxley demonstrated that the action potential could be satisfactorily understood in terms of only two quantities, the Na^+ and K^+ conductances, which they quantitatively described as functions of time and voltage. These discoveries are responsible for much of our present understanding of how voltage-gated channels work: Hodgkin and Huxley postulated gating, demonstrated its voltage dependence, discovered inactivation, and predicted the discovery of gating currents and separate Na^+ and K^+ channel proteins.

This chapter was chiefly devoted to describing these seminal investigations, beginning with a brief description of the action potential. Since the changes in conductance that produce action potentials are functions of both time and voltage, a novel technique was required to study them: the voltage clamp. This technique can be used to measure the membrane current of a cell at a fixed command voltage, and Hodgkin and Huxley used it to record the currents responsible for the generation of the action potential. They postulated that the complicated waveform of the current produced by positive voltage steps was caused by two separate current pathways, one permeable mostly to Na^+ and the other to K^+. From their studies of the voltage and time dependence of the currents came measurements of instantaneous i-V curves and Na^+ current inactivation. Hodgkin and Huxley also used their observations to model the Na^+ and K^+ currents, on which they based their reconstruction of the action potential. The experiments of Hodgkin and Huxley are a landmark in the history of neuroscience and, together with the experiments of Katz and Miledi on synaptic transmission, they initiated the modern era of cellular neurophysiology.

6

The Structure and Function of Voltage-Gated Channels

THE HODGKIN-HUXLEY model was intended to be a quantitative description of the voltage and time dependence of the Na^+ and K^+ conductances. Although Hodgkin and Huxley did not intend for their model to provide any insight into the molecular details of gating, subsequent research has shown that many of their assumptions and conclusions are substantially correct. There is good evidence that Na^+ and K^+ pass through separate channels with different ion selectivity, pharmacology, and structure. Na^+ and K^+ channel genes have been isolated, cloned, and sequenced, and they clearly represent different families of genes coding for distinct though related proteins.

Hodgkin and Huxley suggested that the voltage gating of Na^+ and K^+ channels is caused by the movement of charged groups within the plane of the membrane, and there is now good evidence that this is true. Activation is not, however, caused by the movement of "particles" but rather by voltage-dependent changes in the conformation of the channel proteins. The number of the n or m particles in the Hodgkin and Huxley formulation was assumed to be 4 for the K^+ currents and 3 for the Na^+ currents, since the rising phases of the currents could be best fit with expressions that included the terms n^4 and m^3. Hodgkin and Huxley did not themselves attribute any actual physical meaning to these exponents, and we now know that this conservatism on their part was appropriate: the exponents turn out to be functions of membrane potential. As the holding potential preceding the activating pulse is made increasingly more negative, both Na^+ and K^+ currents become increasingly delayed; as a result, the power of the exponents must be increased to get an adequate fit to the rising phase of the conductance change (see Fig. 6.1). For the K^+ conductance, at very large

Fig. 6.1 Effect of previous hyperpolarization on the time course of the squid axon voltage-gated potassium conductance: the Cole-Moore shift. Superposition of two current traces recorded under voltage clamp from the giant axon of the squid *Loligo pealii*. Membrane potential was held for 10 ms at either −75 mV or −175 mV and then depolarized to +5 mV. The more negative holding potential *(V_H)* produced a marked slowing of the onset of i_K. (From Cole and Moore, 1960, reprinted with the permission of J. W. Moore and of the Biophysical Society.)

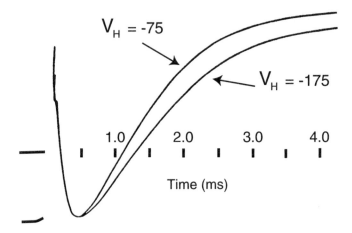

hyperpolarizing potentials the exponent must be made as large as 25 to get an adequate fit (Cole and Moore, 1960).

The explanation for this effect (often referred to as the *Cole-Moore shift*) is unlikely to be a change in the *number* of n or m particles. Suppose, however, that gating is a progression of the channel protein through a series of conformational states,

$$C_1 \rightarrow C_2 \rightarrow C_3 \rightarrow C_4 \rightarrow C_5 \rightarrow O \tag{1}$$

where each C_i is a state for which the pore of the channel is closed and O is the state for which the pore of the channel is open. It is easy to imagine that increasing membrane negativity drives the protein into conformational states like C_1 and C_2, which are further removed from the state that causes opening. With the protein in these "early" states, there is a longer delay in the time required for the channel to pass through the progression of conformational states required for opening.

It may very well be that the basic approach Hodgkin and Huxley used in their model has outlived its usefulness. Alternative models have been shown also to fit voltage-clamp current recordings and to give a better fit to newer measurements of Na^+ channel function—for example, to single-channel recordings. One area of interest, for example, has been the relationship between activation and inactivation. Hodgkin and Huxley assumed that these were separate processes, controlled by different gates (the m and h gates). There is excellent evidence that their assumption is true, as we shall see. On the other hand, in order to simplify their computations, Hodgkin and Huxley assumed that the m and h gates open and close independently of one another. This does *not* seem to be the case. Inactivation occurs with a lag not predicted by the Hodgkin and Huxley model, suggesting that at least a part of the inactivation process cannot occur until activation has taken place. It is now thought that the inactivation gate itself is only weakly voltage-dependent, and that the voltage dependence of the h_∞ curve is due largely to the voltage dependence of activation coupled to inactivation.

In this chapter and the following one, I give some of the experimental results that have led to our present understanding of the structure and function of voltage-gated channels. First I describe basic mechanisms of pore formation, activation, and inactivation. In many respects, these appear to be similar for the Na^+ and K^+ channel families. In the following chapter, I look at voltage-gated channels from another perspective, that of the diversity in their structure and function.

Structure of Na^+ and K^+ Channels

As I described in Chapter 1, the major structural component of Na^+ channels (called the α subunit) was first isolated biochemically in the early 1970s as a protein, about 260 kDa in molecular weight, that bound to the Na^+ channel blocker tetrodotoxin (see Catterall, 1992). Partial primary sequences of this protein were then used to isolate a cDNA clone for the α subunit, first from eel electroplax by Numa and his collaborators (Noda et al., 1984), and later by many other workers in a variety of species (see Catterall, 1992; Kallen, Cohen, and Barchi, 1994; Goldin, 1995). In addition to the α subunit, the assembled channel is thought to contain accessory proteins, called β subunits (see Fig. 6.2A), 30–40 kDa in molecular weight.

Voltage-gated K^+ channels were first isolated entirely by molecular techniques from the fruit fly *Drosophila* (see for example Papazian et al., 1987; Tempel et al., 1987). The methods that were used to clone the first K^+ channel gene (called *Shaker*) are described

Box 6.1

CLONING OF *SHAKER* K⁺ CHANNEL GENE

The diagram to the right presents a simplified description of the genetic methods used to clone the K^+ channel gene *Shaker* from *Drosophila* (Papazian et al., 1987). Mutations in the gene were isolated so they could be used as markers (mutant animals shake their legs during ether anesthesia). The locus of the gene was determined by a combination of classical genetic methods for determining linkage from the frequency of recombination and examination of the giant salivary gland chromosomes of certain classes of mutants in which the genetic lesion was associated with an inversion or translocation of a segment of the chromosome. Mutants were screened and a strain selected in which the mutation was caused by a breakpoint somewhere within the locus of the gene. In the diagram, an inversion of a segment of DNA within a chromosome is depicted, but for *Shaker* the actual mutations that were most helpful were translocations between the X chromosome and other chromosomes. A previously isolated cDNA clone, which had been shown to hybridize to salivary gland chromosomes in the vicinity of the gene of interest, was used to screen a genomic DNA library to find additional clones of DNA fragments in the vicinity of the gene, as if one were following a trail of probes, or taking a "walk" along the chromosome. Each of the overlapping clones was then restriction-mapped so that their order and relative position within the chromosome could be deduced. Probes that bound to both ends of a breakpoint mutation were selected as likely to contain the gene, and these and other overlapping genomic clones were used to isolate cDNA clones, which in turn were sequenced to identify the DNA for the putative protein (Modified from Watson et al., 1992; Papazian et al., 1987.)

in Box 6.1. A large number of K⁺-channel clones have now been isolated from *Drosophila* as well as from amphibians and mammals (see Jan and Jan, 1992, 1994, 1997; Pongs, 1992, 1993; Hoshi and Zagotta, 1993; Chandy and Gutman, 1995). The major component of K⁺ channels (the α subunit) is approximately one-quarter the size of the α subunit of the Na⁺ channel (Fig. 6.2B). β

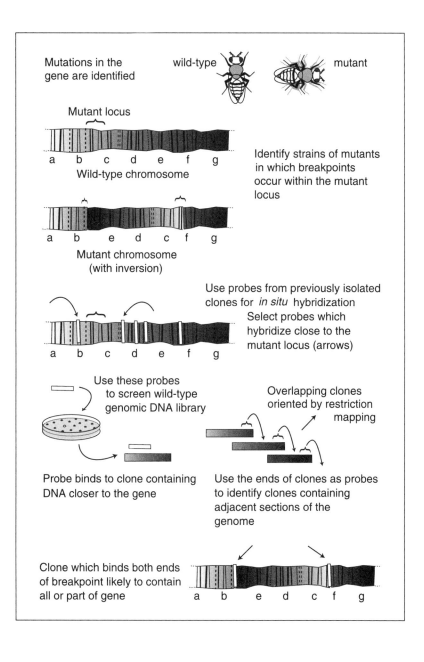

Mutations in the gene are identified

wild-type   mutant

Mutant locus

a b c d e f g

Wild-type chromosome

Identify strains of mutants in which breakpoints occur within the mutant locus

a b e d c f g

Mutant chromosome (with inversion)

Use probes from previously isolated clones for *in situ* hybridization
Select probes which hybridize close to the mutant locus (arrows)

a b c d e f g

Use these probes to screen wild-type genomic DNA library

Overlapping clones oriented by restriction mapping

Probe binds to clone containing DNA closer to the gene

Use the ends of clones as probes to identify clones containing adjacent sections of the genome

Clone which binds both ends of breakpoint likely to contain all or part of gene

a b e d c f g

subunits have also been isolated for K$^+$ channels (see for example Rettig et al., 1994; Isom, DeJongh, and Catterall, 1994).

The α Subunits

The α subunit of Na$^+$ channels is known to contain the binding site for TTX, the selectivity filter, the channel pore, and the structural elements responsible for activation and inactivation. A similar statement can be made for K$^+$ channels: the α subunit contains the binding site or sites for TEA$^+$, the selectivity filter and pore, and the structural elements responsible for activation. As we shall see, some voltage-gated K$^+$ channels show inactivation similar to that first described by Hodgkin and Huxley for Na$^+$ channels, and this property is also determined by the α subunit.

The α subunit of a Na$^+$ channel has four main groupings, called *repeat units,* labeled I–IV in Fig. 6.2A and shown schematically in Fig. 1.7A. These repeat units are 40–60 percent homologous in amino acid composition and appear to be related to one another; perhaps they arise from a common ancestor by gene duplication (Hille, 1989). Hydropathy analysis of the amino acid sequence (see Chapter 1) suggests that each repeat unit has 6 domains, approximately 20 amino acids in length, that are sufficiently hydrophobic to lie within the plane of the membrane. Five of these are quite hydrophobic, but one (S4) is unique in structure, containing mostly hydrophobic residues but also charged residues located every third amino acid. These charged residues are likely to be important in voltage-dependent gating (I shall return to the structure of the S4 domain later in the chapter). The Na$^+$ channel α subunit has several sites for phosphorylation by either cAMP-dependent protein kinase or protein kinase C (see Chapters 12–13), which suggest that these regions of the protein may be intracellular.

The K$^+$ channel α subunit (Fig. 6.2B) resembles one of the four repeat units of the Na$^+$ channel, and this and other evidence (for example MacKinnon, 1991) suggests that K$^+$ channels are composed of four α subunits assembled noncovalently around a central conductance pore (see Fig. 1.7A and Chandy and Gutman, 1995). Hydropathy analysis again suggests that each α subunit has 6 putative transmembrane sequences, and S4 has this same peculiar structure with charged residues located every third amino acid (Fig.

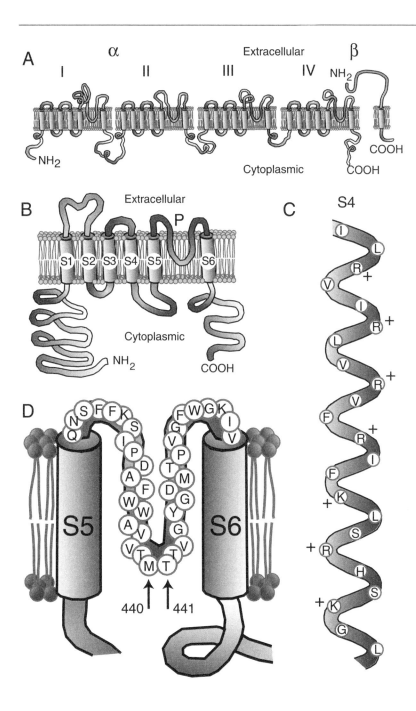

Fig. 6.2 Hypothesized membrane topology of Na$^+$ and K$^+$ channel proteins. **(A)** Voltage-gated Na$^+$ channel. Main α subunit composed of four repeat domains labeled *I–IV*. Amino and carboxyl termini both intracellular. Auxiliary β subunit is hypothesized to have only a single transmembrane domain. **(B)** Voltage-gated K$^+$ channel. Only α subunit is shown. Amino and carboxyl termini both intracellular. Transmembrane domains labelled *S1–S6*. *P,* pore-forming domain. (Parts **(A)** and **(B)** after Isom, DeJongh, and Catterall, 1994.) **(C)** S4 domain expressed by *Shaker* gene, drawn as an alpha helix with amino acids indicated by single-letter code (e.g., *R* = arginine, *K* = lysine; see Stryer, 1995). Seven charged amino acids (indicated by plus signs) are present in every third position of the helix. (Alpha helix after Styer, 1995, sequence for *Shaker* from Tempel et al., 1987.) **(D)** P domain of *Shaker* potassium channel. Individual amino acids in sequence are indicated with single-letter code (see Stryer, 1995). Positions of amino acids 440 (methionine) and 441 (threonine) are indicated. (After Brown, 1993, with sequence for *Shaker* from Tempel et al., 1987).

6.2C). The amino and carboxyl termini of the protein are both likely to be intracellular, as is the region linking S4 and S5, which contains a site for phosphorylation by protein kinase C. In the region linking S1 and S2, two sites can become glycosylated (affixed with sugar), and this part of the protein is therefore probably extracellular. The S5 and S6 linker region contains a sequence known as the *P domain* (also called *H5* or the *SS1–SS2 region*—see Fig. 6.2D), which as we shall see, is the major structural component of the pore of the channel. A similar sequence between S5 and S6 is also present in each of the repeat units of the Na^+ channel.

The β Subunits

The role of the β subunits is not completely understood, but there is evidence for both channel types that β subunits can influence the physiology of the channel, as well as its expression and stability (Isom, DeJongh, and Catterall, 1994; Adelman, 1995). Possible functions for β subunits have been examined by expressing nucleic acid sequences for the α subunits (which are largely responsible for producing the Na^+ or K^+ current) with or without sequences for the β subunits. In some cases, co-expression of the β subunits seems to have little or no effect on currents produced by the α subunits, but in other cases β subunits dramatically alter the voltage dependence or time course of activation or inactivation. For rat Na^+ channel genes, for example, expression of the α subunit alone is sufficient to produce a voltage-gated Na^+ channel, but inactivation is much slower than for neurons *in situ* and is shifted to more positive membrane potentials. If, however, the α subunit gene is expressed together with a β subunit gene, more physiological behavior is observed. Even more dramatic effects have been seen with K^+ channels, for which co-expression of a β subunit gene can accelerate the rate of inactivation for some α subunit K^+ channels by more than 100-fold (Rettig et al., 1994).

Although the contribution of β subunits is of undoubted importance for the physiology of Na^+ and K^+ channels, I devote the remainder of this chapter to exploring the structure and function of the major structural subunits, the α subunits. I begin by asking what part of the protein forms the ion pore, and I then review what is known about the mechanism of channel activation and inactivation. I return to the function of the β subunits in Chapter 7.

The Channel Pore

The α subunit of a Na^+ channel has 1700–2000 amino acids and is a large and complicated molecule. K^+ channel α subunits are considerably smaller but still seem bewildering in their complexity. In spite of the apparent difficulties, the techniques of molecular biology and single-cell recording have made it possible to identify with some confidence certain regions of these proteins, which appear to be mostly responsible for some functions of channel physiology. These experiments have proceeded in the following way. Beginning with the gene for a channel, many groups of investigators have made single-site mutations or have deleted or exchanged parts of the channel gene. The gene is then expressed, often in *Xenopus* oocytes or in a mammalian cell line (Fig. 1.6), and whole-cell or single-channel recordings are made in an attempt to discover alterations in some aspect of channel physiology. Many mutations are unhelpful: the protein either doesn't express functional channels or expresses channels with no detectable change in their properties. Some mutations, on the other hand, produce remarkably specific effects that have made possible the correlation of certain parts of the protein with distinct functions.

Before I begin to describe experiments that have helped to identify the location of the channel pore, it is perhaps useful to ask what sort of change in channel physiology one would expect to result from a mutation in the pore region. One possibility is a change in the conductance of the open channel. One could imagine, for example, that the substitution of a certain amino acid by a larger amino acid could partially occlude the pore, reducing the pore current. On the other hand, one could equally imagine a substitution of an amino acid virtually anywhere in the protein changing the conformation sufficiently to change the pore conductance. What about an amino acid substitution that caused a change in ion selectivity? This would seem a much better indication of the location of the pore, though it is again still possible to imagine that a generalized change in conformation could alter the position of a charged amino acid in the vicinity of the pore sufficiently to change selectivity.

Perhaps the best indication would be the identification of an amino acid at a binding site for a toxin, particularly a toxin like TTX or TEA, both of which are thought to occlude the channel pore. Although again it is possible to imagine a generalized change in conformation that affects toxin binding, one would expect the change in binding affinity to be rather small for such a global change in conformation. If, however, an amino acid were substituted *at the binding site* of the toxin to the channel, much larger changes in binding affinity could occur. It might be useful, therefore, to begin with experiments in which mutations in amino acid sequence resulted in changes in the effectiveness of toxin block, and this is exactly where work did begin to localize the pore.

TTX and STX

Some of the first evidence for the location of the pore came from studies of TTX and STX sensitivity. Recall that these toxins bind with high affinity to Na^+ channels and cause a virtually complete and selective block of the Na^+ current (see Fig. 5.9). Since both of these toxins are charged and polar, they are unlikely to be membrane-permeant and must therefore bind to an external site on the channel protein. Noda and collaborators (Noda et al., 1989) reasoned that since TTX and STX are both positively charged, they might be attracted to an amino acid with a negative charge, like glutamate or aspartate, in the vicinity of the part of the molecule thought to form the pore.

Noda and collaborators therefore made site-directed mutations of a single negatively charged glutamate to the neutral amino acid glutamine in the S5–S6 linker region of repeat I of the Na^+ channel α subunit. The method they used for making the mutations required the synthesis of a primer oligonucleotide with the normal nucleotide sequence except at the location to be mutated (see Watson et al., 1992). The primer oligonucleotide was annealed to a complementary strand of the wild-type DNA, which was then used as a template for the synthesis of the rest of the mutated gene. RNA for normal and mutated Na^+ channel α subunits was injected into *Xenopus* oocytes and recorded with a two-electrode voltage clamp. The substitution of glutamate with a neutral amino acid virtually eliminated the sensitivity of the Na^+ channel to both TTX and STX (Fig. 6.3). Mutations of negatively charged residues at similar positions in the other three repeat domains of the Na^+ channel α subunit had similar effects (Terlau et al., 1991; Kontis and Goldin,

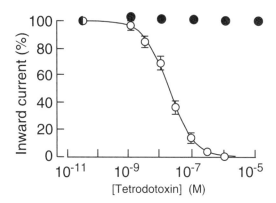

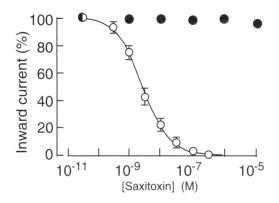

Fig. 6.3 A single point mutation dramatically reduces block of rat Na^+ channels by tetrodotoxin (TTX) and saxitoxin (STX). The negatively charged glutamate 387 was replaced with neutral glutamine (E387Q) in the amino acid sequence of rat sodium channel II (rNaB2). This residue is between S5 and S6 within the pore domain of repeat I. RNAs specific for wild-type and mutant channels were expressed in *Xenopus* oocytes, and whole-cell currents were measured with a two-electrode voltage clamp. Data points show means ± S.D.s (if larger than symbol sizes) for inward currents in the presence of toxins at the indicated concentrations, expressed as a percentage of currents in absence of toxins, for wild-type channels (O) and for mutant E387Q channels (●). (Reprinted from Noda et al., 1989, with the permission of the authors.)

1993). The mutation of other, nearby residues can also affect TTX binding (Satin et al., 1992), indicating that the binding site is likely to consist of several amino acids within the S5–S6 linker.

TEA

Some of the most interesting experiments identifying the pore region of K^+ channel α subunits have been done with site-directed mutations that affect blocking by TEA^+. In Chapter 5, I described the effect of external TEA on K^+ channels (see Fig. 5.9). This block could be altered by site-directed mutations of amino acids lining the P domain in the *Shaker* K^+ channel—for example, at aspartate *(D)* 431 and threonine *(T)* 449 (see Fig. 6.2D and MacKinnon and

Yellen, 1990). Two rat K$^+$ α subunit genes, *Kv1.1* and *Kv1.2,* produce proteins that greatly differ in their sensitivity to external TEA when they are expressed in *Xenopus* oocytes, with Kv1.1 quite sensitive and Kv1.2 almost not at all. This difference seems to be the result of a single amino acid in the S5–S6 linking region, which is tyrosine in Kv1.1 and valine in Kv1.2. Mutation of this amino acid from valine to tyrosine in Kv1.2 produces a protein with an increased TEA sensitivity, similar to the sensitivity of Kv1.1; mutation of tyrosine to valine in Kv1.1 dramatically decreases the TEA sensitivity, nearly to that of Kv1.2 (Kavanaugh et al., 1991).

Perhaps of even greater interest are mutations affecting the block of *internal* TEA and other quaternary ammonium ions (QA). Most voltage-gated K$^+$ channels can be blocked when TEA or QA are placed inside the cell. The binding site is not the same as that for external blocking, and the internal block has some interesting properties (see Armstrong, 1975). For example, blocking can occur only *after* the channel has opened, suggesting that TEA from the internal solution actually enters and occludes the mouth of the open channel. Furthermore, the block can be relieved by high concentrations of external K$^+$, especially at membrane potentials that favor the movement of K$^+$ from outside the channel to the inside. This phenomenon is called *knock-off*: the K$^+$ entering the channel from the outside electrostatically repulses the TEA or QA, knocking the blocking ion off its binding site. It is difficult to imagine how this could occur unless TEA$^+$ and QA$^+$ were actually binding to the pore of the channel.

Two sites in the very middle of the P domain, in the *Shaker* K$^+$ channel's methionine 440 (Choi et al., 1993) and threonine 441 (Yellen et al., 1991), seem to be mainly responsible for TEA$^+$ binding (see Fig. 6.2D). Mutation of either of these sites can reduce the sensitivity of blocking by internal TEA by 10–50-fold, but it has no effect on the sensitivity of blocking by external TEA. Since internal TEA appears to block by entering the channel pore, these two amino acids would seem to be located at a part of the P domain that dips rather deeply into the membrane.

P-domain Exchange

One of the most convincing demonstrations that the P domain forms the channel pore (at least for K$^+$ channels) is the discovery by

Hartmann, Kirsch, Drewe et al. (1991) that exchange of the P domain between two closely related K^+ channels swaps both the amplitude of the single channel conductance and the sensitivity to block by TEA. In these experiments, two K^+ channel α subunit genes, both isolated from rodents, were used to express channel molecules with different properties. The *Kv3.1* gene produces a channel with a single-channel conductance of about 22 pS, which is quite sensitive to block by external TEA but rather insensitive to block by internal TEA. The other, *Kv2.1*, produces a channel with a smaller single-channel conductance—about 8 pS—and is less sensitive than the *Kv3.1* gene product to external TEA but more sensitive to internal TEA.

Hartmann et al. (1991) took most of the S5–S6 linker region from *Kv3.1* and genetically inserted it into the *Kv2.1* gene in place of the *Kv2.1* S5–S6 linker (Fig. 6.4A). This produced a *chimeric* (composite) channel that had most of the properties of Kv3.1: the single-channel conductance was increased nearly to 22 pS (Fig. 6.4B), the sensitivity to external TEA was greatly increased, and the sensitivity to internal TEA was greatly decreased (Fig. 6.4C). Notice that the sensitivity to external TEA is not quite as high in the chimera as in Kv3.1. This may be because sites on the exterior surface of the protein, outside the P domain, also contribute to TEA binding.

Although the experiments of Hartmann et al. provide strong evidence that the P domain forms part of the pore, it is possible that other parts of the channel structure also contribute to permeation (see Kukuljan, Labarca, and Latorre, 1995). It seems likely that the P domain interacts with other parts of the protein, such as the cytoplasmic S4–S5 loop, (Slesinger, Jan, and Jan, 1993) and S6 (Lopez, Jan, and Jan, 1994) to form the actual structure through which ions move when the channel opens.

Activation

One of the most interesting observations Hodgkin and Huxley made was that both g_{Na} and g_K show a remarkably steep dependence of gating on membrane potential: g_{Na} is increased by a factor of e (2.72) by a change in V_m of only 4 mV. This means that the conformational changes that produce channel opening must be exquisitely sensitive to the electric field across the membrane. As this

Fig. 6.4 The P domain confers most of the properties of channel conductance for voltage-gated K[+] channels. Genes for P domains were swapped between mouse *Kv3.1* and rat *Kv2.1* α subunit genes, and mutant and normal channels were then expressed in *Xenopus* oocytes. **(A)** Schematic drawings of Kv2.1, Kv3.1, and chimera. **(B)** *Left:* Representative single-channel currents for three channel types. *Right:* Plots of single-channel current amplitude as a function of membrane voltage for the three channel types. Slopes give single-channel conductances. **(C)** Block of whole-cell currents by TEA. Currents were recorded with a two-electrode voltage clamp. Intracellular TEA was injected into the oocyte from the voltage electrode by application of pneumatic pressure. (After Hartmann et al., 1991.)

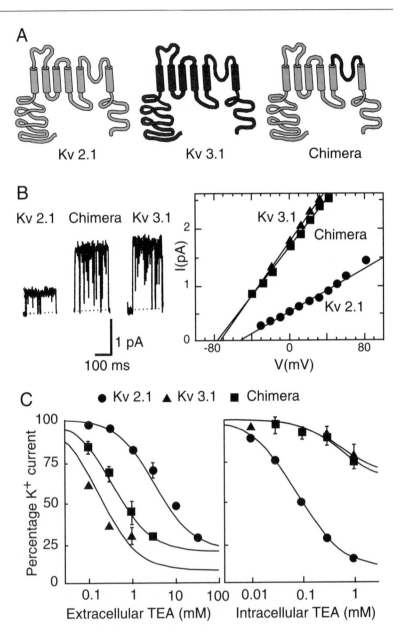

field changes during depolarization, parts of the channel protein must somehow move in response to the change in field, to produce the change in conformation that opens the pore.

Hodgkin and Huxley suggested that the steep dependence of conductance on voltage could be explained if gating were controlled by the movement of charge. This charge would have to be somehow associated with the channel protein itself (e.g., as charged amino acids), so that as the membrane potential changed, the charge would respond by moving across the electric field of the membrane. From the steepness of the voltage dependence of channel opening, Hodgkin and Huxley estimated that at least 6 charges would have to move across the electric field during the opening of a single Na^+ channel. Since gating is the result of membrane depolarization, positive charge would have to move outward or negative charge inward to produce opening.

Gating Currents

If charges actually move as the channels open, then it should be possible to observe the movement as a membrane current. This current would represent a redistribution of charge from one side of the membrane to the other and so would have the characteristics of a capacitive or *displacement* current, but it would have characteristics quite different from the displacement currents described in Chapter 2. There we saw that any change in voltage across the membrane produces a current whose value is given by

$$i = C \frac{dV}{dt} \qquad (2)$$

Provided the capacitance of the lipid bilayer is constant and independent of voltage, this current should be linear and equal in amplitude (though opposite in sign) for positive and negative voltage steps. A displacement current produced by channel gating, on the other hand, should be dramatically asymmetric, since channel gating is voltage-dependent and only depolarizations cause channel opening. Hodgkin and Huxley looked for such an asymmetric displacement current but were unable to see it, probably because (with the techniques available to them) the "gating current" was too small to observe against the background of the linear capacitive current of the membrane and the Na^+ and K^+ ionic currents.

Gating currents were first observed for Na^+ channels in the squid giant axon approximately twenty years after Hodgkin and Huxley's papers were published (Armstrong and Bezanilla, 1973, 1974; Keynes and Rojas, 1974). These currents, though small, were eventually detected as a result of several discoveries and advances in recording techniques. In the first place, the blocking effects of TTX and TEA were discovered. This made it possible to block the large ionic currents that previously obscured the gating currents. Second, techniques were developed for internally perfusing the squid axon, so that the cytoplasm could be replaced almost at will with an artificial solution (Tasaki, Watanabe, and Takenaka, 1962; Baker, Hodgkin, and Shaw, 1962). This made it possible, for example, to remove the K^+ from the internal solution (and the Na^+ from the external solution) as a further means of reducing the ionic currents. Finally, equally important was the development of signal averagers and small laboratory computers fast enough to record the brief displacement currents produced by voltage steps; these were either built by the investigators (Armstrong and Bezanilla, 1973) or cheap enough to be purchased by a single laboratory. These devices made it possible to record currents induced by voltage steps equal in amplitude but opposite in sign, and to *add these currents together*. The linear component of capacitive current disappears with this procedure, revealing the asymmetric component of capacitive current produced by the movement of gating charge.

Fig. 6.5 illustrates the gating current recorded at the onset of a voltage pulse from a squid giant axon and compares this current to the ionic current (Armstrong and Bezanilla, 1973). The gating current was measured in artificial sea water for which all of the Na^+ had been replaced by the largely impermeant cation $Tris^+$ (tris(hydroxymethyl)aminomethane); TTX was also added to the sea water to block any residual Na^+ conductance. The K^+ inside the axon was replaced with Cs^+, which is nearly impermeant and also actually blocks most K^+ channels (Latorre and Miller, 1983). The response of the axon was then measured from a holding potential of -70 mV, first for 2000 pulses $+70$ mV in amplitude (from

$V_m = -70$ mV to 0 mV), and then for 2000 pulses -70 mV in amplitude (from -70 mV to -140 mV). The responses to positive and negative pulses were summed to eliminate the linear component of capacitive current, and the result was averaged to reveal the gating current (Fig. 6.5A). The ionic current in Fig 6.5B is for a single $+70$ mV voltage pulse from a holding potential of -70 mV, from the same axon as in Fig. 6.5A but externally perfused with normal sea water and internally perfused with K^+. Notice that the ionic current is about 300 times larger in amplitude than the gating current.

Some of the most interesting experiments on gating currents have been done with K^+ channels expressed in *Xenopus* oocytes, either by recording from isolated excised patches of membrane or by recording the much larger currents of the whole oocyte with the so-called *cut-open voltage-clamp technique* (see Box 6.2). Fig. 6.6A shows gating currents recorded from an oocyte injected with *Drosophila Shaker* K^+ channel RNA (Bezanilla et al., 1991). Part B of Fig. 6.6 compares the voltage dependence of this gating current with that of the *Shaker* K^+ ionic current. It is significant that considerable charge moves at voltages that produce little or no opening of the channel pore. This reflects charge movement between closed conformations of the channel—say, between C_1 and C_2 or between

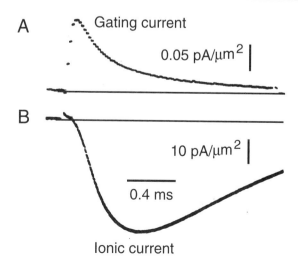

Fig. 6.5 Gating and ionic currents of Na^+ channels recorded from the same squid giant axon. Axon was internally dialyzed and perfused with artificial sea water. **(A)** Gating current. Na^+ in sea water was replaced with impermeant $Tris^+$. Internal (dialysis) solution contained 550 mM CsF (replacement of F^- for Cl^- improved the stability of the recording). Current was averaged from algebraically summed responses to steps of voltage from a holding potential of -70 mV to 0 mV and to -140 mV. **(B)** Ionic current. Axon in sea water was internally perfused with 275 mM KF and 400 mM sucrose. Single trace (not averaged). (From Armstrong and Bezanilla, 1973; reprinted with permission of the authors and of Macmillan Magazines Limited.)

Box 6.2

CUT-OPEN XENOPUS OOCYTE VOLTAGE CLAMP

For the cut-open voltage clamp (Bezanilla et al., 1991; Taglialatela, Toro, and Stefani, 1992), a *Xenopus* oocyte is cut open at the bottom and placed in a small plastic chamber. The chamber has three pools that are sealed to the oocyte with vaseline, where the chamber borders and the oocyte meet. The amplifier labeled *1* measures the membrane potential by measuring the difference between the voltage in the *external* pool and the voltage recorded with an intracellular microelectrode. The voltage is measured backwards: the voltage inside the cell is set to ground, and the voltage of the external solution is taken as $-V_m$. The amplifier labeled *2* compares the voltage inside the cell to ground. It then injects a current into the *internal* pool to keep the voltage recorded by the intracellular microelectrode at the ground potential. A third amplifier (*3*) compares the voltage in the external pool with the negative of the command potential (V_c). Remember that voltage is measured backwards, with the inside of the cell set to ground and the outside to $-V_m$. Any difference between $-V_m$ and $-V_c$ causes a current to flow at the output of *3*, which is then injected into the external pool to clamp the membrane potential of the oocyte to the command potential. The value of this current is measured from the voltage change across the resistor (R) placed between the output of amplifier *3* and the external pool. A fourth amplifier (not shown) clamps the *guard* pool to the same potential as the external pool, to prevent current flow through the vaseline seal. The reason this works is that if the potential between the external and guard pools is the same, then there can be no current flow by Ohm's law from one pool to the other. The inside of the oocyte is perfused with a fine tube, called a canula, which can be used to introduce artificial internal perfusates and to change the solution bathing the inside of the cell membrane.

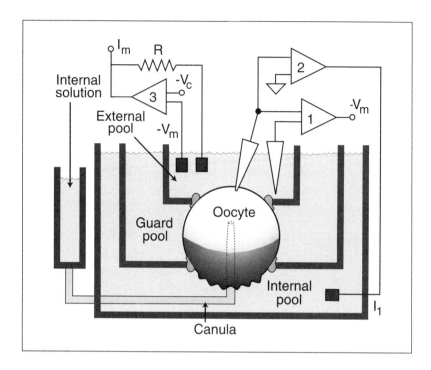

C_2 and C_3 in the scheme described on p. 172—at voltages for which there are few transitions to O.

The measurements of gating currents in Fig. 6.6 were made by replacing Na^+ and K^+ in the internal and external solutions with impermeable ions, virtually eliminating the ionic currents. Essentially identical results have also been obtained from a *Shaker* channel, for which a mutation in the P domain eliminates the conductance of the channel pore (Perozo et al., 1993). In this mutant channel, the gating appears to occur completely normally, even though no ionic current can be recorded.

How Much Charge Moves?

Direct measurement of the gating current should provide an actual value for the number of charges that move during activation. Since current is dq/dt, the gating current can be integrated to calculate the total flow of charge during opening. Once the total charge is known, it is necessary only to know how many channels contribute

Fig. 6.6 Gating currents of *Shaker* K$^+$ channels. *Shaker* cRNA was injected into *Xenopus* oocytes, and currents were recorded with the cut-open voltage-clamp technique (see Box 6.2). **(A)** Gating current recordings for onset of voltage pulse. Na$^+$ in the external solution was substituted with TEA$^+$, and K$^+$ in the internal solution with methylglucamine$^+$. Currents are averages of 10 responses to a series of depolarizing pulses from a holding potential of −80 mV to voltages of −70 mV to +30 mV in steps of 10 mV. Linear component of capacitance subtracted by a method similar in principle to the one used in Fig. 6.5 (see Bezanilla et al., 1991). Only the initial waveform of the current response is shown. (Redrawn from Bezanilla et al., 1991.) **(B)** Comparison of voltage dependence of *Shaker* K$^+$ channel conductance ($G_{(rel)}$, O) and gating charge ($Q_{(rel)}$, ●). Conductance was calculated by dividing the current by the driving force and is given as a fraction of maximal conductance; gating charge was calculated from the integral of the gating current for the duration of the voltage pulse and is also given as a fraction of maximum. Note that gating charge movement can be observed at voltages for which conductance change cannot be detected. (after Bezanilla et al., 1991).

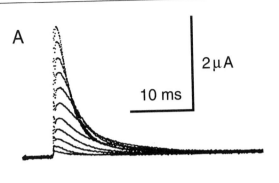

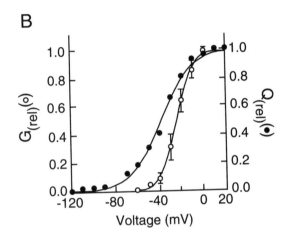

to the gating current in order to calculate the charge that moves per channel.

This problem was approached by Schoppa, McCormack, Tanouye, and Sigworth (1992), using patch recording from *Xenopus* oocytes. *Xenopus* was injected with RNA for *Shaker* K$^+$ channel genes, at a sufficiently high RNA concentration to produce a high density of K$^+$ channels in the membrane; this made it possible to measure gating currents from large excised, inside-out patches (see Fig. 1.4) after TEA was added to the bathing solution to block the ionic currents. Since the patches were inside-out, the TEA block was produced by binding to the internal (cytoplasmic) binding site.

The trick then was to count the channels. This was done by depolarizing the patch and measuring the *variance* of the ionic current. Suppose a patch contains N channels, each with a unitary current of i. If the patch is depolarized to open the channels, then the mean value of the total current I is given by

$$I = Npi \qquad (3)$$

where p is the probability that a channel is open. If each channel opens independently of the others, the distribution of channel openings will be binomial, like the flipping of coins. The variance of the current σ^2 will then be given by

$$\sigma^2 = Ni^2 p(1 - p) \qquad (4)$$

(Neher and Stevens, 1977; Heinemann and Conti, 1992), and if p is eliminated between Eqns. (3) and (4), the variance can be expressed as

$$\sigma^2 = iI - \frac{I^2}{N} \qquad (5)$$

(Sigworth, 1980).

Equation (5) describes a parabola, as demonstrated in Fig. 6.7, where p was varied from 0 to 1 and both σ^2 and I were calculated from Eqns. (3) and (4); σ^2 was then plotted as a function of I. The curve in Fig. 6.7A shows that when the probability of channel opening is low, both σ^2 and I are small since the channel opens rarely. If p is small, then $(1 - p)$ is nearly one, and Eqn. (4) is nearly $\sigma^2 = Ni^2 p$. But since (from Eqn. 3) $p = I/Ni$, for small p we have $\sigma^2 \sim iI$, which means that the variance is nearly linearly proportional to the mean current. Another way of seeing this is to note from Eqn. (5) that $iI \gg I^2/N$ for small I. So if the probability of opening is low, $\sigma^2 \sim iI$, and the variance increases nearly linearly with a slope equal to i, the current of a single channel. This linear region at small p is the initial rising part of the curve in Fig. 6.7A.

As p increases, the variance reaches a maximum value when the probability of opening is exactly one-half. As the probability of opening increases further, the variance of the channel current actu-

Fig. 6.7 Counting charges: estimation of the number of gating charges that move during activation of a single Na^+ channel. **(A)** Graphical solution of Eqn. (5). The variance (σ^2) has been plotted as a function of the mean total current (I) for $0 \leq I \leq iN$ (see Eqn. 3). Calculations are for a membrane containing 100 channels each of unitary current $i = 10$ pA. **(B)** Measurements of variance and mean of current expressed in *Xenopus* oocytes for wild-type *Shaker* K^+ channel truncated near the amino terminus to eliminate voltage-dependent inactivation (see Fig. 6.12). Currents were recorded from large inside-out patches, and mean and variance were calculated as a function of time, as in Sigworth (1980), from 76 responses to the same 160 mV voltage step (from $V_H = -80$ mV to $+80$ mV). Data are from one representative patch and have been fitted with Eqn. (5) for $i = 1.5$ pA and $N = 1500$. **(C)** Charge per channel. Values for N as in **(B)** have been plotted against the maximum value of gating charge (Q_{max}, expressed in femtocoulombs, or 10^{-15} coulomb), determined for the same inside-out patches after K^+ in the bath solution had been replaced by TEA. Gating charge estimated from integral of currents. Solid squares are data points for wild-type *Shaker* channels truncated to remove inactivation. Open symbols are for a mutant of *Shaker* (called *V2*), also truncated but with valine replacing leucine at position 370 in the *Shaker* sequence, near the cytoplasmic end of S4. This single-site mutation alters the voltage dependence of activation of the K^+ currents but does not alter the number of charges that move per channel. The triangle near the origin represents a patch that contained only a single channel. Slope of line represents approximately 12 charges per channel. (Parts **(B)** and **(C)** reprinted from Schoppa et al., 1992, with permission of the authors and the American Association for the Advancement of Science.)

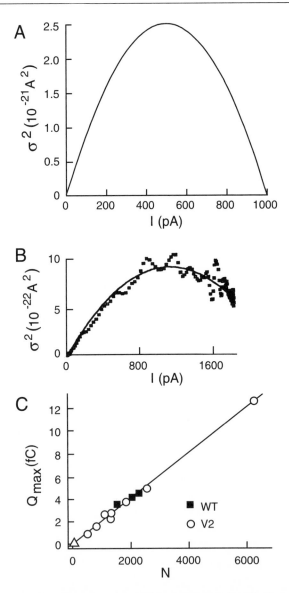

ally decreases, because the channel is open nearly all of the time. In the limit of $p = 1$, the variance is of course zero, because the channel is open continuously and I reaches its maximal value of iN.

From measurements of σ^2 as a function of I, it is possible from the best fit of Eqn. (5) to estimate both i and N. Using this method, Schoppa et al. (1992) estimated the number of channels in the same patches from which they measured the amplitude of the gating currents. They gave a series of depolarizations from a holding potential of -80 mV to zero mV and then calculated for each time point during the voltage step the mean and the variance of the current. This procedure provided a sufficiently large number of data points to produce a curve like the predicted parabola (see Fig. 6.7B). By fitting the data in this figure to Eqn. (5), Schoppa et al. estimated the unitary current to be 1.5 pA and the number of channels in the membrane patch to be about 1500.

Similar measurements from a large number of patches are summarized in Fig. 6.7C, also from Schoppa et al. (1992). The gating charge for a series of different patches is given along the y-axis, plotted as a function of the number of channels estimated to be in each of the patches. The relationship is of course a straight line: the greater the number of channels in the patch, the more the total charge measured from the gating currents. The interesting number is the slope, which gives the number of charges moved per channel. It is about 12–13 elementary charges, twice that estimated by Hodgkin and Huxley. Similar numbers have now been obtained with somewhat different methods both for K^+ (Seoh et al., 1996; Aggarwal and MacKinnon, 1996) and Na^+ channels (Hirschberg et al., 1995), strongly supporting the basic similarity of gating in these two channel types.

Keep in mind that this is 12–13 elementary charges *per channel,* or approximately 3 charges per K^+ channel α subunit (4 of which are required to form a channel), or 3 per Na^+ channel repeat unit. Remember also that the estimate of 12–13 charges from gating current measurements represents 12–13 charges moving *all the way* across the electric field of the membrane, from one side of the membrane dialectric to the other. Gating current measurements cannot distinguish 12–13 charges moving all the way across the electric field from 24–26 charges moving halfway across the field, or 48–52 charges moving one-quarter of the way, and so on.

Which charges move? This would seem on the face of it to be a simple question to ask, and to answer. First look for charged amino acids in the channel structure that are likely to lie within the part of the channel protein that extends through the membrane, and then use the techniques of molecular biology to change these amino acids to other amino acids that are uncharged or oppositely charged. Now ask whether these alterations change gating.

Many of the charged amino acids thought to lie within membrane-spanning domains in Na^+ and K^+ channel α subunits lie within the S4 domain. As already mentioned, the S4 domain has a peculiar structure, consisting mostly of hydrophobic amino acids but with (in most cases) a positively charged lysine or arginine as every third residue (see Fig. 6.2C). If S4 has the geometry of an α helix (often assumed but not really known for certain), the positively charged amino acids would form a gentle spiral through the width of the membrane.

The unusual sequence of S4 has made its positively charged amino acids inevitable candidates for a role in activation, and initial experiments seemed to support this notion (Stühmer et al., 1989). Site-directed mutation of S4 residues of Na^+ channels substituting a charged residue with an uncharged or oppositely charged residue dramatically alter the voltage dependence of gating. When several charged S4 amino acids are altered, the degree of voltage dependence of activation seems to be inversely proportional to the amount of charge removed, as if the S4 helix were moving *en masse* across the membrane (see Fig. 6.8A).

Unfortunately, this simple notion, so appealing when first described, has not been borne out by further experimentation. Similar work on K^+ channels (Papazian et al., 1991) indicated that mutations of some of the S4 residues produced much larger effects than mutations at other points. Furthermore, some changes in the voltage dependence of activation could be produced by amino acid substitutions that replaced one basic amino acid with another basic amino acid—i.e., with no change in the amount of charge of the protein. Other laboratories demonstrated that changes in *uncharged* residues in S4 and in other domains of the channel protein (including the P domain) can also affect the voltage dependence of channel opening (for summaries see Stühmer, 1991; Sigworth, 1993, 1995; Bezanilla and Stefani, 1994). These results are difficult to interpret but seem to suggest that the activation of the channel is a coordinated movement of many parts of the protein and that it is sensitive to changes in conformation in many different regions.

One interesting approach to this problem would be to use the method of Schoppa et al. (1992), described earlier, to estimate the maximum value of the gating charge; and then to ask which amino acids contribute to this charge, after systematic mutation of each of the charged residues in the protein. This approach is not without difficulties of interpretation: it is possible to imagine a change in an amino acid producing a large enough change in the conformation of the protein to alter the gating charge, even though this amino acid itself did not normally move across the membrane field during activation. If, however, replacement of a positive S4 amino acid with a neutral amino acid produced *no* change in the number of charges that move during gating, it would seem safe to conclude that this amino acid could *not* contribute to activation. Amino acid substitutions that *did* affect the total charge would at the very least give an interesting indication of which residues may be involved in the changes in conformation that open the channel.

Studies of this kind (Seoh et al., 1996; Aggarwal and MacKinnon, 1996) suggest that very few of the charged residues of a K^+ channel actually move across the membrane field during activation. Many substitutions do not change the total charge that accompanies gating. Those that do seem to be located near the center of the K^+ channel protein: in the *Shaker* gene, these are the positively charged arginines at 365, 368, and 371 in S4, and the negatively charged glutamate 293 in S2. These experiments seem to suggest that the number of charges that contribute to the gating current is relatively small. If the number of charges that move is small, those charges that *do* move would have to move most of the way across the membrane field. Thus the electric field may be focused within a small region, and only a small change in conformation may be needed to produce activation.

Mechanism of Activation

The original notion that the S4 domain of the α subunit lies entirely within the interior of the protein or lipid and moves with all of its charged amino acids in a coordinated fashion outward across the membrane is unlikely for a number of reasons (see Sigworth, 1993; Bezanilla and Stefani, 1994). It envisages the positive charges as buried within the membrane (see Fig. 6.8A), but positive charges are very unlikely to exist within the hydrophobic interior of protein or lipid in the absence of negatively charged amino acids acting as countercharges to form ion pairs (see Honig, Hubbell, and Flewelling, 1986). Where are the countercharges? Of the 20 common amino acids, only two are negatively charged—aspartate and glutamate—and the *Shaker* sequence has only three of these within

Fig. 6.8 Hypothetical models of Na$^+$ channel activation.

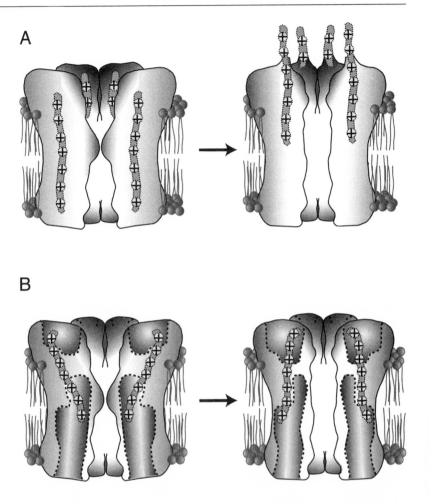

its putative membrane-spanning domains (2 glutamates in S2 and one aspartate in S3). There aren't enough negative charges to act as countercharges for the 7 S4 lysines and arginines proposed to be buried within the *Shaker* protein. In addition, other proteins (like those gated by cyclic nucleotides—see Chapter 16) that have S4 sequences with several charged amino acids show only a weak voltage dependence of gating (see Jan and Jan, 1990; Yau and Chen, 1995). It seems unlikely that the S4 sequence acts as a unit. Proteins don't usually work like this anyway: conformational changes that alter activity are generally rather subtle.

A more likely possibility (Fig. 6.8B), suggested by the experiments I have just described, is that only a few amino acids actually contribute to gating (see Papazian and Bezanilla, 1997). Counter-charges would not be needed if most of the positively charged S4 residues were *not* buried within the hydrophobic interior of the protein but were exposed to the intracellular or extracellular solution within "vestibules" flanking the gating region. Within the gating region, only a few amino acids need move, and they need move only a short distance; but this distance would be sufficient to move charge across the entire width of the membrane field because the field would drop over a physically short distance between the intracellular and extracellular solutions in this region of the protein. This scheme is consistent with the small number of amino acids that appear to contribute to gating (Seoh et al., 1996; Aggarwal and MacKinnon, 1996), as well as with experiments demonstrating that amino acids actually move from one side of the protein to the other when channel opening occurs (Yang and Horn, 1995; Yang, George, and Horn, 1996; Mannuzzu, Moronne, and Isacoff, 1996; Larsson et al., 1996). The diagram in Fig. 6.8B represents the beginning of an emerging consensus of many researchers working in this exciting area, but much more work will have to be done on the structure of these proteins before we understand how depolarization produces the coordinated movement of charge that opens the pore.

Inactivation

Hodgkin and Huxley proposed that activation and inactivation are separate processes, which they modeled as occurring independently of one another. They imagined two gates, an *m* gate resulting in channel activation and pore opening, and an *h* gate producing inactivation. Each gate was supposed to have its own separate voltage dependence and kinetics.

The first experimental evidence that inactivation is separate from activation was the demonstration that the intracellular perfusion of a squid axon with a protease can remove inactivation of the Na^+ current with very little effect on the kinetics of current turn-on (Armstrong, Bezanilla, and Rojas, 1973). In Fig. 6.9A (from Bezanilla and Armstrong, 1977), the currents were recorded in 10 percent Na^+ sea water, and the ionic Na^+ current was sufficiently small in this low-Na^+ extracellular solution that the gating current

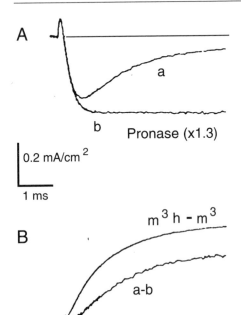

0.2 mA/cm^2

1 ms

Fig. 6.9 Time course of inactivation: block by pronase. **(A)** Effect of pronase on waveform of inward Na$^+$ current recorded from squid giant axon for 70 mV voltage pulse from $V_H = -70$ mV to 0 mV. Axon was bathed in artificial sea water containing 10% of the normal Na$^+$ concentration (replaced with Tris$^+$) and perfused internally with 125 mM CsF and 2 mM NaF (osmolarity adjusted with sucrose). Responses for positive voltage steps have been added to those for negative voltage steps to remove linear component of capacitance. Initial positive deflection is gating current. Control cell *(a)* is inactivated quickly, but inactivation in cell after 15 min dialysis with internal solution containing pronase *(b)* is blocked (Record *b* has been multiplied by 1.3 so that amplitude of gating current equals that in control.) **(B)** Time course of inactivation. Record labeled *a-b* is algebraic subtraction of current records *a* and *b* from **(A)**. This represents the time course of inactivation and is compared with the prediction of the Hodgkin-Huxley model, obtained by subtracting m^3 from m^3h. (From Bezanilla and Armstrong, 1977, reprinted with permission of the authors and of Rockefeller University Press.)

could be seen on the same record as the ionic current (the gating current is the initial upward deflection). After perfusion with a protease called pronase, inactivation nearly disappeared. Pronase also caused the gating current to decline, probably because, in addition to removing inactivation, pronase also digested and disabled a portion of the Na$^+$ channels. The record after pronase in Fig. 6.9A was therefore multiplied by 1.3, so that the gating currents before and after pronase were of the same magnitude.

Experiments with intracellular perfusion of pronase showed that activation and inactivation are separate from one another, but they also confirmed what previous experiments had suggested (see Goldman, 1976): activation and inactivation are *not* independent. When the waveform for the Na$^+$ current before pronase treatment was subtracted from the waveform after pronase treatment, what was left should have been the waveform for inactivation (Fig. 6.9B). In this waveform there is a pronounced delay not predicted from the Hodgkin and Huxley equations. The recording can be much better fit with models that assume that Na$^+$ channels must open before they can inactivate (Goldman, 1976; Bezanilla and Armstrong, 1977). Furthermore, there is little or no gating current associated with inactivation (see for example Armstrong and Bezanilla, 1977). Whatever the change in protein conformation that is responsible for inactivation, this change does not seem to move very much charge from one side of the membrane to the other. If inactivation does not result from movement of charge, then it is difficult to see how it could be voltage-dependent.

These observations led Armstrong and Bezanilla (1977) to propose a model for inactivation usually referred to as the *ball-and-chain* model, shown in simplified form in Fig. 6.10. The important features of this model are as follows. A part of the channel protein located on the cytoplasmic side (and therefore accessible to perfusion internally with pronase) contains a *ball* connected to the rest of the channel protein by a *chain* of amino acids. Opening of the pore produces a change in the conformation of the channel protein, and this new conformation forms a binding site to which the inactivation ball can bind, either by electrostatic or by hydrophobic interactions (or some combination of the two). If opening occurs before inactivation, inactivation must be at least partially coupled to activation. Furthermore, the ball would move from within the cytoplasm to a site at the very cytoplasmic edge of the channel pore. Even if the ball were charged, it would not contribute much to the gating current, since the charge of the ball would not move very far through the electric field across the membrane.

Single-Channel Recordings

Single-channel recordings also provided compelling evidence that activation and inactivation are coupled. The first successful recordings of single Na+ channels were made from rat muscle by Sigworth and Neher (1980), who showed that voltage pulses deliv-

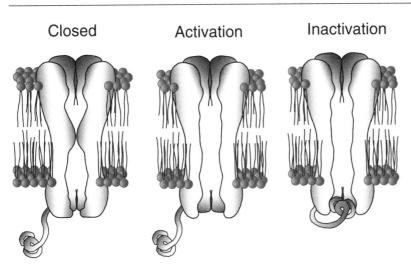

Closed   Activation   Inactivation

Fig. 6.10 "Ball-and-chain" model of voltage-gated sodium or potassium channel inactivation. Activation opens channel and is thought to produce a binding site for the inactivation ball at the cytoplasmic surface of the channel pore. The ball then binds to the site and blocks the channel.

Fig. 6.11 On-cell patch-clamp recordings of single-channel currents of voltage-gated Na$^+$ channels. **(A)** Recording method. Patch-clamp electrode was sealed against a myotube isolated from developing rat muscle. Myotubes were treated with colchicine, which caused them to round up and form spherical "myoballs." Electrode was connected via a silver/silverchloride wire to a patch-clamp amplifier, which was used both to voltage clamp the membrane patch and to record current (see Box 5.1). *R,* feedback resistor, in these experiments 10 GΩ; *V$_{out}$*, output voltage proportional to pipette current; and *V$_c$*, command potential. **(B)** Examples of single-channel currents. Membrane potential held at 30 mV hyperpolarized from resting potential to remove Na$^+$ channel inactivation. Upper trace shows time course of 40 mV change in pipette voltage (*V$_p$*) to a potential 10 mV positive to rest. Records labeled *I$_p$* are nine successive examples of single-channel currents evoked by voltage step. Mean channel current, −1.6 pA. **(C)** Average of 300 current records like those in **(B)**. Note similarity to whole-cell Na$^+$ current waveform (for example, in Fig. 6.5B). (Records in **(B)** and **(C)** redrawn from Sigworth and Neher, 1980 with the permission of the authors and of Macmillan Magazines Limited.)

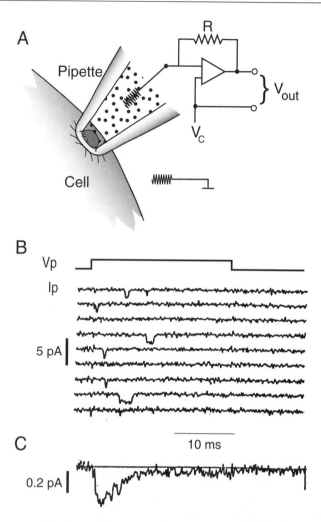

ered to a patch of membrane produce rectangular steps of inward current. These steps are variable in onset and duration and correspond to the opening of channels, each about 18–20 pS in amplitude (Fig. 6.11). When the responses to a large number of identical voltage pulses were averaged, the result was a waveform that looked very much like the waveform of the macroscopic Na$^+$ current, including both activation and inactivation. This similarity indicates that the macroscopic current is the summed average of the currents of many single channels.

Aldrich, Corey, and Stevens (1983) used single-channel recording to analyze two principal components of the opening of Na^+ channels in mammalian cultured cells: the time to first opening, and the duration of channel opening. Na^+ channels open with a variable delay, as can be seen in Fig. 6.11, and then remain open for a time that also varies from one voltage pulse to the next. Aldrich et al. showed that once channels open during a voltage pulse, they close but then very rarely open again. This finding indicates that, at least for mammals, Na^+ channels nearly always close by inactivating, and once inactivated they do not reopen. That is, in the scheme

$$C_1 \to C_2 \to C_3 \to C_4 \to C_5 \to O \to I$$

channels open by moving through the closed states C_1 to C_5 and then to the open state O. They then close mostly by moving from O to I (the inactivated state), from which there is little probability of return until the depolarizing voltage pulse is terminated. If inactivated channels reopened, or if channels closed from O back to C_5, it should be possible to observe reopenings back to O visible as multiple openings within the same trace. These are seldom seen in many mammalian preparations (Fig. 6.11), though they are somewhat more common, for example, for squid Na^+ channels. Na^+ channels therefore close most often by moving from O to I, and the duration of channel opening is a fairly good reflection of the time course of inactivation.

Aldrich, Corey, and Stevens demonstrated that nearly all of the voltage dependence of Na^+ channel behavior lies in the latency to first opening. As the voltage pulse is made larger (more depolarizing), the latency to first opening becomes dramatically shorter (see Fig. 7.1B in Chapter 7). The reason for this is that depolarization accelerates the activation of the channel, so with larger depolarizations channels move more quickly from C_1 to O. Once the channels open, they remain open for a variable length of time before they inactivate, and this time seems not to depend very much on voltage (see Fig. 7.1C). Since for the most part the rate of channel closing reflects the time course of channel inactivation, inactivation does not depend very much on membrane potential. The apparent acceleration of inactivation at depolarized potentials seems mostly due to the acceleration of activation.

Molecular Biology: K+ Channels

A dramatic confirmation of the coupling of inactivation to activation and of the ball-and-chain model came from a study not of Na+ channels, but rather of inactivation in K+ channels. Some K+ channels inactivate (see Chapter 7), and the most famous of these is the channel of the *Shaker* gene, which has a rapid inactivation in many respects similar to that of Na+ channels. This fast inactivation is due entirely to a stretch of amino acids at the amino-terminal end of the protein (see Fig. 6.2B), which appears actually to form a physical ball and chain much like the one Armstrong and Bezanilla first postulated.

The role of the amino terminus in *Shaker* inactivation was first demonstrated by Hoshi, Zagotta, and Aldrich (1990), who made deletion mutations in *Shaker* channel genes by digesting away a part of the DNA of the *Shaker* clone with a nuclease. The remaining DNA was then used to make cRNA, which was expressed in *Xenopus* oocytes (Fig. 1.6). Single-channel recordings of wild-type *Shaker* K+ channels from inside-out patches show inactivation quite similar to recordings for Na+ channels, with only occasional multiple openings. The likeness can be appreciated by comparing the trace in Fig. 6.12A labeled *ShB* with the records in Fig. 6.11. Mutations that removed a part of the sequence *after* amino acid 28 produced little change in inactivation (e.g., *ShBΔ28–34*, lacking amino acids 28 through 34). On the other hand, deletions that removed any significant number of the first 20 or so amino acids, such as *ShBΔ6–60*, lacking amino acids 6 through 60, have a pronounced effect (Fig. 6.12A). Since inactivation in *Shaker* channels resembles Na+ channel inactivation, with the time course of channel closing mostly reflecting the time course of inactivation (Zagotta, Hoshi, and Aldrich, 1989; Zagotta and Aldrich, 1990), the prolonged duration of openings in these channels with amino acids deleted indicates that inactivation has virtually disappeared. These experiments provide compelling evidence that the first 20 amino acids are at least part of the inactivation particle that blocks the channel in the Armstrong and Bezanilla model.

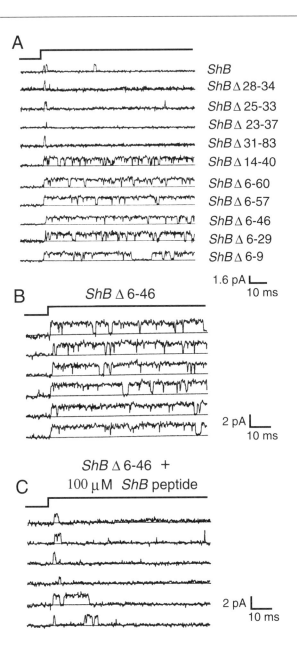

A

ShB
ShBΔ28-34
ShBΔ25-33
ShBΔ23-37
ShBΔ31-83
ShBΔ14-40
ShBΔ6-60
ShBΔ6-57
ShBΔ6-46
ShBΔ6-29
ShBΔ6-9

1.6 pA
10 ms

B   ShB Δ 6-46

2 pA
10 ms

ShB Δ 6-46 +
C   100 μM ShB peptide

2 pA
10 ms

Fig. 6.12 Role of the amino terminus in *Shaker* channel inactivation. **(A)** *Shaker* wild-type cRNA *(ShB)* and cRNA with deletions *(ShBΔ28–34,* e.g.) near the amino terminus were injected into *Xenopus* oocytes, and recordings of K[+] single-channel currents were made from inside-out patches. Openings were evoked by voltage steps from −100 mV to +50 mV (voltage waveform shown at top). (From Hoshi, Zagotta, and Aldrich, 1990; reprinted with permission of the authors and the American Association for the Advancement of Science.) **(B)** and **(C)** Restoration of inactivation by exposure to amino-terminal peptide. Openings evoked by 170 mV steps from $V_H = -120$ mV to +50 mV (voltage waveforms shown above current traces). Records in **(B)** are representative currents from one patch after expression with *ShBΔ6–46,* which nearly eliminated rapid inactivation. Records in **(C)** are from same patch as in **(B)** after perfusion of the cytoplasmic surface of the patch with 100 μM of the *ShB* peptide, consisting of the first 20 (amino-terminal) amino acids of the *Shaker* sequence. (From Zagotta, Hoshi, and Aldrich, 1990; reprinted with permission of the authors and the American Association for the Advancement of Science.)

Remarkably, inactivation can be restored to a mutant channel simply by exposing the cytoplasmic surface of the channel to synthetic peptide (Zagotta, Hoshi, and Aldrich, 1990). (See Fig. 6.12B and C.) The records in Fig. 6.12B labeled *ShBΔ6–46* were recorded from an inside-out patch taken from a *Xenopus* oocyte, for a *Shaker* mutant lacking amino acids 6–46. The openings are prolonged, as for the deletion mutants in Fig. 6.12A. When a synthetic peptide with the sequence of the first 20 amino acids was added to the medium bathing the cytoplasmic face of the channel, inactivation was restored.

The discovery that the amino terminus of the *Shaker* protein is largely responsible for fast inactivation provides a remarkable confirmation of the ball-and-chain model and represents one of the greatest contributions that the techniques of molecular biology have made to our understanding of channel structure. One word of caution is, however, in order. *Shaker* channels from which the amino terminus is removed still inactivate, though much more slowly than normal. This slower form of inactivation is sometimes referred to as *C-type* or *P-type* inactivation, since it has been shown to be affected by mutations in the region of the protein near the C-terminus (in S6) and near the P domain (see Chandy and Gutman, 1995; Kukuljan, Labarca, and Latorre, 1995). There is still much about the structure of the K^+ channel protein and the nature of inactivation that we do not understand.

Na⁺ Channel Inactivation

Since internal perfusion of an axon with protease can remove the inactivation of Na^+ currents, it seems reasonable to suppose that cytoplasmic regions of the Na^+ channel must also play an important role in the mechanism of channel turn-off. Considerable evidence suggests that the segment of the Na^+ channel which links repeat units III and IV is essential for inactivation. Antibodies directed against this region slow inactivation (Vassilev, Scheuer, and Catterall, 1988), and deletion of this linking unit nearly eliminates inactivation altogether (Stühmer et al., 1989). Mutations of three hydrophobic amino acids within the III/IV repeat unit have particularly marked effects (West et al., 1992; Kellenberger et al.,

1997). It is of some interest that, so far, only a single candidate in-activation region has been discovered for the Na^+ channel. It may be relevant to note that an assembled K^+ channel (with four α sub-units) has four amino-terminal inactivation balls, but only a single ball is required to block the channel (MacKinnon, Aldrich, and Lee, 1993).

For K^+ channels, the inactivation ball sitting in the channel pore can actually be "knocked off" by the entry of K^+ into the channel from the external medium, much as for internal TEA (Armstrong, 1975). We know this because Demo and Yellen (1991) have shown that recovery from inactivation is speeded when the external solution is high in K^+. This finding suggests that there may be some dif-ferences in the mechanism for inactivation between Na^+ and K^+ channels. If Na^+ channels were inactivated by blocking with a sim-ple ball and chain, the cytoplasmically attached ball would be ex-pected to be swept away by the large influx of Na^+ from the exter-nal solution during normal channel activation. Ironically, the ball-and-chain model, first proposed for Na^+ channels, seems more ap-propriate for *Shaker* and its relatives. The nature of Na^+ channel inactivation is still unclear.

Summary

Hodgkin and Huxley proposed that action potentials are generated by voltage-gated Na^+ and K^+ currents produced by ions flowing through separate channels, each channel with its own voltage de-pendence and kinetics. We now know this to be true. The genes for Na^+ and K^+ channel proteins have been isolated, cloned, and se-quenced; they represent members of a large family of voltage-gated channels.

The channel proteins consist of a large α subunit, which contains the channel pore and the protein domains mostly responsible for activation and inactivation; in addition, there are smaller β sub-units, which can alter the function of the α subunits. The channel pore appears to be formed mostly by a sequence of amino acids called the P domain, which dips into the membrane and forms the regions through which ions move.

Hodgkin and Huxley proposed that the opening of voltage-gated channels is produced by the movement of charges from one side of the membrane to the other. There is considerable evidence that this is also true. The movement of charge has been measured as a gating current, and approximately 12–13 charges move all the way across the membrane field during the activation of a single channel. Considerable effort is now directed at understanding which charges move, and how charge movement in one part of the protein causes pore opening in another part.

Hodgkin and Huxley showed that Na$^+$ channels undergo activation and then inactivation, and they modeled these events as separate and independent. If activation and inactivation are independent, then any closed or open state can inactivate, since the h (pore-closing) gate would be able to move from activated to inactivated independent of movement of the m (pore-opening) gates. Evidence from macroscopic currents, gating currents, and single-channel recordings all indicate that activation and inactivation are not independent but are, rather, coupled. That is, in many cases the channel opens before inactivation occurs,

$$C_1 \rightleftharpoons C_2 \rightleftharpoons C_3 \rightleftharpoons C_4 \rightleftharpoons C_5 \rightleftharpoons O \rightleftharpoons I$$

The opening of the channel reveals a binding site, to which an inactivation particle or "ball" binds and occludes the channel.

The scheme pictured above for which the channel must open before it can inactivate is a *strictly coupled* model. Although it is probably a better representation of channel activation and inactivation than the Hodgkin-Huxley model, it is also unlikely to be completely accurate. We know, for example, that weak, slow depolarizations inactivate the Na$^+$ conductance, even though such changes in potential produce little measurable inward current. This phenomenon, called *accommodation,* is responsible for the failure of slow depolarizations to excite spiking in axons. If an excitatory depolarization occurs too slowly, the channels inactivate before sufficient activation can occur to permit the axon to reach threshold. It would therefore seem that, at least in some circumstances, channels can inactivate directly from closed states with a significant probability.

A more realistic view of activation and inactivation is probably something between the Hodgkin-Huxley model and the strictly coupled model, perhaps something like this:

$$
\begin{array}{ccccccc}
 & & \text{I} \rightleftharpoons \text{I} \rightleftharpoons \text{I} & & \\
 & & \updownarrow \quad \updownarrow \quad \updownarrow & & \\
\text{C}_1 \rightleftharpoons \text{C}_2 \rightleftharpoons \text{C}_3 \rightleftharpoons \text{C}_4 \rightleftharpoons \text{C}_5 \rightleftharpoons \text{O}
\end{array}
$$

This is a *partially coupled* model (see for example Horn and Vandenberg, 1984; Zagotta and Aldrich, 1990; Vandenberg and Bezanilla, 1991). Inactivation can occur from some but not all closed states, as well as from the open state. In this model, the inactivated state is labeled *I* as if all inactivated states had the same conformation. This may not be true: different inactivated states may represent different conformations of the channel molecule. We don't really know how many distinct changes in conformation the channel passes through on its way from closed to open to inactivated. The greatest challenge for the future is to understand how the various kinetic states of voltage-gated channels correspond to different structural states of the proteins. We still have only a rudimentary understanding of the three-dimensional structure of channels, and until our knowledge of structure dramatically improves, we are left only to guess how activation and inactivation actually occur.

7

The Diversity of
Voltage-Gated Channels

A SINGLE ORGANISM has not one kind of Na$^+$ channel but at least 8–10, and at least 20–25 different kinds of K$^+$ channels. In addition, neurons contain a variety of voltage-gated Ca^{2+} channels, and channels selective for Cl$^-$. The wide diversity of different channel types is on the one hand confusing, since we know so little about what these different channels do; but on the other hand, it is tremendously important, since different channels have different physiological properties that are likely to have dramatic effects on action potential threshold, firing rates, and the voltage and time dependence of synaptic transmitter release.

I: Na$^+$ CHANNELS

In the rat there are at least nine genes for Na$^+$ channel α subunits (see Kallen, Cohen, and Barchi, 1994; Goldin, 1995). At least four have been shown to be expressed in brain (*rNaB1–3* and *NaCh6*—see Schaller et al., 1995), and at least two in peripheral neurons (Akopian, Sivilotti, and Wood, 1996; Toledo-Aral et al., 1997). In addition, two are expressed in skeletal muscle *(rNaSk1–2)* and one in glia (*rNaG1*—Gautron et al., 1992). All of these genes code for proteins with a similar structure. The sequences for the pore domain and for regions thought to be important for activation and inactivation (S4 and the III/IV linker) are highly conserved within the Na$^+$ channel α subunit family, and it seems likely that the pore structure and the mechanisms of activation and inactivation are similar for all of these proteins.

In addition to the variability introduced by different genes, there is evidence that the mRNA from at least one of the brain genes *(rNaB2)* can be alternatively spliced into at least two different messages, and splicing seems to be regulated during development (Sarao et al., 1991). The α subunits of Na^+ channels can be post-translationally modified, particularly by phosphorylation. Furthermore, Na^+ channels in brain appear to be associated with two auxiliary subunits, called β_1 and β_2, which could conceivably occur in alternate forms. It seems possible that a single α gene could be associated with different β genes in different tissues, and this could have important effects on the kinetics and voltage dependence of activation and inactivation (Isom, DeJongh, and Catterall, 1994).

Why are there so many different Na^+ channel types? Our knowledge on this point remains rather sketchy. One reason may be *spatial:* different Na^+ channel subunits seem to be localized to different parts of the nervous system, for reasons that are still unclear. Another explanation may be *temporal:* one form of Na^+ channel α-subunit gene in brain *(rNaB3)* seems to be expressed mainly in embryos and its gene product is considerably less abundant in adult (see Kallen, Cohen, and Barchi, 1994), except after injury (Waxman, Kocsis, and Black, 1994). In skeletal muscle, rNaSk2 is found almost exclusively in embryonic and denervated muscle; whereas in adults, the predominant form of the Na^+ channel α subunit in muscle is rNaSk1.

If different Na^+ channel genes are regulated so that they are expressed in different tissues or at different stages in development, it would seem reasonable to suppose that their gene products have functional differences that are important for the physiology of the organism. This seems to be true, at least in some cases. The different skeletal muscle Na^+ channels, for example, show differences in kinetics and voltage dependence (Pappone, 1980): activation in the embryonic form (rNaSk1) occurs at more hyperpolarized potentials, with slower turn-on and decay, than in the adult form (rNaSk2). The embryonic form is also considerably less sensitive to TTX than the adult form, though the functional consequences of this difference are unknown. Changes in Na^+ channel expression may have important effects on the physiology of muscle contraction and behavior, since mutations in skeletal muscle Na^+ channel genes can have serious consequences (see Box 7.1).

Dorsal root ganglion cells also contain TTX-sensitive and TTX-insensitive forms of Na^+ channels (see for example Elliott and

Box 7.1

Na⁺ CHANNELS AND DISEASE

The cloning of voltage-gated Na⁺ channels has not only increased our understanding of channel function, it has also provided new information about some forms of the muscle disease *myotonia congenita*. Myotonia congenita is an inherited disease in which skeletal muscle relaxes slowly and poorly after contraction, often producing long-lasting spasms. One form of this disease, fortunately rather rare, is called *paramyotonia congenita* or *Eulenberg disease,* and was discovered by the German physician Albert Eulenberg in 1886. Symptoms begin from infancy and are often precipitated by brief exposure to cold. They include spasms of the facial and distal muscles, with involuntary grimacing, closing of the eyelids, and clenching of the hands.

Paramyotonia congenita can apparently be caused by an autosomal dominant single-site mutation of the gene for the Na⁺ channel protein (see Ji et al., 1995). Mutations at several different sites can produce the phenotype, but if genes containing these mutations are expressed in a cell line, the Na⁺ currents recorded from these cells show a common defect: inactivation is 2–5 times slower. The currents in the figure below (reprinted with permission from Ji et al., 1995) were recorded from tsA 201 cells, transfected with DNA either for the wild-type human skeletal muscle SkM1 channel or for the SkM1 mutation R1448H channel (arginine substituted with histidine at amino acid 1448, at the extracellular end of the fourth membrane-spanning region in the fourth repeat domain). Inactivation proceeds more slowly for the mutant protein. Single-channel recordings, shown below the whole-cell currents, demonstrate that R1448H channel openings are prolonged and multiple, again reflecting slower inactivation. The slower inactivation of the Na⁺ channel produces hyperexcitability of the muscle, which is probably directly responsible for the muscle spasms experienced by patients.

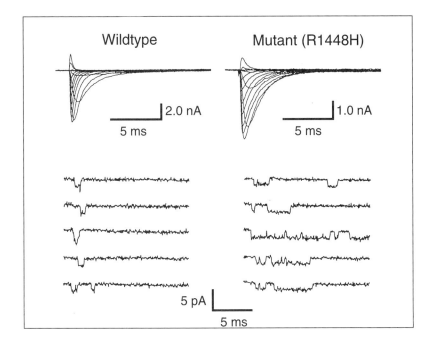

Elliott, 1993). The TTX-insensitive current turns on and decays more slowly and is activated at more depolarized membrane potentials than the TTX-sensitive current. The TTX-insensitive current also recovers from inactivation much more rapidly, which could affect the maximum rate of action potential firing frequency.

One of the most remarkable examples of differences between Na^+ channel properties in different cell types comes from the study of Barres, Chun, and Corey (1989), who compared Na^+ currents in a form of glial cell (the type-1 astrocyte from optic nerve) with Na^+ currents in the neurons whose axons pass next to these glial cells (the retinal ganglion cells). Many studies have shown that glial cells contain Na^+ channels, typically at lower density than nerve cells (Sontheimer and Ritchie, 1995). Barres and colleagues demonstrated that the Na^+ channels in the type-1 astrocytes are much slower in kinetics than those of retinal ganglion cells (Fig. 7.1A). Following the lead of Aldrich, Corey, and Stevens (1983), they analyzed the statistics of single-channel records from both cell types into two probability histograms, one for the latency to first opening and the other for the open-time duration (see Chapter 6 and Fig.

Fig. 7.1 Sodium currents from astrocytes and retinal ganglion cells. **(A)** Comparison of waveform of currents. Upper traces are whole-cell voltage-clamp recordings from type-1 astrocyte dissociated from optic nerve of rat; middle traces, whole-cell currents from retinal ganglion cell; lower traces, waveform of voltage steps. Currents have been superimposed from responses to a series of depolarizing steps from $V_H = -100$ mV. Note the much slower time course of astrocyte currents. **(B)** First-latency distributions for sodium channels recorded from on-cell patches. Only patches thought to contain a single active channel were included in the analysis. Cells were bathed in high-K^+ solution, to bring the resting potential of the cell to zero. This was done so that the potential across the membrane of the patch in the on-cell recording could be accurately known from the potential at the pipette (see Fig. 6.11A). Membrane potential is given in the lower right-hand corner of each graph in mV. Ordinate gives probability that a channel will have opened by the time shown on the abscissa, for traces that did record channel openings (traces without openings were not included). Dotted lines are astrocytes, solid lines ganglion cells. **(C)** Open-time distributions, recorded from single channels in on-cell patches as in **(B)**. Ordinate gives the probability that the channel remained open for a time shorter than the time shown on the abscissa. For example, at t =1 ms the ordinate gives the probability that the channel remained open for 1 ms or less. Since Na^+ channels usually close by inactivating (see Chapter 6), the open-time distribution reflects the time course of inactivation, with dotted lines for astrocytes and solid lines for ganglion cells. Note that voltage has little effect on the open-time distribution for either cell. (From Barres, Chun, and Corey, 1989; reprinted with permission of the authors and of Cell Press.)

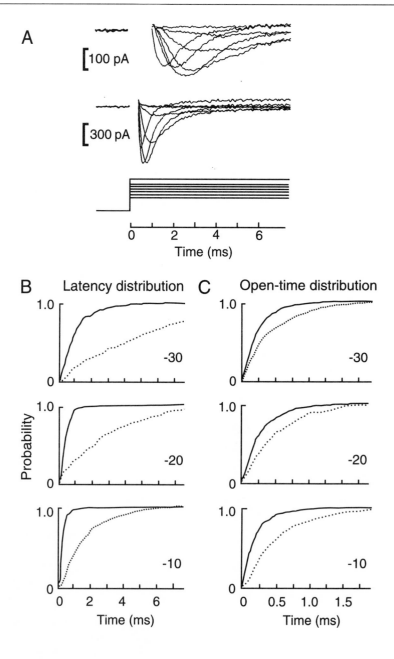

6.11B). These are shown for several voltages in Figs. 7.1B and C. The histograms are quite different for the astrocyte (dotted lines) and the ganglion cell (solid lines). The first-latency distribution is voltage-dependent, with channel opening occurring much faster at more depolarized voltages; however, for the glial cell, channel opening is consistently slower. The open-time distribution, on the other hand, is rather insensitive to voltage. Open times are consistently longer for the glial cells, reflecting a slower time course of inactivation.

We do not yet know enough about Na^+ channels to know whether the differences in kinetics illustrated in Fig. 7.1 are typical of different cell types throughout the nervous system, or whether the cells studied in these experiments represent an extreme case. It is still uncertain why glial cells even have Na^+ channels, since these cells do not seem to produce action potentials. We must also always ask whether the properties of Na^+ channels in particular experiments are affected by the conditions of recording. Na^+ channels in inside-out patches might be less likely to be phosphorylated than channels *in situ*. It nonetheless seems clear that the nervous system expresses many different kinds of Na^+ channels, some of which have dramatically altered properties. How these differences affect function is still a subject for much future investigation.

II: K^+ CHANNELS

Potassium channels are found in nearly every cell in the body and are remarkable for their diversity (Latorre and Miller, 1983; Rudy, 1988). They are the beetles of membrane channels: one can't help wondering why God made so many different kinds. Nearly all have a similar selectivity for ions, with K^+ much more permeable than Na^+. Many can be blocked by quaternary amines, such as TEA, or by 4-aminopyridine and related compounds; and nearly all can be blocked by external Ba^{2+} and internal Cs^+. They differ in almost every other way: voltage dependence, time course of inactivation, mechanism of activation, and sensitivity to Ca^{2+} and to toxins. This diversity, which has profound implications for the electrical properties of nerve cells, is often produced by changes in only a few amino acids, making these proteins particularly intriguing and among the most actively investigated of all the channels in the nervous system.

Delayed Rectifiers and *A* Currents

The K$^+$ conductance Hodgkin and Huxley discovered in the squid giant axon is usually referred to as the *delayed rectifier*. It is *delayed,* because activation of g_K is slower than activation of g_{Na}, for the squid giant axon and for nerve cells in general. It is a *rectifier,* because like any rectifier in an electronic circuit, current passes more readily in one direction than in the other. What makes the delayed rectifier rectify has little to do with the mechanism of permeation, since the instantaneous *i–V* curve (and the *i–V* curve of the single channels) for the squid giant axon K$^+$ conductance is very nearly linear, at least in symmetrical K$^+$ solutions. The squid giant axon K$^+$ conductance is said to rectify primarily because conductance is gated by voltage: the channel opens to allow current to flow only when the membrane potential is depolarized.

Hodgkin and Huxley did not observe any inactivation of the delayed rectifier of the squid giant axon during the relatively short time scale of the voltage pulses used in their experiments (see Chapter 5). Subsequently, others have shown (see for example Chabala, 1984) that when longer voltage pulses are used, inactivation *can* be observed in squid, though it is very slow (the time constant can be several seconds). This is a general feature (perhaps *the* distinguishing feature) of the subset of K$^+$ channels called delayed rectifiers, that inactivation occurs very slowly or not at all.

Many nerve cells (and muscle cells in insects) have voltage-gated K$^+$ currents that are also activated by depolarization but, unlike the delayed rectifier, are rapidly inactivated. These currents were first discovered in the cell bodies of molluscs (Hagiwara, Kusano, and Saito, 1961; Conner and Stevens, 1971a–c; Neher, 1971) and are often referred to as *rapidly inactivating K$^+$ currents* or *A currents*. Rapidly inactivating K$^+$ currents are quite variable in their properties, though they have in common that the time constant of inactivation is generally 10–100 ms—slower than for g_{Na} but considerably faster than for delayed rectifiers. In many cases, they also activate more rapidly than delayed rectifiers.

The most famous rapidly inactivating K$^+$ current is the *Shaker* current, so named because it is the current that is deficient in the

Shaker mutant of *Drosophila*. When *Shaker* mutants are exposed to ether, instead of becoming immobile, as wild-type flies do, they begin to shake vigorously because their muscle membranes have too little K^+ conductance and are electrically unstable. Physiologically, the muscles of mutant flies lack a voltage-gated, rapidly inactivating K^+ current, some of whose properties were already described in Chapter 6.

The cloning of the *Shaker* gene (Box 6.1) not only provided our first view of the structure and function of K^+ channels (see Fig. 6.2B), it also made possible the isolation of other similar genes, first in *Drosophila*, then in mouse (see Chandy and Gutman, 1995; Jan and Jan, 1997). The *Drosophila* nervous system has at least 4 voltage-gated K^+ α subunit genes, called *Shaker, Shal, Shab,* and *Shaw,* which when expressed produce K^+ channels with similar ion selectivity and voltage dependence but different TEA sensitivity and time course of inactivation (see Fig. 7.2). Mammals have at least 16 α subunit genes closely related to the 4 *Drosophila* genes, and the *Drosophila* genes can be used to define 4 *subfamilies* of α subunit genes in mammals, with at least 7 genes related to *Shaker (Kv1.1–*

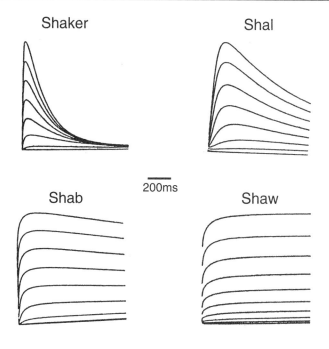

Fig. 7.2 Diversity of voltage-gated K^+ channels from *Drosophila*. RNAs for *Shaker, Shal, Shab,* and *Shaw* genes were injected into *Xenopus* oocytes, and currents were recorded with a two-electrode voltage clamp in response to 1 s voltage pulses from $V_H = -90$ mV to membrane potentials from between -80 mV and $+20$ mV in steps of 10 mV. Peak currents ranged from 0.4 to 1.5 µA. (Reprinted from Wei et al., 1990, with permission of the authors and of the American Association for the Advancement of Science.)

Fig. 7.3 Diversity of mammalian voltage-gated K⁺ channels. RNAs for the genes *Kv1.1–Kv1.4* cloned from rat brain were injected into *Xenopus* oocytes, and currents were recorded from large on-cell patches. Voltage steps were 3.2 s long, from $V_H = -80$ mV to a test potential of 0 mV. Note difference in rates of inactivation. (Modified from Stühmer et al., 1989.)

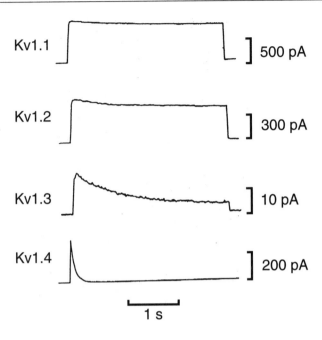

Kv1.7), 2 to *Shab (Kv2.1* and *Kv2.2),* 4 to *Shaw (Kv3.1–Kv3.4),* and 3 to *Shal (Kv4.1-Kv4.3).* All of these genes code for proteins that are closely related in sequence and structure and especially highly conserved within the putative membrane-spanning regions (S1–S6) and in the P domain. They can, however, show considerable variability within the amino- and carboxyl-terminal regions.

As in *Drosophila,* the channels produced by expression of different α subunit genes produce channels with different properties. The currents illustrated in Fig. 7.3 were recorded from *Xenopus* oocytes after expression of four different but closely related rat genes, all from the *Shaker* subfamily (Stühmer et al., 1989). These currents have a similar selectivity for K⁺ but differ in their voltage dependence, time course of activation, single-channel conductance, and sensitivity to TEA.

Besides the variability due to the large number of α subunit genes, additional variability in K⁺ channel properties can arise from alternative splicing (see for example Luneau et al., 1991), posttranslational modification, association with different β subunits (Rettig et al., 1994; Heinemann et al., 1996)—which may also be alternatively spliced (McCormack et al., 1995)—and *heteromeric assembly*. Heteromeric assembly is the assembly of K$^+$ channels from more than one *different* α subunit. Recall that each functional K$^+$ channel consists of 4 α subunits, which may or may not be identical. There is considerable evidence for both *Drosophila* and mammals that α subunits from within the same family can join to form *heteromeric channels* (see for example Christie et al., 1990; Isacoff, Jan, and Jan, 1990; Weiser, et al., 1994).

A typical example of such evidence is given in Fig. 7.4. In this experiment (from Weiser et al., 1994), a *Xenopus* oocyte was injected with a small quantity of RNA complementary to *Kv3.4* DNA, and a small, rapidly inactivating current was observed (Fig. 7.4A). A 4–5 times larger amount of the RNA complementary to the *Kv3.1* DNA was then injected into another oocyte, and a much larger, slowly inactivating current was recorded (Fig. 7.4B). When both RNAs were injected together, the current recorded could not be described as the sum of the currents in Figs. 7.4A and B. It inactivated with a time constant more rapid than for *Kv3.1* but slower than for *Kv3.4,* and its waveform could not be obtained by summing the homomeric currents in any combination. Experiments like those in Fig. 7.4 indicate that heteromeric combinations *can* form, and considerable morphological information suggests that they *do* form (see for example Sheng et al., 1993; Weiser et al., 1994), though we are still far from knowing what combinations are permissible in which cells, and why.

The assembly of a large number of α (and β) subunits, alternatively spliced and combined to form different homomeric and heteromeric combinations, permits a staggering variety of voltage-gated K$^+$ channels with varying voltage dependence and time course of inactivation. Different subunits are found in different cell types (Sheng et al., 1993; Weiser et al., 1994) and may be localized to particular regions of a single cell (Sheng et al., 1994). Many neurons have been shown to have more than one kind of K$^+$ channel, and slowly inactivating and rapidly inactivating conductances are often found in the same cell (see Rudy, 1988).

Function of Voltage-Gated K$^+$ Currents

Although we are very far from understanding the function of these many different channel types, we can say something of a general

Fig. 7.4 Formation of heteromeric voltage-gated K$^+$ channels. Currents recorded with two-electrode voltage clamp from *Xenopus* oocytes. **(A)** Oocyte injected with cRNA for *Kv3.4* alone. **(B)** Oocyte injected with cRNA for *Kv3.1* alone. **(C)** Oocyte injected with cRNA for both *Kv3.4* and *Kv3.1*. (Modified from Weiser et al., 1994.)

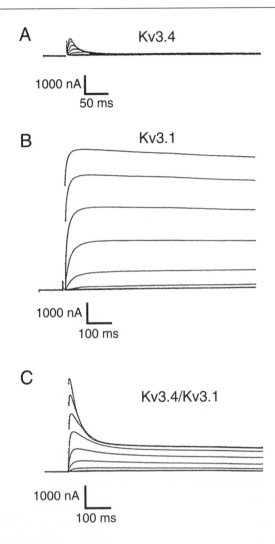

nature about the role of delayed rectifiers and *A* currents in nerve cell physiology. Slowly inactivating K$^+$ currents are mostly responsible for the falling phase of the action potential, in squid giant axon and in most neurons in the central nervous system. K$^+$ currents with intermediate rates of inactivation (sometimes called *D currents*) may also contribute to action potential repolarization (Storm, 1987, 1988; Wu and Barish, 1992).

Rapidly inactivating K$^+$ currents, on the other hand, seem to play a different role. Since they activate and inactivate rapidly, they may produce a membrane-potential-dependent change in K^+ conductance that regulates the excitability of the neuron. This change in conductance could have the effect of controlling the spread of action potentials locally within axons or dendrites (Hoffman et al., 1997; Debanne et al., 1997). In addition, as Conner and Stevens (1971c) first pointed out, A currents can control the interval between spikes in a neuron that fires repeatedly.

Fig. 7.5A presents a calculation that Conner and Stevens first made on a model neuron, for three cases for which the same amount of Na^+ and delayed-rectifier K^+ current was used. For the first *(A1)*, no A current was added, and to the others some *(A2)* or a bit more A current *(A3)* was included. In each case, the neuron was stimulated with the same depolarizing current pulse, and the resulting voltage response of the model cell has been plotted. As the amount of A current added to the model cell is increased, the delay before the first spike and the interval between successive spikes (the *interspike interval*) are both increased. The reason for this is as follows. When the stimulating current is first turned on, the cell depolarizes, and if no A current is present a spike is rapidly generated *(A1)*. If A current is added to the model cell, the depolarization rapidly activates the A current, and the cell K^+ conductance increases, preventing the cell from reaching spike threshold. After the A current has substantially inactivated, the first action potential is generated. The more the A current added to the model cell, the longer the time before enough of the K^+ conductance declines to permit the net current to become inward and the first spike to be produced.

As the neuron then depolarizes during the rising phase of the first action potential, the Na^+ channels inactivate, the delayed rectifier is activated, and the membrane potential hyperpolarizes back down toward the K^+ equilibrium potential. This hyperpolarization causes the delayed-rectifier channels to close, and in the absence of an A current a new spike is soon generated by the maintained depolarization produced by the current injection. If an A current is present, however, the hyperpolarization following a spike has an additional effect: it removes the inactivation of the A current, just as hyperpolarization removes inactivation of Na^+ currents (see Fig. 5.14). The continued injection of current depolarizes the neuron, but the A current is ready to be activated and counters the effect of

Fig. 7.5 Contribution of *A* currents to length of interspike interval. Calculations were performed on model neuron in the program Nodus™. **(A)** Cell was constructed with Na[+] currents, delayed-rectifier K[+] currents, and *A* currents, as in Conner and Stevens (1971c), with parameter values given in De Schutter (1986). Responses in *A1* are for a cell with no *A* current, and *A2* and *A3* are for addition of *A* currents with g_{max} equal to 50 and 90 mS/cm[2]. Responses are to stimulation with 0.5 nA current pulse. **(B)** Calculations as in **(A)**. For each panel, g_{max} for the *A* current was equal to 50 mS/cm[2], and responses are to stimulation with 1.0 nA current pulse (twice that used for *A1–A3*). Plot in *B1* is for cell with *A* current having the same kinetic parameters as for the model cell in parts *A2* and *A3*. For *B2*, α_h and β_h for the *A* current were multiplied by 0.5 (increasing the time constant of inactivation at any given voltage twofold). For *B3*, α_h and β_h for the *A* current were multiplied by 0.25 (increasing the time constant of inactivation at any given voltage fourfold). For definition of α_h and β_h, see Eqn. (20) in Chapter 5. (Calculations courtesy of M. C. Cheney.)

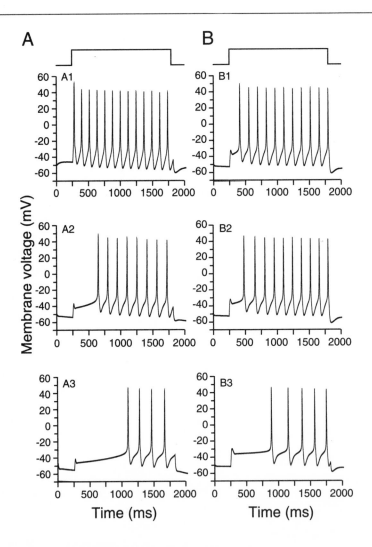

the applied current, preventing the membrane potential from depolarizing further. Eventually, the *A* current inactivates, and the applied current now generates another spike. The more *A* current the neuron contains, the longer the delay before the generation of a new spike (and the greater the interval between the spikes).

In much of the older literature, the physiology of voltage-gated K[+] currents is presented as if there were only two types: the delayed-rectifier currents responsible for spike repolarization, and *A* currents responsible for setting the interspike interval. Expression of the many different K$^+$ channel genes and recordings from many different cells in different parts of the nervous system now inform us that life is not so simple: delayed rectifiers and *A* currents are extremes with many intermediate classes. Fig. 7.5B gives calculations for model cells constructed as in Fig. 7.5A, all with the same *amount* of rapidly inactivating K$^+$ current, but with an altered *time constant* of inactivation. These parameters change the delay before the first spike and the interspike interval, since slowing the rate of inactivation slows the decay of K$^+$ conductance. Since K$^+$ currents with a variety of rates of inactivation are present in neurons (see for example Ficker and Heinemann, 1992), they provide a multiplicity of mechanisms for altering the rate of spike firing. The challenge for the future is to understand why we need all these different K$^+$ channels, why they are distributed within the central nervous system in so selective a fashion, and what they do.

Ca^{2+}-Activated K$^+$ Channels

Ca^{2+}-activated K$^+$ conductances were discovered by Meech and Strumwasser (1970), who showed that injection of Ca^{2+} into the large neurons of the mollusc *Aplysia* produces membrane hyperpolarization and a decrease in resistance. Meech and Standen (1975) subsequently demonstrated (in neurons of another mollusc, *Helix aspersa*) that this hyperpolarization is produced by an increase in K$^+$ conductance.

The properties of this conductance were studied in some detail by Gorman and Hermann (1979), who penetrated *Aplysia* neurons with several electrodes so that the cells could be injected with Ca^{2+} under voltage clamp (see Fig. 7.6A). The advantage of injecting the Ca^{2+} in this way is that the current used to inject the Ca^{2+} from the Ca^{2+}-containing electrode is balanced by an equal but opposite current from the current electrode of the voltage clamp, so that no net current is introduced into the cell during the Ca^{2+} injection. This has the consequence that Ca^{2+} injections did not change the membrane potential, which means that the effects of Ca^{2+} injection (and Ca^{2+} concentration increase) can be separated from any electrical effects produced by passing current through the Ca^{2+} electrode.

Gorman and Hermann found that the amplitude of the K$^+$ cur-

Fig. 7.6 Ca^{2+}-activated K$^+$ currents in *Aplysia* neurons. **(A)** Method of recording and Ca^{2+} injection. Pipette for Ca^{2+} injection was filled with 0.1 M CaCl$_2$ and connected to a circuit that injected a constant current (double circles). Pipettes and amplifiers to right were standard two-electrode voltage clamp. Abbreviations: V_m, membrane potential; *FBA,* feedback amplifier (for voltage clamp); V_c, command potential; and *gnd,* ground (earth). **(B)** Responses at top are representative records of *Aplysia* neuron for Ca^{2+} injections 10 s in duration with injection currents of 50, 100, and 200 nA. Bars beneath records show timing and duration of injections. Graph plots means ± S.E. for peak amplitude of current produced by Ca^{2+} injection as a function of injection current for constant-duration (10 s) injection. Holding potential (V_H) was −50 mV. **(C)** Peak K$^+$ current for Ca^{2+} injections of same duration (10 s) and injection current (200 nA) but with injection electrode positioned at different depths within the cell. Electrode was first placed to produce maximum outward current (this is the zero point on abscissa), presumably near the cell membrane. Electrode was then advanced in 20 μm intervals into the cell interior. Representative records are placed near data points, illustrated for same cell. Bars beneath records show timing and duration of injections. (Parts **(B)** and **(C)** redrawn from Gorman and Hermann, 1979.)

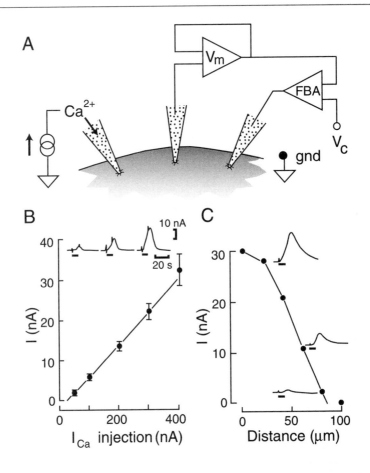

rent is directly proportional to the size of the Ca^{2+} injection (Fig. 7.6B). Since the voltage of the cell was held by the voltage-clamp circuitry at a constant value of −50 mV during the injection, these experiments indicated that Ca^{2+} itself could gate the conductance change. Furthermore, in a parallel series of experiments, Gorman and Thomas (1980a,b) used the Ca^{2+}-sensitive dye arsenazo III (see Chapter 13) to show that Ca^{2+} injections produce increases in intracellular Ca^{2+} concentration that are linearly proportional to the amplitude of the injection. This would suggest that changes in Ca^{2+} concentration are responsible for the increase in K$^+$ conductance, as would be expected if Ca^{2+} were binding directly to the channel, or to some other protein that gates the channel.

Gorman and Hermann (1979) also found that the amplitude of

the response depended upon where in the cell the Ca^{2+} injection occurred (see Fig. 7.6C). The Ca^{2+} injection electrode in these experiments was first positioned in the cell where it produced the maximal K^+ current, usually very near the plasma membrane. As the electrode was then advanced into the cell, the response to the injection declined. Since Ca^{2+} is highly buffered and diffuses slowly (see Chapter 4), this experiment indicated that the Ca^{2+} concentration increase must occur very near the membrane in order to be effective, presumably adjacent to the K^+ channels.

Just two years after Gorman and Hermann's experiments, single-channel recordings of Ca^{2+}-activated K^+ conductances were made by Alain Marty (1981) from chromaffin cells and by Barrett, Magleby, and Pallotta (1982) from rat skeletal muscle. In both sets of experiments, isolated inside-out patches of membrane were pulled from the cell (see Fig. 1.4), so that the membrane could be voltage-clamped and the cytoplasmic surface of the channel exposed to solutions of varying Ca^{2+} concentration. As the Ca^{2+} concentration was increased, both the frequency and duration of opening of the channels increased (see Fig. 7.7A). When, for the skeletal muscle channels, the current of an open channel was measured in internal and external solutions both containing the same concentration of K^+ (144 mM) and then plotted as a function of the patch potential (Fig. 7.7B), the i–V curve was linear, with a slope of 230 pS. This is about 10 times larger than the single-channel conductance of a typical delayed rectifier (for example squid axon—see Bezanilla and Correa, 1995).

Since the experiments on both chromaffin cells and skeletal muscle were done with isolated (inside-out) patches, Ca^{2+} can apparently gate channels in the absence of any cytoplasmic enzymes or other factors, suggesting that Ca^{2+} binds directly to the channel. In addition to their sensitivity to Ca^{2+}, Ca^{2+}-activated K^+ conductances in *Aplysia* neurons (Gorman and Thomas, 1980b), chromaffin cells (Marty, 1981), and skeletal muscle (Barrett, Magleby, and Pallotta, 1982) are also quite sensitive to voltage. In skeletal muscle, the probability of opening of the channels is low at negative membrane potentials (see Fig. 7.8). At positive membrane potentials, on the other hand, Ca^{2+} can cause the channel to be open nearly all of the time. The probability of opening seems to depend upon both Ca^{2+} and voltage in some coordinated fashion, not yet completely understood.

Fig. 7.7 Ca^{2+}-activated K^+ currents: single-channel recordings from skeletal muscle. **(A)** Recordings from inside-out patches pulled from the surface membrane of embryonic rat myotubes. Both pipette and bathing solutions contained the same (144 mM) K^+ concentration. Free Ca^{2+} in the pipette solution (exposed to the external surface of the membrane of the patch) was 0.01 μM. Concentration of Ca^{2+} in bath (exposed to the cytoplasmic surface of the membrane of the patch) is noted above each record. Ca^{2+} was buffered with EGTA to produce the desired free-Ca^{2+} concentration (see Chapter 13). Membrane potential was +20 mV, and openings are indicated by upward deflections. Records indicate that three channels were active in this patch, whose current level appears to the left of the records as follows: c, level with all channels closed (zero current); o_1, level with one channel open; o_2, two channels open; and o_3, all three channels open. **(B)** Plot of single-channel current as a function of membrane potential, with Ca^{2+} in the bathing medium (facing cytoplasmic side of membrane) set to 1 μM (circles) or 1 mM (triangles). Line is for conductance of 230 pS. (Reprinted from Barrett, Magleby, and Pallotta, 1982, with permission of the authors and of the Physiological Society.)

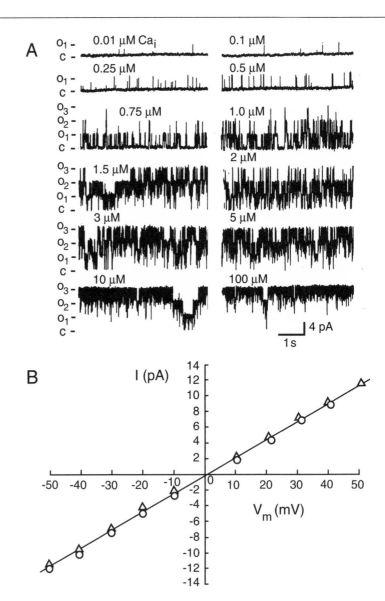

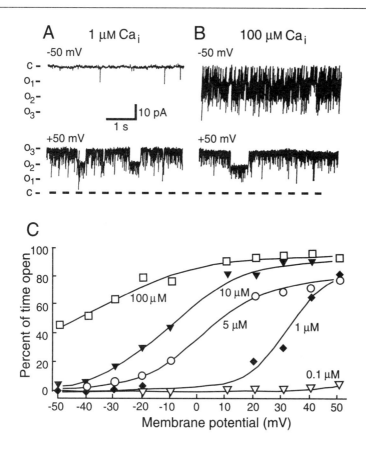

Fig. 7.8 Effect of membrane potential on activity of Ca^{2+}-activated K^+ channels. Inside-out recordings as in Fig. 7.7. **(A)** Free-Ca^{2+} concentration bathing cytoplasmic surface of membrane, 1 μM. Channel activity recorded at two membrane potentials (−50 and +50 mV), as indicated. Note that at −50mV, channel openings are downward (channel currents are negative), whereas at +50mV channel currents are upward (positive)—see Fig. 7.7B. **(B)** As in **(A)**, but internal free-Ca^{2+} concentration was 100 μM. **(C)** Plot of percentage of time channels were open as a function of membrane potential, at five cytoplasmic free-Ca^{2+} concentrations, as indicated near each curve. (Reprinted from Barrett, Magleby, and Pallotta, 1982, with permission of the authors and of the Physiological Society.)

Different Kinds of Ca^{2+}-Activated K^+ Currents

The very large Ca^{2+}-activated channels—which have been observed in chromaffin cells, skeletal muscle cells, and many other cell types including neurons—have been called *BK* channels (sometimes also *maxi-K* or *Big Brother*). These channels constitute a very diverse group (Blatz and Magleby, 1987; Latorre et al., 1989) having similar ion selectivity (with $K^+ \gg Na^+$), and in many cases they can be blocked by charybdotoxin (CTX), a toxin from the scorpion, *Leiurus quinquestriatus* (Miller et al., 1985), and by iberiotoxin from another scorpion, *Buthus tamulus* (Galvez et al., 1990). In spite of these similarities, the channels vary widely in their Ca^{2+} dependence and sensitivity to block by TEA.

In place of or in addition to BK channels, many cells also have Ca^{2+}-activated K^+ channels with a smaller unitary conductance (10–50 pS), called *SK* channels. This group of channels seems also rather diverse in its properties (Latorre et al., 1989; Sah, 1996) but in some cases can be distinguished from BK channels by an insensitivity to charybdotoxin and sensitivity to the bee venom toxin apamin. SK channels seem to be less voltage-dependent and more sensitive to intracellular Ca^{2+} than BK channels, though there is considerable variability within both groups. Both SK and BK channels are found in skeletal muscle (Blatz and Magelby, 1987), where they are clearly gated by different $[Ca^{2+}]_i$ and may have different functions.

We know only a little about the structure of Ca^{2+}-activated K^+ channels (see Ganetzky et al., 1995). The first Ca^{2+}-activated K^+ channel α subunit gene to be cloned was that coded by the gene for the *Drosophila slowpoke (slo)*. Animals with defective *slo* gene products have uncoordinated and sluggish movements, and the defect seems to be attributable to a specific loss of a Ca^{2+}-activated K^+ conductance.

The gene product coded by the *slo* locus was shown to be a protein similar in many respects to the α subunit of voltage-gated K^+ channels, but with some important differences (Atkinson, Robertson, and Ganetzky, 1991). The protein is nearly twice as large as the *Shaker* protein. The amino-terminal half looks very much like any other potassium channel α subunit, with six putative transmembrane domains, a clearly evident S4 sequence, and a P domain similar in amino acid composition to that of *Shaker* and the other *Drosophila* K^+ channels (*Shab, Shaw,* and *Shal*). The carboxyl-terminal half of the *slo* gene product is much larger and not homologous to that of any other K^+ channel α subunit. Between the end of S6 and the COOH terminus, there may be as many as 850 amino acids whose conformation is unknown, perhaps including membrane-spanning domains. Mammalian genes homologous to *slo* have been identified in several species, and these are similar: they are at least 50 percent larger than voltage-gated K^+ channel α subunit genes, with a large carboxyl-terminal region of unknown structure, which contains at least part of the site of Ca^{2+} sensitivity (Wei et al., 1994).

Both *Drosophila* and mammalian genes can be alternatively

spliced to produce many variants (Atkinson, Robertson, and Ganetzky, 1991; Adelman et al., 1992; Butler et al., 1993), and β subunits have been characterized (Knaus et al., 1994; Tseng-Crank et al., 1996) that, when expressed with α subunits, alter the kinetics and both the Ca^{2+} and voltage dependence of the current (McManus et al., 1995; Tseng-Crank et al., 1996). Alternative splicing of the α subunit and modulation of β subunit expression could conceivably be responsible for some of the variety of properties of Ca^{2+}-activated K^+ channels found in different cell types.

The *slo* gene and its mammalian relatives produce only BK channels. The gene for a protein having many of the properties of an SK channel has also been cloned (Köhler, Hirschberg, Bond, et al., 1996) and appears to have a structure similar to that of BK channels, with 6 putative transmembrane domains, a P domain, and a long carboxyl-terminal tail. These channels represent yet another family of K^+ channel proteins, whose structure, function, and relationship to other channel types are topics of active investigation.

Function of Ca^{2+}-Activated K^+ Channels

Ca^{2+}-activated K^+ channels function much like voltage-gated K^+ channels: as the cell is depolarized, they open and allow the outward flow of K^+. In most neurons $[Ca^{2+}]_i$ increases during depolarization, because depolarization activates voltage-gated Ca^{2+} channels (see Section III of this chapter). Thus Ca^{2+}-activated K^+ channels can be activated during the time course of an action potential and contribute to spike repolarization (Storm, 1987; Sah, 1996). If $[Ca^{2+}]_i$ were buffered strongly inside the cell, so that Ca^{2+} is rapidly bound and slowly released, $[Ca^{2+}]_i$ might increase and decrease with a slower time course than the time course of voltage change. This would have the effect that Ca^{2+}-activated channels could be used by neurons to produce slow changes in K^+ conductance and membrane excitability.

Ca^{2+}-activated K^+ conductances, particularly those of the SK variety, are often responsible for producing a slow hyperpolarization following an action potential. Fig. 7.9A reproduces two recordings from a frog motoneuron (from Barrett and Barrett, 1976), the first in normal external solution and the second in low-Ca^{2+} solution. A single spike is followed by a brief negativity, like that

Fig. 7.9 Role of Ca^{2+}-activated K$^+$ conductance in producing after-hyperpolarizations. Intracellular recordings from motoneurons in the frog spinal cord. **(A)** An action potential was evoked by injection of a brief pulse of depolarizing current. Full amplitude of spike cannot be seen in this recording (note voltage scale). Spike was then followed by rapid hyperpolarization (probably due to a delayed-rectifier current) and a much slower after-hyperpolarization in cells in normal Ringer solution (*left*). The slow after-hyperpolarization was abolished when cell was bathed in solution containing low Ca^{2+} (*right*). **(B)** Repetitive discharge of motoneuron in normal Ringer solution to step injection of current (time course of injection indicated by lowermost trace). Note the slow decrease in rate of spike firing, called *spike accommodation*. (Modified from Barrett and Barrett, 1976.)

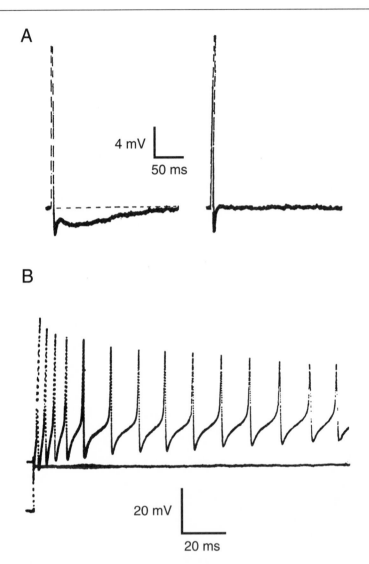

in Fig. 5.1B, shown here on a much slower time scale and probably produced by a voltage-gated delayed-rectifier K$^+$ conductance. This "dip" is then succeeded by a much slower wave of hyperpolarization, which is abolished in low-Ca^{2+} solution (Fig. 7.9A, *right*) since it is likely to be produced by Ca^{2+}-activated K$^+$ channels.

Although in some cells spike firing produces sufficient entry of Na^+ to activate the Na^+/K^+ ATPase and hyperpolarize the cell membrane (see Chapter 4 and Fig. 4.6), in many cells the increase in Na^+ is too small (or the resistance of the cell too low) for activation of the pump to have much of an effect on membrane potential. This is particularly true of cells with relatively large cell bodies, like motoneurons, which nevertheless often have prominent slow after-hyperpolarizations produced by Ca^{2+}-activated K^+ conductances (see Sah, 1996). Since the buildup of Ca^{2+} occurs slowly, it can increase with successive action potentials to produce a gradually increasing permeability to K^+. This can have the effect of gradually hyperpolarizing the cell and slowing down the rate of action potential production, an effect often referred to as *spike adaptation*. Fig. 7.9B illustrates spike adaptation occurring in a frog motoneuron, and other experiments indicate that adaptation of this sort is mostly due to a slow buildup of Ca^{2+} and increase in the Ca^{2+}-activated K^+ conductance.

Inward Rectifiers

A group of K^+ channels quite unlike the ones so far described was discovered unexpectedly by Bernard Katz (1949). Katz bathed a skeletal muscle in high-K^+ solution, anticipating that with the K^+ concentration nearly symmetric on the two sides of the muscle membrane, the conductance of the membrane would also become symmetric. To his surprise, this did not happen: the membrane became much more conductive for inward currents when the voltage was made negative than for outward currents when the muscle membrane potential was made positive. Katz called this rectification *anomalous*, because current flow was larger for hyperpolarizations than for depolarizations, unlike that of voltage-gated K^+ conductances like delayed rectifiers. I prefer a somewhat more recent nomenclature, however, and refer to this channel as the *inward rectifier*.

Inward rectifiers have been observed in neurons (see Llinás, 1988), but they have been studied in more detail in other cell types, such as skeletal muscle (Adrian, 1969) and the eggs of tunicates and starfish (Hagiwara and Jaffe, 1979). Some characteristic features of these conductances are illustrated in Fig. 7.10. Part A of this figure plots (for a starfish egg) current-voltage curves for three different extracellular K^+ concentrations. Notice first that the currents are quite small in the outward direction but large in the inward direction, as Katz first observed. Notice also that the current reverses near E_K and is quite selective for K^+ (see also Latorre and Miller, 1983; Rudy, 1988). Finally, observe that the shape of the current-voltage curve and of the curve relating conductance to voltage (Fig. 7.10B) seems to depend not upon voltage per se but rather upon the equilibrium potential for potassium (see Hagiwara and Takahashi, 1974; Hagiwara, Miyazaki, and Rosenthal, 1976). As external K^+ is altered, the conductance-voltage curve slides along the voltage axis, by an amount determined approximately by the shift in E_K. Experiments in both starfish (Hagiwara and Yoshii, 1979) and muscle (Leech and Stanfield, 1981) have shown that this peculiar shift in voltage dependence happens only when *external* K^+ is changed: internal K^+ has little effect.

Fig. 7.10 Dependence of inward rectification on voltage and external K^+ concentration. Recordings from a two-electrode voltage clamp of intact egg of starfish *Mediaster aequalis*. **(A)** Current-voltage curve for steady-state current (I_S) at three different external K^+ concentrations, indicated by labels adjacent to the curves. Note shift in reversal potential. **(B)** Steady-state chord conductance of inward rectifier as a function of membrane potential, calculated from data in **(A)** as $g_K = I_S / (V_m - V_0)$, where V_0 is the reversal potential from graph in **(A)**. Curves are shown for three K^+ concentrations, and values of reversal potentials are indicated by arrows. (Reprinted from Hagiwara and Yoshii, 1979, with permission of M. Yoshii and the Physiological Society.)

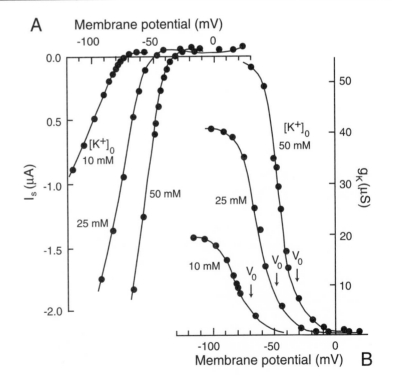

The shift in the voltage dependence of conductance as a function of external K^+ is not observed for delayed rectifiers and A currents and seems to indicate that inward rectifiers are not gated by voltage per se but rather by some other mechanism that is affected by the external K^+ concentration. Suppose, for example, that the cytoplasm (or the channel itself) contained a positively charged particle that could enter the channel pore from the inside and block the current (Hagiwara and Takahashi, 1974; Armstrong, 1975; Hille and Schwarz, 1978; Standen and Stanfield, 1978). Suppose in addition that this particle could be knocked off by K^+ entering the pore from the outside but not by K^+ attempting to enter the pore from the inside. Then outward currents would be small, since the particle would occlude the pore; inward currents, however, could be large, since K^+ coming into the channel from the outside could knock the particle off and keep it from occupying its blocking site by electrostatic repulsion. The larger the external K^+ concentration, the greater the probability that the channel would be unblocked and conduct current.

There is now excellent evidence that the peculiar voltage dependence of the inward rectifier is in large part the result of such a block by cytoplasmic particles, and at least two kinds of particles have been discovered: Mg^{2+} and cytoplasmic polyamines, such as spermine and spermidine. Blocking by Mg^{2+} was first discovered for inward rectifiers in the heart (Matsuda, Saigusa, and Irisawa, 1987; Vandenberg, 1987), but similar experiments have now been done on cloned and expressed inwardly rectifying channels (Nichols, Ho, and Herbert, 1994). Removal of Mg^{2+} from the internal surface of the plasma membrane (in an inside-out patch) is sufficient for some inwardly rectifying channels to remove completely the rectification of the i–V curve: inward currents are nearly unaffected, but outward currents become much larger, and the i–V curve becomes nearly linear (see for example Vandenberg, 1987; Nichols, Ho, and Herbert, 1994).

For some cells, Mg^{2+} removal has little or no effect on inward rectification (see for example Silver and DeCoursey, 1990). Although inward rectifiers in these cells were once postulated to have *intrinsic* voltage dependence, it would now seem that most of this apparently intrinsic voltage gating is actually due to blocking by another group of particles, cytoplasmic polyamines (Ficker et

Fig. 7.11 Inward rectification can be produced by block by polyamines. *HRK1* genes for inwardly rectifying K$^+$ channels were expressed in *Xenopus* oocytes. Membrane potential of oocyte was brought to near 0 mV by perfusion with high-K$^+$ solution. **(A)** Recording on slow time base of currents from oocyte patch in response to voltages of −50 and +50 mV. Voltage protocol is shown in lowermost trace in **(B)** and was repeated at 3 s intervals. Recordings are for on-cell patch, which was excised (to form inside-out patch) at arrow. Horizontal line through record indicates zero current level, with inward currents downward and outward currents upward from this line. Numbers refer to recordings in **(B)**. **(B)** Recordings from same preparation as in **(A)**, but with faster time scale. Note that excision of patch produced slow increase in the amplitude of the outward current in response to positive voltage step. **(C)** Recordings as in **(A)** and **(B)**, 3 min after formation of inside-out patch in control intracellular bathing solution (*left*) and for bathing solution containing 25 µM (*center*) or 1 mM (*right*) spermidine. Note selective block of outward currents. Pipette and bathing solutions contained 140 mM KCl. Voltage protocol is indicated in upper right. (Reprinted from Lopatin, Makhina, and Nichols, 1994, with permission of the authors and of Macmillan Magazines Limited.)

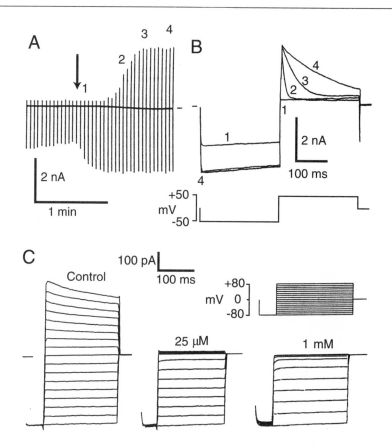

al., 1994; Lopatin, Makhina, and Nichols, 1994; Fakler, Brändle, Bond et al., 1994). A typical result is given in Fig. 7.11 (from Lopatin, Makhina, and Nichols, 1994), for an inwardly rectifying current recorded from an oocyte injected with cRNA for one of the inward rectifier genes (*HRK1* or *Kir2.3*)—I shall describe the molecular biology of inward rectifiers shortly. Recordings were first made on-cell from large membrane patches, with the K$^+$ concentration in the pipette approximately equimolar with that inside the cell ($E_K \sim 0$ mV). The voltage was stepped from a holding potential of 0 mV first to −50 mV and then to +50 mV (see lowermost trace in Fig. 7.11B), and the current responses that were recorded are shown on a slow time base in Fig. 7.11A. The inward currents are large and the outward currents small. The patch was then pulled off the oocyte (arrow in Fig. 7.11A), and the inside surface of the membrane was bathed in high-K^+, zero-Mg^{2+} solution. With time, outward currents appeared, and after a sufficiently long perfusion of the inside surface of the membrane with the bathing medium, the i–V curve became nearly linear, as illustrated by currents recorded from a similar patch 3 minutes after isolation (Fig. 7.11C, *left*). The block of the outward currents can be restored by moving the patch back toward the oocyte, treating the patch with an oocyte-conditioned medium, or adding spermine or spermidine (without Mg^{2+}) to the medium bathing the internal surface of the membrane patch (Fig. 7.11C, *center* and *right*).

These experiments and similar results from other laboratories (Ficker et al., 1994; Fakler, Brändle, Bond, et al., 1994) indicate that inward rectification in the absence of Mg^{2+} can be produced with concentrations of cytoplasmic polyamines similar to those actually found within cells (Ficker et al., 1994). Inward rectification would therefore seem to be produced by blocking either by Mg^{2+} or by polyamines, or by both together, though the contribution of other blocking particles or of part of the protein of the inward rectifier itself cannot at present be excluded.

Cloning of Inward Rectifiers: Structure and Function

The cloning and sequencing of several inwardly rectifying K^+ channel genes has greatly increased our understanding of these proteins (see for example Ho et al., 1993; Kubo, Baldwin, et al., 1993; Kubo, Reuveny, et al., 1993; Dascal et al., 1993; Ashford et al., 1994; Spauschus et al., 1996). A large number of related genes have now been described (see Doupnik, Davidson, and Lester, 1995; Nichols and Lopatin, 1997), at least some of which can undergo alternative spicing. Like voltage-gated and Ca^{2+}-activated K^+ channels, the inward rectifiers can be posttranslationally modified by direct phosphorylation (Fakler, Brändle, Glowatzki, et al., 1994). The variety of channel properties is further increased by heteromeric assembly of two or more different channel types into a single functional unit (Krapivinsky et al., 1995; Kofuji, Davidson, and Lester, 1995; Spauschus et al., 1996).

The proteins coded by inward-rectifier genes are much smaller than voltage-gated K^+ channel proteins and appear to have only

Fig. 7.12 Hypothesized membrane topology of inward rectifier K$^+$ channel protein. (Redrawn from Ho et al., 1993.)

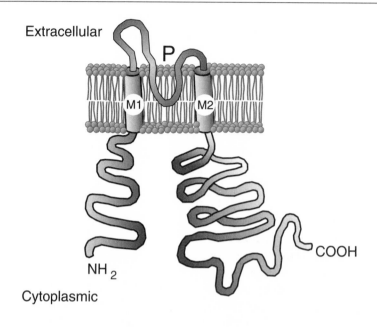

two domains long enough and sufficiently hydrophobic to traverse the membrane (M1 and M2—Fig. 7.12). These domains show some homology to S5 and S6 of voltage-gated K$^+$ channels (Jan and Jan, 1994, 1997), as if the inward rectifier were derived from an ancestral gene from which the carboxyl-terminal third of the voltage-gated K$^+$ channel gene was also derived. Although the exact conformation of the inward-rectifier protein is not yet known, the amino and carboxyl termini have numerous consensus sites for phosphorylation and are probably intracellular. The M1-M2 linker region has a potential site for glycosylation and is probably at least partially extracellular. The M1-M2 linker also has a sequence with high homology to the Na$^+$ and K$^+$ channel P domain, which may dip into the membrane and form part of the channel pore. It is likely that a functional channel is formed from 4 subunits, like the one shown in Fig. 7.12 (Yang, Jan, and Jan, 1995b).

The similarity of the sequence of the P domain of inward rectifiers to that of voltage-gated Na$^+$ and K$^+$ channels strongly suggests that this domain forms part of the channel (see Box 7.2). There is evidence that the properties of the pores of inward rectifiers are also strongly influenced by the carboxyl-terminal part of the pro-

Box 7.2

ATOMIC STRUCTURE OF THE PORE OF A POTASSIUM CHANNEL

The low molecular weight and relative simplicity of inwardly rectifying K^+ channels make them excellent targets for structural studies. The smallest pore-forming K^+ channel proteins appear to be found in prokaryotes. The genome of the soil bacterium *Streptomyces lividans,* for example, contains a gene for a protein of only 160 amino acids, smaller even than the inward rectifiers of neurons. This protein (called $K_{Cs}A$) has only two trans-membrane α-helical domains (see Fig. 7.12) on either side of a clearly recognizable P domain, remarkably similar in its amino acid sequence to the P domain of the *Shaker* α subunit (Schrempf et al., 1995). When expressed, $K_{Cs}A$ forms channels selective for K^+.

After deleting the cytoplasmic terminal region of the protein to make it even smaller and simpler, Doyle et al. (1998) determined the structure of the *Streptomyces lividans* channel with X-ray crystallography at a resolution approaching 3.2 Å. This structure has many interesting features. When viewed from above (i.e. from the extracellular medium), the channel shows a fourfold symmetry produced by four $K_{Cs}A$ proteins that form the tetrameric structure of the channel. In the middle of this structure, there is a clearly identifiable pore large enough for a potassium ion to enter. When viewed from the side, the pore of the channel is surrounded by amino acids of the P domain and by α-helices in the shape of an inverted teepee. The ion channel is fairly wide near the center and at the cytoplasmic end of the protein but is more narrow near its extracellular orifice.

The narrow part of the pore near the extracellular surface is particularly interesting, since it may form the "selectivity filter" which determines the ion selectivity of the channel. This part of the pore is lined by amino acids from the P domain, whose carbonyl oxygens probably face the middle of the channel. Potassium ions from the extracellular solution surrounded by a shell of oxygens from hydrating water molecules may pass into the pore by replacing this shell of water with the carbonyl oxygens of the pore amino acids. The fixed diameter of this region of the

continued

> pore may be responsible for allowing K^+ to permeate but not the smaller Na^+ ion, since Na^+ may not be able to fit into the coordination sites of the carbonyl oxygens lining the channel. This narrow part of the channel is only 12 Å long and contains at least two binding sites for K^+. Potassium ions may bind to these sites sequentially as they pass through the channel, and the mutual repulsion between ions in these sites may speed the passage of ions through this part of the pore to permit rapid conduction through the channel.
>
> Since the structure of the P domain of the *Streptomyces lividans* channel is so similar to that of *Shaker* and other K^+ channel pore-forming subunits, it is possible, even likely that inferences about the structure of the pore in this protein will be applicable to other K^+ channels and even to Na^+ and Ca^{2+} channels. The results of Doyle et al. (1998) provide our first glimpse of the structure of a voltage-gated channel, and the methods they exploited give promise of a much more detailed understanding of ion selectivity and perhaps eventually of other properties of channel proteins.

tein (Taglialatela et al., 1994; Yang, Jan, and Jan, 1995a). Block by Mg^{2+} and polyamines is critically influenced by residues both on M2 (Lu and MacKinnon, 1994; Wible et al., 1994; Stanfield et al., 1994) and on the carboxyl terminus (Pessia et al., 1995; Yang, Jan, and Jan, 1995a).

Function of Inward Rectifiers

Inward rectifiers play many roles. In skeletal muscle, an inward rectifier is apparently the K^+ conductance responsible for the resting K^+ permeability that sets the value of the membrane potential (Katz, 1949; Hodgkin and Horowicz, 1960). Inward rectifiers are present in kidney (Ho et al., 1993) and in heart (Ashford et al., 1994), where they appear to contribute to K^+ transport and to the generation and modulation of the heart beat. Some inward rectifiers are blocked by internal ATP (Ashcroft, 1988). ATP-sensitive inward rectifiers are found in many tissues but are especially prominent in pancreatic β cells, where they help regulate the glucose-dependent secretion of insulin (see Babenko, Aguilar-Bryan, and Bryan, 1998).

In nerve cells, much as in skeletal muscle, inward rectifiers have been postulated to be responsible for setting the resting membrane potential. A cell with a large population of inwardly rectifying K^+ channels would have a stable resting permeability to K^+, which would be reduced by depolarization and so not interfere with the generation of action potentials. On the other hand, many neurons seem not to show much inward rectification under resting conditions, and it is still unclear for many cells what channels are responsible for the resting K^+ conductance. The most important neuronal inward rectifiers may in fact be a family of channels regulated by G proteins (see Doupnik, Davidson, and Lester, 1995; Jan and Jan, 1997). These channels have been shown to be coupled to a variety of transmitter receptors and to modulate changes in K^+ permeability produced by substances like dopamine, opioids, somatostatin, serotonin, and adenosine. I shall describe these channels and their second messenger pathways in more detail in Chapter 12.

III: Ca^{2+} CHANNELS

Ion channels selectively permeable to divalent ions are found in many cells in the body, including most if not all neurons. Like inwardly rectifying K^+ channels, channels selective for Ca^{2+} were discovered by accident. Paul Fatt and Bernard Katz (1953) were recording intracellularly from the muscle fibers of the crayfish, in order to study neuromuscular transmission. Intracellular recording was at this time a relatively new technique, and the experiments of Fatt and Katz were one of the first attempts to insert *two* microelectrodes into the same cell, one to apply current and the other to measure voltage. The large muscle fibers of crayfish were ideal for this purpose.

In preliminary experiments stimulating the muscle with depolarizing currents, Fatt and Katz noticed that in normal Ringer the fiber produced variable responses, and in many cases they observed only small, nonconducting action potentials. In order to see if these small spikes were Na^+-dependent, like those in squid axon, they replaced all of the Na^+ in the bath with choline, TEA, or tetra-butylammonium (TBA). Much to their surprise, the action potentials became larger and very prolonged, lasting up to 15–20 s. These results showed that the action potentials in crayfish muscle are produced not by Na^+ but by the entry (or exit) of some other ion.

Although it was initially possible to imagine that the ion producing the action potential was TEA or choline, this seemed unlikely for TBA, action potentials could be recorded even after the TBA was removed from the bathing solution; that is, the effect of the TBA was partially reversible. Since TBA also produced a depolarization of the resting potential and a decrease in the muscle membrane conductance, Fatt and Katz made the more likely suggestion that spikes became larger because choline, TEA, and TBA all block the muscle's K^+ conductance, with a relative effectiveness of TBA > TEA > choline. We now know this to be the case.

Later experiments by Fatt and Ginsborg (1958) demonstrated that although the spikes remained in zero-Na^+ solution, they were abolished when Ca^{2+} was removed from the Ringer. Ba^{2+} and Sr^{2+} could substitute for Ca^{2+}, and the amplitude and duration of the spike increased with increasing divalent ion concentration (Fig. 7.13). Similar Ca^{2+}-dependent action potentials were subsequently shown to be present in a wide variety of organisms and cell types, usually after exposure to a K^+ channel blocker such as TEA. In many preparations, Ca^{2+} spikes can also be evoked by exposure to extracellular Ba^{2+}, which both substitutes for Ca^{2+} in carrying current through the Ca^{2+} channels and blocks K^+ conductances; or by injection of the Ca^{2+} chelator EGTA (see Chapter 13 and Fig. 13.1) into the cell cytoplasm, to reduce activation of the Ca^{2+}-dependent K^+ conductance and increase the driving force for Ca^{2+} entry (Hagiwara and Naka, 1964). During the 1960s and 70's, Ca^{2+}-dependent action potentials were studied in considerable detail, particularly by the laboratory of Susumu Hagiwara (see Hagiwara 1973, 1975).

Voltage-clamp recordings from large cells—like barnacle muscle, snail neurons, and egg cells—provided the first information about the biophysics of voltage-gated Ca^{2+} currents (Hagiwara and Byerly, 1981). Ca^{2+} channels are activated by depolarization, with

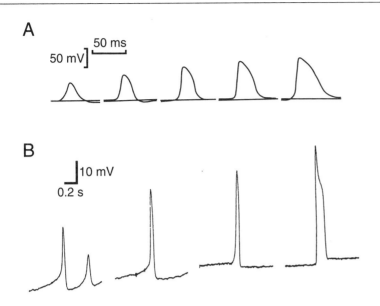

Fig. 7.13 Ca^{2+} spikes: dependence of amplitude on divalent ion concentration. **(A)** Action potentials recorded with intracellular micropipette from crayfish muscle fiber in different concentrations of extracellular Sr^{2+}, evoked by brief stimulating pulse. Sr^{2+} concentrations were as follows *(left to right):* 5 mM, 10 mM, 20 mM, 40 mM, and 80 mM. (Redrawn from Fatt and Ginsborg, 1958.) **(B)** Action potentials recorded with intracellular microelectrodes from rod photoreceptors from the toad *Bufo marinus*. Ringer solution contained 12 mM TEA and 1.8 mM Ca^{2+} *(record to left)*; or 12 mM TEA and 1.8 mM Ca^{2+} plus 3.6 mM, 7.2 mM, or 28 mM Sr^{2+} *(records to right)*. (Reprinted from Fain, Gerschenfeld, and Quandt, 1980, with permission of the authors and of the Physiological Society.)

a voltage dependence and kinetics of activation similar to though distinct from those of Na^+ channels. Many Ca^{2+} channels inactivate, although the time course of inactivation is quite variable from one cell type to another.

Recordings from the early experiments also gave the first indication that there are different types of Ca^{2+} channels (Hagiwara, Ozawa, and Sand, 1975), for which there is now abundant evidence (see Bean, 1989; Hess, 1990; Dunlap, Luebke, and Turner, 1995). Subsequently, voltage-gated Ca^{2+} channels were isolated biochemically (Catterall, Seagar, and Takahashi, 1988) and their genes cloned and sequenced (Tanabe et al., 1987), first from skeletal muscle. Skeletal muscle clones were then used to isolate a family of Ca^{2+} channel genes from many species, including human. Several different channel genes have now been isolated, and these appear to code for proteins with different activation and inactivation kinetics, single-channel conductance, and pharmacology (Zhang et al., 1993; Hofmann, Biel, and Flockerzi, 1994; Dunlap, Luebke, and Turner, 1995; Stea, Soong, and Snutch, 1995; Perez-Reyes and Schneider, 1995).

Structure and Diversity of Voltage-Gated Ca²⁺ Channels

The α subunit of Ca^{2+} channels is similar in structure to the α subunit of Na^+ channels, having four repeat units each consisting of 6 transmembrane domains (Fig. 7.14). Each repeat unit has a highly charged S4 domain and a P domain. As for Na^+ and K^+ channels, the α subunit is most responsible for voltage-dependent activation, permeation, and channel pharmacology.

Ca^{2+} channels also have a variety of auxiliary subunits. In skeletal muscle the auxiliary subunits are called β, α_2–δ, and γ, and genes for these proteins have all been cloned and studied in some detail (see Isom, DeJongh, and Catterall, 1994; Hofmann, Biel, and Flockerzi, 1994; Stea, Soong, and Snutch, 1995). The β subunit appears to be located mostly intracellularly and to bind to an identified cytoplasmic binding site on the α subunit (Pragnell et al., 1994). The α_2 and δ subunits are distinct proteins in muscle, connected by a disulphide bridge. Both δ and γ subunits have sequences that are thought to cross the membrane. Neuronal channels also contain auxiliary subunits, and the genes for several proteins similar to the skeletal muscle β and α_2–δ have been cloned from brain. With only a few exceptions, however, we have little information about which auxiliary subunits are associated with which α subunits.

Several different α subunit genes have been isolated, one *(α_{1S})* apparently expressed only in skeletal muscle and the rest expressed in a variety of tissues, including brain. Many of these genes have been shown to be alternatively spliced, and the number of different α subunit messages is likely to be several times larger than the number of genes. The α_{1S}, α_{1C}, and α_{1D} genes are more closely related to one another than the other α subunit genes, and they code for proteins that form channels with a similar pharmacology: all are sensitive to a group of organic compounds called dihydropyridines (DHPs), such as nimodipine, nitrendipine, and BAY K 8644. Channels expressed from these genes all tend to have a similar physiology, showing voltage activation at relatively depolarized voltages and slow inactivation. These channels are often referred to as *L-type* channels.

The α_{1B} gene (Williams et al., 1992) forms proteins for Ca^{2+} channels that are selectively blocked by a protein toxin called ω-

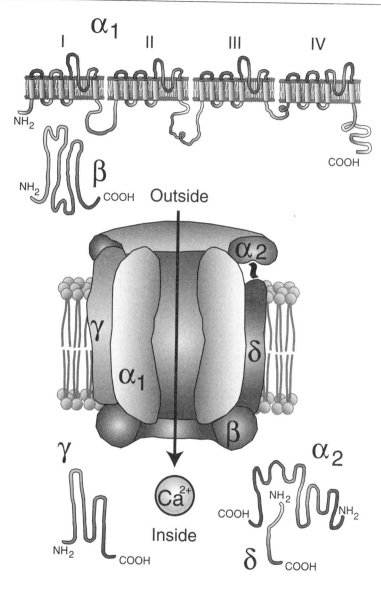

I   II   III   IV

α_1

NH₂

COOH

β

NH₂   COOH

Outside

α_2

γ   δ

α_1

β

γ   α₂

NH₂   COOH

Ca²⁺

Inside   COOH   NH₂   NH₂

δ   COOH

Fig. 7.14 Proposed structure of Ca^{2+} channel and membrane topology of each of subunits. (Redrawn from Hofmann, Biel, and Flockerzi, 1994, with reference also to Isom, DeJongh, and Catterall, 1994.)

conotoxin GVIA, from the venom of the marine snail *Conus geographus* (Kerr and Yoshikami, 1984). These channels are usually referred to as *N-type* and were first identified in cells of the dorsal root ganglion (Fox, Nowycky, and Tsien, 1987). N-type channels have now been recorded from cells in many regions of the brain

(Westenbroek et al., 1992). They appear to play an important role in the release of synaptic transmitter (Dunlap, Luebke, and Turner, 1995).

The mRNA from α_{1A} and α_{1E} cDNA can also be made to express Ca^{2+} channel proteins, but it is not yet clear whether these channels correspond to any of the Ca^{2+} currents that have been recorded from actual cells in the nervous system. The channels produced from α_{1A} mRNA (Sather et al., 1993; Stea et al., 1994), for example, are insensitive to DHPs and to ω-conotoxin GVIA but can be blocked by a toxin from the funnel web spider, ω-Aga-IVA. This toxin has been shown to block a Ca^{2+} channel variety called *P-type* (Mintz et al., 1992), first described from recordings from Purkinje cells (Llinás et al., 1992). However, the P-type channels in the CNS are in general much more sensitive to ω-Aga-IVA than are channels expressed from α_{1A} mRNA. This has led some investigators to suggest that channels expressed from α_{1A} mRNA are not P-type channels but are more closely related to neuronal channels termed *Q-type*—for example, those of cerebellar granule cells (Randall and Tsien, 1995). Q-type channels are relatively insensitive to ω-Aga-IVA but can be blocked by another *Conus* neurotoxin, called ω-conotoxin MVIIC.

Channels produced from α_{1E} mRNA (Soong et al., 1993; Ellinor et al., 1993; Schneider et al., 1994) are relatively insensitive to all known blocking compounds, except for divalent ions like Ni^{2+} and Cd^{2+}. There is some support for the notion that α_{1E} mRNA codes for channels sometimes called *R-type,* which are also relatively insensitive to blocking compounds, except for divalent cations. A recently cloned gene, α_{1G}, may code for a channel which is a member of a group of Ca^{2+} channels known as *T-type* (Perez-Reyes et al., 1998), which are low-threshold, rapidly inactivating Ca^{2+} channels found in cardiac and skeletal muscle and in many neurons (Bean, 1989; Hess, 1980; Huguenard, 1996).

At present we do not have a coherent view of how the many physiological types of Ca^{2+} channels are produced from the genes so far isolated, perhaps because (1) we do not have all the genes, (2) we have not studied all of the alternatively spliced forms of these genes, and/or (3) we do not yet know which auxiliary subunits go with which α subunits in actual neurons. The importance of auxiliary subunits, and in particular the β subunit, cannot be over-emphasized. Co-expression of β subunit mRNA with α subunit mRNA increases the peak amplitude of the Ca^{2+} current, at least in part because the β binds to the α subunit and increases the probability of channel opening (Neely et al., 1993). Co-expression of the β subunit can also dramatically alter the physiological properties of the Ca^{2+} current, and different β subunits can have different effects. The absence of a β subunit, as the result of mutation or gene knockout, can have serious consequences for the behavior of the organism, in some cases producing pronounced lethargy, ataxia, and seizures (Burgess et al., 1997).

At least 4 different β subunit genes have been identified (Stea, Soong, and Snutch, 1995; Dunlap, Luebke, and Turner, 1995). These, like the α subunits, have been shown to be alternatively spliced. The variable effects of different β subunits on Ca^{2+} channel properties can be seen from the results in Fig. 7.15, for which α_{1A} mRNA was injected into *Xenopus* oocytes with RNA from several different β genes (Stea et al., 1994). Co-injection with β RNA produced a consistent negative shift in the current-voltage curve (Fig. 7.15A) and a shift in steady-state inactivation (Fig. 7.15B), in most cases to more hyperpolarized membrane potentials but to more depolarized membrane potentials for β_{2a}. The time constant of inactivation (Figs. 7.15C and D) was either faster or slower, depending upon the β RNA injected. These results suggest that great care should be taken in any attempt to associate particular Ca^{2+} channel α subunit genes with native channels of a particular physiology. They also emphasize the large variety in physiological properties that can be achieved with different combinations of α and auxiliary subunits.

There is now general agreement for the classification of DHP-sensitive channels as L-type and their association with the α_{1S}, α_{1C}, and α_{1D} genes. There is also agreement that the α_{1B} gene codes for N-type channels with a high sensitivity to ω-conotoxin GVIA. However, there is no consensus about which Ca^{2+} channels are produced by the other genes, or about which of these genes (if any) codes for Ca^{2+} channel types that have been termed P, Q, R, and T (Bean and Mintz, 1994). Since many Ca^{2+} channel types have been shown to contribute to the release of synaptic transmitter, often with several different varieties in the same cell (Dunlap, Luebke, and Turner, 1995), and since these proteins are important targets for synaptic modulation (see Chapter 12), it is imperative that we identify and characterize the different proteins in

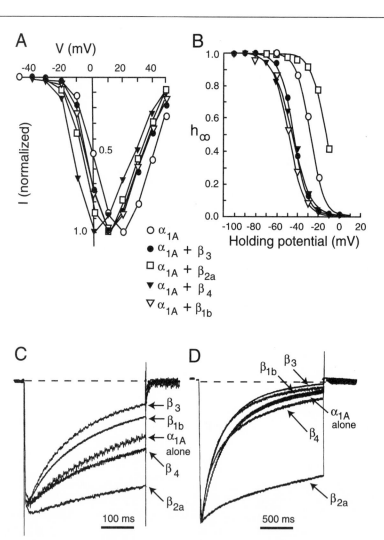

Fig. 7.15 Effect of the expression of genes for different β subunits on Ca^{2+} channel currents. The RNAs for α_{1A} alone and α_{1A} in combination with RNA for a Ca^{2+} channel β subunit were injected into *Xenopus* oocytes, and recordings were made with a two-electrode voltage clamp. **(A)** Voltage dependence of peak Ca^{2+} current, normalized to the maximum current for each recording condition (i.e., for each different RNA injection). Note consistent shift of curve to more negative voltages produced by β co-expression. **(B)** Steady-state inactivation as a function of voltage (h_∞ curve). Note again shift to negative voltages for all β RNAs except β_{2a}. **(C)** Waveform of current responses to 400 ms test pulse from V_H of -100 mV to test voltage of $+10$ mV. **(D)** Same as **(C)** but test pulse was 2 s. (Reprinted from Stea et al., 1994, with permission of the authors and of the National Academy of Sciences.)

nerve terminals responsible for Ca^{2+} influx during membrane depolarization.

Structure and Function: Permeation

Since the overall structure of a Ca^{2+} channel α subunit appears to be similar to that of a Na^+ channel α subunit, with 4 repeat units each similar to a voltage-gated K^+ channel α subunit, it would not be too surprising if Ca^{2+} channels behaved much like Na^+ and K^+ channels. Ca^{2+} channels have highly charged S4 domains, as noted above, and these are probably at least in part responsible for voltage-dependent activation. Gating current measurements from Ca^{2+} channels from cut-open oocytes (Neely et al., 1993) indicate that about 10–12 charges move during Ca^{2+} channel activation (Noceti, Toro, and Stefani, 1996), similar to the value for K^+ channels.

Ca^{2+} channels have a recognizable P domain between S5 and S6 in each repeat unit, and several studies indicate that this domain plays an important role in ion permeation. Ion permeation through Ca^{2+} channels has some rather peculiar features: Ca^{2+} channels are highly selective for divalent cations and quite impermeant to monovalent cations, provided divalent cations are present in the external medium. If, however, the external divalents are reduced to below 1 μM, monovalent ions become quite permeable (Almers, McCleskey, and Palade, 1984). The reason for this seems to be that the mouth of the Ca^{2+} channel contains high-affinity binding sites for divalent cations, and Ca^{2+} must bind to these sites before Ca^{2+} can pass through the channel (Almers and McCleskey, 1984). When Ca^{2+} is present, these binding sites are occupied sufficiently frequently by Ca^{2+} to prevent the movement of monovalent ions through the channel. When Ca^{2+} is removed from the external solution, monovalent ions are free to enter and permeate the channel. Divalent cations that block Ca^{2+} channels (such as Cd^{2+} and Co^{2+}) also bind to these same sites, often with higher affinity than Ca^{2+}, and so they prevent other ions (including Ca^{2+}) from permeating.

The sites to which Ca^{2+} and other divalent cations bind have been identified as 4 negatively charged glutamates, present in analogous positions in each of the P domains of the 4 repeat units of the Ca^{2+} channel (Heinemann et al., 1992; Yang et al., 1993; Kim et al., 1993). Mutation of any of these glutamates produces a change in divalent cation binding. Na^+ channels also have negatively charged glutamates or aspartates in the P domain in analogous positions, but only in repeats I and II and not in III and IV. In repeat III, for example, a Na^+ channel may have a positively charged lysine, and in repeat IV an uncharged alanine. If these lysine and alanine codons in the Na^+ channel gone are replaced with codons for glutamate and the cRNA is then injected into *Xenopus* oocytes, the permeation properties of the channel expressed are not those of a Na$^+$ channel but those of a Ca^{2+} channel. These experiments provide additional evidence that the P domain of Na$^+$ and Ca^{2+} channels plays a central role in determining ion selectivity.

Structure and Function: Inactivation

Two kinds of inactivation have been described for Ca^{2+} channels: one apparently produced by voltage and another produced by Ca^{2+} itself, which enters the channel and then blocks it (Eckert and Chad, 1984). Some channels (e.g., those formed from α_{1E}) appear to inactivate almost exclusively by a voltage-dependent mechanism. Surprisingly, the III-IV connecting loop, which appears to play a role in inactivation for Na$^+$ channels (see Chapter 6), may not be essential for voltage-dependent inactivation for Ca^{2+} channels (Zhang et al., 1994). β subunits also make an important contribution to the voltage dependence of inactivation (Olcese et al., 1994—see Fig. 7.15).

Ca^{2+}-dependent inactivation was first demonstrated in the unicellular organism *Paramecium* (Brehm and Eckert, 1978) but was subsequently observed in many cell types, including neurons (Eckert and Chad, 1984). It has two distinguishing characteristics: (1) inactivation is much larger when the current is carried by Ca^{2+} than when it is carried by Sr^{2+} or Ba^{2+}; and (2) the strength of inactivation does not depend upon voltage per se but rather upon the value of the current—in other words, the greater the current, the greater the entry of Ca^{2+} and block of the channel. This second characteristic is often used to identify Ca^{2+}-dependent inactivation, since the amplitude of the current through Ca^{2+} channels increases as the membrane is depolarized and then decreases again as the voltage approaches the Ca^{2+} equilibrium potential. As a consequence, Ca^{2+}-dependent inactivation also increases and then decreases.

The results in Fig. 7.16 are from recordings by Eckert and Tillotson (1981) from *Aplysia* neurons. In these experiments, inactivation was induced by a conditioning prepulse *(P1)* of variable voltage preceding a fixed test pulse *(P2)*, much as in the experiments described in Chapter 5 for the Na$^+$ channels of squid giant axon (see Figs. 5.13 and 5.15). For squid Na$^+$ channels, inactiva-

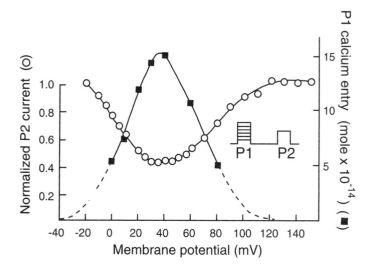

Fig. 7.16 Ca^{2+}-dependent inactivation of Ca^{2+} channels. Recordings were made with a two-electrode voltage clamp from neurons in the visceral ganglion of *Aplysia californica*. Neurons were filled with Cs^+ to block outward K^+ currents and bathed in artificial sea water containing 410 mM $Tris^+$ and 100 mM $CaCl_2$ (with no NaCl) to enhance amplitude of Ca^{2+} currents. Voltage protocol is shown in inset: a conditioning pulse *P1* was given for 200 ms to voltages whose values are given on the abscissa. After an interval of 400 ms, a second, test pulse *P2* was given, also 200 ms in duration, to a fixed voltage of +20 mV. Circles mark the peak amplitude of current recorded to pulse *P2* normalized to the maximum value of peak current, as a function of conditioning voltage *P1*. Squares plot the integral of current during pulse *P1*, also as a function of the amplitude of *P1*. Integrals were estimated by cutting the current records from chart paper and measuring the mass of the paper on a balance. $V_H = -40$ mV. (Reprinted from Eckert and Tillotson, 1981, with permission of D. L. Tillotson and the Physiological Society.)

tion varies as a simple function of the conditioning pulse, increasing with depolarization (Fig. 5.15B). For *Aplysia* Ca^{2+} current, on the other hand, the voltage dependence is more complex. The squares in Fig. 7.16 plot the integral of the Ca^{2+} current waveform for the conditioning pulse. The integral of the current waveform is proportional to the amount of Ca^{2+} entering the cell. The circles give the amplitude of the response to the test pulse, *P2*. The circles and squares have a similar but opposite dependence upon voltage: as the amount of Ca^{2+} entering the cell during *P1* increases, the amplitude of *P2* decreases. Voltage steps to very depolarized or very hyperpolarized potentials produced little if any inactivation, since at these voltages little Ca^{2+} entered the cell.

Ca^{2+}-dependent inactivation has so far been observed only for L-type channels. The mechanism of Ca^{2+}-dependent inactivation has been the subject of considerable debate but now seems to be due to binding of Ca^{2+} directly to a region of the α subunit (Neely et al., 1994; Imredy and Yue, 1994). For channels formed from the α_{1C} gene, the Ca^{2+}-binding domain has been located between the end of the last membrane-spanning sequence (S6) of the fourth repeat unit and the carboxyl terminus of the protein (deLeon et al., 1995).

IV: Cl⁻ Channels

In addition to transmitter-activated channels that are Cl⁻-permeable, such as GABA and glycine receptors (see Chapter 10), many if not all neurons have other kinds of channels selectively permeable to Cl⁻ (see Foskett, 1998). These channels come in a great variety: there are small-conductance Cl⁻ channels and large-conductance channels. There are channels that are activated by hyperpolarization and channels that are activated by depolarization (Chesnoy-Marchais, 1990; Franciolini and Petris, 1990; Blatz, 1994; Weiss, 1994; Franciolini and Adams, 1994). There are Cl⁻ channels with a very large unitary conductance that have the highest probability of opening when the membrane potential is zero and are closed by changes of membrane potential in either direction (Blatz, 1990). Other Cl⁻ channels show complicated patterns of voltage gating, called "double-barreled": the channel appears to have two separate pores for Cl⁻ gated together by hyperpolarization to bring the channel into a mode permissive for channel opening (Miller and Richard, 1990). A second gating process favored by depolarization then opens each of the two pores independently. Finally, there are Cl⁻ channels that are primarily gated by an increase in intracellular Ca^{2+}. Ca^{2+}-dependent Cl⁻ channels were first observed in vertebrate photoreceptors (Bader, Bertrand, and Schwartz, 1982) but have now been found in a variety of cell types, including dorsal root ganglion cells and spinal cord neurons (Mayer, Owen, and Barker, 1990).

What are all these Cl⁻ channels doing? The fair answer is that we do not know. In skeletal muscle, Cl⁻ is distributed passively across the plasma membrane (see Chapter 4), and Cl⁻ channels present in muscle at high density make an important contribution to the resting membrane conductance (Hodgkin and Horowicz, 1960). Mutations in the skeletal muscle chloride channel gene *(ClC-1)* can produce congenital myotonia (see Jentsch et al., 1995), similar (though not identical) in its symptoms to myotonia produced by Na^+ channel defects (as described in Box 7.1).

Most neurons probably also have a small contribution from the Cl⁻ gradient to the resting membrane potential (see Chapter 3). Ca^{2+}-dependent Cl⁻ channels can produce after-hyperpolarizations (or after-depolarizations) following the entry of Ca^{2+} during an ac-

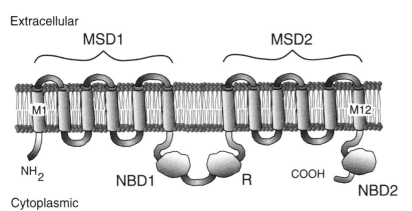

Extracellular

MSD1   MSD2

M1   M12

NH$_2$ NBD1   R   COOH   NBD2

Cytoplasmic

Fig. 7.17 Hypothesized membrane topology of the cystic fibrosis transmembrane conductance regulator (CFTR). *MSD*, membrane-spanning domain; *NBD*, nucleotide-binding domain; *R*, regulatory region. (After Welsh et al., 1994.)

tion potential (Mayer, Owen, and Barker, 1990), though it is unclear how large these responses are under physiological conditions. In many cells chloride channels play an important role in regulatory responses to osmotic swelling (Strange, Emma, and Jackson, 1996).

The Cl$^-$ channel that is best known and was the first whose gene was cloned and sequenced is not a skeletal muscle or neuronal channel but a channel found in many epithelia, called the *cystic fibrosis transmembrane conductance regulator,* or CFTR (Welsh et al., 1994; Hanrahan et al., 1995). The structure of this molecule resembles none of the other ion channels I have so far described. There appear to be five large domains (see Fig. 7.17): first a region called membrane-spanning domain one (MSD1), consisting of 6 putative membrane-spanning sequences; followed by two cytoplasmic regions, one that binds nucleotides (NBD1) and another that is regulatory (R), both of which contain multiple sites for phosphorylation; and then a second membrane-spanning domain (MSD2) and a second nucleotide binding region (NBD2) near the carboxyl terminus.

When the gene for CFTR was first cloned, it was thought by many to be a transporter, not a channel, since its structure is much more similar to that of the Na$^+$/K$^+$ ATPase (see Fig. 4.1) or the Na$^+$/Ca^{2+} countertransporter (Fig. 4.8) than to that of any of the voltage-gated channels. The evidence, however, is now very strong that CFTR does form a voltage-independent channel selective for anions and regulated by phosphorylation and ATP. This protein has been the focus of intense interest, since it is the protein whose defect is in most cases responsible for the inherited disorder of the respiratory system called *cystic fibrosis*. However, CFTR has been found mostly in membranes of epithelial cells, and there is little evidence so far that it plays an important role in the physiology of nerve cells.

Some progress has been made identifying and cloning other Cl⁻ channels, including two (called ClC-0 and ClC-2) found in cells in the brain (Jentsch, 1994; Petris, Trequattrini, and Franciolini, 1994). These channels, and the related protein ClC-1 whose gene was cloned from muscle, appear to lack the nucleotide-binding and regulatory domains of CFTR but are thought to have 8–10 transmembrane sequences, and they also look more like transporters than channels. The relationship between these two groups of proteins may be closer than once thought, since it is now apparent that some transporters have an additional role as membrane channels. Glutamate transporters, for example, which transport glutamate from the extracellular space into the cell cytoplasm, are also permeable to Cl⁻ (Fairman, Vandenberg, Arriza, et al., 1995; Wadiche, Amara, and Kavanaugh, 1995). This Cl⁻ permeability may play an important role in the physiology of certain neurons, particularly in the retina (Eliasof and Werblin, 1993; Grant and Dowling, 1995; Grant and Werblin, 1996).

The study of the structure and function of Cl⁻ channels has barely begun. A few channel genes have been cloned, but many more still remain to be investigated. Many studies have shown that Cl⁻ channel activity can be recorded from nerve cell membrane, and the properties of these channels have in some cases been studied in considerable detail. These observations have given only a rudimentary idea of the role these channels play in the normal physiology of the cell.

Summary

There is an immense variety of different channel types in neurons. This is a consequence first of the many different families of channels. Although there is apparently only one family of genes for voltage-gated Na$^+$ channel α subunits, there are several members of this family, and these genes can be alternatively spliced and expressed with different auxiliary proteins (β subunits) to produce a large variety of channel types. For K$^+$ channels, the diversity is much greater. There are several channel families, including the voltage-gated (delayed rectifier and *A* current) family, the Ca^{2+}-dependent K$^+$ channels, and the inward rectifiers. Again, within each family several genes may be alternatively spliced and expressed with alternative auxiliary proteins. Voltage-gated Ca^{2+} channels and Cl$^-$ channels are also quite variable in their structure and physiological characteristics.

This diversity of channel types clearly has important physiological consequences, which we are only just beginning to understand. It is responsible for differences in properties like the voltage-dependence of activation and inactivation, activation and inactivation time course, single-channel conductance, and pharmacology. Different channels are expressed in different cell types, and channels of one kind may be expressed preferentially in dendrites and those of another kind near the cell body. It seems likely that there are good reasons why one channel is expressed here and another there. Unfortunately, for the most part, these explanations still elude us.

This chapter presents only a partial description of the different kinds of channels present in neurons. Of those omitted are several interesting kinds of K$^+$ channels, including Na$^+$-activated K$^+$ channels (Bader, Bernheim, and Bertrand, 1985), the *Ether-à-go-go* channel (Warmke, Drysdale, and Ganetzky, 1991; Brüggemann et al., 1993; Ganetzky et al., 1995), and outward rectifiers, which, like inward rectifiers, derive their voltage sensitivity from channel block rather than voltage-dependent gating (Ketchum et al., 1995). Also not described here are proton channels (Thomas and Meech, 1982; DeCoursey and Cherny, 1994) and a current called i_f or i_h, which is activated by hyperpolarization, as are inwardly rectifying K$^+$ currents, but is readily permeable to both Na$^+$ and K$^+$ (Bader, Bertrand, and Schwartz, 1982; Mayer and Westbrook, 1983; Schlichter, Bader, and Bernheim, 1991; DiFrancesco, 1994; Pape, 1996). No mention has been made of *persistent* Na$^+$ currents, which resemble voltage-gated Na$^+$ currents and are blocked by

TTX but do not inactivate (Crill, 1996). I have also left out a description of a very important Ca^{2+} channel called i_{CRAC}, which is more selectively permeable to Ca^{2+} than voltage-gated Ca^{2+} channels are and is not gated by voltage (Hoth and Penner, 1992). The i_{CRAC} channels may be gated by a cytosolic intracellular messenger and appear to open for the refilling of intracellular Ca^{2+} stores after these have been depleted by intracellular Ca^{2+} release. A fuller description of these channels appears in Chapter 13.

The diversity of ion channel types is one of the most puzzling and intriguing aspects of the molecular physiology of neurons. This diversity is characteristic not only of voltage-gated channels but also of transmitter ligand-gated channels (Chapters 9 and 10) and metabotropic receptors (Chapter 11). As we learn more about how different channel types are distributed and what these channels do, we may begin to understand why so many different types are needed.

Synaptic Transmission and Ligand-Gated Channels

8

Presynaptic Mechanisms of Synaptic Transmission

Part Three of this book describes the fundamental basis of nerve cell communication: the physiology of synaptic transmission. Synapses are the basic building blocks for neural integration. Understanding how they work is absolutely essential for understanding how signals travel from one cell to another, and how they are processed within the central nervous system. Synapses are also the sites of activity for mechanisms of neuromodulation that strengthen or weaken neural activity during learning and memory. Finally, synapses are important clinically. The proteins responsible for releasing transmitter and the receptors to which transmitters bind are common targets of psychoactive drugs used clinically to treat mental disorders.

Although many different kinds of cellular communication in the CNS have been postulated or described, I shall confine discussion to the two most common forms: electrical synapses at gap junctions and chemical synapses of the usual sort, for which the chemical transmitter is contained within membranous vesicles and is released by a Ca^{2+}-dependent mechanism at specialized sites within the presynaptic terminal.

I: GAP JUNCTIONS

Electrical synapses are formed by gap junctions, which are well-organized regions of contact between adjacent cells. In transmission electron microscopy, gap junctions appear as closely opposed regions of plasma membrane separated by a small but regular gap of 1–2 nm (see Fig. 8.1A). They can also be recognized in freeze-fracture replicas as plaques of membrane particles in each of the

Fig. 8.1 Electron microscopy of gap junctions. **(A)** Thin-section transmission electron micrograph. Note that normal extracellular space *(arrows)* is replaced by a dense band that contains the external domains of the connexin molecules. Scale bar, 0.1 μm (100 nm). **(B)** Freeze-fracture replica of gap junction. Note again reduction in the width of extracellular space *(arrows)*. Fracture plane passed from the external (exoplasmic) leaflet (E face) of the plasma membrane of one cell to the internal (protoplasmic) leaflet (P face) of the membrane of the neighboring cell. Junction is composed of aggregates of cell-to-cell channels that fractured, leaving particles about 8 nm in diameter on the P face with complementary pits on the E face. Scale bar, 0.1 μm (100 nm). (Micrographs courtesy of G. A. Zampighi.)

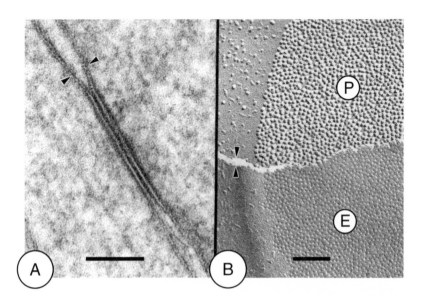

adjoining cells (Fig. 8.1B), which represent the molecular components of the junction itself.

Gap junctions are formed by protein molecules called *connexins* that are located in the membranes of both the connecting cells; these molecules span the gap between the cells to connect their cytosolic interiors (for reviews, see Bennett and Spray, 1985; Bennett, Barrio, Bargiello, et al., 1991; Dermietzel and Spray, 1993; Beyer, 1993; Ransom, 1995; Paul, 1995; Wolburg and Rohlmann, 1995; White, Bruzzone, and Paul, 1995; Goodenough, Goliger, and Paul, 1996). Connexins form a multigene family of related proteins, and as many as 13 different connexins have been identified in a single species. They all appear to have a similar topology, as revealed by antibody-binding experiments (see Milks et al., 1988; Yeager and Gilula, 1992) and structural studies (see for example Unwin and Zampighi, 1980; Unwin, 1989; Unger et al., 1999). Each connexin molecule has four highly conserved membrane-spanning regions. One of these (called M3), containing polar basic and acidic amino acids separated by aromatic residues, has been proposed to form the channel wall. The two extracellular loops, also highly conserved, contain cysteine residues that probably act as anchors fixing connexin molecules from adjacent cells into position to form the channel. Both the amino and carboxyl ends of the protein face the interior of the cell. The carboxyl terminus is generally much longer and shows the greatest variability with tissue and species, and both amino and carboxyl termini appear to have sites that can be phosphorylated. For those genes which have been sequenced (see Beyer, 1993), the whole of the connexin protein coding sequence is contained within a single exon; alternatively spliced connexin proteins have not yet been described.

It is likely that gap junctions are formed when connexins from the adjacent membranes of the two cells meet and form some kind of tight, noncovalent association. The membrane of each cell at the junction is thought to contain a unit of connexin molecules called a hemichannel (or *connexon*), consisting of six connexin proteins arranged in an hexagonal array, much like an elongated donut. Two hemichannels from adjacent cells meet to form a continuous structure (Unger et al., 1999), which encloses a pore connecting the cytoplasm of the two cells (Fig. 8.2B). The channel running through the middle of the gap junction is apparently about 1.6 nm in diameter and is readily permeable to Na^+, K^+, and Cl^-. As a result, gap junctions facilitate the passage of current between cells, which means that changes in voltage can spread decrementally from one cell to another. Gap junctions are also permeable to many other substances, including Ca^{2+}, H^+, nucleotides, IP_3, and other second messengers (see Chapters 11–13), and so they probably allow the transmission of intracellular chemical signals between cells.

Different connexin proteins have different distributions in body tissues and distinct physiological properties. Several different types have been found to occur among cells in the brain, including connexins 26, 31, 32, 37, 43, and 45 (the number indicates the approximate molecular weight in kilodaltons). Most of these form junctions between glial cells; connexin 32 has been reported to occur at junctions between neurons, and other connexins may also participate in neuronal gap junctions (see for example O'Brien et al., 1998). In most cases, junctions are thought to be formed by hemichannels composed of the same connexin molecule (homotypic junctions), but several cases of *heterotypic* junctions have

Fig. 8.2 Structure of connexins. **(A)** Hypothetical membrane topology of connexin 43. (After Yeager and Gilula, 1992.) **(B)** Connexins are assembled into hexameric hemichannels (connexons) in both the presynaptic and postsynaptic cell, and these line up to form complete channel. (After Makowski et al., 1977.)

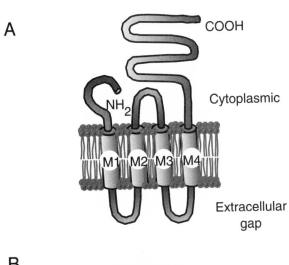

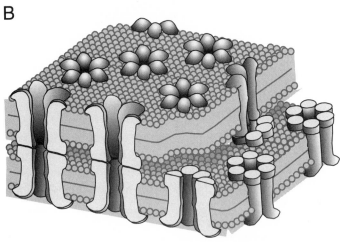

now been reported (Barrio et al., 1991; Elfgang et al., 1995; Konig and Zampighi, 1995). The role of heterotypic junctions in the nervous system is still unclear.

Electrical Synapses

Since gap junctions permit the flow of current from one cell to another, they act as a conduit for the passage of electrical signals between cells. Gap junctions and cellular coupling are quite common throughout the body among cells of the same tissue type, for example between liver cells and between epithelial cells lining the trachea. Gap junctions were once thought to be rare in the nervous system, but they have now been identified between many cell types, for example in the retina (Vaney, 1994) and spinal cord (Rash et al., 1996). In some cases, gap junctions are small and highly localized; in others they connect arrays of cells in extensive, tightly coupled networks. When neurons have been found with gap junctions between them, and when the physiology of these cells has been investigated in detail, in every case the cells have been shown to be coupled by *electrical* (or *electrotonic*) synapses. Electrical synaptic communication is rapid, since there is no measurable latency for signal to travel from presynaptic to postsynaptic cell. It is also usually considered more reliable than chemical transmission, since no release of transmitter is required.

The physiology of electrical synapses is best studied in preparations consisting of pairs of large, tightly coupled cells. Electrodes are placed in both cells (on both sides of the junction) and current is passed from one cell to the other. Experiments of this kind have shown that currents passed into one cell produce a change in voltage in the adjacent, electrically coupled cell. In most cases, the conductance of the junction is symmetric: currents can be passed in either direction across the junction with equal ease. There are some electrical synapses, however, for which current passes much more easily in one direction than the other. These are called *rectifying synapses,* and I shall have more to say about them later in the chapter.

Voltage-Clamping Gap Junctions

Although much has been learned about the properties of electrical synapses by passing current into cells and recording voltages, a much more quantitative approach is to voltage-clamp both cells and record currents. This approach was first used by Spray, Harris, and Bennett (1981) on blastomeres from amphibian embryos. Pairs of coupled cells were removed from the embryos and were each penetrated with two microelectrodes, one to record voltage and the other to apply current (see Fig. 8.3A). The leads from the two electrodes were connected to voltage-clamp circuits similar to the one used by Hodgkin and Huxley. The voltage electrodes were led into voltage preamplifiers (labeled V_a and V_b), whose outputs went to one of the inputs of the feedback amplifiers (labeled *FBA* in Fig. 8.3A). The other inputs to the feedback amplifiers were the command voltages, labeled V_{ca} for cell A and V_{cb} for cell B. The circuit included amplifiers used to measure the currents injected through the two current electrodes, only one of which is shown (whose output is labeled i_a).

I shall simplify the circuit just as I did for the experiments of Hodgkin and Huxley. First I shall assume that the feedback amplifiers work quickly and efficiently, so that the voltage recorded from cell A is just $V_a = V_{ca}$, and the voltage from cell B is $V_b = V_{cb}$. I also ignore series resistances and membrane capacitance. The resulting circuit is shown in Fig. 8.3B, where V_a and V_b are the membrane voltages of cells A and B, at the two nodes (i.e., the two points of intersection) of the circuit on either side of the junctional conductance (g_j).

The current flowing across g_j is said to be positive when it flows from cell A to cell B. This means that the junctional voltage across g_j can be given as $V_j = V_a - V_b$, and the junctional current as $i_j = g_j(V_a - V_b)$. It isn't important whether we define positive current as A→B or as B→A, but we have to adopt some convention so that we can write the equations for the currents.

The currents injected by the current electrodes of the voltage-clamp circuits are called i_a and i_b. Ordinarily these would also be the membrane currents of cells A and B. In the case of coupled cells, however, some of the current injected into cell A passes through the junctional conductance to cell B and vice versa. This has the effect that the currents injected into cells A and B are given by

$$i_a = g_a V_a + g_j(V_a - V_b), \quad i_b = g_b V_b - g_j(V_a - V_b) \qquad (1)$$

Let us suppose that we begin by setting the command potentials and therefore the membrane potentials of the two cells to the same

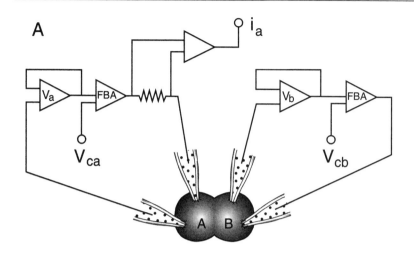

A

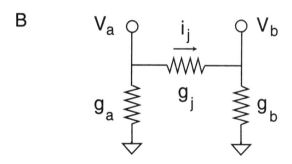

B

Fig. 8.3 Voltage-clamping gap junctions. **(A)** Two electrically coupled blastomeres from amphibian embryos were each impaled with two microelectrodes, one for recording voltage and the other for applying current. The voltages for each of the cells were measured by voltage amplifiers (V_a and V_b) and are set separately to command voltages (V_{ca} and V_{cb}). The current emerging from the feedback amplifiers *(FBA)* was measured by placing a resistor between the output of the feedback amplifier and the current-passing pipette. The voltage drop across this resistor is proportional to the current by Ohm's law, and this voltage is measured and recorded (shown in figure only for i_a). (After Spray, Harris, and Bennett, 1981.) **(B)** Simplified circuit diagram for recording in **(A)**.

values near the normal resting potential. Then $V_a = V_b$, and we shall call these potentials V_a^0 and V_b^0. Since there is no potential difference between the cells, there can be no current flowing across the junctional resistance, and the currents are

$$i_a^0 = g_a V_a^0, \quad i_b^0 = g_b V_b^0 \tag{2}$$

Suppose we now hold V_b at V_b^0 but change V_a to some new value, which we call V_a. The currents flowing into the two cells can now be written from Eqn. (1) as

$$i_a = g_a V_a + g_j(V_a - V_b^0), \quad i_b = g_b V_b^0 - g_j(V_a - V_b^0) \qquad (3)$$

If we define $\Delta i_a = i_a - i_a^0$ and $\Delta i_b = i_b - i_b^0$, then

$$\Delta i_a = g_a V_a + g_j(V_a - V_b^0) - g_a V_a^0 \qquad (4)$$

But

$$\Delta i_b = -g_j(V_a - V_b^0) = -g_j V_j = -i_j \qquad (5)$$

This means that if we change the command voltage only for cell *A* but measure the current injected by the voltage clamp into cell *B*, the current at cell *B* gives the negative of the current flowing through the junctional conductance. One way to think about this is to realize that when the voltage of cell *A* is changed, any current flowing across the junction into cell *B* from cell *A* will fall across g_b and change the membrane potential in cell *B*, unless the feedback amplifier injects current into cell *B* equal but opposite in sign to the current coming into the cell through the gap junction.

Since it is possible to pass currents in both directions, the junctional conductance can be measured as a function of junctional voltage. When Spray and colleagues did this experiment, they obtained an unexpected result. The junctional conductance at steady state is symmetrical but highly voltage-dependent. In Fig. 8.4A, the steady-state junctional conductance (labeled g_∞) is plotted as a function of the *transjunctional voltage* (V_j). As long as the voltage of the two cells is nearly the same, the junctional conductance is high; but if the voltage of one cell becomes very different from the other, the junctional conductance goes to zero and the cells electrically disconnect. This may be a useful property of junctions in embryonic tissue, because cells that are connected share intracellular messengers. Cells may have to change potential and close their gap junctions in order to differentiate.

Voltage Dependence of Gap-Junctional Conductance

Using techniques like those pioneered by Spray and colleagues, other researchers have measured the conductance of electrical syn-

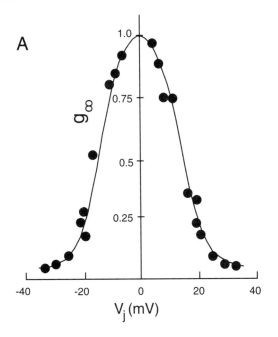

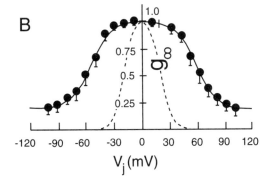

Fig. 8.4 Voltage dependence of gap-junctional conductance. Conductance measured with double voltage clamp, as in Fig. 8.3. **(A)** Steady-state conductance of amphibian blastomeres as a function of transjunctional voltage (V_j). Conductances have been normalized to apparent conductance at 0 mV. Curve through data is Boltzmann relation (see Spray, Harris, and Bennett, 1981); conductance was assumed to be symmetrical with voltage, decreasing with the same function for positive and negative transjunctional voltage changes. (After Spray, Harris, and Bennett, 1981.) **(B)** Steady-state conductance of junctions formed by connexin 32. *Xenopus* oocytes were injected with RNA for connexin 32, and coupled pairs were formed by apposing two oocytes at their vegetal poles. Cells were voltage-clamped as in Fig. 8.3. Data points show mean conductance and error bars standard deviations for steady-state conductance normalized to conductance at 0 mV and plotted as a function of transjunctional voltage (V_j). Curve through data is Boltzmann relation, assumed to be symmetrical for positive and negative transjunctional voltage changes. Dotted curve is curve from part **(A)**, repeated here for comparison. (After Barrio et al., 1991.)

apses in many different preparations. Although junctions between embryonic cells are markedly voltage-dependent, those between liver and heart cells and between neurons are much less so. For most nerve cells for which the voltage dependence of coupling has been measured, the coupling conductance is much less dependent on voltage, and junctional current varies nearly linearly with junctional voltage at least for voltages within the physiological range.

A particularly useful approach for investigating the physiology of gap junctions has been to inject RNA for one or more of the gap-junctional proteins into two adjacent *Xenopus* oocytes (Dahl et al., 1987—see Ebihara, 1992), and then to push the oocytes up against one another so that they touch. The paired oocytes can be made to express the connexins appropriate for the injected RNA and to form electrical junctions with one another. Since the oocytes are also able to express native connexins, it is helpful if the synthesis of the native protein is suppressed by injecting antisense RNA for the native proteins along with the RNA for the foreign connexins (Barrio et al., 1991). In this way, the oocyte can be made to produce junctions containing a well-defined homotypic or heterotypic protein composition.

Using oocyte expression, several laboratories have characterized the voltage dependence of homotypic junctions formed by most of the cloned connexins, as well as heterotypic junctions for several combinations (see White, Bruzzone, and Paul, 1995). A typical example is given in Fig. 8.4B (from Barrio et al., 1991), for homotypic junctions formed with connexin 32, the protein that has been identified as forming gap junctions between at least some kinds of neurons. The data points in this figure give the steady-state conductance, which is much less voltage-dependent than g_j for *Xenopus* embryos (the curve in Fig. 8.4A has been replotted as the dashed curve in Fig. 8.4B). For a V_j of 50 mV on either side of zero, g_j declines precipitously for junctions from *Xenopus* embryos but is nearly independent of voltage for junctions made with connexin 32. These results are consistent with many reports that neuronal gap-junctional conductance is nearly voltage-independent (see Fig. 8.7A).

Rectifying Electrical Synapses

In some cases, neurons are connected by *rectifying synapses,* electrical synapses for which the junctional conductance is not only voltage-dependent but also asymmetric, meaning that current passes more easily in one direction than the other. The most famous of these is the crayfish giant motor synapse, first studied by Furshpan and Potter (1959). At the giant motor synapse, the lat-

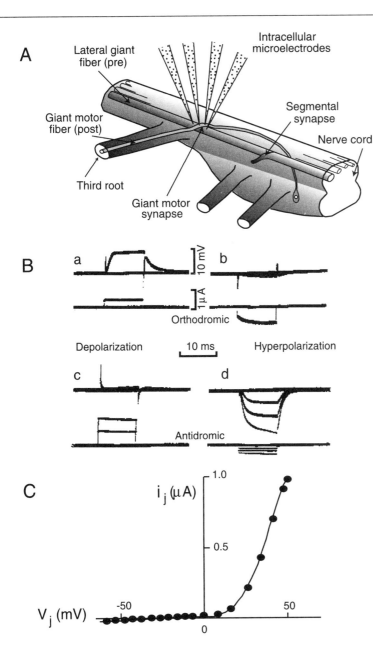

A

Lateral giant
fiber (pre)

Intracellular
microelectrodes

Giant motor
fiber (post)

Segmental
synapse

Nerve cord

Third root

Giant motor
synapse

Giant motor
synapse

B

a 10 mV

b

1 µA

Orthodromic

Depolarization   10 ms   Hyperpolarization

c

d

Antidromic

C

i_j (µA)

1.0

0.5

V_j (mV)

-50   50

0

Fig. 8.5 The rectifying electrical junction at the crayfish giant motor synapse. **(A)** Anatomy of the synapse and method of recording. The giant motor synapse is formed between lateral giant fibers (which are *pre*synaptic) and giant motor fibers (which are *post*synaptic) in the abdominal nerve cord. Two microelectrodes are placed on both sides of the synapse as shown, one to pass current and the other to record voltage. (After Furshpan and Potter, 1959.) **(B)** Effect of injected currents on transsynaptic voltages. Upper two sets of traces (*a* and *b*) are for current injected into the presynaptic lateral giant fiber, with voltage measured in the postsynaptic giant motor fiber. This is the normal direction for synaptic transmission and has been labeled *orthodromic*. The lower two sets of traces (*c* and *d*) are for current applied in the opposite direction, into the postsynapic side of the synapse with voltage measured presynaptically; these have been labeled *antidromic*. For each set of traces, voltage is shown above and current below (scales given only for *a* and *b*). For orthodromic stimulation, an outward current injected presynaptically produces a large voltage change (*a*), but an inward current (*b*) has little effect. For antidromic stimulation, only inward currents are effective (*d*). (From Furshpan and Potter, 1959, reprinted with permission of the authors and the Physiological Society.) **(C)** Double voltage-clamp measurements of junctional conductance of crayfish rectifying synapse, plotted as a function of transmembrane voltage. (Reprinted from Giaume, Kado, and Korn, 1987, with permission of the authors and of the Physiological Society.)

eral giant fiber makes a large electrical synapse onto the giant motor fiber (see Fig. 8.5A), which is used by the crayfish in a rapid escape response. Both fibers are large enough to be penetrated with microelectrodes. The injection of depolarizing current into the presynaptic fiber causes a depolarization of the postsynaptic fiber, but hyperpolarizing current has little or no effect (Fig. 8.5B). Conversely, hyperpolarizing current injected into the postsynaptic fiber hyperpolarized the presynaptic fiber, but depolarizing currents produced little if any voltage change.

This junction was subsequently studied using methods similar to those of Spray and colleagues—that is, by voltage-clamping both presynaptic and postsynaptic cells (Giaume, Kado, and Korn, 1987). These experiments show that the rectification of synaptic transmission observed by Furshpan and Potter is in fact due to a nonlinear junctional conductance. When the junctional voltage is positive (i.e., $V_{pre} > V_{post}$), the junctional current is large. If the junctional voltage is negative, the junctional current is near zero (Fig. 8.5C).

Rectifying synapses have been observed in several preparations, but it is unclear how common they are in the central nervous system. They may serve to limit the sign or direction of signals passed across the synapse. The mechanism is still unknown but may result from some form of heterotypic channel, with different connexin subunits contributed by the presynaptic and postsynaptic cells (Barrio et al., 1991).

Modulation of Electrical Synapses

Gap-junctional resistance can be altered in several ways. Rose and Loewenstein (1976) showed that increases in intracellular Ca^{2+} close the junctions, though it is now apparent that at least for some kinds of gap junctions rather high Ca^{2+} concentrations are required (Spray et al., 1982). Gap junctions are also sensitive to pH (Turin and Warner, 1980) and can be blocked by extracellular (but not intracellular) application of aliphatic alcohols, such as heptanol and octanol (see Ramón, Zampighi, and Rivera, 1985).

The conductance of electrical synapses can also be modulated by second messengers, presumably via direct phosphorylation of the gap-junctional proteins at sites located at the cytoplasmic surface of the protein (see Goodenough, Goliger, and Paul, 1996). Although effects of second messengers on junctional resistance have been observed for many cell types, the clearest case reported for neurons is the modulation of the junctional resistance between retinal horizontal cells by dopamine.

Retinal horizontal cells are connected by an extensive network of gap junctions. The connections are so extensive that when a single cell is injected with a dye or marker, such as Lucifer Yellow™ or biocytin, which can pass through gap junctions in many tissues, interconnecting cells are stained (Fig. 8.6). If, however, the retina is perfused with dopamine, the diffusion of the dye is greatly restricted as a result of a decrease in the gap-junctional conductance.

The physiology of the dopamine modulation can best be studied in isolated pairs of cells, voltage-clamped as in Spray, Harris, and

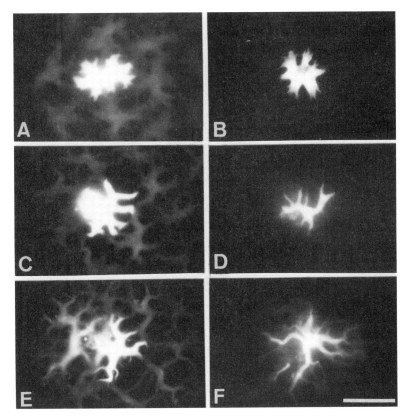

Fig. 8.6 Effect of dopamine on gap-junctional coupling of retinal horizontal cells: dye coupling. A horizontal cell in the retina of the fish *Eugerres plumieri* was penetrated with an intracellular micropipette containing 6% of the dye Lucifer Yellow™, and the dye was injected into the cell by passing negative current. The dye then diffused into neighboring cells through the gap junctions. The retina was fixed in paraformaldehyde and examined in the light microscope. Scale bar, 50 µm. *A, C,* and *E* are representative experiments in control solution (normal Ringer), and *B, D,* and *F* cells in solution containing 10–25 µM dopamine. (Reprinted from Negishi et al., 1988, with permission of the authors and of the journal *Biomedical Research.*)

Fig. 8.7 Effect of dopamine on gap-junctional coupling of retinal horizontal cells: measurements of conductance. Recordings were made from pairs of horizontal cells, dissociated from the retina of the catfish, *Ictalurus punctatus*. Junctional conductance was measured as in Fig. 8.3, but cells were voltage-clamped with whole-cell patch clamp rather than with separate current and voltage electrodes (see Box 5.1). **(A)** Junctional current plotted as a function of junctional voltage, corrected for pipette series resistance, for cells in control solution *(squares)*, with slope equal to the junctional conductance of 11.3 nS; and for cells after addition to bathing medium of 1 μM dopamine *(triangles)*, with the conductance now equal to 1.0 nS. **(B)** Dose-dependent reduction of junctional conductance by dopamine, for cell pair different from the one in **(A)**. Junctional conductance is graphed as a function of time in control solution and after perfusion with 1–100 nM dopamine. Dopamine exposures are indicated by bars. (Reprinted from DeVries and Schwartz, 1989, with permission of the authors and the Physiological Society.)

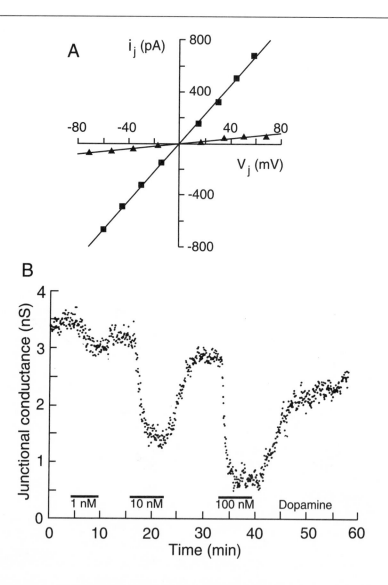

Bennett (1981). Such experiments were first done by Lasater and Dowling (1985), who showed that dopamine and cAMP decrease g_j. The data in Fig. 8.7, from a later study by DeVries and Schwartz (1989), illustrate the current-voltage curve of the junction in the absence and presence of 1 μM dopamine (Fig. 8.7A) and the concentration dependence of dopamine (Fig. 8.7B). Similar effects are seen for intracellular application of cAMP. Dopamine apparently activates a D_1 receptor, which in turn stimulates an adenylyl cyclase (see Chapter 12). The cyclase increases the cAMP concentration, and cAMP probably activates protein kinase A (DeVries and Schwartz, 1992) to phosphorylate the gap-junctional connexin molecules.

The dopamine modulation of horizontal cell junctional conductance may be quite important, as it regulates the region of the retina over which the horizontal cell is receptive for different conditions of illumination. Dopamine has also been shown to modulate gap junctions between retinal amacrine cells (Hampson, Vaney, and Weiler, 1992; Mills and Massey, 1995) and between developing cortical pyramidal cells (Rörig, Klausa, and Sutor, 1995).

We are accustomed to thinking of electrical synapses as fast and highly dependable connections used in situations (such as escape responses) where speed and reliability are essential. As gap junctions are beginning to be discovered in the central nervous system with greater abundance than previously thought (see for example Rash et al., 1996), and as we begin to learn how they can be modulated, our ideas about electrical connectivity are beginning to change. Unfortunately, we still know too little about the physiology and molecular biology of these synapses and their connexin proteins to be able to make any general statements about their role in neural processing.

II: CHEMICAL SYNAPSES AND THE Ca^{2+} HYPOTHESIS

Although electrotonic gap junctions are found in many areas of the central nervous system, most synapses in the brain use chemical transmitters for signaling. Chemical transmission provides a more versatile control of the sign and amplitude of signal transfer than electrical transmission. Chemical transmitters can produce signals that are excitatory or inhibitory, and signals that are fast and brief or slow and long-lasting. This variety provides a wealth of possibilities for neural integration. Nearly every step in the process of chemical transmission can be modulated, from the depolarization of the presynaptic terminal to the production of a postsynaptic response. As will be described later in the book (Chapters 11–14), nerve cells contain elaborate chemical mechanisms involving second messengers and protein kinases and phosphatases, which ultimately have the effect of phosphorylating and dephosphorylating proteins. These mechanisms are probably responsible in one form or another for strengthening certain pathways and weakening others, as must somehow occur during learning and memory. Chemical synapses are also the sites of many important drugs for treating psychic disorders, such as depression and schizophrenia.

At most chemical synapses, transmission is thought to occur according to the following scheme. An action potential invades the presynaptic terminal, and depolarization causes the opening of Ca^{2+} channels in the terminal plasma membrane. Ca^{2+} enters the terminal cytosol, and the increase in intracellular Ca^{2+} concentration facilitates the fusion of vesicles containing transmitter to the presynaptic cell membrane by a process known as exocytosis. The vesicles release their contents into the synaptic cleft, transmitter diffuses across the extracellular space to the postsynaptic membrane, and the binding of transmitter to receptors in the plasma membrane of the postsynaptic cell directly or indirectly changes the conductance of that membrane.

Chemical synapses come in a variety of forms (see Heuser and Reese, 1977). We have already seen that specialized regions of contact occur on the spines of pyramidal cells (see Fig. 1.1C). Similar specializations on areas of closely apposed membrane are seen at high density throughout the central nervous system (Fig. 8.8A). Such synapses have a variety of specialized components (Fig. 8.8B). There are synaptic vesicles in the presynaptic cell, some apparently randomly arranged within the cytoplasm and some clustered and apparently "docked" along the presynaptic membrane adjacent to the postsynaptic cell. Near the docked vesicles is a region of the presynaptic membrane often referred to as the *active zone,* consisting of rows of membrane particles observed in freeze-fracture replicas (see Figs. 8.8C and 8.9B). These particles are in part probably Ca^{2+} channels and Ca^{2+}-dependent K^+ channels (see for example Roberts, Jacobs, and Hudspeth, 1990; Robitaille et al., 1993) but may also include other components of the release machinery. In transmission micrographs, there are often regions of electron density at the active zone of presynaptic cells, probably indicating spe-

A

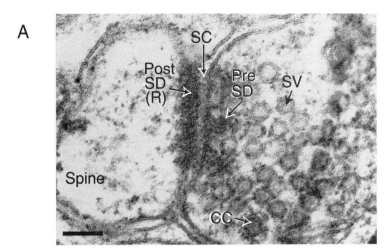

B

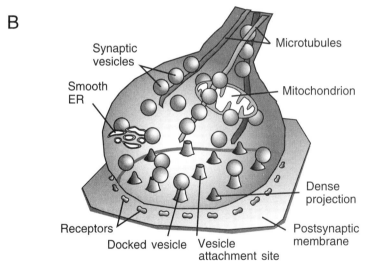

Fig. 8.8 Anatomy of chemical synapses.
(A) Electron micrograph of synapse from central nervous system. (Courtesy G. A. Zampighi.) Presynaptic cell containing synaptic vesicles is to right and postsynaptic spine to left. *Post SD (R),* postsynaptic densities (receptors); *SC,* synaptic cleft; *Pre SD,* presynaptic densities; *SV,* synaptic vesicle; *CC,* clathrin-coated vesicle (see Fig. 8.20). **(B)** Schematic diagram of synaptic ending in CNS. (After Gray, 1987.) **(C)** Freeze-fracture micrograph of presynaptic membrane in region of synapse (active zone) for mechanoreceptive hair cell from the frog sacculus (see Chapter 15). Note regular array of particles, which probably represent channels or other proteins that are a part of the release mechanism. Scale bar, 100 nm. (From Roberts, Jacobs, and Hudspeth, 1990, reprinted with permission of the authors and the Society for Neuroscience.)

Fig. 8.9 Neuromuscular junction. **(A)** Transmission micrograph of synapse between motor axon and muscle. Axon forms presynaptic boutons (see Fig. 8.10A), which lie in invaginations of the muscle membrane, called *gutters.* Opposed to the boutons are numerous outpocketings of muscle membrane called *postsynaptic folds* (*PSF*), whose apices form the postsynaptic active zones containing acetylcholine receptors. *SchC,* Schwann cell; *M,* mitochondria; *SC* (*BL*), synaptic cleft containing basal lamina; *BL,* extracellular basal lamina filling spaces between synaptic folds; *ASV,* agranular synaptic vesicles (within circle). Scale bar, 0.5 μm (500 nm). (Courtesy of G. A. Zampighi.) **(B)** High-magnification freeze-fracture micrograph of presynaptic active zone of frog neuromuscular junction. Note regular array of particles, which probably represent channels or other proteins that are a part of the release mechanism. Scale bar, 0.1 μm (100 nm). (From Heuser et al., 1979, reprinted with permission of the authors and of Rockefeller University Press.)

A

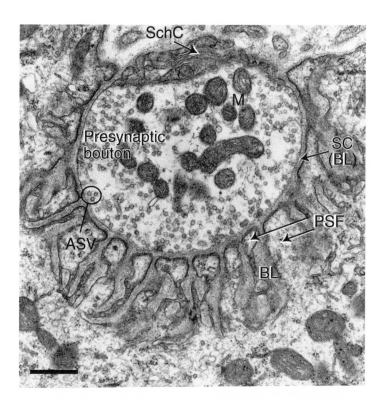

B

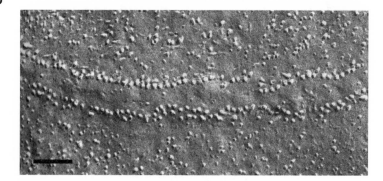

cialized protein components that play some role in release. The postsynaptic membrane also exhibits a region of increased electron density, and between the presynaptic and postsynaptic cells there is a fairly well-defined gap called the synaptic cleft.

One highly specialized synapse has served as a useful preparation for investigating the nature of chemical transmission, the neuromuscular junction between peripheral nerve and skeletal muscle (Fig. 8.9). This synapse has many of the same components as chemical synapses in the central nervous system but is more easily accessible, allowing the structural relationships to be visualized more clearly. Much of our understanding of the physiology of synaptic transmission has come from experiments with this preparation and with another synapse, one that is less accessible but particularly large, the giant synapse of squid, described later in this chapter.

The Ca^{2+} Hypothesis

The suggestion that Ca^{2+} is the intermediate link between presynaptic depolarization and the release of synaptic transmitter is known as the Ca^{2+} hypothesis. Although initially a subject of intense debate when first proposed by Bernard Katz and his colleagues (see Katz, 1969), the Ca^{2+} hypothesis is now almost universally accepted as the explanation for how transmitters are released at most chemical synapses in the central nervous system.

The first evidence that Ca^{2+} is required for neurotransmitter release was actually obtained by Sydney Ringer (of Ringer's solution) and F. S. Locke (of Locke's solution), who showed over one hundred years ago that some Ca^{2+} must be added to the bathing medium for the maintenance of transmission between nerve and skeletal muscle. As soon as it became possible to do intracellular recording from muscle, several studies demonstrated that Ca^{2+} facilitated and Mg^{2+} blocked transmission at the neuromuscular junction (see for example del Castillo and Katz, 1954a).

These early studies showed that Ca^{2+} was necessary but not what it did. The first evidence for a direct role for Ca^{2+} in release was obtained by Katz and Miledi (1965a), who used the method of focal recording at the neuromuscular junction. They placed an extracellular electrode up against a frog muscle, close enough to the synapse to record extracellular synaptic potentials produced by local currents (Fig. 8.10A). Since the resistance of the extracellular

Fig. 8.10   Ca^{2+} is required for transmitter release at the neuromuscular junction. **(A)** Focal recording. Microelectrode is placed extracellularly, close to the position of nerve contact at the motor endplate. (After Fatt and Katz, 1952.) **(B)** Focal recording measures the voltage drop produced by extracellular current moving between the ground electrode and the recording pipette. Since current moves inward into the muscle membrane during the synaptic response, extracellular current will converge in the vicinity of synapse as it flows into the muscle. Recording pipette will measure a negativity with respect to the ground electrode, since current will be moving away from the ground electrode and toward the recording pipette. **(C)** Focal recordings of endplate potentials made from frog neuromuscular junction in Ca^{2+}-free Ringer. Synapse stimulated by shock to nerve, with timing indicated on traces to left by initial positive spikes. These are then followed by presynaptic action potentials *(arrows)*. Focal pipette contained 0.5 M CaCl$_2$, and constant negative current was passed through pipette to retard leakage of Ca^{2+} onto the synapse. At beginning of experiment, negative current was adjusted to block transmission completely by inhibiting all movement of Ca^{2+} out of the pipette. In the absence of Ca^{2+}, no responses were recorded (traces labeled *No Ca^{2+}*). The current was decreased, and synaptic responses could be observed (*Some Ca^{2+}*). A further decrease in current increased response amplitude (*More Ca^{2+}*), and the current was then increased back to its initial value (*No Ca^{2+}*). Individual responses are superimposed at left; averages of 600 traces for each condition are shown to the right. Time calibration applies only to traces on left. (From Katz and Miledi, 1965a, with permission of the authors and the Royal Society of London.)

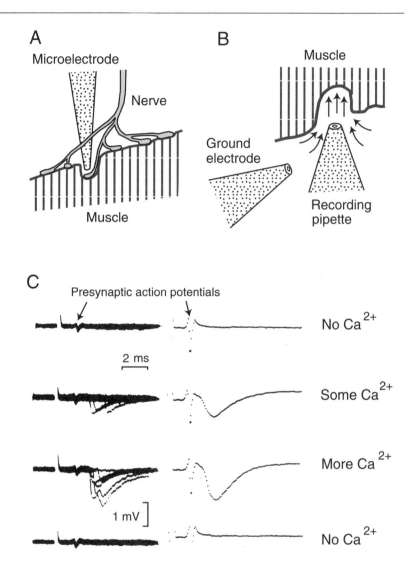

fluid is rather low, the voltage change produced by extracellular current flow is not very large (typically less than 1 mV) and can be detected only if the density of current is fairly high. This means that an extracellular pipette can record extracellular synaptic potentials only if the pipette is close to the postsynaptic membrane (generally within a few μm) and in the region where the postsynaptic conductance change is occurring. The sign of these extracellular potential changes is negative, since the electrode is placed where the current density (and therefore the extracellular potential drop) is highest, just outside the region of postsynaptic membrane. At this position, the loops of extracellular current converge before they move through endplate channels into the muscle (Fig. 8.10B), and the pipette records a change in voltage negative with respect to a more remotely placed ground electrode.

In normal Ringer solution, focal postsynaptic potentials (PSPs) can be routinely recorded from the neuromuscular junction after stimulation of the peripheral nerve with a brief electric shock. When the bathing medium lacks Ca^{2+}, PSPs can be recorded only when Ca^{2+} is allowed to leak out from the recording pipette. In the experiment of Fig. 8.10C, for example, recordings were made in Ca^{2+}-free Mg^{2+} Ringer, but the recording pipette contained 0.5 M $CaCl_2$. For the uppermost trace, a negative current was passed through the pipette sufficient to prevent Ca^{2+} from leaking out. The current was then reduced in two stages to allow the Ca^{2+} to leak out; the current was increased again to prevent Ca^{2+} leakage (lowermost trace). Individual records are shown to the left, and averages of recordings to the right. The brief positive-going potential at the beginning of the records to the left is an artifact produced by stimulation of the peripheral nerve; the negative-going potential immediately following this artifact (arrows) was produced by extracellular currents generated by the action potential as it invaded the presynaptic terminal. Notice that even though action potentials invaded the terminal in all of the records, postsynaptic responses were recorded only in the presence of extracellular Ca^{2+}.

Ca²⁺ Entry and the Release of Transmitter

Focal recordings indicated that Ca^{2+} is somehow directly involved in the process that causes transmitter release. This method can also provide an accurate measurement of the time course of release. From recordings like those shown in Fig. 8.10C, it is possible to measure the time between the arrival of the action potential at the terminal and the production of a postsynaptic response. This interval, called the *synaptic delay*, is variable from one recording to the next as successive stimuli are given to the same preparation; it is also a function of temperature, decreasing rather steeply as the temperature is increased. Even at high temperatures, however, it is never smaller than 500 μs (Katz and Miledi, 1965b). The delay cannot be primarily due to the diffusion of transmitter across the synaptic cleft or to the binding of the transmitter to the receptor, because if the transmitter (in this case acetylcholine) is delivered to the muscle from a pipette even from a much greater distance than the synaptic cleft, delays as short as 100–200 μs can be observed. Most of the delay must be caused by Ca^{2+} entry into the pre-synaptic terminal and Ca^{2+}-mediated release of the transmitter.

Some insight into the role Ca^{2+} is playing can be obtained by examining the dependence of release on extracellular Ca^{2+} concentration ($[Ca^{2+}]_o$). The first quantitative measurements of this kind were made by Dodge and Rahamimoff (1967), who measured and plotted the amplitude of the endplate potential (EPP) at the frog neuromuscular junction as a function of $[Ca^{2+}]_o$. The initial rising phase of this curve was sigmoidal and could be well fit by a straight line when the log of the EPP amplitude (denoted *epp*) was plotted as a function of the log of $[Ca^{2+}]_o$. Suppose, for small EPP amplitudes, the amplitude is proportional to $[Ca^{2+}]_o$ raised to some power, *m*:

$$epp = K[Ca^{2+}]_0^m \tag{6}$$

where K is a constant of proportionality. By taking the logs of both sides of Eqn. (6), we obtain

$$\log_{10}(epp) = \log_{10}(K) + m\log_{10}([Ca^{2+}]_0) \tag{7}$$

Thus by plotting the $\log_{10}$ of EPP amplitude versus the $\log_{10}$ of Ca^{2+} concentration, *m* can be obtained from the slope. In the experiments of Dodge and Rahamimoff, *m* was 3.78. Provided $[Ca^{2+}]_i$ in the presynaptic terminal is proportional to $[Ca^{2+}]_o$, this result suggests that more than three Ca^{2+} must bind for transmitter to be released.

The Input-Output Relation of a Synapse

In order to obtain more precise information about the control of transmitter release and the role of Ca^{2+} entry into the presynaptic cell, it would be helpful to record from both the presynaptic and postsynaptic cells simultaneously. For technical reasons (small cell size), this has not been possible at the neuromuscular junction until very recently (Yazejian et al., 1997). Many of the most important experiments on the physiology of chemical transmission were instead performed on a different synapse, the giant synapse of the squid stellate ganglion.

The first recordings from the squid giant synapse were made by Ted Bullock and Susumu Hagiwara (1957). They placed electrodes in the main processes of the presynaptic and postsynaptic nerves (Fig. 8.11A). Subsequently, Katz and Miledi (1967) discovered that more accurate measurements of the voltage dependence of transmission could be obtained if the pipettes were placed in the fine processes of the nerves, as close to the synapse as possible. They blocked action potential propagation with TTX and injected current directly into the presynaptic process. They measured the amplitude of the postsynaptic response as a function of presynaptic potential, and an example of this curve, usually referred to as the *input-output relation,* is given in Fig. 8.11B. One important feature of this curve is that little postsynaptic response is produced until the presynaptic terminal is depolarized 25–30 mV from the resting membrane potential.

Katz and Miledi reasoned that the voltage dependence of synaptic transfer must reflect the voltage dependence of Ca^{2+} channels in the presynaptic membrane. Since some kinds of Ca^{2+} channels become activated only at rather depolarized potentials, the increase in transmitter release at potentials 25–30 mV depolarized from resting potential probably reflects the degree of depolarization necessary to produce a significant increase in the probability of opening of the Ca^{2+} channels. The data in Fig. 8.11B indicate that significant release of transmitter occurs only at rather depolarized presynaptic potentials, but the value of this potential range may have been overestimated in these experiments as a result of the difficulty of measuring and controlling the voltage just at the region of presynaptic membrane where release occurred.

Voltage-Clamping the Squid Giant Synapse

To understand the physiology of synaptic transmission in greater detail, it would be useful to obtain a better control of the voltage

Fig. 8.11 The squid giant synapse. **(A)** Anatomy of synapse. The squid giant synapse occurs between the presynaptic second-order giant fiber *(Presynaptic)* and the postsynaptic third-order giant *(Postsynaptic nerve)*. Because of the large size of these nerve fibers, it is possible to place microelectrodes both presynaptically and postsynaptically, fairly close to the site of junctional contact. (After Bullock and Hagiwara, 1957.) **(B)** Input-output curve for squid giant synapse. Recordings as in **(A)**, but presynaptic terminal was penetrated with two microelectrodes, for passing current and for measuring voltage (as illustrated above graph). Positive currents passed into the presynaptic terminal produced depolarizations, which are plotted on the abscissa relative to the resting membrane potential. Postsynaptic responses, on the ordinate, are also plotted relative to resting membrane potential. In the inset at left, the foot of the curve is given with a larger scale for the ordinate. (After Katz and Miledi, 1967.)

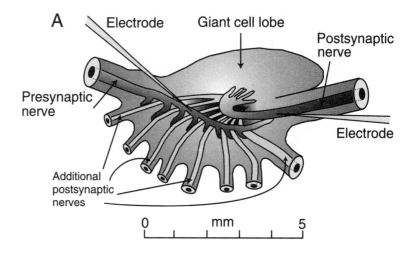

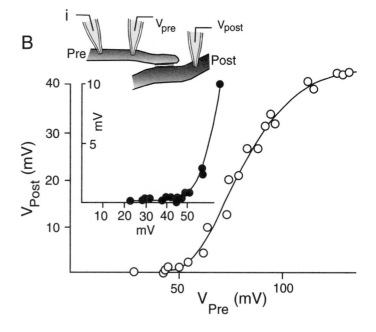

of the presynaptic membrane. This could be achieved, at least in theory, by voltage-clamping the presynaptic fiber. One could then measure the net movement of Ca^{2+} into the presynaptic terminal by measuring the time integral of the presynaptic Ca^{2+} current. The increase in Ca^{2+} could also be measured with Ca^{2+}-sensitive photoproteins or dyes (see Chapter 13) and could be compared with the increase in the conductance of the postsynaptic fiber, which could also be measured under voltage clamp.

A first step toward this aim was taken by Rudolfo Llinás and co-workers (1981a,b), who voltage-clamped the presynaptic terminal of the squid giant synapse either by inserting two electrodes into the terminal, one to pass current and the other to measure voltage; or by using the three-electrode voltage-clamp method first devised by Adrian, Chandler, and Hodgkin to voltage-clamp muscle fibers (1970). To isolate the Ca^{2+} current from other voltage-gated conductances, Llinás and colleagues added TTX to the bath to block the voltage-gated Na^+ current, and they added 3-aminopyridine to the bath and injected TEA into the presynaptic terminal to block the voltage-gated K^+ current.

Llinás and colleagues showed that the Ca^{2+} current in the presynaptic terminal is a function of presynaptic voltage (Fig. 8.12A), much as is true for other voltage-gated Ca^{2+} channels. Furthermore, the dependence of the Ca^{2+} current on presynaptic potential was very similar to the dependence of postsynaptic voltage on presynaptic potential (Fig. 8.12B). Both displayed a significant increase at a presynaptic potential about 20 mV depolarized from rest. This is less than the depolarization Katz and Miledi reported to be necessary for measurable synaptic transmitter release, but the lower level may have been the result of more uniform depolarization of the terminal in the experiments of Llinás and colleagues. The voltage clamp used in their experiments may not have achieved a complete control of the voltage in the presynaptic terminal because of the difficultly of clamping an elongated structure with microelectrodes; but voltage control was probably significantly better than in any previous experiments on this preparation.

The experiments of Llinás and co-workers were extended by Augustine, Charlton, and Smith (1985a,b), who voltage-clamped both the presynaptic and postsynaptic terminals, and in addition measured the increase in Ca^{2+} concentration in the presynaptic ter-

Fig. 8.12 Comparison of calcium currents with postsynaptic responses in the squid giant synapse. **(A)** Voltage dependence of presynaptic Ca^{2+} current. Ca^{2+} current measured in voltage-clamped presynaptic terminals in bathing solution containing TTX to block Na^+ currents and 5 mM 3-aminopyridine to inhibit K^+ currents. K^+ currents were further diminished by intracellular injection of TEA. Ordinate plots peak amplitude of Ca^{2+} current as a percentage of the maximum value of peak current, recorded from 8 synapses. Abscissa gives voltage of presynaptic depolarization from a holding potential of -70 mV; thus, a depolarization of 60 mV corresponds to a presynaptic voltage of -10 mV. (Replotted from Llinás, Steinberg, and Walton, 1981a.) **(B)** Postsynaptic voltage as a function of presynaptic voltage. Recordings as in **(A)**, but an additional pipette was inserted in the postsynaptic process close to synapse, to record voltage. Ordinate is postsynaptic response for 7 synapses, normalized to the maximum response recorded in each preparation. Abscissa as in **(A)**, voltage of presynaptic depolarization from a holding potential of -70 mV. (Replotted from Llinás, Steinberg, and Walton, 1981b and used with the permission of the authors and of the Biophysical Society.)

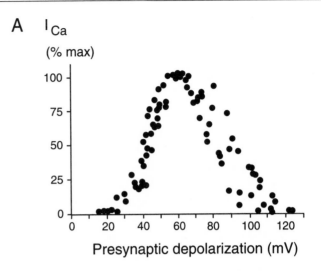

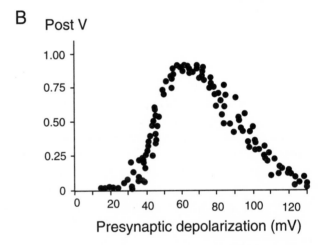

minal with an indicator dye called Arsenazo III (see Chapter 13). They found that presynaptic depolarization produces an increase in Ca^{2+} current and in Ca^{2+} concentration. The integral of i_{Ca} shows the same dependence on presynaptic potential as the change in $[Ca^{2+}]_i$, and postsynaptic conductance increases approximately as the third power of the presynaptic intracellular Ca^{2+} concentration (provided the change in Ca^{2+} is not too large). These measurements provide strong evidence that Ca^{2+} entry is directly related to the release of transmitter and that the relationship between transmitter release and Ca^{2+} concentration is not a linear relation but rather a power relation, as Dodge and Rahamimoff first demonstrated.

Ca^{2+} Not Voltage Causes Release

Experiments with voltage-clamped synapses provided strong evidence that the entry of Ca^{2+} through Ca^{2+} channels in the presynaptic terminal triggers transmitter release. Some have argued, however, that these experiments do not show that Ca^{2+} and release are causally related. Perhaps depolarization instead of or in addition to elevated Ca^{2+} is needed to evoke release (Hochner, Parnas, and Parnas, 1989).

One way of showing that a change in $[Ca^{2+}]_i$ is both necessary and sufficient to produce release might be to change the $[Ca^{2+}]_i$ without changing the presynaptic voltage. This could be done with a caged-Ca^{2+} compound. Caged compounds contain an agent (such as Ca^{2+} or a nucleotide like ATP) in a protected form, so that it is either tightly bound or inactive (see Chapter 13). When the caged compound is illuminated with bright light, a photochemical reaction releases the agent into the cytosol or extracellular medium.

Mulkey and Zucker (1991) recorded from the neuromuscular junction of the crayfish in a bathing solution containing high concentrations of Co^{2+} and Mg^{2+}, to block Ca^{2+} entry through Ca^{2+} channels (see Chapter 7). After injection of the caged-Ca^{2+} compound DM-nitrophen into the presynaptic terminal, Mulkey and Zucker flashed a light to release Ca^{2+} into the presynaptic terminal cytoplasm (see Fig. 13.4A). A postsynaptic response was recorded, even without a change in presynaptic voltage. Furthermore, as long as the entry of Ca^{2+} through voltage-gated Ca^{2+} channels was blocked, changes in presynaptic voltage were without effect if no Ca^{2+} was released with the caged compound.

Where Are the Ca^{2+} Channels?

This question has been addressed in several ways. At the neuromuscular junction (Robitaille, Adler, and Charlton, 1990; Cohen, Jones, and Angelides, 1991), the Ca^{2+} channels (which at this synapse are N-type) were localized with ω-conotoxin conjugated to a fluorescent dye, or with ω-conotoxin and a fluorescently tagged antibody that bound to ω-conotoxin. The Ca^{2+} channels are in rows with the same spacing as active zones at the presynaptic terminal, just adjacent to the postsynaptic receptors. A similar conclusion was reached with atomic force microscopy of chick ciliary ganglion synapses labeled with ω-conotoxin tagged with gold particles (Haydon, Henderson, and Stanley, 1994).

For the squid giant synapse, the location of Ca^{2+} channels has been determined from dye measurements of the increase in intracellular Ca^{2+}. The presynaptic terminal of the squid axon giant synapse was loaded with Ca^{2+}-fluorescent indicators, either the high-affinity dye fura-2 (Smith et al., 1993) or the low-affinity n-aequorin-J, a chemically modified form of the jellyfish luminescent protein aequorin (Llinás, Sugimori, and Silver, 1992). These two Ca^{2+} indicators gave different results. Fura-2 indicated a generalized increase in Ca^{2+} throughout the presynaptic terminal of the synapse, though the increase was highest near the region of the synapse. The generalized increase in Ca^{2+} can be understood from the high affinity of this dye: the dye fluorescence increases as a function of $[Ca^{2+}]_i$ in the range of a few tens to hundreds of nanomolar. Thus diffusion of Ca^{2+} from its points of entry throughout the terminal could have provided a sufficiently large change in Ca^{2+} concentration to have permitted a widespread change in terminal fluorescence. Measurements with n-aequorin-J, on the other hand, showed a discrete, punctate Ca^{2+} increase. Since n-aequorin-J has a relatively low affinity (it only fluoresces at $[Ca^{2+}]_i$ exceeding 100 μM), these measurements suggest that Ca^{2+} may rise to quite high concentrations in very localized regions at the synapse.

Ca^{2+} Domains

Much evidence strongly suggests that the Ca^{2+} channels are highly localized near the presynaptic membrane (see for example Robitaille, Adler, and Charlton, 1990; Roberts, Jacobs, and Hudspeth, 1990; Cohen, Jones, and Angelides, 1991; Smith et al., 1993; Issa and Hudspeth, 1994). Since Ca^{2+} is rapidly buffered in the cytosol and diffuses less readily than if free in solution (see Chapter 4), it is reasonable to suppose that Ca^{2+} entry at the presynaptic terminal produces a sharp gradient of Ca^{2+} concentration.

There may be quite high concentrations for a short period of time very near the membrane (Llinás, Sugimori, and Silver, 1992), where the machinery for vesicle release is located (Burgoyne and Morgan, 1995). Regions of high Ca^{2+} near Ca^{2+} channels have been given the name *Ca^{2+} domains* (Chad and Eckert, 1984). Theoretical calculations suggest that the Ca^{2+} concentration can rise to several hundreds of micromolar or even millimolar during the time necessary for the release of a synaptic vesicle (100–200 μs), but only in a restricted area close to the Ca^{2+} channel (see for example Allbritton, Meyer, and Stryer, 1992; Roberts, 1993, 1994).

Some of the best evidence for Ca^{2+} domains has come from studying the effect on transmitter release of introducing Ca^{2+} buffers into the cytosol of presynaptic terminals. When the Ca^{2+} buffer EGTA (see Fig. 13.1) is injected into the presynaptic terminal of the squid giant synapse, there is virtually no effect on transmitter release (Adler et al., 1991). This is a surprising finding, since EGTA is a high-affinity buffer that would be expected to bind Ca^{2+} entering the terminal through the Ca^{2+} channels. The key to understanding this result is to recognize that EGTA, though of high affinity, has a relatively slow rate of Ca^{2+} binding (see Chapter 13). A different result was obtained with the Ca^{2+} buffer BAPTA (see Fig. 13.1), which has a Ca^{2+} affinity similar to that of EGTA but a much higher rate of Ca^{2+} binding. BAPTA can substantially suppress transmitter release. Apparently Ca^{2+} entering the synaptic terminal through the Ca^{2+} channels is available to trigger release for only a short period, and EGTA cannot bind Ca^{2+} fast enough to have any effect on release. Since the time course of Ca^{2+} action is very short, Ca^{2+} is unable to diffuse far from the site of Ca^{2+} entry.

How Much of a Change in Ca^{2+} Concentration Is Needed to Release a Vesicle?

Probably the best answer to this question has been given by Gary Matthews, Erwin Neher, and their colleagues for the synaptic terminals of retinal bipolar cells (von Gersdorff and Matthews, 1994a; Heidelberger et al., 1994; summarized in Matthews, 1996). The terminals of these cells are sufficiently large that recordings can be made with patch-clamp electrodes (Fig. 8.13A), either from dissociated bipolar cells or from detached terminals. Depolarization

Fig. 8.13 Amplitude of Ca^{2+} change required to trigger release: recordings from retinal bipolar cell synaptic terminals. **(A)** Preparation. *Left:* Dissociated bipolar cell from goldfish retina. *Right:* Synaptic terminal isolated from bipolar cell, with patch pipette for whole-cell recording. **(B)** Measurement of Ca^{2+} and capacitance. At arrow in trace at bottom of figure, the membrane potential was depolarized from $V_H = -60$ mV to a test potential of 0 mV for 250 ms, producing the inward current shown in the boxed inset above. Graphs show time dependence of change in capacitance and in Ca^{2+} in response to this depolarization. Capacitance was determined from the impedance of the cell to a sinusoidal command voltage under voltage clamp. Ca^{2+} was measured with a fluorescent dye (see Chapter 13). **(C–E)** Whole-cell recordings were made from synaptic terminals at times indicated by arrows (*Break-in*), with pipettes containing the indicated free-Ca^{2+} concentrations. Capacitance measured as in **(B).** Note that only the recording with a pipette containing 52 μM free Ca^{2+} produced a measurable increase in capacitance. (From von Gersdorff and Matthews, 1994a, reprinted with permission of the authors and of Macmillan Magazines Limited.)

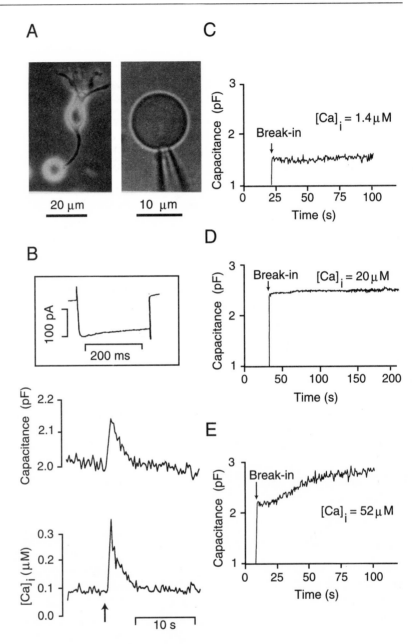

of an isolated terminal produces an inward Ca^{2+} current that is non-inactivating and known from other evidence to be sensitive to dihydropyridine and therefore L-type (Fig. 8.13B, upper trace). The entry of Ca^{2+} produces a marked increase in *cell capacitance*, due to the fusion of transmitter vesicles to the presynaptic membrane (Fig. 8.13B, lower trace). This increase in capacitance was associated with a generalized increase in cytoplasmic Ca^{2+} of about 0.3 μM measured for the whole of the cytosol, but the increase in the region near the membrane was probably much higher.

To show how large a change in Ca^{2+} is necessary to trigger release, two methods were used. In the first (von Gersdorff and Matthews, 1994a), a patch pipette was filled with a solution containing a free-Ca^{2+} concentration of a known value, and the capacitance was measured just after a whole-cell recording was established (i.e., just after *break-in*). As the Ca^{2+}-containing solution entered the cell, it produced a uniform increase in Ca^{2+} throughout the cytosol. No change in capacitance (and therefore no transmitter release) was observed unless the Ca^{2+} concentration was raised above 20–50 μM (Fig. 8.13C–E). This would suggest that the change in Ca^{2+} required at the release site was at least tens of micromolar.

The change in Ca^{2+} concentration was also estimated in a second series of experiments (Heidelberger et al., 1994), in which the synaptic terminal was filled with the caged-Ca^{2+} compound DM-nitrophen (Fig. 13.4A), as in the experiments of Mulkey and Zucker (1991). Flashes of light were used to release Ca^{2+}, and the Ca^{2+} concentration achieved by illumination of DM-nitrophen was measured with the low-affinity Ca^{2+} indicator dye Furaptra (see Chapter 13). The rate of vesicle release (measured from the increase in capacitance) increased as the Ca^{2+} concentration increased. A half-maximal rate was estimated to occur at a Ca^{2+} concentration of the order of 100–200 μM.

These experiments indicate that the presynaptic terminal of a bipolar cell is a highly organized structure, with Ca^{2+} channels positioned quite close to the release machinery such that large changes in Ca^{2+} concentration are required to trigger release. Considerable evidence suggests that this may be true at other synapses as well, particularly for those mediating fast chemical transmission with transmitters such as acetylcholine and glutamate. Lando and

Zucker (1994) found that the synaptic release produced by an action potential could be mimicked by flash photolysis of caged Ca^{2+}, but only if the $[Ca^{2+}]_i$ reached tens of micromolar.

The high Ca^{2+} concentration required for release at fast chemical synapses may have important consequences. First, the high concentration needed may reduce the amount of cross-talk between different regions of active zone. Ca^{2+} entering through a particular Ca^{2+} channel may need to travel a short distance to reach a release site (Borst and Sakmann, 1996) but would release vesicles only over a restricted region of the terminal; the smaller amounts of Ca^{2+} that spread over larger distances may be without effect on release at adjacent sites. Second, the high Ca^{2+} concentration required for release may have the effect of increasing the temporal fidelity of transmission. If a high Ca^{2+} concentration is required to trigger release, the affinity of Ca^{2+} binding to the control site must be low. In this case, Ca^{2+} would bind and dissociate rapidly from its binding site, and the time course of Ca^{2+} action would more faithfully reflect the time course of Ca^{2+} entry.

III: Quantal Release, Synaptic Vesicles, and the Mechanism of Exocytosis

When the first intracellular recordings were made from skeletal muscle by Paul Fatt and Bernard Katz (1951, 1952), a curious thing was observed. If a microelectrode was inserted in the vicinity of the neuromuscular junction, small spontaneous depolarizations were recorded. These miniature endplate potentials (MEPPs) seemed to be due to release of transmitter (in this case, acetylcholine, or ACh), since they were blocked by curare, which blocks the binding of ACh to its receptor. The MEPPs were present only if the pipette was in the vicinity of an endplate. Furthermore, if the Ca^{2+} in the bath was reduced, the normal endplate potential (EPP) also became smaller, because Ca^{2+} influx into the terminal and the probability of release of synaptic vesicles decreased. The smallest EPPs recorded in low-Ca^{2+} medium were identical in amplitude and waveform to the spontaneous MEPPs (Fig. 8.14). Also observed in

Fig. 8.14 Intracellular recordings of endplate potentials (synaptic responses) from frog neuromuscular junction. Presynaptic stimulation was given at arrows. Recordings were made in bathing solution containing 25% of the normal Ca^{2+} concentration to reduce the probability of transmitter release and decrease the size of the postsynaptic response. Records from top to bottom are repetitions of the same presynaptic stimulus under the same conditions from the same preparation. There is an apparent step-like variability in the amplitude of the response. (Modified, with contrast reversed, from Fatt and Katz, 1952.)

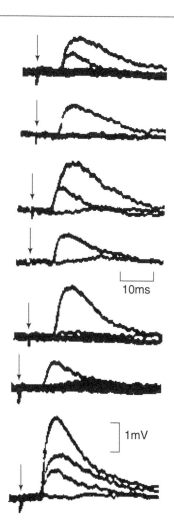

low-Ca^{2+} medium were responses that appeared to consist of the sum of 2 or 3 MEPPs.

The Quantal Theory of Transmitter Release

These observations suggested that MEPPs might represent spontaneously occurring, irreducible units of transmitter release, which Katz and his colleagues called "quanta." If during nerve-evoked stimulation transmitter is also released in similar irreducible units, the endplate potential might be composed of the summation of many such units, each having the same amplitude as a miniature potential. The quantal composition of the EPP would be difficult to observe under normal conditions, at least at the neuromuscular junction, since so many quanta would be summing to form the response. In low-Ca^{2+} medium, the number of quanta might be sufficiently small so that the contributions of individual quanta could be observed.

We can summarize these ideas in the following way. Let $<epp>$ represent the mean amplitude of the endplate potential, $<mepp>$ the mean amplitude of a miniature endplate potential, n the total number of release sites in the presynaptic membrane capable of responding to stimulation, and p the probability that nerve stimulation leads to the release of a quantum of transmitter at a release site. The mean endplate potential is then given by $<epp> = np<mepp>$. Under normal conditions, p and consequently $<epp>$ are rather large, but in low Ca^{2+} or high Mg^{2+}, p and $<epp>$ become small, and $<epp>$ may be of the same order of magnitude as $<mepp>$.

If each quantum of transmitter is released independently of the others (i.e., if the probability of release at each release site is independent of release at other sites), then the number of quanta released should follow a binomial distribution. Each of the release sites can be thought of as a coin that when flipped comes up as "heads" with a probability p. When the presynaptic terminal is stimulated, all of the coins are flipped simultaneously. The probability p_i of observing i heads when n coins are flipped is given by

$$p_i = \binom{n}{i} p^i (1-p)^{n-i} = \frac{n!}{(n-i)!\,i!} p^i (1-p)^{n-i} \qquad (8)$$

This is also the expression that gives the probability of observing i quanta when there are n release sites, when the probability of release is the same at each release site and is equal to p. If, for example, n is 4 and p is 0.46 (experiment 49 of Korn et al., 1982, for inhibitory synaptic input to a goldfish Mauthner cell), then the probabilities of observing no release (p_0) and of observing 1–4 quanta (p_1–p_4) can be calculated from Eqn. (8) to be 0.085, 0.29, 0.37, 0.21, and 0.045.

For the neuromuscular junction, n is very large. There are several hundred active zones like those shown in Fig. 8.9, each of which can serve as a release site for one or more vesicles (see Korn and Faber, 1991). Furthermore, in low-Ca^{2+} solution, the probability of release at any one active zone is very small. Thus, to continue our analogy, the number of coins is very large, but the probability of any one coin turning up "heads" is very small. This means that for transmission at the neuromuscular junction in low-Ca^{2+} solution, the statistics of release can be described by the Poisson distribution, as an approximation of the binomial distribution for large n and small p.

Following del Castillo and Katz (1954b), we call m the ratio of $<epp>$ to $<mepp>$, that is,

$$m = \frac{<epp>}{<mepp>} = np \qquad (9)$$

If the EPP is made up of the sum of many MEPPs, we can think of m as the mean number of MEPPs (that is, of quanta) produced by stimulation. It is often referred to as the *quantal content* and can also be thought of as the mean number of release sites activated by stimulation. The probability of observing an EPP composed of i quanta is given by the Poisson distribution as

$$p_i = \frac{m^i}{i!} e^{-m} \qquad (10)$$

Del Castillo and Katz (1954b) tested the applicability of the Poisson distribution for transmitter release in a low-Ca^{2+} Ringer solution using two different approaches. They first used Eqn. (10) to estimate the value of the mean quantal content *(m)*. To obtain m from Eqn. (10), they measured the frequency with which a nerve impulse failed to evoke a response. Eqn. (10) predicts that the probability of observing a failure (i.e., p_0) is just $(m^0/0!)e^{-m}$. Since $m^0/0!$ is 1 (0! is 1 by definition), $p_0 = e^{-m}$, and $m = \ln(1/p_0)$. Del Castillo and Katz then compared this value to the one estimated from Eqn. (9) by dividing the mean amplitude of the EPP ($<epp>$) by the mean amplitude of the MEPP ($<mepp>$). These estimates agreed closely.

Del Castillo and Katz also attempted to measure directly the frequency of occurrence of EPPs consisting of n quanta, for n equal to 0, 1, 2, 3, and so on. They constructed a histogram of the amplitudes of the EPPs for a large number of responses and then attempted to fit this histogram with the Poisson distribution. This is not as easy as it may seem. The difficulty is that the amplitudes of the MEPPs (and therefore presumably of the quantal units that sum to produce the EPPs) are not entirely constant but vary from one MEPP to the next (Fig. 8.15A), perhaps because different vesicles contain different amounts of transmitter or because the concentration of receptors in the postsynaptic membrane is not uniform.

The distribution of MEPPs at the neuromuscular junction is nearly Gaussian, with a mean equal to $<mepp>$ and a variance equal to σ^2 (Fatt and Katz, 1952). If evoked and spontaneous responses are produced by identical mechanisms, EPPs consisting of only one quantum will also have a Gaussian distribution, with a mean equal to $<mepp>$ and a variance equal to σ^2, while EPPs consisting of two quanta will be Gaussian with mean $2<mepp>$

Fig. 8.15 Statistics of transmitter release. **(A)** and **(B)** Intracellular recordings from frog neuromuscular junction in 25% Ringer solution. Histogram in **(A)** plots the number of spontaneous MEPPs (ordinate) as a function of their amplitude (abscissa) and therefore indicates the extent of variability in the size of the MEPPs. The scale on the abscissa is given in units normalized to the mean amplitude of the MEPP, $<mepp>$, which was 0.875 mV. This amplitude is at the point labeled I. Histogram in **(B)** plots the number of EPPs evoked by presynaptic stimulation (as in Fig. 8.14), again in units normalized to the mean value of the MEPP. Thus, 0 corresponds to no response (failure), I to response of same amplitude as the mean of a single MEPP, II to two MEPPs, and so on. Arrows indicate number of failures predicted from Eqn. (10). Continuous curve calculated from Poisson distribution, on the assumption that quanta of postsynaptic response have the same mean amplitude and variance as MEPPs. Values of mean amplitude and variance of MEPPs were estimated from distribution in **(A)**. (Redrawn from del Castillo and Katz, 1954b.) **(C)** Whole-cell recordings of postsynaptic currents from neurons ("bushy cells") in anteroventral cochlear nucleus, recorded in response to stimulation of auditory nerve in thin slices of rat brain perfused with 100 μM Cd^{2+} (to reduce probability of transmitter release). Number of quantal units for each response is shown to right of traces. Timing of presynaptic stimulation indicated by stimulation artifact *(arrow)*. Lowermost trace is average of 298 responses. **(D)** Response amplitude histograms, as in **(B)** for cell in **(C)** and for two other cells. Ordinate gives number of responses, and abscissa gives response amplitude in units of the mean amplitude of the mEPSC. Open bars are observed number of responses, solid bars are predictions of Poisson equation for value of m given for each histogram. N is the total number of traces for each experiment. (Parts **(C)** and **(D)** reprinted from Isaacson and Walmsley, 1995, with permission of the authors and of Cell Press.)

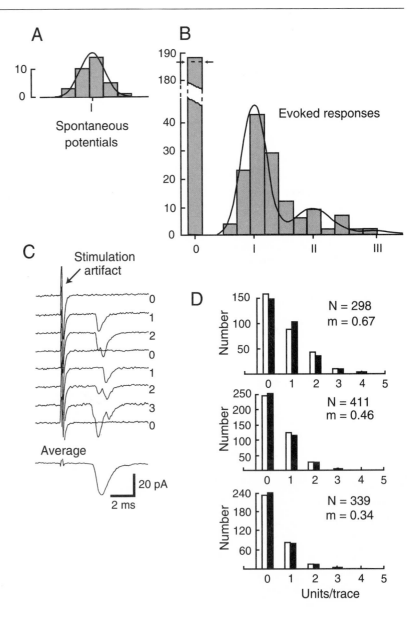

and variance $2\sigma^2$, and so on. The variance must be multiplied by 2 because we have assumed that the release of quanta occurs independently at different release sites; and for independent variables, the variance of a sum is equal to the sum of the variances.

Del Castillo and Katz attempted to fit the histogram of EPP amplitudes by first constructing a Gaussian to fit the amplitude distribution for MEPPs and then multiplying the mean and variance of this Gaussian by 2 for $n = 2$, by 3 for $n = 3$, and so on. Each of these Gaussians was then multiplied by a factor proportional to the probability of occurrence of an EPP consisting of n quanta (i.e., by p_i), obtained from the Poisson equation. Although the fit of these Gaussians to the data was reasonably good (Fig. 8.15B), the variance of MEPP amplitude was rather large. A more convincing demonstration was given in a subsequent study from Katz's laboratory for mammalian neuromuscular junction (Boyd and Martin, 1956).

Transmission at Central Synapses

Since transmission at synapses in the CNS seems similar to that at the neuromuscular junction, it is reasonable to suppose that chemical transmission in the CNS is also quantal. This postulate has been difficult to prove. Especially good evidence exists for one synapse, that of auditory nerve fibers onto neurons in the anteroventral cochlear nucleus (Isaacson and Walmsley, 1995). These synapses, called the endbulbs of Held, are much larger than most CNS synapses and, like the neuromuscular junction, may contain hundreds of release sites. In the presence of Cd^{2+} (to reduce the Ca^{2+} current and probability of release), evoked responses have a quantal distribution (Fig. 8.15C) that is well described by the Poisson distribution (Fig. 8.15D).

At other synapses in the CNS, transmission is also thought to be quantal, but this is still not certain (see Korn and Faber, 1991; Lisman and Harris, 1993; Bekkers, 1994; Stjärne et al., 1994). Numerous difficulties face the experimenter who wishes to understand transmission, for example at synapses in the hippocampus. A single presynaptic cell may make many synapses onto a postsynaptic neuron, and each synaptic bouton may have more than one release site. Are all of these boutons and release sites equivalent? If some occur at distances further away from the cell body than others, they may produce smaller currents or voltages at the site of recording, as a result of passive spread (Chapter 2). Different terminals may have dramatically different probabilities of release (Rosenmund, Clements, and Westbrook, 1993; Hessler, Shirke, and Malinow, 1993; Isaac, Nicoll, and Malenka, 1995; Murthy, Sejnowski, and Stevens, 1997). Furthermore, the areas of postsynaptic membrane may be quite variable, in that activation produces a larger postsynaptic potential (PSP) at some synapses than at others (Lisman and Harris, 1993). These parameters may in part be responsible for the large variability of MPSPs at central synapses, though MPSPs seem to be variable even at a single synaptic bouton (Liu and Tsien, 1995), perhaps as a result of variability in the amount of transmitter contained in different synaptic vesicles (Frerking, Borges, and Wilson, 1995) or channel noise produced by postsynaptic receptors (Faber et al., 1992).

The neuromuscular junction and the endbulbs of Held are very large synapses containing many release sites and a large number of postsynaptic receptors, but a more typical synapse in the CNS is quite small and may contain only one or a few release sites. Theoretical calculation and much experimental evidence suggests that the release of a single vesicle at such a synapse may be sufficient to produce a millimolar increase in the concentration of transmitter in the synaptic cleft and to saturate the postsynaptic receptors at that synapse (see Clements, 1996; Chapters 9 and 10). Since one neuron may make many such synapses with a single postsynaptic cell, the units of quantal release may actually be single synaptic terminals (Korn et al., 1982). This is not to say that multiple vesicle release does not occur (see for example Tong and Jahr, 1994), but in most cases a single vesicle may be sufficient for nearly complete activation of the receptors in the postsynaptic membrane adjacent to each synapse. The summed synaptic potential would then consist of "quantal" components produced by activation at each of the individual terminals (Forti et al., 1997). Though transmission at central synapses is likely to be quantal in one form or another, there remain many unanswered questions about the relationship between miniature synaptic potentials and evoked responses and about the details of the statistics of release.

Transmitter Is Released from Vesicles

The first electron micrographs of the nervous system showed presynaptic terminals filled with vesicles (De Robertis and Bennett, 1955; Palay, 1956—see also Couteaux and Pecot-Déchavassine, 1970), and these vesicles were immediately hypothesized to contain synaptic transmitter. With the development of techniques for isolating and purifying presynaptic vesicles from brain (see for example Whittaker, Michaelson, and Kirkland, 1964), the evidence rapidly became overwhelming that vesicles do indeed contain chemicals such as acetylcholine (ACh), catecholamines, γ-aminobutyric acid (GABA), and neuropeptides at high concentration. Furthermore, specific mechanisms were discovered for the synthesis, transport, and recycling of the vesicles, as well as for the transport of transmitter into the vesicles (see Kelly, 1993).

That vesicles probably function in transmitter release gradually became clear from two kinds of observations. The first, largely biochemical, were made initially on adrenal medullary cells rather than on neurons. Adrenal medullary cells contain large *dense-core* vesicles (sometimes called granules) that, in addition to the transmitter epinephrine, contain ATP and several different proteins, including *chromogranins*. When stimulated, these cells release epinephrine, but ATP and chromogranins can also be detected in the venous effluent leading away from the adrenal medulla. The key observation is this: the ratio of epinephrine concentration to ATP concentration (or of epinephrine concentration to chromogranin concentration) in the venous effluent was very similar to the ratios measured biochemically from isolated vesicles (Douglas and Poisner, 1966; Schneider, Smith, and Winkler, 1967). It is difficult to see how this could occur unless vesicles were responsible for release.

The second group of observations in support of vesicular release were morphological. When the neuromuscular junction is exposed to lanthanum ions (La^{3+}) or to black widow spider venom, there is a massive increase in the frequency of MEPPs recorded from the muscle, produced by an avalanche of quantal release. Examination of the structure of the neuromuscular junction in the electron microscope revealed that both La^{3+} (Heuser and Miledi, 1971) and black widow spider venom (Clark, Hurlbut, and Mauro, 1972) produce a massive depletion of synaptic vesicles, leading eventually to their complete disappearance from the terminal. Subsequently, depletion was shown also to occur just as the result of high rates and/or long durations of stimulation (see for example Ceccarelli, Hurlbut, and Mauro, 1972; Heuser and Reese, 1973).

A role for vesicles in transmitter release was conclusively demonstrated by fast-freezing the neuromuscular junction in the act of transmitter release (Heuser et al., 1979; Heuser and Reese, 1981). Heuser, Reese, and their colleagues attempted to catch vesicles in the act of fusing to the presynaptic membrane with a special apparatus, constructed to stimulate a muscle held on a moveable plate. The plate together with the tissue was allowed to fall against a copper block, cooled to 4°K with liquid helium. A mechanical trigger was provided so that the muscle was electrically stimulated just before freezing occurred. To increase the mean quantal content (i.e., m) and therefore the probability of observing vesicles in the act of release, the muscle and nerve were soaked in solution containing the K$^+$ channel blocker 4-aminopyridine (4-AP) just before the muscle was mounted on the moveable plate. 4-AP increased the probability of vesicle release by prolonging the presynaptic action potential and increasing the length of time during which Ca^{2+} entered the presynaptic terminal through voltage-gated Ca^{2+} channels. Frozen muscles were removed after freezing and thin-sectioned. Alternatively, the tissue was freeze-fractured and etched, and replicas were formed by coating with platinum-carbon. The sections and replicas were observed in the electron microscope.

Figure 8.16A is a thin section from a stimulated muscle at an active zone. There are two outpocketings of the presynaptic membrane of the same size and curvature as vesicles; these appear to represent vesicles caught in the act of releasing their transmitter. There are in addition numerous bulges in the presynaptic membrane, which may represent vesicles that fused and are in the process of flattening. Figure 8.16B is an external view of the inside half of the presynaptic membrane (the protoplasmic or P face) at an active zone, from a freeze-fractured replica. This micrograph is similar to that in Fig. 8.9B, which also shows the P face of an active zone but in an unstimulated muscle. Stimulation causes the appearance of numerous indentations along the edge of the active zone.

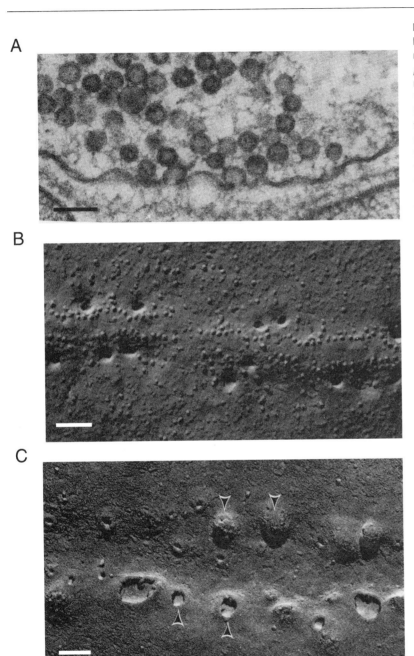

A

B

C

Fig. 8.16 Stimulation produces vesicle release at the frog neuromuscular junction. Cutaneous pectoris muscle from the frog *Rana pipiens* was dissected together with motor nerve and placed in Ringer solution containing 1 mM 4-aminopyridine to reduce voltage-gated K^+ conductance and prolong the decay of action potentials at the presynaptic terminal. Muscle was mounted on a special freezing apparatus so that tissue could be fast-frozen at a fixed time after stimulation of the nerve. Scale bars, 0.1 μm (100 nm). **(A)** Thin-section transmission electron micrograph of terminal at active zone, frozen 5.2 ms after motor nerve stimulation. Note bulges in plasma membrane, probably due to fusion of synaptic vesicles. **(B)** Freeze-fracture view of internal leaflet (protoplasmic or P face) of neuronal (presynaptic) plasma membrane at active zone. Tissue frozen 3.7 ms after nerve stimulation. **(C)** Freeze-fracture view of external leaflet (exoplasmic or E face) of neuronal (presynaptic) membrane. Tissue frozen 20 ms after nerve stimulation. The bulges at the top of the figure are synaptic vesicles, attached to the plasma membrane *(downward arrow heads)*. The pits shown below have been formed as the result of fracturing the tissue across the "neck" of the vesicle *(upward arrow heads)*. (Reprinted from Heuser and Reese, 1981, with permission of the authors and of Rockefeller University Press.)

The number of indentations increased with increasing concentration of 4-AP (Heuser et al., 1979), and their time dependence was consistent with the time course of the EPP.

That these indentations were really caused by vesicle fusion is supported by freeze-fracture micrographs of the exoplasmic or E face (the inner view of the external surface of the membrane). The E face of a nerve terminal, stimulated 20 ms before freezing, is shown in Fig. 8.16C. The bulges at the top of the figure are actually synaptic vesicles, attached to the plasma membrane. The pits below have been formed as the result of fracturing the tissue across the "neck" of the vesicle. These pits in all probability are the holes through which transmitter has left the vesicles and diffused out into the synaptic cleft.

The Mechanism of Exocytosis

The evidence is now overwhelming that synaptic transmitter at the great majority of synapses in the central nervous system is released from vesicles, and that these vesicles are responsible for the quanta observed electrophysiologically. The question now remains, how does vesicle release occur? The membrane of the presynaptic terminal is complicated in structure. In an unstimulated cell, vesicles are arrayed along the active zone, "docked" in place by some interaction between the terminal membrane and the membrane of the vesicle (Fig. 8.9). The opening of Ca^{2+} channels causes the intracellular Ca^{2+} concentration to rise to very high levels in the vicinity of the membrane, and this somehow triggers the fusion of vesicles with the plasma membrane.

A large body of evidence indicates that vesicle fusion at the synaptic terminal is similar in mechanism to fusion occurring in other places within the cell, for example between the cisternae of the Golgi stack. In the Golgi apparatus (Rothman, 1994; Rothman and Wieland, 1996), fusion is mediated by a specific interaction between proteins called *SNAP receptors,* or *SNAREs.* There are complementary SNAREs on both the vesicle membrane and its target membrane, the v-SNARE and t-SNARE. The SNAREs presumably provide specificity for the vesicle-target interaction. The binding of the SNAREs to one another then allows the binding of cytoplasmic proteins called *SNAPs* (soluble NSF attachment proteins), which facilitate the binding of another cytosolic protein, an ATPase called the *N*-ethylmaleimide-sensitive factor, or *NSF*. The formation of the SNARE-SNAP-NSF complex activates NSF to hydrolyze ATP, and this somehow leads to fusion.

For synaptic vesicles, similar events seem to occur (see Bajjalieh and Scheller, 1995; Scheller, 1995; Schweizer, Betz, and Augustine, 1995; Südhof, 1995; Tingley, 1995; Zucker, 1996; Geppert and Südhof, 1998). Since work on Golgi vesicle fusion and synaptic vesicle fusion proceeded largely independently, an entirely different nomenclature has emerged for the synaptic proteins. There is evidence that the synaptic vesicle protein *VAMP* (also called *synaptobrevin*) is a v-SNARE. There are apparently two t-SNAREs at the active zone embedded in the plasma membrane, called *syntaxin* and *SNAP-25*. (Note: SNAP-25 is synaptosomal associated protein–25 kDa and is in no way related to the SNAP protein of the SNARE-SNAP-NSF complex.) VAMP, syntaxin, and SNAP-25 can form a complex (called the 7S complex), apparently in the form of a slender rod (see Fig. 8.17 and Hanson et al., 1997; Sutton et al., 1998). The aggregation of these three proteins and the formation of the 7S complex are known to be absolutely required for exocytosis, since various toxins (botulinum and tetanus toxins), which are proteases, cleave these proteins and inhibit exocytosis. In sufficient quantity, these toxins can kill an organism by causing complete paralysis of transmission.

What happens after the formation of the 7S complex is still uncertain. One possibility is that, after the binding and attachment of the vesicle to the active zone ("docking"), a further series of reactions must occur to make the vesicle competent for rapid, Ca^{2+}-sensitive membrane fusion (Schweizer, Betz, and Augustine, 1995; Südhof, 1995). These reactions are sometimes referred to as *priming*. The proteins α-SNAP and/or β-SNAP (which *are* true SNAP proteins) are thought to bind to the 7S particle, apparently forming a cylindrical structure with the SNARE-containing rod at its core (Hanson et al., 1997). This then leads to the binding of the soluble NSF protein and the formation of the 20S complex, just as for the Golgi apparatus. The NSF protein hydrolyzes ATP, somehow completing the priming of the vesicle. Another possibility is that the 7S

Fig. 8.17 A possible molecular mechanism for vesicle fusion. The plasma membrane at the synapse is known to contain two proteins, synapsin and SNAP-25, which form a rod-like t-SNARE complex with a high α-helical content *(top left)*. A synaptic vesicle containing VAMP (or synaptobrevin), which is a v-SNARE, and the Ca^{2+}-regulated protein synaptotagmin (as well as other proteins not illustrated) approaches the membrane, and VAMP complexes with the t-SNAREs. This forms the so-called 7S complex. The soluble proteins NSF and SNAP may then bind to the 7S complex, perhaps as multimeric cylinders enclosing the rod-shaped 7S complex. Together these proteins form the 20S complex. At some point the vesicle protein synaptotagmin may also become associated with this complex. The addition of ATP causes the release of NSF and SNAP, leaving the vesicle closely apposed to the membrane and "primed" for release. Alternatively, the 7S complex itself may mediate release, and the NSF and SNAP proteins may bind at a later stage to reactivate the release machinery. Addition of Ca^{2+} triggers membrane fusion and the release of transmitter by a process that may involve synaptotagmin, but the detailed mechanism of Ca^{2+}-dependent release is still unclear.

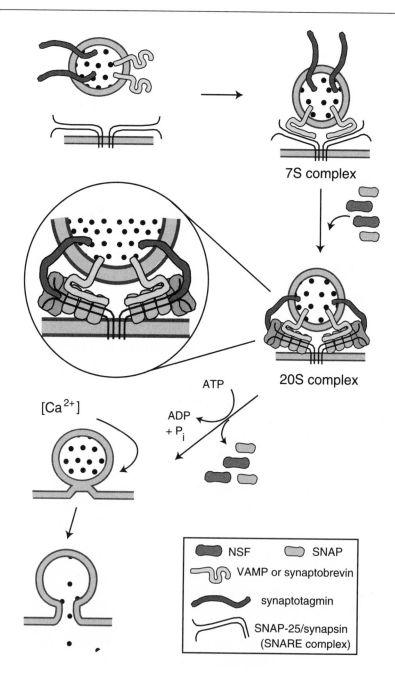

complex itself mediates fusion, and that the SNAP and NSF proteins only bind *after fusion* to reactivate the fusion machinery (see Geppert and Südhof, 1998).

After priming, the vesicle must actually fuse to the plasma membrane and release its contents into the synaptic cleft. This process is highly Ca^{2+}-dependent, as we have seen, and a protein called *synaptotagmin* may somehow become associated with the other fusion proteins and be responsible for the Ca^{2+} dependence of release (Littleton and Bellen, 1995; Südhof and Rizo, 1996; Geppert and Südhof, 1998). This protein binds Ca^{2+} and phospholipids and can undergo a Ca^{2+}-dependent change in conformation. In transgenic mice in which one of the genes for synaptotagmin *(synaptotagmin I)* is knocked out, Ca^{2+}-triggered rapid transmitter release is impaired (Geppert et al., 1994). Certain mutations of synaptotagmin in *Drosophila* cause a change in the *stoichiometry* of Ca^{2+} dependence (Littleton et al., 1994). Nevertheless, the exact role of synaptotagmin is still a subject of considerable controversy (see for example Scheller, 1995; DeCamilli and Takei, 1996).

We still have no details of the mechanism by which a change in Ca^{2+} concentration produces vesicle fusion. Several studies indicate that Ca^{2+} channels are closely associated with the proteins mediating vesicle release (see for example Rettig et al., 1996), and the probability of opening of Ca^{2+} channels may even be regulated in some way by these proteins (Bezprozvanny, Scheller, and Tsien, 1995). How these complex interactions are controlled to produce vesicle fusion is still not understood, and regulators of vesicle release (including munc 18, complexin, and the small-molecular-weight G-protein RAB3—see Geppert and Südhof, 1998) may play an essential role in this process.

Formation of the Fusion Pore

The fusion of the vesicle begins with the formation of a metastable complex of lipid and protein at the site of vesicle release, from which a channel (called a *fusion pore*) forms between the vesicle and the plasma membrane. This process has been studied in considerable detail, especially in mast cells (see Almers, 1990; Monck and Fernandez, 1992, 1994; Lindau and Almers, 1995). Mast cells, which are found in connective tissue, secrete histamine during the inflammatory response. They are an ideal preparation for studying vesicle-mediated secretion because of the large diameter of their vesicles. Although it is possible that some features of vesicle secretion differ in mast cells and neurons, the mechanism of fusion pore formation is likely to be similar.

In mast cells, the initial size of the fusion pore has actually been measured. It was possible to do so because in a mouse line called *beige,* the mast cell vesicles are so large that fusion of a single vesicle produces a significant change in the area of the plasma membrane and can be visualized as a step change in capacitance (see Fig. 8.19A). Furthermore, as the vesicle membrane fuses, charge flows. The reason for this is that the potential across the vesicle membrane is not the same as that across the plasma membrane (Fig. 8.18A). The vesicle membrane contains proton transporters that accumulate H^+ inside the vesicle interior. Fusion of the vesicle membrane with the plasma membrane allows the H^+ to flow out of the vesicle, and charge continues to flow through the fusion pore until the potential across vesicle and plasma membranes is the same (Breckenridge and Almers, 1987; Almers, 1990; Spruce et al., 1990).

The waveform of the current flow through the fusion pore from a typical recording is as in Fig. 8.18B (from Spruce et al., 1990). The current is initially large and then goes to zero as the potentials across the vesicle and plasma membranes reach the same value. The value of the charge q carried by the current can be obtained as a function of time (Fig. 8.18C) by integrating the current waveform, since $i = dq/dt$ (see Chapter 2). Furthermore, since $dV/dt = i/C$,

$$\frac{dV}{dt} = \frac{dq}{dt} \cdot \frac{1}{c} \quad \text{and} \quad \Delta V = \frac{\Delta q}{c} \tag{11}$$

Therefore the change in charge can be used together with the size of the vesicle capacitance (measured as in Fig. 8.19A) to calculate the change in the membrane potential (Fig. 8.18D). Finally, since $g = V/i$, the conductance of the fusion pore can be calculated from the ratio of the voltage difference and the current (Fig. 8.18E). It is initially 200–300 pS, about the size expected for a pore of 10–20 Å.

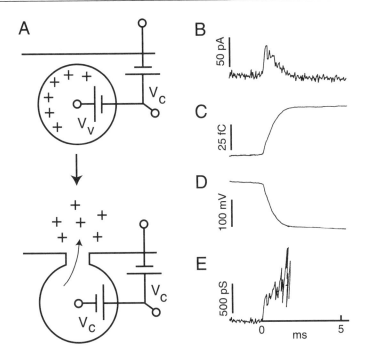

Fig. 8.18 Measuring currents through the fusion pore. **(A)** The electrical properties of a large vesicle in a mast cell from a *beige* mouse. V_c is the potential across the cell membrane and is also the command potential of the voltage-clamp amplifier in a whole-cell patch-clamp recording. The potential across the vesicle membrane is V_v. For a vesicle at rest *(upper diagram)*, V_v is not the same as V_c because vesicles contain proton pumps that accumulate protons (and therefore excess positive charge) within the vesicle interior. After fusion of vesicle and plasma membranes *(lower diagram)*, positive charge flows out through the fusion pore, and this equilibrates V_v and V_c. (From Breckenridge and Almers, 1987, reprinted with permission of the authors and of Macmillan Magazines Limited.) **(B)** Change in current recorded during a fusion event, equal to the current flowing through the fusion pore during vesicle fusion. Mast cell was whole-cell patch-clamped with pipette containing 20 μM GTPγS (to stimulate vesicle fusion). **(C)** Charge moving through fusion pore. Time integral of current transient shown in **(B)**. **(D)** Time dependence of potential driving current through fusion pore (i.e., $V_C - V_V$), calculated from $\Delta V = \Delta q/C$. Charge from **(C)** was subtracted from its final value and divided by capacitance of vesicle (286 fF, measured as in Fig. 8.13 and Fig. 8.19A). From an initial value of 138 mV, ΔV declined to zero as vesicle and cell membrane potentials equilibrated. **(E)** Time dependence of conductance of fusion pore, calculated from $g = i/(V_C - V_V)$ by dividing trace in **(B)** from that in **(D)**. Conductance increased abruptly as fusion pore opened, then grew more gradually. Large fluctuations are noise due to small value of current measurements in **(B)**. Parts **(B)**–**(E)** reprinted from Spruce et al., 1990, with permission of the authors and of Cell Press.)

The conductance of the pore than increases, presumably as the pore widens.

When the fusion events in mast cells are monitored by measuring the change in capacitance that occurs as the vesicles fuse to the plasma membrane (as for bipolar cells—see Fig. 8.13), the fusion events appear as increases in capacitance (Fig. 8.19A), large enough in mast cells to be visualized as individual step-like events because of the large surface area of the vesicles. These events provide an actual measure of the time course of fusion. Most of the step increases in capacitance are irreversible, but occasionally a transient event occurs, indicating that a vesicle fuses and then unfuses (Spruce et al., 1990). When this happens, the capacitance is often less than it was initially (Fig. 8.19B), as if the vesicle carried off some of the plasma membrane with it (Monck and Fernandez, 1992). This is evidence that the formation of the fusion pore causes lipid to move from the plasma membrane into the vesicle. This flux of lipid may be as large as a million lipid molecules per second and may be responsible for the widening of the vesicle that eventually

Fig. 8.19 Reversible vesicle fusion. **(A)** Capacitance measurements from mast cell of normal mouse recorded with whole-cell pipette containing GTPγS. Capacitance measured as in Fig. 8.13; scale in *femto* farads (= 10^{-15} F). Upward steps are increases in capacitance caused by fusion of single vesicles to membrane. Though most capacitance increases are irreversible, a few are not *(arrows)*. These "steps down" indicate fusion events that initiate but do not go to completion. **(B)** Reversible fusion of giant vesicle from *beige* mouse mast cell. Several incomplete fusion events probably occurred in the same vesicle. In each case the capacitance of the plasma membrane actually decreases after fusion reversal (note difference in dotted and dashed lines indicated by arrows), showing that the vesicle has picked up lipid from the plasma membrane. **(C)** Model of reversible fusion. (Reprinted from Monck and Fernandez, 1992, with permission of the authors and of Rockefeller University Press. See also Monck, de Toledo, and Fernandez, 1990.)

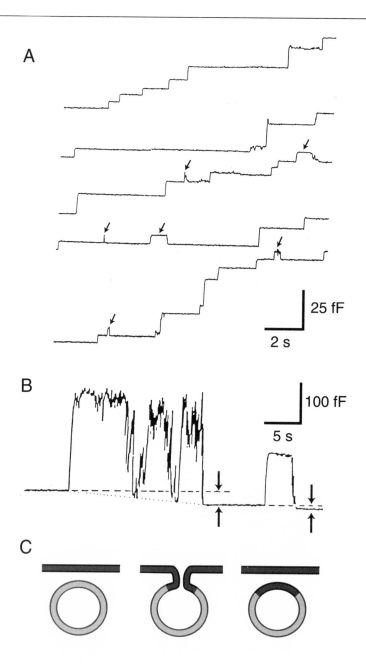

A

25 fF

2 s

B

100 fF

5 s

C

leads to the release of transmitter molecules into the extracellular space.

There are at present two theories about how fusion pores form (see Betz and Angleson, 1998). According to the first (Lindau and Almers, 1995), the pore is formed by protein, much as ion channels are constructed. The protein components would come, presumably, from both the vesicle and the plasma membrane and perhaps are brought into register and set for fusion during or after priming of the vesicle. It is possible that fusion is facilitated by proteins known as cysteine string proteins (Gundersen, Mastrogiacomo, and Umbach, 1995; Buchner and Gundersen, 1997), which are known to be present in synaptic vesicles (Mastrogiacomo et al., 1994).

A second theory (Monck and Fernandez, 1994) proposes that the fusion pore is predominantly lipidic. The plasma membrane first dimples out toward the vesicle, facilitated by a protein scaffolding holding the plasma membrane in place (see for example Chandler and Heuser, 1980). The lipid bilayers of the vesicle and plasma membrane then fuse spontaneously to form the fusion pore. At present, too little information is available to distinguish between these hypotheses.

Endocytosis

Depolarization and Ca^{2+} entry cause an increase in the capacitance of a terminal that—even for irreversible fusion—is transient: the capacitance increases as vesicles fuse to the presynaptic membrane, and the capacitance then declines, presumably as the result of retrieval of membrane back into the cytoplasm (see Fig. 8.13B). Membrane retrieval is called *endocytosis*. In bipolar cells, a weak stimulus is followed by rapid endocytosis, which is approximately exponential with a time constant equal to about 1.5–2 s (von Gersdorff and Matthews, 1994a). Larger stimuli produce a much more prolonged decrease in capacitance, with a time constant in the tens of seconds. This longer time course may be due at least in part to inhibition of endocytosis by the large increase in intracellular Ca^{2+} produced by strong stimuli (von Gersdorff and Matthews, 1994b; but see also Ryan, Smith, and Reuter, 1996; Wu and Betz, 1996).

The time course of vesicle renewal has also been studied with extracellular marker molecules that are taken up into the cytoplasm when endocytosis occurs. The protein horseradish peroxidase (HRP), for example, when placed in the perfusion medium, is taken up into presynaptic terminals of motor fibers at the neuromuscular junction when the muscle is stimulated (Heuser and Reese, 1973). The HRP first makes its appearance in "coated vesicles," whose extracellular surface contains an electron-dense material. These vesicles (see Fig. 8.20) then enter the population of synaptic vesicles, from which HRP can be released back into the extracellular space by further stimulation.

Another method for studying membrane endocytosis employs fluorescent dyes (Betz, Mao, and Bewick, 1992; Smith and Betz, 1996). The dye FM1-43, for example, if placed in the external solution, will partition reversibly into the outer leaflet of the cell plasma membrane. The dye then becomes localized in the synaptic vesicle membrane after endocytosis, clearly labeling vesicles even after the dye in the external solution and plasma membrane has been washed out. The dye in the vesicles can be released by further stimulation, much as HRP is released. The advantage of FM1-43 is that measurements can be made repeatedly from living tissue, either at the neuromuscular junction (Betz and Bewick, 1993) or at synapses between cultured neurons (Ryan et al. 1993; Ryan and Smith, 1995; Ryan, Smith, and Reuter, 1996). These measurements show that membrane can be endocytosed with a time constant of about 20 s and vesicles then reformed and made ready for release within about 1 min (see Betz and Angleston, 1998). This duration includes the time necessary for membrane retrieval, as measured by the change in cell capacitance, and the time necessary for formation of competent vesicles, filled with transmitter. Although vesicles can also be formed by synthesis and transport from the cell body (Kelly, 1993), the greater part of vesicle turnover (at least for rapid transmission mediated by transmitters like glutamate and GABA) occurs locally within the presynaptic terminal.

How does endocytosis occur? One mechanism requires the recruitment to the plasma membrane of "adaptor proteins" (see De Camilli and Takei, 1996). These proteins form a lattice that promotes the assembly of a *clathrin cage* (see Fig. 8.20), an hexagonal structure formed from monomers of the protein clathrin. It is the

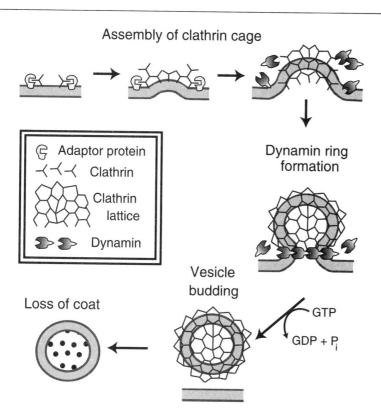

Assembly of clathrin cage

Fig. 8.20 Proposed molecular mechanism of endocytosis.

Dynamin ring formation

Adaptor protein

Clathrin

Clathrin lattice

Dynamin

Vesicle budding

Loss of coat

GTP

GDP + P$_i$

formation of this cage that seems to provide the guiding structure for membrane invagination. As the clathrin cage is forming around the membrane, oligomers of another protein, *dynamin,* assemble as a ring at the neck of the vesicle. Dynamin is a GTPase, and GTP hydrolysis apparently drives the budding off of the vesicle from the membrane to form the coated vesicles, which (as Heuser and Reese, 1973, noticed) accumulate after stimulation at the neuromuscular junction. The coated vesicles appear then to lose their coats and enter the vesicle pool, perhaps via the formation of a further membrane inclusion called an *endosome* (Heuser and Reese, 1973; but see De Camilli and Takei, 1996).

Although the formation of coated vesicles is probably the major pathway for vesicle retrieval, other pathways have been proposed. It is conceivable that some vesicles may release transmitter during the transient formation of a fusion pore, as in Fig. 8.19. Partial release of this kind, sometimes referred to as "kiss and run," has been demonstrated for mast cells (Alvarez de Toledo, Fernandez-Chacon, and Fernandez, 1993; see Fig. 8.19B) and may occur at the neuromuscular junction as well (Henkel and Betz, 1995). New powerful techniques may enable us to resolve these issues and eventually understand the rapid and reliable recirculation of vesicle membrane at the presynaptic terminal.

Summary

There are two major forms of synaptic contacts in the central nervous system: gap junctions, or electrical synapses, and chemical synapses. Gap junctions are assemblies of connexin molecules that form a pore providing direct communication of the cytoplasm of presynaptic and postsynaptic cells. Although gap junctions used to be considered static structures useful for rapid transmission at specialized synapses, we now know that this is an oversimplification. Gap junctions are much more abundant than previously thought and have been found in many parts of the nervous system. Furthermore, electrical transmission can be modulated by chemical transmitters. Gap junctions are often found in close proximity to chemical synapses (see Rash et al., 1996), and this arrangement of dual synaptic input raises interesting possibilities for synaptic modulation (Korn and Faber, 1979), especially on fine dendrites. The activation of a chemical synapse could produce a large change in the conductance of a fine dendrite in the vicinity of the gap junction, which could greatly influence the efficiency of transmission across the electrical synapse. Chemical transmission could also alter the gap-junctional conductance. Effects of this kind have been shown to occur, but we have little idea how general such mechanisms may be. Despite many years of careful experimentation, we are still very far from understanding the role of gap junctions in the central nervous system.

The more common form of synapse in the CNS is the chemical synapse, mediated by vesicle release. In contrast to the progress made in our knowledge of the gap junction, our understanding of how chemical transmission occurs has grown tremendously. We know, for example, that at most chemical synapses, transmitter release is dependent upon the influx of Ca^{2+}. Voltage-gated Ca^{2+}

channels appear to form a macromolecular complex in the presynaptic membrane, probably together with Ca^{2+}-dependent K^+ channels (whose function is still not understood). These channels are located near "active zones," specialized regions of presynaptic membrane that appear to contain the proteins responsible for vesicle attachment and fusion. The entry of Ca^{2+} causes an increase, by several hundred micromolar, in the intracellular free Ca^{2+} concentration, but the increase is localized to a microdomain in the vicinity of the plasma membrane. This then triggers the actual fusion of the vesicle to the presynaptic membrane and the release of transmitter. Many of the proteins that participate in vesicle docking and release have been identified, and we seem close to gaining a detailed molecular understanding of how this process occurs.

As we identify the interactions between proteins that produce vesicle fusion, we may also discover important targets for the modulation of transmitter release. It is quite possible that phosphorylation (say) of t-SNAREs or NSF proteins, or of the putative Ca^{2+} sensor synaptotagmin, could have a dramatic effect on the probability of release at a synaptic terminal. These proteins, together with the receptors I describe in the following two chapters, may very well hold the key to answering the question how certain synapses or pathways are facilitated during learning and other forms of complex processing. We address these questions more directly in Chapter 14.

9

Excitatory Transmission

NEUROTRANSMITTERS in the central nervous system can act in two ways. Some directly gate the opening and closing of receptors that are themselves ion channels. Receptors that are ion channels (called *ligand-gated receptors* or *ionotropic receptors*) make up at least three major families of proteins, and they include nicotinic acetylcholine (ACh) receptors, $GABA_A$ receptors, glycine receptors, many glutamate receptors, several receptors for ATP, a least one receptor for serotonin (5-hydroxytryptamine, 5-HT), and receptors for histamine in invertebrates (see Fig. 9.1).

A second kind of chemical communication, often called *metabotropic transmission* also uses a chemical transmitter (sometimes called a *neuromodulator*) that is released at synapses or simply into the extracellular space. The transmitter in this case alters the properties of the postsynaptic cell indirectly, by binding to a receptor that leads to activation of a G protein (see Chapter 11), which may gate channel opening or activate enzymatic pathways leading to changes in the concentrations of small-molecular-weight second messengers such as cAMP, cGMP, and Ca^{2+}. These substances then gate ion channels or have some other effect on the physiology of the postsynaptic cell (see Fig. 11.1). Receptors that transduce via G proteins (called *G-protein-coupled* or *metabotropic receptors*) include muscarinic ACh receptors, $GABA_B$ receptors, many serotonin, histamine, and glutamate receptors, all known dopamine, adenosine, and norepinephrine receptors and most receptors for neuroactive peptides.

In this chapter and the one following, I describe the structure and function of ligand-gated receptors and the excitatory and inhibitory responses they produce. Metabotropic receptors and neuromodulation will be the subject of Chapters 11–14.

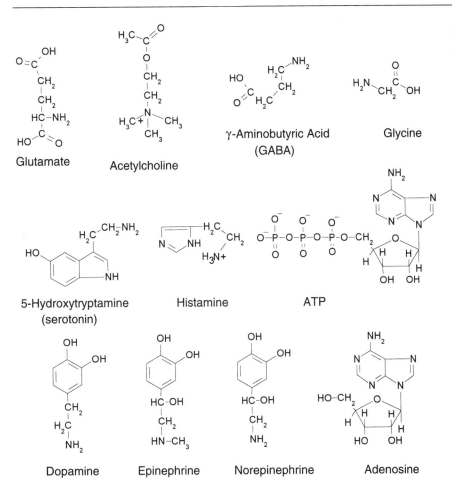

Fig. 9.1 Chemical structure of common neurotransmitters and neuromodulators.

I: Acetylcholine and Cholinergic Transmission

The most thoroughly studied synapse in the nervous system is the motor endplate, the synapse between motoneurons and skeletal muscle (see Fig. 8.9). Dale and his colleagues (Dale, Feldberg, and Vogt, 1936) first showed that motoneurons release ACh, which binds to nicotinic ACh receptors. These receptors are themselves ion channels, whose opening produces the endplate potential.

The nicotinic ACh receptor at the vertebrate endplate is the best understood of all synaptic receptors. It is called *nicotinic* because nicotine—along with a variety of other compounds, such as carbacol and suberyldicholine—will activate the receptor; these agents are called *agonists*. Nicotinic ACh responses at the motor endplate can be blocked by a variety of *antagonists,* including curare, prepared from the vines *Stychnos* or *Chondrodendron* and used by South American Indians as an arrow poison, and α-bungarotoxin, a toxin from the venom of the snake *Bungarus multicinctus.*

The ACh receptor of the motor endplate was the first of the specialized membrane proteins of excitable cells to be isolated and sequenced, and the first whose single-channel activity was recorded with patch-clamp techniques. The study of this receptor is an excellent example of the way molecular biology, biophysics, and neurophysiology can be combined to provide detailed knowledge of the function of a membrane protein.

The Structure of the Acetylcholine Receptor at the Endplate

The ACh receptor at the motor endplate is a complex formed by five transmembrane proteins surrounding a central region (Fig. 1.7B) that forms the ion-permeation pathway of the channel (Stroud, McCarthy, and Shuster, 1990; Karlin, 1993; Lindstrom, 1995). The proteins that form the ACh receptor were first isolated biochemically from the electric organ of the ray *Torpedo,* with a method similar to that used for Na^+ channels. The electric organ contains a large number of synapses similar to (and evolved from) neuromuscular endplates, and ACh receptors are quite abundant in this tissue. The receptors from these organs were assayed by binding to the high-affinity antagonist α-bungarotoxin, and four homologous proteins (called α, β, γ, and δ) with molecular weights ranging from 50 to 65 kDa were subsequently purified, and their genes cloned and sequenced. They all have a similar composition, with 35–50 percent homology in amino acid composition. Each has a large amino-terminal segment located on the extracellular side of the membrane (see Figs. 9.2 and Fig. 9.3C). Hydropathy analysis suggests that there are four transmembrane regions, which have been given the names M1–M4, followed by a small carboxyl-terminal region probably located extracellularly.

The ACh receptor is the only ligand-gated receptor for which de-

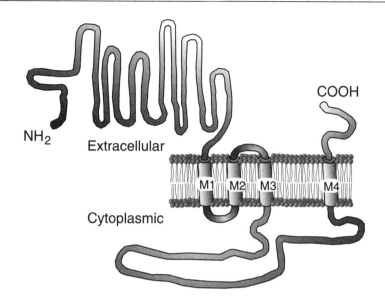

Fig. 9.2 Hypothesized membrane topology of acetylcholine receptor subunits. *M1* through *M4* are the transmembrane domains suggested by hydropathy analysis. (After Stroud, McCarthy, and Shuster, 1990.)

tailed structural information is presently available. Preparations of native *Torpedo* electroplax vesicles form tubular crystals containing several thousand receptors in a regular array. High-resolution electron micrographs are then used for analysis, much as in X-ray crystallography. The regularity of the electron-microscopic images of the crystals has so far been sufficient to obtain electron-density maps at a resolution of 0.9 nm (9 Å—Unwin, 1993a, 1995)—not enough to identify individual amino acids but adequate for visualizing much of the three-dimensional structure.

Maps of electron density (Fig. 9.3) show that the receptor has a cross-sectional diameter of approximately 8 nm and is about 12.5 nm long, with about 55 percent of its mass on the extracellular side of the membrane, 25 percent within the membrane, and 20 percent intracellular. The cytoplasmic side of the receptor is associated with another protein, called the 43K protein, whose function may be structural. The electron density indicated by the dashed box in Fig. 9.3A is presumed to be due mostly to this protein. The extracellular aspect of the ACh receptor extends 6 nm from the surface of the lipid bilayer and consists of large, claw-like extensions of mass, thought to be formed mostly by the amino-terminal regions of each of the homologous monomers. In the middle of these extensions is a region of minimal electron density (Fig. 9.3A, vertical arrow), probably representing the extracellular vestibule of the channel. A cross-section of the electron-density map in this region of the protein (Fig. 9.3B) clearly demonstrates the pentameric structure of the receptor, revealing the extracellular vestibule in the middle, and shows another interesting feature. The receptor protein (which for *Torpedo* receptors has a stoichiometry of $\alpha_2\beta\gamma\delta$) has two α

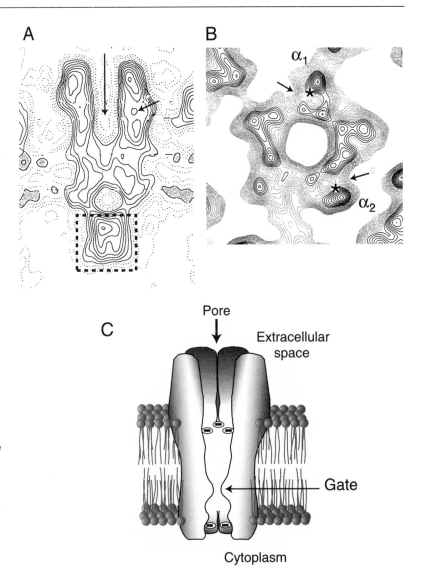

Fig. 9.3 Electron-density maps obtained from electron microscopy of tubular "crystals" of acetylcholine receptors from postsynaptic membranes of the electric organ of the ray *Torpedo marmorata*. **(A)** Side view of electron density showing receptor extending through membrane from extracellular *(top)* to intracellular *(bottom)*. Long, vertical arrow marks vestibule on extracellular side of receptor, probably directly above the channel pore. Shorter arrow may represent approximate location of one of the binding sites for ACh. Box outlines electron density in part contributed by the so-called 43K protein, which is not part of the receptor itself but may play some role in anchoring the receptor to the membrane. **(B)** Slice through **(A)**, 30 Å above bilayer surface in region of possible binding sites for ACh. Note fivefold axis of symmetry of electron density, formed by pentameric structure of protein. Each subunit has three peaks of electron density, formed by rods that may be α helices running approximately perpendicular to plane of section. Locations of two α subunits are shown, determined in other experiments from binding to specific markers (see Kubalek et al., 1987). Stars are hypothesized binding sites of the receptor blocker α-bungarotoxin on the two α subunits, and arrows point to clefts that may be part of the binding sites for ACh. **(C)** Model of ACh receptor based on electron-density maps like those in **(A)** and **(B)**. Negative charges in vestibules of pore at both extracellular and cytoplasmic surfaces facilitate permeation of positive ions through channel. (Parts **(A)** and **(B)** relabeled from Unwin, 1993a and used with the permission of the author, Macmillan Magazines Limited, and Academic Press Limited; **(C)** modified from Unwin, 1993b.)

subunits, which have been identified by labeling with specific markers after crystal formation (Kubalek et al., 1987). Both α subunits have cavities within their extracellular "claws" (arrows, Fig. 9.3B), which have been hypothesized to form the binding sites for acetylcholine. The position of one of these cavities is also indicated by the shorter arrow in Fig. 9.3A.

ACh Binding

Although there is as yet no actual evidence that ACh binds within these cavities, it does seem likely that the binding site lies at least in part within the extracellular amino-terminal region of the α subunits. The evidence for this (see Karlin, 1993; Lindstrom, 1995; Karlin and Akabas, 1995) has come in part from *affinity labeling* of the protein, with reagents that bind to the ACh binding site and then react to form chemical bonds with amino acids in the vicinity; and in part from molecular techniques, such as the formation of chimeras (as in the experiment of Fig. 6.4) and site-directed mutagenesis. The binding site is thought to be formed by a conserved pair of cysteine residues, at positions 192 and 193 of the α subunit (for *Torpedo*), and other amino acids in the vicinity, including several aromatic amino acids such as tryptophan and tyrosine. There is some evidence that both binding sites may span more than one subunit, with one binding site including one α and the δ (Czajkowski and Karlin, 1991) and the other binding site the other α and the γ (see Karlin and Akabas, 1995).

Since the binding sites are formed at least in part by α subunits, and since there are two α subunits per receptor, it would not be too surprising if there were two binding sites. Evidence for two binding sites for ACh was actually first obtained by Katz and Thesleff (1957), who noticed that the amplitude of the response at the neuromuscular junction increases nonlinearly with increasing ACh concentration, as would be expected if more than one ACh molecule could bind to receptors. An experiment of a similar kind is shown in Fig. 9.4 for the cholinergic response of a cell from the medial habenula of the rat CNS. In this experiment (Lester and Dani, 1995) the receptors were stimulated with nicotine, and the response amplitude increased with increasing nicotine concentration in a clearly nonlinear fashion (Fig. 9.4A). A plot of log response versus log nicotine concentration gives a slope of approximately 2,

Fig. 9.4 Dose-response relation for nicotinic currents recorded with whole-cell patch-clamp ($V_H = -49$ mV) from neurons dissociated from rat habenula nucleus. Nicotine was applied from a linear array of glass microbarrels, positioned about 100 μm from the neuron. **(A)** Responses to 1–8 μM ACh. Bars indicate duration of drug exposure. The increase in current is clearly nonlinear. **(B)** Dose-response curve. The ordinate plots the log of the current, normalized to the response recorded at 2 μM; the abscissa is the log of nicotine concentration in μM. Data are means ± S.D., with numbers of trials at each concentration given in parentheses next to each data point. (Reprinted from Lester and Dani, 1995, with permission of the authors and of the American Physiological Society.)

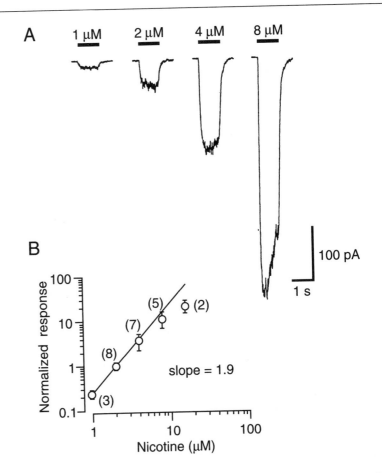

indicating that, for small nicotine concentrations, the response increases approximately as the square of the nicotine concentration (see Eqns. 6 and 7 of Chapter 8). This is consistent with at least two molecules of nicotine or ACh being required for activation. Similar results have been obtained for GABA, glycine, serotonin, and glutamate receptors, indicating that most if not all ligand-gated receptors have more than one binding site.

The Channel

The first information about the channel was obtained from measurements of ion selectivity. Recall that the change in current produced by an agonist for a ligand-gated channel is given by

$$\Delta i = \Delta g(V_m - E_{rev}) \tag{1}$$

where Δg is the change in conductance, V_m is the membrane potential, and E_{rev} is the reversal potential. The reversal potential is the membrane voltage for which agonist produces no change in current, since when V_m is equal to E_{rev}, Δi is zero regardless of the size of the conductance change. At the reversal potential there is no net current flowing through the open ACh channels, and the value of the reversal potential is therefore given by the GHK voltage equation (see Chapter 3),

$$E_{rev} = \frac{RT}{F} \ln \frac{P_{Na}[Na^+]_o + P_K[K^+]_o + P_{Cl}[Cl^-]_i}{P_{Na}[Na^+]_i + P_K[K^+]_i + P_{Cl}[Cl^-]_o} \tag{2}$$

Suppose the reversal potential for the ACh response of a muscle fiber is first measured with Na^+ as the only permeant ion in the bath, and it is found to be ψ_1. Suppose the Na^+ is then replaced with another monovalent ion, X^+, and the new reversal potential is found to be ψ_2. Provided no change occurs in intracellular ion concentrations (a good bet, since muscle fibers are such large cells), then

$$\psi_2 - \psi_1 = \frac{RT}{F} \ln \frac{P_X[X^+]_o}{P_{Na}[Na^+]_o}, \tag{3}$$

and P_X/P_{Na} can be estimated from the change in reversal potential (see also Chapter 3).

The first attempts to measure reversal potentials of endplate currents from voltage-clamped muscle fibers were made by Takeuchi and Takeuchi (1959) with a two-electrode voltage clamp, a method insufficient to permit a true "space clamp" throughout the entire length of the muscle fiber but probably good enough to clamp the endplate region directly adjacent to the presynaptic terminal. A true reversal potential could not be measured in these experiments, since holding potentials that depolarized the membrane enough to reverse the endplate potential (EPP) caused contraction of the muscle, which dislodged the microelectrodes. Nevertheless, reversal potentials estimated by extrapolation suggested that the end-

Fig. 9.5 Ion selectivity of ACh receptors at the neuromuscular junction: currents measured in response to brief applications of ACh. Recordings were made from frog muscle, voltage-clamped with the vasoline-gap technique. Traces are superimposed current responses at membrane voltages in the vicinity of the reversal potential, in external solutions containing 114 mM of the indicated monovalent ion substituted for Na^+. Traces with the notation *2x* were recorded at a gain half as large as the one indicated by the current scale to left (currents were twice as large as scale indicates). Solution inside the muscle was 115 mM NaF. (From Adams, Dwyer, and Hille, 1980, reprinted with permission of the authors and of Rockefeller University Press.)

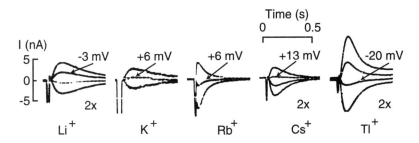

plate ACh receptor is permeable to both Na^+ and K^+ (Takeuchi and Takeuchi, 1960), and even to Ca^{2+} (Takeuchi, 1963).

A more thorough study of the ion selectivity of the muscle ACh receptor was made by Hille and his colleagues (Dwyer, Adams, and Hille, 1980; Adams, Dwyer, and Hille, 1980), using an improved method of voltage clamp called the *vasoline gap* (see Hille and Campbell, 1976). This method provides a better control of the voltage of the muscle fiber and permits solutions to be introduced into the fiber cytoplasm, so that the intracellular ion concentrations can be kept nearly constant even when large changes are made in the composition of the Ringer solution in the bath. Furthermore, intracellular Ca^{2+} can be buffered inside the cell to prevent muscle contraction.

Some permeability ratios P_X/P_{Na} for the ACh receptor at the frog neuromuscular junction (X^+ given in parentheses) are: 1.4 (Cs^+), 1.3 (Rb^+), 1.1 (K^+), and 0.9 (Li^+). (See Fig. 9.5.) Small organic cations are highly permeable (hydroxylamine$^+$ is nearly twice as permeant as Na^+), but the permeability is smaller for Tris$^+$ and choline$^+$ and decreases as the size of the cation increases. The diameters of the largest permeant ions indicate that the channel diameter at its narrowest region is unlikely to be less than 0.6–0.7 nm (6–7 Å). As in the experiments of Takeuchi (1963), a significant permeability was measured for Ca^{2+}, with P_{Ca}/P_{Na} between 0.15 and 0.25. Anions were not measurably permeant.

The channel seems to be formed at least in part by the M2 membrane-spanning regions of the receptor subunits (see Fig. 9.2), which may form a ring of α-helical "barrels" lining the channel (see Lester, 1992; Lindstrom, 1995; Karlin and Akabas, 1995). The evidence for this proposal comes in part from affinity labeling with reagents that block the channel pore and from site-directed mutagenesis (see Stroud, McCarthy, and Shuster, 1990; Lester, 1992; Unwin, 1993b; Karlin, 1993; Lindstrom, 1995).

The narrowest region of the pore may be near the cytoplasmic end of M2. Studies measuring both channel conductance (Villarroel et al., 1992) and relative permeability for bulky organic cations such as $Tris^+$ (Cohen et al., 1992) indicate that the greatest effects on ion flow and permeability are produced by mutation of amino acids near the cytoplasmic side of the α helix. This conclusion is also supported by Akabas et al. (1994), who systematically changed each of the amino acids in M2 to a cysteine residue and then tested the accessibility of these residues to charged, water-soluble reagents added to the bathing medium. This technique is described in detail in Chapter 10 (see Fig. 10.3 and accompanying discussion).

The regions of the protein on either side of M2 at the extracellular and cytoplasmic vestibules of the channel contain negatively charged amino acids, which may facilitate the entry of positively charged Na^+ and K^+ ions into the channel pore by electrostatic attraction (see Fig. 9.3C). When these negatively charged amino acids are removed by site-directed mutagenesis, the conductance of the channel is decreased (Imoto et al., 1988). This effect is quite specific: the removal of charge from the extracellular side decreases the conductance only for inward current flow, and the normally nearly linear i–V curve of the ACh-gated response becomes outwardly rectifying. Negatively charged amino acids at the cytoplasmic vestibule may also be important for the permeability of the receptor to Ca^{2+} (Bertrand et al., 1993).

Gating

The opening of the channel is a chemical reaction in which the receptor changes conformation from a closed state, which has little or no ion permeability, to an open state, which under physiological conditions permits the inward flow of about 10^7 ions per second (see Lingle, Maconochie, and Steinbach, 1992; Edmonds, Gibb, and Colquhoun, 1995a). A single vesicle containing about 10^4 molecules of transmitter (ACh) is released at the motor endplate and transiently increases the concentration of ACh in the synaptic cleft to ~1 mM (see Edmonds, Gibb, and Colquhoun, 1995a). Diffusion and binding of ACh to the receptor are thought to occur rapidly, and ACh then diffuses away from the site of release and is rapidly hydrolyzed by the enzyme *acetylcholine esterase,* which is located extracellularly in the vicinity of the synapse.

The kinetics of channel opening were first investigated by Katz and Miledi (1972), who noticed that when ACh was applied to an endplate with a pipette, so that transmitter was present continuously at a constant concentration, the amplitude of the endplate potential showed small fluctuations. They reasoned that these fluctuations were caused by random openings and closings of ACh receptors, and they showed that the time course of the noise produced by these fluctuations could give useful information about the duration of channel opening.

The rationale for their approach is roughly as follows. If the channel on average is open for only a short time, then the noise should be dominated by high-frequency components, since the response in the presence of continuous ACh should fluctuate with high frequency as the channel rapidly flickers between the open and closed states (see for example Fig. 1.8). If on the other hand the open time is long, fluctuations in the EPC should be much slower.

Katz and Miledi determined that the mean time of opening of the ACh channels at the motor endplate is surprisingly short, of the order of 1 ms. Using similar techniques, Anderson and Stevens (1973) demonstrated that the mean open time of the channel is a function of voltage and increases as the membrane potential is hyperpolarized, confirming earlier experiments of Magelby and Stevens (1972). Several other interesting features of ACh receptors were also deduced from noise measurements (summarized in Neher and Stevens, 1977). The mean open time is a function of the agonist used to open the channel. It is long for suberyldicholine, intermediate for ACh, and short for carbacol. Presumably different agonists bind to the receptor with different affinities, as is reflected in the difference in the amount of time the opening lasts. The open time even for the same agonist can also vary for ACh receptors in different tissues; for example, it is longer for channels in embryonic skeletal muscle than for channels at the adult endplate. The reason for this we now know: in mammals embryonic channels are mostly $\alpha_2\beta\gamma\delta$, whereas channels at the adult endplate contain a subunit called ε and are mostly $\alpha_2\beta\varepsilon\delta$ (Mishina et al, 1986). Substitution of γ with ε alters both the open time and conductance of the receptor, at least in part as a result of changes in amino acids in the M2 domain (Herlitze et al., 1996).

Single-Channel Recordings

The first successful recordings of the electrical activity of single ACh receptors with patch-clamp techniques quickly confirmed most of the conclusions of noise measurements (Neher and Sakmann, 1976). In addition, single-channel recordings also revealed that the ACh receptor is much more complicated than the noise measurements appeared to indicate. Single-channel currents, for example, do not consist of simple openings and closing like Na^+ channels (see Fig. 6.11) but rather show clusters or *bursts* of openings. The mean duration of these bursts varies with membrane potential and with the agonist used to activate the channel, much as the open time determined from noise.

In order to summarize the evidence from single-channel recordings that has led to our present understanding of the gating of the ACh receptor, it is helpful to begin with a model of transitions between conformations of the receptor, including conformations with no ACh molecules bound, with one bound, and with two (Fig. 9.6A). The letter C in Fig. 9.6A is used to denote the receptor in a closed state and O the receptor in an open state. A is the agonist (e.g., ACh). Thus CA is a closed receptor with one molecule of ACh bound, and OA_2 is an open receptor with two ACh's bound. The α's, β's, and k's are rate constants.

If it were possible to assign values to all of the rate constants in Fig. 9.6A, and if we could be sure that the open and closed states in this model comprise *all* of the possible states of the channel, we would have a complete kinetic description of channel gating. This would be an important achievement, essential for understanding how changes in receptor structure produce opening of the channel. Unfortunately, technical difficulties limit the temporal resolution of single-channel recordings and make it impossible to detect very brief openings and closings. The model in Fig. 9.6 is certainly an

Fig. 9.6 Mechanism of acetylcholine receptor gating. **(A)** Kinetic scheme of gating, diagramming physiologically observable open and closed states of channel and transitions between these states. *C* and *O* by themselves indicate closed and open states with no agonist (ACh) molecule bound, whereas *CA* and *OA* indicate one agonist molecule bound, and *CA$_2$* and *OA$_2$* indicate two molecules bound. The *k*'s, α's, and β's are rate constants for the indicated transitions. **(B)** Single-channel recording of ACh receptor current. On-cell recording from frog muscle with pipette containing 100 nM of the ACh agonist suberyldicholine. *C* indicates approximate zero current level (channel closed) and *O* the most commonly observed current value for the open channel at the holding potential used in the experiment. Arrows indicate rapid closings ("gaps") within larger "burst." These gaps probably represent rapid transitions from *OA$_2$* to *CA$_2$* and then back to *OA$_2$*. (Part **(B)** reprinted from Colquhoun and Sakmann, 1985, with permission of the authors and of the Physiological Society.)

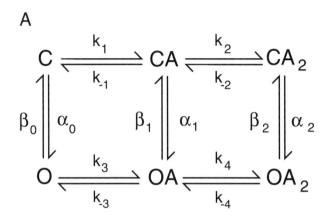

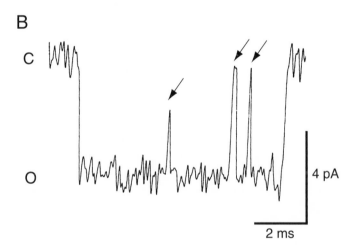

oversimplification, and it is still unclear how many states the channel can enter (Hamill and Sakmann, 1981; see Sachs, 1983).

In spite of these limitations, some interesting things emerge from the model. To focus on the essentials, I ignore transitions between

OA_2, OA, and O, since open states bind ACh much more tightly than closed states (see for example Jackson, 1988). This means that open receptors are unlikely to dissociate from agonist directly but are much more likely first to close to CA_2, CA, or C, and then dissociate from the agonist. I also ignore transitions from C to O and from CA to OA. Transitions from C to O reflect spontaneous openings in the absence of transmitter, which are observable but very infrequent (Jackson, 1984). Transitions from CA to OA reflect openings with only a single ACh bound. These openings are shorter and much more infrequent than openings with two ACh's bound (see Lingle, Maconochie, and Steinbach, 1992) and are unlikely to make an important contribution to the endplate current under physiological conditions.

During the normal postsynaptic response at the motor endplate, most of the conductance change is caused by openings of doubly liganded receptors, and the scheme in Fig. 9.6A can be simplified to:

$$C \underset{k_{-1}}{\overset{k_1}{\rightleftharpoons}} CA \underset{k_{-2}}{\overset{k_2}{\rightleftharpoons}} CA_2 \underset{\beta_2}{\overset{\alpha_2}{\rightleftharpoons}} OA_2$$

The effect of ACh on the single-channel current often looks like the response in Fig. 9.6B, from Colquhoun and Sakmann (1985). The change in current can best be described as a burst of openings, on average several milliseconds long but whose exact length is random. The burst consists of openings interrupted by brief closings (arrows in Fig. 9.6B), which probably represent rapid transitions from OA_2 to CA_2 and back again. Thus the channel with two ACh's bound opens rapidly and then flickers between OA_2 and CA_2. The burst terminates when one of the two ACh's falls off a CA_2 to form CA. Subsequent rebinding of a second ACh to reform CA_2 and reopen the channel could conceivably take place but is unlikely, since the concentration of ACh in the cleft declines so rapidly by diffusion and hydrolysis during the normal endplate response that, by the time the average burst has ended, little ACh would be present in the synaptic cleft to rebind.

How Does Channel Opening Occur?

Single-channel recordings show that the binding of ACh produces conformational changes in the receptor that lead to channel opening. Binding of ACh to the extracellular domain must somehow be communicated to the parts of the protein that line the pore. One of the most interesting attempts to understand the nature of channel opening was made by Unwin (1995), who examined the structure of *Torpedo* receptors in crystalline tubules rapidly frozen after a brief exposure to droplets of ACh. The intention of these experiments was to freeze the receptor in its open configuration, so that a comparison could be made of the open and closed receptor conformations. The result of this comparison suggests that binding of ACh produces changes in the conformation of both α subunits, as well as a small rotation of α subunit extracellular domains. This rotation produces a twisting of the molecule, which is communicated to all of the α helices lining the pore, presumably the α helices of M2 for the five receptor monomers. The most remarkable observation of this study was that ACh binding causes the lower (cytoplasmic) halves of these α helices to rotate, so that instead of pointing inward as in the closed configuration, they rotate to the side, opening up the middle of the protein (Fig. 9.7). This movement of the protein may in some way contribute to the opening of the channel. It is tempting to suppose that this movement of M2 *is* channel opening, frozen in the act. This would be premature, however, since it is presently unclear how these observations can be reconciled with other studies that appear to place the narrowest region of the channel at the cytoplasmic extremity of M2 (see Karlin and Akabas, 1995).

Desensitization

In addition to the changes produced by channel opening, the ACh receptor undergoes at least one other important kind of conformational state. If high concentrations of ACh are applied to a muscle fiber for a sufficiently long period of time, the response to ACh becomes smaller—a phenomenon called *desensitization,* first described by Katz and Thesleff (1957). Although there is little consensus how desensitization is produced (see Edmonds, Gibb, and

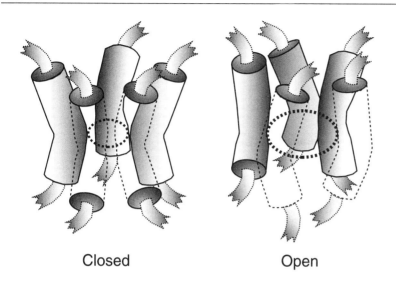

Closed   Open

Fig. 9.7 Change in conformation of the acetyl-choline receptor during channel opening. Model is based on change in structure of channel, as deduced from electron micrographs of tubular vesicles (as in Fig. 9.3) in the presence and absence of ACh. Diagram shows only changes in the conformation of membrane-spanning rods, thought to be the M2 domains of each of the subunits lining the channel pore. Conformational change produced by ACh is characterized by outward rotation of the lower halves of the rods, which may be responsible for channel opening. (After Unwin, 1995; used with the permission of the author and of Macmillan Magazines Limited.)

Colquhoun, 1995a), there is agreement that for the ACh receptor desensitization occurs slowly—too slowly to take place within the time course of the endplate potential. As we shall see, this may not be true for all ligand-gated receptors. For some glutamate receptors, desensitization occurs much more rapidly, and there is increasing evidence that it may have an important effect on the waveform of the response, at least at some synapses.

Neuronal Nicotinic ACh Receptors

Once the genes for the α, β, γ, δ, and ϵ monomers of muscle ACh receptors were identified and cloned, these genes were used to construct probes or primer sequences to identify genes coding homologous proteins from neuronal cDNA libraries (Boulter et al., 1986; see Patrick et al., 1987). These efforts led to the identification of a large number of homologous proteins that appear, at least in part, to form the nicotinic ACh receptors of the central nervous system (see Sargent, 1993; McGehee and Role, 1995; Sivilotti and Colquhoun, 1995; Lindstrom, 1995; Vidal and Changeux, 1996). There are at least eight genes for proteins analogous to *Torpedo* α subunits, called α_2–α_9. These proteins may contain binding sites for ACh and function somewhat as the α subunits of muscle proteins,

Fig. 9.8 Physiological properties of some combinations of neuronal ACh receptors, based on measurements from *Xenopus* oocytes after injection of cRNA as indicated at top. Data are for genes from rat except for α_7 (which is from chick). Lines labeled λ, τ_o give in schematic form the mean single-channel conductance and open time for the most commonly observed open state of the channel expressed by the genes. Expressed (and native) neuronal ACh channels typically have more than one open state, and a more complete compilation is given in McGehee and Role (1995). Data labeled *EC 50* give the concentration of agonist (here ACh) required to produce a response that is 50% of the maximal response. For *Agonist potency profile*, abbreviations are as follows: *N,* nicotine; *D,* 1,1-dimethyl-4-phenylpiperazinium iodide (DMPP); *A,* acetylcholine; and *C,* cytisine. (Reprinted with updates and modifications from McGehee and Role, 1995, with the help and permission of the authors and of Annual Reviews, Inc.)

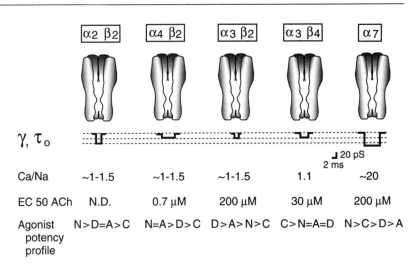

	$\alpha2$ $\beta2$	$\alpha4$ $\beta2$	$\alpha3$ $\beta2$	$\alpha3$ $\beta4$	$\alpha7$
Ca/Na	~1-1.5	~1-1.5	~1-1.5	1.1	~20
EC 50 ACh	N.D.	0.7 μM	200 μM	30 μM	200 μM
Agonist potency profile	N>D=A>C	N=A>D>C	D>A>N>C	C>N=A=D	N>C>D>A

though the evidence for this is incomplete (especially for α_5 and α_6). Some of these α's (e.g., α_7–α_9) can produce functional ACh receptors when expressed alone as homomers (see for example Couturier et al., 1990), but most α's form functional receptors only when expressed together with other proteins, of which there are at least three, called β_2, β_3, and β_4. The β's are homologous to the neuronal α proteins and to one another, but the relationship is not particularly close: different β's are as different from one another as they are from the α's. The number of different neuronal α and β proteins may be further increased by alternative splicing (see for example Connolly, Boulter, and Heinemann, 1992). By analogy to muscle ACh receptors, it is usually assumed that α's and β's associate as pentamers ($2\alpha{:}3\beta$ or $3\alpha{:}2\beta$), and there is evidence at least for some receptors that this is the case (see for example Cooper, Couturier, and Ballivet, 1991).

When different α and β combinations are expressed in *Xenopus* oocytes, they produce ACh receptors with strikingly disparate properties (see Fig. 9.8). Single-channel conductances and mean open times differ, as do the relative orders of the potencies of different agonists. There are also surprisingly large differences in Ca^{2+} permeability, with the α_7 homomeric receptor having a P_{Ca}/P_{Na} perhaps as high as 20 (Séguéla et al., 1993).

Large differences are also seen in the properties of ACh responses recorded from actual neurons (Sargent, 1993; McGehee and Role, 1995), suggesting that different cells have receptors composed of different subunits. The $\alpha_4\beta_2$ combination is thought to be the predominant nicotinic receptor in the brain (Whiting and Lindstrom, 1987; Flores et al., 1992). The subunit α_5, which does not form receptors either by itself or in combination with any of the β subunits, can combine with both α_4 and β_2 to form functional channels (Ramirez-Latorre et al., 1996). Cells of the ciliary ganglion may assemble receptors containing α_5 together with α_3 and β_4, which appear to be located predominantly at synapses. These cells seem also to form other receptors containing α_7 at nonsynaptic locations (Vernallis, Conroy, and Berg, 1993).

The protein sequences of neuronal ACh α subunits indicate that $\alpha_2-\alpha_6$ are more closely related to one another than to $\alpha_7-\alpha_9$, suggesting that α subunits may fall into at least two subgroups (see Ortells and Lunt, 1995; Le Novère and Changeux, 1995). These two subgroups can also be distinguished by their pharmacology. The snake toxin α-bungarotoxin, which is a potent and irreversible blocker of the ACh receptor from muscle, has provided an especially useful tool for studying the function and distribution of neuronal ACh receptors, since receptors made from $\alpha_2-\alpha_6$ appear to be largely insensitive to α-bungarotoxin, whereas $\alpha_7-\alpha_9$ receptors can be blocked, often at very low concentrations. The responses of α_7 homomeric receptors, for example, can be dramatically reduced by an α-bungarotoxin concentration in the nanomolar range (Couturier et al., 1990; Zhang, Vijayaraghavan, and Berg, 1994; Zhang, Coggan, and Berg, 1996).

There is some evidence that receptors that are sensitive to α-bungarotoxin and those that are not may play somewhat different roles in synaptic function. The CNS contains large numbers of high-affinity binding sites for α-bungarotoxin (see for example Clarke et al., 1985), probably reflecting the distribution of $\alpha_7-\alpha_9$ receptors. There are also large numbers of high-affinity binding sites for ACh and nicotine, which may reflect at least in part the distribution of $\alpha_2-\alpha_6$. There is surprisingly little overlap in these distributions. There is some evidence that receptors composed of $\alpha_7-\alpha_9$ are particularly prevalent at *nonsynaptic* locations, perhaps in part on presynaptic terminals (Role and Berg, 1996).

Physiology of Neuronal ACh Responses

Neuronal ACh receptors are activated by nicotine and carbacol, as are muscle ACh receptors. In addition, certain agonists, such as suberyldicholine, are generally more effective for muscle; and others, such as 1,1-dimethyl-4-phenylpiperazinium iodide (DMPP), seem more effective for neuronal responses. Some neuronal receptors that are insensitive to α-bungarotoxin can be blocked by another *Bungarus* toxin, called variously κ-bungarotoxin, toxin F, or neuronal bungarotoxin. Other blockers selective for at least some neuronal receptors are the compounds hexamethonium and decamethonium.

Like ACh receptors (AChR's) in muscle, neuronal ACh receptors form channels that are selective for cations. For muscle, the *i–V* curve of the ACh response is nearly linear under physiological conditions, but most if not all neuronal responses, including α-bungarotoxin-sensitive currents (Zhang, Vijayaraghavan, and Berg, 1994), show prominent inward rectification (see Sargent, 1993). In the experiments shown in Fig. 9.9, for example, inward currents were much larger than outward currents regardless of the direction of the Na^+ gradient. The Na^+ gradient was changed by altering either the intracellular or extracellular Na^+ concentration by replacement with an uncharged compound (mannitol or glucose), so that the reversal potentials for Na^+ and for Cl^- were shifted in opposite directions. For example, for $[NaCl]_o = 142$ mM and $[NaCl]_i = 55$ mM (third column of responses in Fig. 9.9A), E_{Na} can be calculated to be $+23$ mV and E_{Cl}, -23 mV. The current-voltage curves in Fig. 9.10B indicate that the reversal potential of the response shifted in the appropriate direction for a cation-selective conductance, and by about the right amount. Regardless of the ionic conditions, outward currents were small or undetectable.

There are indications in some systems that at least part of the inward rectification of neuronal ACh responses is due to Mg^{2+} block, as is true for some K^+-selective inward rectifiers (see Chapter 6), but considerable inward rectification remains even in zero-Mg^{2+} solution (Mathie, Colquhoun, and Cull-Candy, 1990; Sands and Barish, 1992). It has been proposed that the Mg^{2+}-insensitive component of rectification is caused by an intrinsic voltage dependence

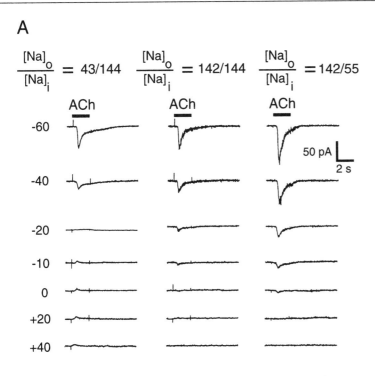

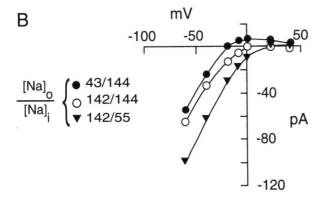

Fig. 9.9 Inward rectification of current through neuronal ACh receptors in retinal ganglion cells. Whole-cell patch-clamp recordings were made from dissociated cells from the retina of the goldfish. **(A)** Current responses recorded under voltage clamp from three different cells, with extracellular and intracellular (pipette) Na^+ concentrations indicated for each cell above each column of records. Acetylcholine was applied by rapid perfusion for 2 s at the time indicated by the bars above the records. Numbers to left give membrane potentials. **(B)** Current-voltage relations for responses shown in **(A)**. Peak amplitude of current response is plotted against command potential of voltage clamp. (From Yazejian and Fain, 1993, reprinted with permission of the authors and of Cambridge University Press.)

of channel gating, but other explanations have not as yet been excluded.

Function of Nicotinic ACh Transmission in the CNS

Although the role of ACh in the brain is poorly understood, its importance has always been realized: addiction to nicotine is one of the gravest health problems we face as a society, causing many more premature deaths than any communicable disease (including AIDS). Nicotine produces increased arousal and attention and can influence both learning and memory, and these effects are probably produced mostly if not entirely by activation of ACh receptors. Inherited or engineered deficiencies in neuronal nicotinic ACh receptor subunits have been shown to produce severe behavioral effects, including epilepsy in humans (Steinlein et al., 1995) and abnormal learning in mice (Picciotto et al., 1995).

Although in some parts of the nervous system ACh functions as a classical neurotransmitter, released onto receptors located either within or just adjacent to postsynaptic membrane (see for example Masland, 1988; Lipton, Aizenman, and Loring, 1987; Yazejian and Fain, 1993; Zhang, Coggan, and Berg, 1996), there is increasing evidence that an even more important function of ACh may be to modulate the release of other transmitters presynaptically (Wonnacott, 1997). Presynaptic nicotinic receptors have been shown to accentuate the release of glutamate and dopamine (see for example Wonnacott et al., 1990). It is possible that the high Ca^{2+} permeability of some of the neuronal nicotinic receptors is in some way responsible for these effects (McGehee et al., 1995).

Some new and interesting effects of ACh on neuronal activity have been revealed by direct recording from CNS neurons (see McGehee and Role, 1995). One particularly interesting study of this kind (Gray et al., 1996) was of the effect of nicotine on spontaneous transmitter release for pyramidal cells in the rat hippocampus. Recordings were made of miniature excitatory postsynaptic currents (mEPSCs) with whole-cell voltage clamp from brain cells bathed in TTX (to block Na^+ channels) and Cd^{2+} (to block Ca^{2+} channels). EPSCs were recorded in the absence of nicotine (Fig. 9.10A, upper trace), produced by the spontaneous release of glutamate (the predominant excitatory transmitter in hippocampus).

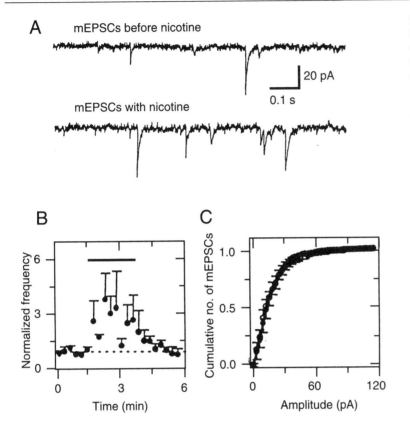

Fig. 9.10 Effect of nicotine on miniature EPSCs, recorded from rat hippocampal pyramidal cells with whole-cell voltage clamp. **(A)** Recordings from CA3 pyramidal cell from rat brain slice perfused with 1 μM TTX and 200 μM Cd^{2+}. EPSCs were recorded before *(above)* and after *(below)* puffing of 20 μM nicotine onto the dendrites of the cell. Note the increase in frequency of miniature EPSCs produced by nicotine. **(B)** Frequency of EPSCs from whole-cell recordings from hippocampal pyramidal cell in tissue culture in presence of 0.5–1.0 μM TTX. Application of 0.5 μM nicotine *(bar)* produced an increase in frequency. **(C)** Cumulative amplitude distributions of EPSPs before *(open circles)* and after *(filled circles)* nicotine administration, from recordings, as in **(B)**. The ordinate plots the probability of observing an EPSC less than or equal to the amplitude given on the abscissa. For example, the probability was about 0.8 of seeing an EPSC less than or equal to 30 pA in amplitude. The cumulative amplitude distributions (and hence the probabilities of observing EPSCs of a given size) were the same before and after nicotine, indicating that the effect of nicotine was predominantly to increase the frequency of release rather than to change the amplitude of the EPSC. (From Gray et al., 1996, reprinted with permission of the authors and of Macmillan Magazines Limited.)

These EPSCs could be completely blocked by glutamate antagonists, such as CNQX (see Section II of this chapter). Nicotine increased the frequency of the glutamate EPSCs (Fig. 9.10A, lower trace), probably by increasing the probability of vesicle release. Plotting normalized frequency of EPSCs as a function of time (Fig. 9.10B) shows the large increase in frequency produced by nicotine. The amplitude of the synaptic currents remained unaffected (Fig. 9.10C). These data provide compelling evidence for a presynaptic effect of nicotine at excitatory synapses in the hippocampus, and it would be easy to imagine a role for such an effect on arousal, learning, or memory.

Despite interesting indications provided by experiments like those in Fig. 9.10, the role of nicotinic receptors in the central nervous system is still under debate. Presynaptic actions are undoubt-

edly important, though it is not yet clear whether the increase in release is produced by depolarization of the synaptic terminals or
more directly, by Ca²⁺ entry (McGehee et al., 1995; Gray et al.,
1996). Some evidence exists that there may be a subdivision of
function, with some kinds of nicotinic receptors more important at
postsynaptic sites and others at presynaptic locations, but much
more information is required before these hypotheses can be confirmed. Possible differences in receptor location could turn out to
be of considerable practical importance. Since different receptors
may have a somewhat different pharmacology, it may be possible
to target drugs to receptors at specific places, and nicotinic agonists
and antagonists may in this way emerge as important drugs in the
treatment of nervous disorders and addiction.

II: Glutamate and Glutamatergic Transmission

Glutamate is the most common excitatory synaptic transmitter in
the CNS. There are three major classes of ligand-gated glutamate channels, called AMPA (α-amino-3-hydroxy-5-methyl-4-
isoxazoleproprionic acid), kainate, and NMDA (N-methyl-D-
aspartate—see Fig. 9.11). Much is now known about the molecular
biology and structure of these receptors and the responses they produce (see Hollmann and Heinemann, 1994; Sprengel and Seeburg,
1995). In addition, some progress has been made understanding
how activation of the receptors produces postsynaptic responses
(see Jahr, 1994; Edmonds, Gibb, and Colquhoun, 1995b; Jones
and Westbrook, 1996; Clements, 1996).

AMPA and Kainate Receptors

The genes of glutamate receptors (GluRs) proved much more difficult to clone than those of ACh receptors, since there was no
highly selective and specific ligand like α-bungarotoxin that could
be used to identify the receptor proteins during biochemical isolation. Furthermore, the concentration of glutamate receptors in the
brain is much lower than that of ACh receptors in electroplax.
Consequently, the first glutamate receptor genes were cloned by

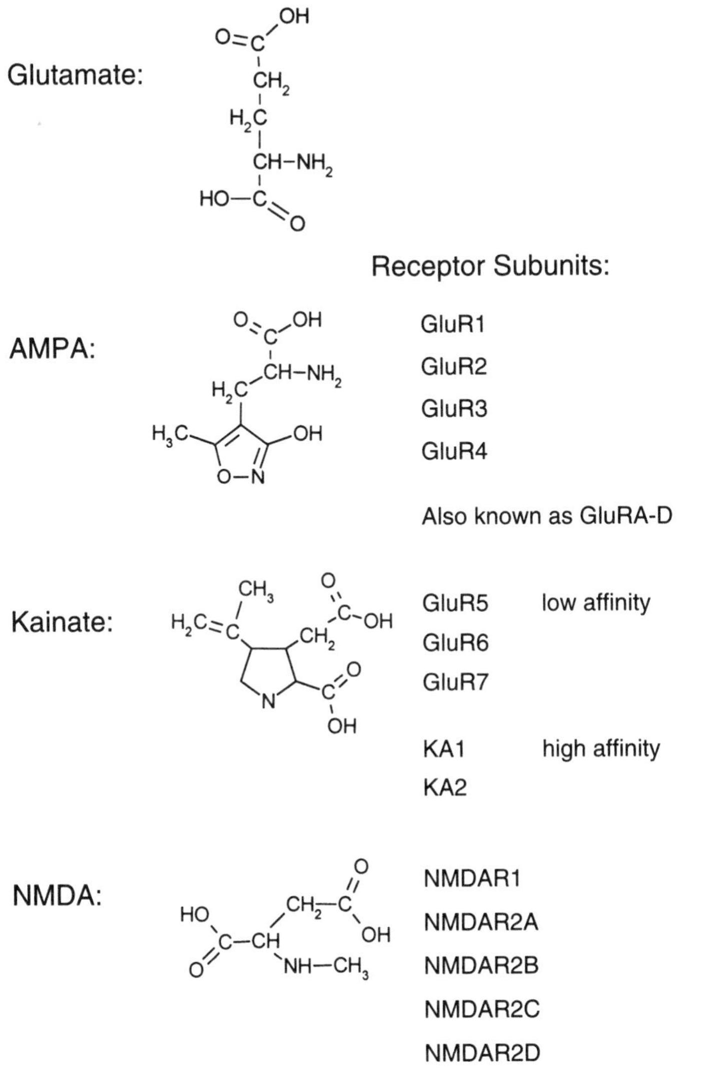

Glutamate:

Receptor Subunits:

AMPA:

GluR1

GluR2

GluR3

GluR4

Also known as GluRA-D

Kainate:

GluR5   low affinity

GluR6

GluR7

KA1   high affinity

KA2

NMDA:

NMDAR1

NMDAR2A

NMDAR2B

NMDAR2C

NMDAR2D

Fig. 9.11 Glutamate and its receptors. The structure of glutamate is compared to that of agonists used to separate ionotropic glutamate receptors into three classes: the AMPA receptors (GluR1–4), the kainate receptors (GluR5–7 and KA1–2), and the NMDA receptors.

the laborious procedure of expression cloning (Hollmann et al., 1989). RNA transcribed from cDNA from a rat brain library was injected into *Xenopus* oocytes, and the oocytes were tested with the glutamate agonist kainate (see Box 9.1). When a response was detected, the cDNA library used to produce the RNA was subdivided into successively smaller numbers of clones until one clone was found that consistently directed the synthesis of a glutamate receptor. Subsequently this clone, called *GluR1,* was used to produce primers for PCR amplification, leading to the isolation of three additional closely related genes, *GluR2–4* (or *GluRB–D*—Keinänen et al., 1990).

AMPA Receptors

The *GluR1–4* gene products produce ligand-gated channels that can be activated by glutamate. Since the distribution of the mRNA for these receptors mostly matches that for [^{3}H]AMPA binding sites throughout the CNS (Keinänen et al., 1990), these gene products are usually referred to as AMPA receptors. Members of the AMPA receptor family have about 900 amino acids (ACh receptor subunits have only about 500) and are 68–73 percent identical to one another in sequence. Their sequence identity with ACh receptors is generally less than 20 percent and not significantly higher than expected for two random sequences. Thus GluR1–4 constitute a family separate and only very distantly (if at all) related to ACh receptors.

Hydropathy analysis first suggested that glutamate receptors may have four hydrophobic segments long enough to span the membrane, and this was originally used as evidence to suggest that the conformation of glutamate receptors may be similar to that for ACh receptors: four transmembrane regions with the amino terminus and the carboxyl terminus both extracellular. There is now considerable evidence that this is not the case (see Wo and

---

Box 9.1

EXPRESSION CLONING OF GLUTAMATE RECEPTORS

The method used to clone the first gene for AMPA receptors, based on the description in Hollman et al. (1989), is illustrated on the facing page. Records of responses were taken from the same paper. A similar method was used to clone the first NMDA receptor (Moriyoshi et al., 1991).

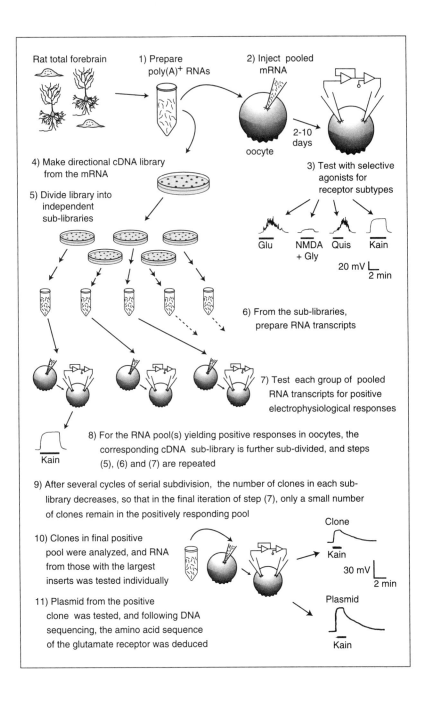

Rat total forebrain

1) Prepare
   poly(A)⁺ RNAs

2) Inject pooled
   mRNA

2-10
days

oocyte

3) Test with selective
   agonists for
   receptor subtypes

Glu   NMDA   Quis   Kain
         + Gly

20 mV
         2 min

4) Make directional cDNA library
   from the mRNA

5) Divide library into
   independent
   sub-libraries

6) From the sub-libraries,
   prepare RNA transcripts

7) Test each group of pooled
   RNA transcripts for positive
   electrophysiological responses

Kain

8) For the RNA pool(s) yielding positive responses in oocytes, the
   corresponding cDNA sub-library is further sub-divided, and steps
   (5), (6) and (7) are repeated

9) After several cycles of serial subdivision, the number of clones in each sub-
   library decreases, so that in the final iteration of step (7), only a small number
   of clones remain in the positively responding pool

10) Clones in final positive
    pool were analyzed, and RNA
    from those with the largest
    inserts was tested individually

Clone

Kain

30 mV
         2 min

11) Plasmid from the positive
    clone was tested, and following DNA
    sequencing, the amino acid sequence
    of the glutamate receptor was deduced

Plasmid

Kain

Oswald, 1994; Hollmann, Maron, and Heinemann, 1994; Bennett and Dingledine, 1995). Four segments do appear to lie within the plane of the membrane, but only three of these appear to reach from one side of the membrane to the other.

Some of the evidence for this revised structural model comes from Hollmann, Maron, and Heinemann (1994), who engineered cDNA for the GluR1 receptor to contain sites for glycosylation (sugar addition) at different points along the channel sequence. The DNA was then used to produce RNA, which was expressed in *Xenopus* oocytes. The resulting protein was extracted from the oocytes, and glycosylation was detected as a change in the molecular weight of the receptor protein, indicated by the change in the mobility of the protein during SDS-polyacrylamide gel electrophoresis. Since glycosylation occurs only on amino acids folded in the protein in such a way that they would be exposed to the extracellular medium, the presence or absence of a sugar group on the expressed GluR1 indicated whether or not that part of the protein was folded to face the outside of the membrane.

The results of these experiments are shown in Fig. 9.12A. The round lollipop shapes are the glycosylation sites native to the protein; these were removed in most of the genetically engineered mutants. The filled diamonds are engineered sites that were glycosylated, and the empty diamonds, sites not glycosylated. Clearly the amino terminus is glycosylated and so is probably extracellular, as for the ACh receptor. The hydrophobic (and therefore putatively transmembrane) domain TMDI apparently threads its way across the membrane from outside to inside, since sites immediately C-terminal to TMDI are *not* glycosylated and so are probably intracellular. This seems to be true for sites on both sides of TMDII, indicating that this sequence, though hydrophobic, is unlikely to extend all the way across the membrane. TMDIII, on the other hand, does appear to be a transmembrane sequence, since sites C-terminal to TMDIII *are* glycosylated. Thus the long loop between TMDIII and TMDIV appears to be extracellular. At some point near TMDIV, the protein reenters the membrane, and the carboxyl terminus is intracellular.

A structure consistent with these findings is given in Fig. 9.12B. Notice that TMDII is drawn as forming a loop within the membrane, much like the P domain of K$^+$ channels (see Chapter 6). The

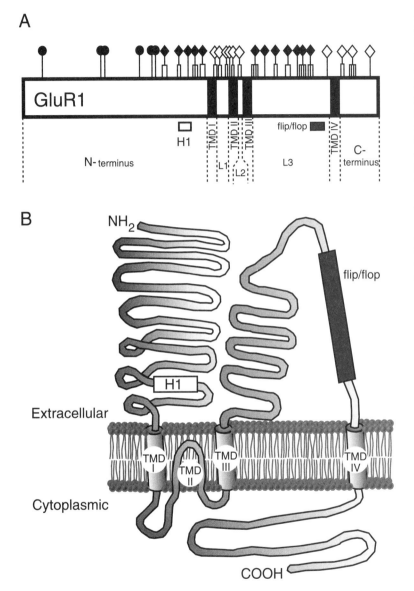

Fig. 9.12 Membrane topology of AMPA-type glutamate receptor. **(A)** Glycosylation was used to determine which parts of the GluR1 protein sequence are located on the extracellular side of the plasma membrane. *GluR1* cDNA shown here, was engineered to remove endogenous glycosylation sites (marked by round lollipop shapes) and to add consensus glycosylation sequences at various positions along the protein coding sequence. DNA was then transcribed to produce cRNA, which was expressed in *Xenopus* oocytes (~20 oocytes per engineered sequence). Protein was extracted from the oocytes, and glycosylation was detected from a change in mobility of the protein with SDS-polyacrylamide gel electrophoresis. Filled diamonds mark sites that, after expression, were glycosylated; empty diamonds are sites that were not glycosylated. *TMDI–IV,* putative transmembrane domains I–IV; *L1–L3,* loops connecting putative transmembrane domains; *H1* hydrophobic domain; *flip/flop,* site of alternate splicing of AMPA receptors. **(B)** Proposed topology of GluR1 receptor based on data in **(A).** (After Hollmann, Maron, and Heinemann, 1994.)

structure of TMDII in the membrane is still not entirely clear, but the notion that it may form a loop is attractive since, as we shall see, TMDII (also known as M2) probably forms at least part of the pore of the receptor channel. Although initially supposed to be pentameric like acetycholine receptors (Ferrer-Montiel and Montal, 1996), more recent experiments indicate that glutamate receptors may be tetrameric unlike any of the other ionotropic receptors (Rosenmund et al., 1998; Laube et al., 1998), more closely resembling voltage-gated channels in their quaternary structure.

Flip-flop

AMPA receptors exist in four forms, GluR1–4, coded for by four different genes. Their variety and the diversity of their physiology is further increased by alternative splicing. The carboxyl tails of some AMPA receptors are alternatively spliced, and the different molecules produced may play a role in altering receptor modulation or the targeting of the receptor to different parts of the cell. In addition, there are two modules, each containing 38 amino acids, that can be alternatively expressed at a site immediately preceding TMDIV. These two modules are usually referred to as *flip* and *flop* (Sommer et al., 1990; see Fig. 9.12B). All of the four AMPA genes can be alternatively spliced with these two modules, and expression of *flip* and *flop* seems to be different in different parts of the nervous system and to be regulated during development. There is also some evidence that receptors containing the *flop* module may desensitize more rapidly than those containing *flip* (Mosbacher et al., 1994; Lambolez et al., 1996; but see also Angulo et al., 1997).

mRNA Editing

The amino acid sequence of AMPA receptors can also be altered by mRNA editing (see Seeburg, 1996; Simpson and Emeson, 1996). At least two sites can be edited: one, called the Q/R site, lies within M2 (Sommer et al., 1991); and another, called the R/G site, lies just in front of (amino-terminal to) the *flip/flop* domain (Lomeli et al., 1994). Editing in both cases appears to occur by a similar mechanism. In the mRNA in the nucleus, an adenosine may be deaminated to form inosine, which is read in the ribosome as a guanosine (Yang et al., 1995; Rueter et al., 1995; Melcher et al., 1995). At the Q/R site, for example, newly transcribed mRNA for all the GluR1–4 AMPA receptors has a glutamine (Q) codon, CAG. The adenosine may be deaminated to form inosine, which is read as guanosine, so that the codon of the mRNA effectively becomes CGG, which encodes the amino acid arginine (R). At the R/G site, a codon for an arginine (R) may be similarly converted to be read as a codon for a glycine (G). The deamination in both cases seems to be highly dependent upon the three-dimensional structure of the mRNA and to be mediated by specific mRNA deaminases present in the nucleus (see for example Melcher et al., 1996).

Editing of mRNA can have important effects on the physiology of the AMPA receptors. The R/G site, for example, can be edited in *GluR2–4* (but apparently not in *GluR1*) and seems to alter the time course of desensitization, which in edited channels can have a slower onset and/or a faster recovery (Lomeli et al., 1994). The Q/R site can be edited only in *GluR2* and can affect both the voltage dependence of channel opening and the Ca^{2+} permeability of the receptor.

Nearly all of the *GluR2* expressed in the brain is expressed with the Q/R site in edited form, with a positively charged arginine replacing a neutral glutamine. Homomeric GluR2 channels or heteromeric channels containing GluR2 (for example GluR1/GluR2 combinations) produce current-voltage curves that are outwardly rectifying at large depolarizations but nearly linear within the physiological range of voltages (see Fig. 9.13A). Channels formed from homomeric GluR1, GluR3, or GluR4 (and heteromeric combinations not including GluR2) have a highly inwardly rectifying current-voltage curve (see Fig. 9.13C), probably at least partly because they are blocked by polyamines (Bowie and Mayer, 1995; Donevan and Rogawski, 1995).

If GluR2, whose RNA is normally edited to contain an arginine at the Q/R site, is engineered to contain a glutamine instead, the current-voltage curve becomes inwardly rectifying (Fig. 9.13B). Conversely, if GluR4 is engineered to contain an arginine, the curve becomes nearly linear in the physiological range (Fig. 9.13D). Thus the alteration of a single amino acid can have a profound effect on the conductance of the channel (Verdoorn et al., 1991), suggesting that the Q/R site may be close to or within the channel pore.

Fig. 9.13 Effect of mRNA editing at Q/R site on current-voltage curves of AMPA receptor responses. Human embryonic kidney cells were transfected with wild-type and mutant GluR2 and GluR4 DNA, and recordings were made with whole-cell patch-clamp. Current-voltage curves were constructed by applying voltage ramps at the command voltage input of the voltage clamp. Data obtained in the absence of the agonist were subtracted from data in the presence of the agonist. **(A)** Wild-type (edited) GluR2, with arginine at the Q/R site. **(B)** GluR2 with glutamine at Q/R site. **(C)** Wild-type (unedited) GluR4, with glutamine at Q/R site. **(D)** GluR4 with arginine at Q/R site. (Reprinted from Verdoorn et al., 1991, with permission of the authors and of the American Association for the Advancement of Science.)

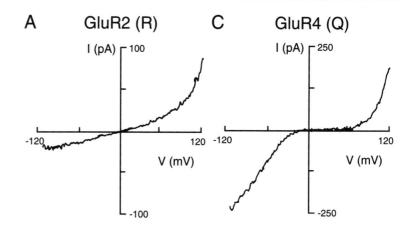

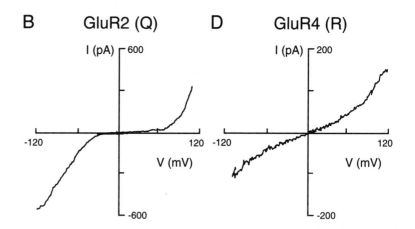

The Q/R site also seems to control the Ca^{2+} permeability of the cell (Hollmann, Hartley, and Heinemann, 1991). Homomeric or heteromeric channels containing edited GluR2 have very little Ca^{2+} permeability (P_{Ca}/P_{Na} of 0.01 to 0.05), whereas channels without GluR2 are quite Ca^{2+} permeable (P_{Ca}/P_{Na} of about 1 to 3—see for example Burnashev, Monyer, et al., 1992; Burnashev et al., 1995). Since in the CNS GluR2 appears to be nearly always edited, the Ca^{2+} permeability of AMPA receptors in particular neurons seems to reflect the GluR2 content of those neurons, with high GluR2 content correlated with low Ca^{2+} permeability (Geiger et al., 1995).

Agonist Specificity and Pharmacology

Homomeric AMPA receptors can be produced by expression of the cRNA from a single gene, but receptors can also be formed from heteromeric assemblies, and heteromeric receptors may be the most common forms in the central nervous system (see for example Craig et al., 1993). Despite this diversity, expressed and native AMPA receptors share many common physiological features. All produce rapidly desensitizing responses to the agonists quisqualate (Quis), AMPA, and L- and D-homocysteate (L-HCA and D-HCA) but very slowly or nondesensitizing responses to kainate (see Fig. 9.14A). AMPA receptors also show rapidly desensitizing responses to glutamate, and the desensitization for many receptor subtypes can be rather effectively blocked by the compound cyclothiazide (CTZ—see Fig. 9.14C). AMPA receptors can be blocked competitively by a variety of organic compounds, including kynurenic acid and the quinoxalinediones CNQX and DNQX (Honoré et al., 1988); they can be blocked noncompetitively by the selective antagonists GYKI 52466 and GYKI 53655 (Donevan and Rogawski, 1993; Zorumski et al., 1993; Paternain, Morales, and Lerma, 1995; Wilding and Huettner, 1995).

Kainate Receptors

After AMPA receptor genes were cloned, their sequences were used for low-stringency hybridization and as probes for PCR amplification to search for further members of the glutamate receptor family. Two further subfamilies of glutamate receptors were isolated, which have been called *kainate* receptors (see Fig. 9.11). The members of the first group, *GluR5–7*, share 75–80 percent sequence identity to one another but only about 40 percent identity with *GluR1–4* (see Hollmann and Heinemann, 1994). The second, called *KA1* and *KA2*, again share about 70 percent sequence identity with one another but only about 40 percent with the AMPA and GluR5–7 proteins. Both groups of receptors are called kainate receptors because the distribution of their mRNA in the brain overlaps that of binding sites for [^{3}H]kainate but is very different from that for [^{3}H]AMPA.

Although not as extensively investigated as AMPA receptors, kainate receptors are probably similar in structure. *GluR5* and *GluR6*, for example, both can be edited at a Q/R site in M2 (Sommer et al., 1991; Köhler et al., 1993), though the editing is less complete than it is for *GluR2*. Recordings from edited forms of GluR5 and GluR6 show altered rectification and single-channel conductance (Swanson et al., 1996), suggesting that, as for the AMPA receptors, the M2 sequence may line the conductance pathway. *GluR6* can also be edited at two further sites in the M1 domain, and these also alter the properties of the channel. Splice variants have been reported for both *GluR5* and *GluR6*. Neither alternative splicing nor mRNA editing has been observed for *KA1* or *KA2*.

Fully functioning glutamate receptors can be formed by homomeric expression of either *GluR5* or *GluR6* but not, for some reason, of *GluR7*. *KA1* and *KA2* gene products do not form channels by themselves but can form channels when co-expressed with *GluR5* or *GluR6* (see for example Herb et al., 1992). There is no evidence that any of the kainate channel subunits can associate with GluR1–4 (see for example Puchalski et al., 1994). Thus the AMPA and kainate receptor proteins appear to form mutually exclusive subsets of glutamate receptors, with associations permitted only between members of the same subfamily. The mechanisms responsible for this selectivity are not presently known.

Ligand-gated channels formed from kainate receptor subunits respond to many of the same agonists and antagonists as AMPA channels (see Fig. 9.14). For example, both kainate and AMPA receptors give rapidly desensitizing responses to glutamate, which are blocked by CNQX and DNQX. In spite of these similarities, there are some characteristic differences. First, responses of kainate receptors to kainate densensitize rapidly (Fig. 9.14B). Recall that AMPA receptors show little desensitization with kainate as an agonist (Fig. 9.14A). Some kainate receptor combinations do not respond to AMPA, but others do (Fig. 9.14B). Cyclothiazide, which blocks desensitization of AMPA receptors, has little effect on kainate receptor desensitization; but the lectin concanavalin A has

A AMPA receptors

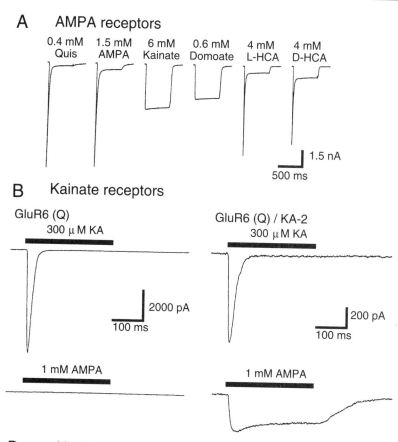

B Kainate receptors

Desensitization: selective block by cyclothiazide and ConA

C GluR1

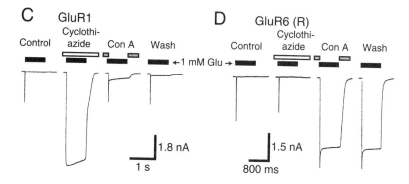

D GluR6 (R)

Fig. 9.14 Agonist specificity and pharmacology of AMPA and kainate receptors. **(A)** Whole-cell patch-clamp recordings of AMPA receptor responses from dissociated mouse hippocampal neurons. Agonists applied from microbarrels of glass tubing whose position was controlled by a stepping motor (similar to method in Fig. 9.15A). Current traces are responses to near-saturating doses of quisqualate (*Quis*), AMPA, kainate, domoate, L-homocysteate (*L-HCA*), and D-homocysteate (*D-HCA*), at the indicated concentrations. Note rapid desensitization for Quis and for AMPA (also for glutamate—not shown) and slow desensitization for kainate and domoate. (Reprinted from Patneau and Mayer, 1991, with permission of the authors and of Cell Press.) **(B)** Whole-cell patch-clamp recordings from human embryonic kidney (293) cells, transfected with DNA for indicated rat brain receptor proteins. *GluR6* (Q) is *GluR6* with Q at the Q/R site. Note that AMPA has no effect on GluR6 expressed by itself but does activate channels produced by co-expression of GluR6 and KA2. (Reprinted from Herb et al., 1992, with permission of the authors and of Cell Press.) **(C)** and **(D)** Pharmacology of desensitization. Transfection as in **(B)** of *GluR1* **(C)** and *GluR6* with arginine at Q/R site **(D)**. Recordings with whole-cell patch clamp, drugs applied as in **(A)**. *Con A* is concanavalin A, which was applied at a concentration 0.3 mg per ml. Cyclothiazide concentration was 100 µM. Dark bars indicate application of 1 mM glutamate. Note the selective effect of cyclothiazide on desensitization for GluR1 channel, and of Con A for GluR6 channel. (Reprinted from Partin et al., 1993, with permission of the authors and of Cell Press.)

just the opposite effect and produces a dramatic block of desensitization of kainate receptors (Fig. 9.14D). The different waveforms of responses to kainate, and the different effects of CTZ and con A on receptor desensitization have been useful in distinguishing AMPA and kainate receptors responses in the CNS.

Also useful has been the development of new antagonists, such as GYKI 52466 and GYKI 53655, which are selective blockers of AMPA receptors. Since many CNS neurons have large AMPA receptor responses, it is often difficult to detect and study the contributions of kainate receptors unless the AMPA component of the response can be blocked. Although in some cells rapidly desensitizing responses to kainate have been observed even without blocking AMPA responses (Huettner, 1990; Lerma et al., 1993), such reports have been rare. In the presence of GYKI 53655, responses similar to those in Fig. 9.14B are more frequently observed (Wilding and Huettner, 1997; Li et al., 1999). Responses mediated by kainate receptors and particularly enhanced by high-frequency stimulation have been recorded from hippocampal cells in slices (Vignes and Collingridge, 1997; Castillo, Malenka, and Nicoll, 1997) and are probably present in many regions of the brain.

Kainate receptors are found in many parts of the CNS (see for example Herb et al., 1992) and probably have important physiological effects. In addition to their evident role in some synapses as postsynaptic receptors, perhaps responding selectively to repetitive activation, kainate receptors appear also to be present presynaptically. There is evidence that kainate receptors may regulate the release of both glutamate (Chittajallu et al., 1996) and GABA (Clarke et al., 1997; Rodríguez-Moreno, Herreras, and Lerma, 1997). With the further development and use of selective agonists and antagonists, we may acquire a clearer notion of the role of kainate receptors in brain processing.

NMDA Receptors

The most easily distinguished class of iontotropic glutamate receptors is the one selectively activated by N-methyl-D-aspartate, or NMDA (see Fig. 9.11), some of whose properties were described in Chapter 1. These receptors can of course also be activated by glutamate, as well as by aspartate and homocysteate, but they are quite insensitive to AMPA, quisqualate, and kainate. They are blocked selectively by a variety of competitive antagonists, for example AP5, also known as APV (2-amino-5-phosphonopentanoic acid), and AP7 (2-amino-7-phosphonoheptanoic acid); as well as by several classes of noncompetitive antagonists. The selectivity of these agonists and antagonists makes NMDA receptors the easiest to identify among the classes of glutamate-gated ion channels (see Hollmann and Heinemann, 1994; McBain and Mayer, 1994; Sprengel and Seeburg, 1995).

The first NMDA receptor (called NMDAR1 or NR1) was isolated and sequenced by expression cloning (Moriyoshi et al., 1991), the method used for *GluR1*. Expression of the *NR1* receptor cRNA produced responses to glutamate with many of the characteristics of NMDA receptors recorded from intact CNS neurons. Low-stringency hybridization and PCR with probes from *NMDAR1* DNA were then used to isolate 4 additional clones, called *NMDAR2A–D* or *NR2A–D,* which share considerable sequence identity with one another but much less with the NR1 receptor (Meguro et al., 1992; Monyer et al., 1992; Kutsuwada et al., 1992). Unlike *NR1, NR2A–D* gene products appear not to form channels when their cRNA is injected into *Xenopus* oocytes, either singly or in combinations, say, of *NR2A* with *NR2B*. When however the RNA of one of the *NR2* genes is expressed together with that of *NR1*, the efficiency of channel expression is much higher than for *NR1* alone, and channels are formed with somewhat different properties (see for example Monyer et al., 1992; Kuner and Schoepfer, 1996). Many NMDA receptors may therefore be heteromers consisting of both NR1 and NR2 subunits.

NR1 expression is widely distributed throughout the central nervous system and may be present in almost every cell in the CNS. *NR2* gene expression, on the other hand, is quite variable from region to region, and this variability may play an important role in the regulation of NMDA receptor properties in different parts of the nervous system and during development (Monyer et al., 1994). Additional receptor diversity is produced by a large number of alternatively spliced gene products, which can alter the pharmacological and physiological properties of the receptor (Zukin and

Bennett, 1995) and may play some role in the targeting of receptors to synaptic sites in the plasma membrane (Ehlers, Tingley, and Huganir, 1995).

The structure of NMDA receptor proteins is probably similar to that of other glutamate receptors (Fig. 9.12B). The amino terminus and M3-M4 loop appear to be extracellular, and the carboxyl terminus is probably intracellular (Hirai et al., 1996). There are four hydrophobic sequences (called M1–M4), which are probably mostly contained within the membrane. The position analogous to the Q/R site in the M2 domain of NMDA receptors is not edited but is occupied by an asparagine in both the *NR1* and *NR2* gene families. This asparagine appears to play an important role in both Mg^{2+} block and Ca^{2+} permeability of NMDA receptors (Burnashev, Schoepfer, et al., 1992), which I described in Chapter 1. Together with other adjacent amino acids, this asparagine may also help determine the ion selectivity of the channel pore (Wollmuth et al., 1996). It therefore seems likely that, as for AMPA and kainate receptors, the M2 sequence forms part of the ion channel.

Glycine

One of the most remarkable features of the native NMDA receptor in the central nervous system is that it is poorly if at all activated by glutamate alone but requires the simultaneous presence of glycine as a co-agonist. This was discovered by Jon Johnson and Philippe Ascher (1987), who were recording with whole-cell patch-clamp from cultured neurons from mouse brain. They were measuring the responses of these cells by applying NMDA from a double-barreled pipette while perfusing the bath with an extracellular bathing medium (see Fig. 9.15A). They noticed that the size of the response of the cells to NMDA from the pipette depended on the rate at which they perfused the cells with the bathing medium. The slower the rate of bath perfusion, the larger the response to NMDA, as if a substance necessary for producing the response to NMDA was generated by the cultured cells and normally present in the spaces between cells but was washed away when the perfusion rate was too high. Furthermore, the response to NMDA could be potentiated (made larger) by co-perfusion with culture medium (see traces

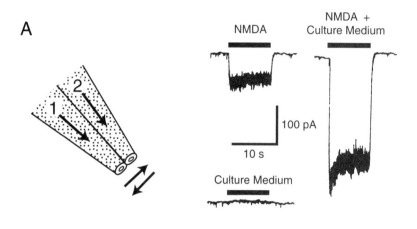

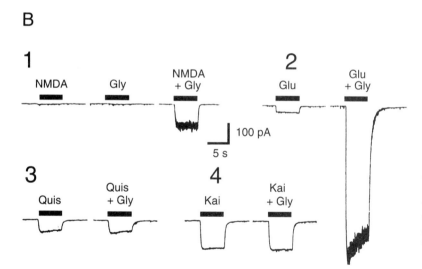

Fig. 9.15 Dependence of NMDA-type glutamate response on extracellular glycine. **(A)** *Left:* A double-barreled tube containing control solution in barrel 1 and test solution with agonist in barrel 2 was mounted on a micromanipulator and rapidly moved from side to side under visual control. The pipettes were positioned above the cell from which recordings were made, and the micromanipulator was moved to apply the drug-containing solution. Solutions were fed into barrels 1 and 2 from independent reservoirs by gravity. Solutions were free of Mg^{2+}, to enhance amplitude of NMDA responses (see Fig. 1.8). *Right:* Whole-cell recording from cultured embryonic mouse CNS neuron, $V_H = -50$ mV. NMDA (50 μM) produced small response, which was significantly enhanced by co-perfusion with culture medium taken from CNS neuron cultures after 2–8 hours of incubation. Culture medium alone had no effect. Timing and duration of exposure to NMDA and culture medium indicated by horizontal bars. **(B)** Effect of glycine on NMDA receptor response. Recording conditions as in **(A)**. Timing of drug applications indicated by horizontal bars. *1:* Response to 10 μM NMDA is significantly enhanced by 1 μM glycine, though glycine by itself produced no response. *2:* Response to 10 μM glutamate also greatly enhanced by 1 μM glycine. *3* and *4:* Responses to 2 μM quisqualate (*Quis*) and 10 μM kainate (*Kai*) were not significantly potentiated by 1 μM glycine (these responses were probably produced by AMPA receptors). (Reprinted from Johnson and Ascher, 1987, with permission of the authors and of Macmillan Magazines Limited.)

in Fig. 9.15A). After a few simple biochemical tests, they determined that the active component was a small-molecular-weight metabolite, which they subsequently identified as glycine.

If both glycine and glutamate must bind to the NMDA receptor for opening to occur, one could reasonably ask, is the NMDA receptor a glutamate receptor or a glycine receptor? Or both? Since at least in some cases NMDA receptors have been found postsynaptically at the same synapses as AMPA receptors, it seems likely that glutamate is the transmitter released from the presynaptic terminals at these synapses. Furthermore, it seems likely that under most conditions the glycine binding site is occupied, since its affinity is in the nanomolar range, and there are probably a few *micromolar* glycine normally present in the cerebrospinal fluid. There remains the possibility that under some conditions glycine concentrations are modulated in CNS and can regulate NMDA channel activity (see for example Lukasiewicz and Roeder, 1995; Supplisson and Bergman, 1997). Indeed, if this were not the case, there would be little need for a glycine binding site on the NMDA receptor in the first place.

NMDA Receptor Antagonists

Antagonists for the NMDA receptor come in two varieties: competitive antagonists, which bind to glutamate or glycine binding sites, and noncompetitive antagonists, which bind somewhere else (see McBain and Mayer, 1994). I have already described two of the most important competitive antagonists for glutamate, AP5 and AP7. The binding of *glycine* to the NMDA receptor can also be competitively antagonized by several drugs, for example 7-chlorokynurenic acid or 5,7-dichlorokynurenic acid.

A large number of clinically important drugs, such as ketamine, phencyclidine (PCP or "angel dust"), and MK-801, are noncompetitive antagonists of the NMDA receptor, binding neither to the glutamate nor to the glycine binding site. Instead, they appear to bind to and block the channel. A particularly interesting and useful noncompetitive antagonist is MK-801, which acts as a trapping blocker: it binds within the pore of the open channel and then remains trapped within the pore when the channel closes (Huettner and Bean, 1988). When MK-801 is applied in the absence of NDMA, no block occurs, since the channel remains closed and MK-801 cannot enter the pore to block (Fig. 9.16A). When NMDA and MK-801 are applied together, the channel opens and is rapidly blocked, a phenomenon often referred to as *use-dependent block* (Fig. 9.16B). Since the channel closes with the blocker inside, the block is very long-lived and is relieved only by prolonged application of agonist (Fig. 9.16C). The long-lasting action of trapping

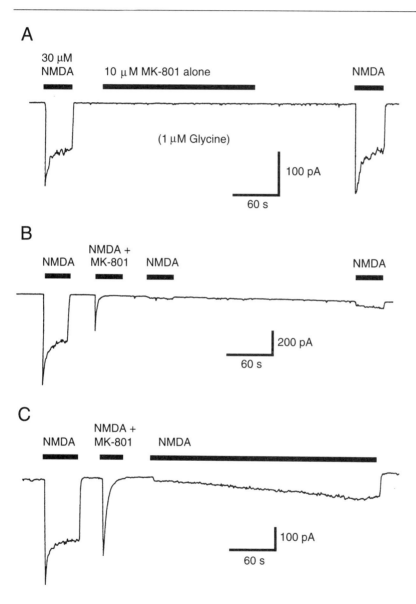

Fig. 9.16 Block of NMDA receptor response by MK-801. Whole-cell patch-clamp recordings from neurons dissociated from embryonic rat visual cortex grown in primary culture. Solutions were applied from microbarrels as in Figs. 9.14 and 9.15 and were Mg^{2+}-free to enhance amplitude of NMDA responses. Glycine was also added at a concentration of 1 μM. $V_H = -70$ mV. **(A)** Application of 10 μM MK-801 did not block responses to 30 μM NMDA if the MK-801 was applied in the absence of NMDA. **(B)** Application of MK-801 in the presence of NMDA, at same concentrations as in **(A)**, produced rapid blocking, which outlasted MK-801 application; response recovered very slowly. **(C)** Time course of recovery of NMDA response from MK-801 block was accelerated if NMDA was applied continuously during recovery period (concentrations were NMDA, 30 μM; MK-801, 20 μM). (Reprinted from Huettner and Bean, 1988, with permission of the authors.)

blockers like MK-801 and PCP may in part be responsible for their dramatic neuropharmacologic effects (see Chapter 1).

NMDA receptors are also affected by a variety of agents that seem not to bind to either the glutamate or glycine binding sites or to enter the pore. These include Zn^{2+} and other heavy-metal cations (e.g., Cd^{2+}), which appear to bind to a site near the external surface of the membrane (Westbrook and Mayer, 1987; Peters, Koh, and Choi, 1987). Zn^{2+} is of special interest, since it is present in rather high amounts in some areas of the CNS and may be released in a selective manner (Assaf and Chung, 1984; Howell, Welch, and Frederickson, 1984).

Gating of Glutamate Receptors and Glutamatergic Transmission

At many glutamate synapses in the CNS, more than one kind of receptor is present in the postsynaptic membrane, and an excitatory postsynaptic potential (EPSP) can have a complicated waveform. Since AMPA and kainate receptors are both selectively blocked by CNQX, and NMDA receptors are selectively blocked by AP5, the non-NMDA and NMDA components of the EPSP can be isolated and studied independently from one another (see for example Keller, Konnerth, and Yaari, 1991). Remarkable differences in their waveform have been found (Fig. 9.17). Responses mediated by non-NMDA receptors have a rapid onset and decay, whereas NMDA-mediated responses are much slower.

The waveform of receptor activation depends upon several factors (see Jahr, 1994; Edmonds, Gibb, and Colquhoun, 1995b; Jones and Westbrook, 1996; Clements, 1996). The time course of the rising phase is a function of the rate of glutamate binding and the latency to the first opening of the channel once glutamate is bound. The time course of the falling phase depends upon the rate of transmitter clearance from the cleft and the rate of *deactivation* or closing of the channel following transmitter removal. The falling phase may also be influenced by delayed openings of the channel. Since for glutamate receptors the rate of desensitization is much faster than for ACh receptors, channel desensitization may also affect the time course of response decay.

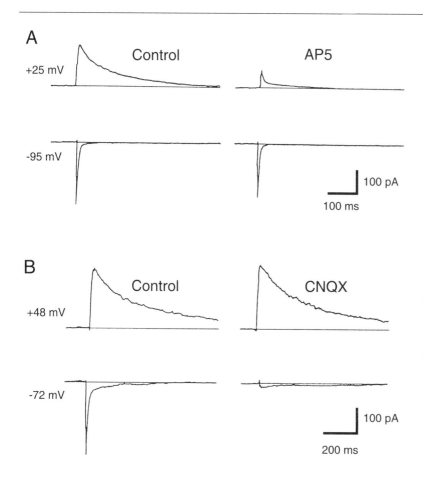

Fig. 9.17 Isolation of contributions from NMDA and non-NMDA receptors to EPSPs in hippocampal granule cells. Recordings were made with whole-cell patch-clamp from granule cells in rat hippocampal slices, and EPSPs were evoked by stimulating presynaptic neurons with extracellular current application with a stimulation pipette near the outer border of the dentate granule cell layer. Since NMDA responses are largely blocked at hyperpolarized membrane potentials by voltage-dependent block by Mg^{2+} (see Fig. 1.8), responses recorded at negative membrane potentials were produced mostly by AMPA and kainate receptors, whereas those at positive membrane potentials had a large component produced by NMDA receptors. Receptor components were isolated by selective block with AP5 and CNQX. **(A)** Non-NMDA receptor's component of EPSP revealed by block of NMDA component with AP5 (50 μM). **(B)** NMDA receptor's component revealed by block of AMPA and kainate components with CNQX (5 μM). Note much slower time course of decay of NMDA component. (Reprinted from Keller, Konnerth, and Yaari, 1991, with permission of the authors and of the Physiological Society.)

Transmission Mediated by NMDA Receptors

The release of glutamate from a presynaptic terminal causes a brief increase in transmitter concentration in the synaptic cleft to ~1 mM (Clements et al., 1992; Clements, 1996). At glutamate synapses, there is no enzyme like acetylcholine esterase adjacent to the synapse to hydrolyze the transmitter. Instead, the glutamate concentration decreases by diffusion and by binding to and uptake by transporters, which remove the glutamate from the cleft by transporting it into glial cells or back up into the synaptic terminal (see Lester et al., 1994; Borowsky and Hoffman, 1995). The rate of glutamate decrease in the cleft may be rapid at some synapses (Clements et al., 1992) but more prolonged at others (Barbour et al., 1994; Otis, Wu, and Trussell, 1996), and the glutamate removal rate may be markedly affected by the activity of transporters and the geometry of the extracellular space.

It is likely that glutamate binds rapidly to the receptors but that channel opening occurs more slowly: just how slowly is still uncertain (see Jahr, 1992; Edmonds and Colquhoun, 1992; Dzubay and Jahr, 1996). The slow rate of channel opening may simply be a consequence of the complicated kinetics of the receptor, which has many open and closed states (Gibb and Colquhoun, 1992); it may also be influenced by glycine binding or by the rate of removal of Mg^{2+} block.

The decay of the NMDA receptor response is also slow (see Fig. 9.17B), so slow that it is unlikely to be determined by the rate of clearance of transmitter from the cleft. This was demonstrated in the following way (Lester et al., 1990). Whole-cell recordings were made presynaptically and postsynaptically from two neurons in a culture of hippocampal cells, so that one cell could be stimulated and the response of the other cell recorded. CNQX was used to block the AMPA component of the response, so that the NMDA component could be studied in isolation; and Mg^{2+} was removed from the bathing solution. A double-barrel pipette (as in Fig. 9.15A) was used to apply either Mg^{2+} or AP5 rapidly during the response. Mg^{2+} produces a rapid block of the NMDA channel as soon as it is applied (see Fig. 9.18A), because Mg^{2+} enters the channel pore and blocks the channel (see Chapter 1). This means that block can occur at any time during the response, since during this time the channel must be open and Mg^{2+} can enter. The results with AP5 are very different. Since AP5 is a competitive inhibitor, it blocks by preventing glutamate from binding. AP5 has no effect if delivered after the beginning of the response (see Fig. 9.18B), presumably because at that point the glutamate has already bound to the receptor. Only when AP5 is present just before synapse activation does any block occur (Fig. 9.18B, bottom record).

These experiments indicate that glutamate need be present for only a brief time during synapse activation but probably then remains bound to the NMDA receptor for the duration of the EPSP.

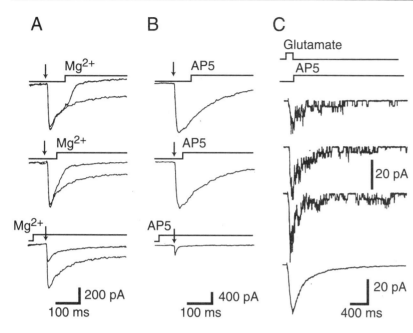

A

B

C

Fig. 9.18 Slow decay of NMDA receptor response is predominantly the result of slow unbinding of agonist. **(A)** Whole-cell patch-recordings were made simultaneously from two neurons in primary cultures of embryonic rat hippocampus. Stimulation of one neuron (arrow) was used to evoke EPSP in second neuron. Recordings were made in zero-Mg^{2+} Ringer containing 5 µM CNQX, to isolate and enhance NMDA response. At time indicated by step above each set of records, medium containing 100 µM Mg^{2+} was rapidly perfused onto the cell. Each set of records shows two EPSPs superimposed: the larger response is a control, without Mg^{2+} perfusion; the smaller (or more rapidly terminating) response shows the effect of Mg^{2+} addition. Note that Mg^{2+} addition is effective throughout the time course of the NMDA response. **(B)** Recording and stimulation conditions as in **(A)**, but cells were rapidly perfused with medium containing 100 µM AP5 instead of Mg^{2+}. Block occurred only when AP5 was present just before synapse stimulation. **(C)** Single-channel recordings from outside-out patches taken from cultured hippocampal neurons as in **(A)** and **(B)**. External solution was Mg^{2+}-free and contained a cocktail of channel blockers, including 2 µM CNQX. Brief (100 ms) application of 100 µM glutamate produced long-lasting channel activity, which was unaffected by subsequent application of 100 µM AP5. Figure shows three representative traces and ensemble average of 130 trials. (Traces relabeled from Lester et al., 1990.)

This conclusion is further supported by the observation that a short pulse of glutamate to an NMDA receptor in an outside-out patch produces a long-lasting current, which is not blocked by the subsequent addition of AP5 (Fig. 9.18C). The very slow decay of the NMDA receptor response would therefore appear to be mostly due to the very slow unbinding of glutamate.

One important difference between NMDA receptors and AMPA receptors is the large difference in their binding affinities for agonist. NMDA receptors are half-maximally activated at a glutamate concentration of a few micromolar, whereas for AMPA receptors half-activation occurs at 0.5–1 mM. This large difference in affinities is probably attributable to a large difference in the rate of glutamate unbinding (the k_{off}) and probably explains why the decay of NMDA-mediated responses is so slow. When, for example, NMDA receptors in outside-out patches are exposed to agonists that bind less tightly to the receptor (e.g., L-cysteate), receptor activation decays more quickly (Lester and Jahr, 1992); and EPSPs with more rapidly decaying NMDA components can be produced by introducing a lower-affinity agonist into the presynaptic terminal as a substitute (or "false") transmitter (Pan, Tong, and Jahr, 1993).

The general picture we have for NMDA receptor activation is therefore much like the one we have for ACh receptors. At least two glutamates (and two glycines) bind, and, in the absence of block by Mg^{2+}, the channel then flickers between open and closed states until one of the agonist molecules falls off the channel. Since the affinity of the channel for glutamate (and glycine) is high, transmitter stays bound for a relatively long time. To understand in detail how the waveform of the response is produced, we would need to know how many open and closed states the channel has, how rapidly the channel moves between these states, and how rapidly and from what kinetic states the channel desensitizes. The role of desensitization is of particular interest for NMDA receptors, since it is rapid enough to contribute to the waveform of the response (see for example Lester and Jahr, 1992), and since there is evidence that several different kinds of desensitization may have different effects on the physiology of glutamate transmission (see McBain and Mayer, 1994).

Transmission Mediated by non-NMDA Receptors

Under most conditions at most of the glutamate synapses so far investigated, the great majority of the current that enters the postsynaptic membrane during glutamate receptor activation is carried by AMPA receptors. The reason for this is that most NMDA receptors are blocked at resting membrane potentials by Mg^{2+} (see Chapter 1), and kainate responses in many cases seem to be rather small. Despite their importance, AMPA receptors are still poorly understood. With their low affinity for glutamate, they seem to be optimized for rapid channel opening and closing and for the rapid transmission of neural information. Unhappily for the physiologist, activation, deactivation, and desensitization all occur so rapidly that they are often difficult to distinguish. Furthermore, the kinetics of AMPA receptor activation seem to be quite variable from synapse to synapse, so conclusions drawn from one preparation may not apply to others.

The opening of AMPA channels is so fast that it is probably limited by the rate of glutamate binding to the receptor. What happens next is mostly a matter of conjecture. In some cases (e.g., synapses onto cerebellar granule cells—Silver, Colquhoun, Cull-Candy, and Edmonds, 1996), deactivation is so rapid and desensitization so slow that desensitization is unlikely to occur during the time course of an EPSP. Most of the decay of the EPSP seems therefore to be due to glutamate unbinding and deactivation (channel closing)—much as I described for ACh receptors. Even for such rapid synapses, the EPSP does have a slow tail (Silver et al., 1996), probably caused by a slow component of glutamate removal from the synaptic cleft (Barbour et al., 1994; Otis, Wu, and Trussell, 1996).

For other synapses, AMPA receptor deactivation is sufficiently slow and desensitization sufficiently rapid that desensitization may actually affect the EPSP waveform (Trussell and Fishbach, 1989; Hestrin, 1993; Otis, Zhang, and Trussell, 1996). Desensitization seems to have a profound effect on the amplitude of the EPSP when the synapse is stimulated several times at closely spaced intervals (Trussell and Fishbach, 1989; Otis, Zhang, and Trussell, 1996). Since the time course of desensitization can be altered by editing at the R/G site and perhaps by alternative splicing of the *flip* or *flop* modules, there can be tremendous variety in the waveforms of glutamate responses at different synapses in the CNS (see for example Angulo et al., 1997). We know this variety is present, but we still have very little idea which forms of AMPA receptors are expressed on which neurons, and why.

One way of determining the role of receptor subunits in setting the waveform of the EPSP is to record the glutamate response and determine the AMPA subunit composition *in the same cell,* with the technique of *single-cell PCR* (see Sucher and Deitcher, 1995; Ozawa and Rossier, 1996). A patch-clamp pipette is used to make a whole-cell recording from a cell, generally from one in a brain slice. During the recording, the cytoplasm of the cell is dialyzed into the pipette, and at the end of the recording, further suction is applied to bring the remaining cytoplasm into the pipette interior. The contents of the pipette are then removed, and the RNA extracted. The RNA is used to make cDNA, which is amplified with PCR by the use of primers specific for the different channel subunits. This technique has been used in several studies in an attempt to correlate AMPA receptor subunit composition with the kinetics and ion permeability of the receptor (see for example Geiger et al., 1995; Lambolez et al., 1996; Angulo et al., 1997). Single-cell PCR may eventually provide an explanation of the molecular variety of AMPA responses and help us understand the role of the receptor subunits in establishing the properties of excitatory input in different parts of the CNS.

Summary

Neural transmission in the CNS can occur in two ways. Transmitter released at synapses can activate receptors called ligand-gated channels, which directly alter the conductance of the postsynaptic membrane. Alternatively, chemicals (sometimes called neuro-modulators) released from presynaptic terminals can bind to metabotropic receptors, which activate G proteins. Ligand-gated receptors are most commonly used at synapses that mediate the rapid transfer of information between presynaptic and postsynaptic cells. The most common ligand-gated receptors in the CNS appear to be those normally activated by glutamate and acetylcholine, which are excitatory, and GABA and glycine, which mediate inhibition.

Of the excitatory ligand-gated channels, the actylcholine (ACh) receptor at the muscle endplate has been the most extensively studied. It is a pentamer formed by five homologous subunits. Each subunit has a large amino-terminal region, which for one of the subunits (called α) probably contains at least part of the ACh binding site. Each subunit contains four transmembrane domains, one of which (M2) probably lines the interior of the channel. The channel formed by the M2 domains apparently narrows near its cytoplasmic end to a diameter of 0.6–0.7 nm, limiting the size of the ions that can permeate the receptor. Although the muscle ACh receptor is cation-selective, it is poorly selective among different monovalent cations and is also permeable to divalent cations, including Ca^{2+}. The binding of two ACh molecules to the receptor leads to a change in conformation and opening of the channel. The receptor can then flip back and forth between open and closed states for as long as two ACh molecules remain bound.

ACh receptors are found in neurons, too. A large number of homologous receptor subunits form functional cholinergic receptors in the CNS. Functional synapses containing ACh receptors have been described in many parts of the brain, but the abundance of subunits seems to be much greater than can be accounted for by the few reports of cholinergic EPSPs. The function of neuronal ACh receptors is still largely unknown, though some evidence suggests that these receptors may be active primarily at presynaptic locations.

Another major group of excitatory channels are the glutamate receptors. Glutamate and ACh receptors appear to constitute unrelated families of proteins. The glutamate receptors have a different structure, for example: there are four hydrophobic domains, but only three span the membrane. Moreover, glutamate receptors may be tetrameric rather than pentameric. Glutamate receptors fall into three subfamilies: the AMPA receptors, which are the workhorses of the group, carrying most of the current at glutamate receptors in the brain; the NMDA receptors, which show voltage-dependent block by Mg^{2+} and high permeability to Ca^{2+} and which may play a special role in certain CNS functions, such as synapse modification (see Chapters 1 and 14); and the kainate receptors, which are now being observed at increasing numbers of CNS preparations and whose role is beginning to be clarified. Glutamate is the most important excitatory transmitter in the central nervous system, and the structure and function of glutamate receptors is a rapidly evolving subject of considerable importance.

Other groups of excitatory receptors have been omitted from this chapter. $5\text{-}HT_3$ (serotonin) receptors are a relatively recent addition to the group of ligand-gated channels; they are closely related to ACh receptors in structure and function (Jackson and Yakel, 1995; Lambert, Peters, and Hope, 1995). Also not mentioned are the P_{2X} receptors, a family of ligand-gated receptors for ATP (Surprenant, Buell, and North, 1995; Séguéla et al., 1996; Soto et al., 1996; Collo et al., 1996). P_{2X} receptors, with no sequence homology to either the ACh or glutamate receptors, appear to have quite a different structure, with only two transmembrane domains. In some respects they resemble the inwardly rectifying K^+ channels (see Chapter 7), except that most of the mass of inward rectifiers is inside the membrane, whereas most of the P_{2X} receptors' mass is outside. I have also omitted discussion of histamine receptors in invertebrates and the recently described ligand-gated channels for the peptide FMRFamide (Lingueglia et al., 1995). As more is discovered about these proteins, so variable in their structure, we may obtain a better understanding of the mechanisms they share for transducing excitatory responses.

10

Inhibitory Transmission

THE OUTPUT OF a neuron is determined not only by excitatory synapses from neurons releasing ACh and glutamate but also by a large and physiologically important *inhibitory* input. The most important sources of inhibition in the CNS are mediated by γ-aminobutyric acid (GABA) receptors and glycine receptors. These two receptor classes apparently comprise all of the inhibitory ligand-gated channels of vertebrates, and together they are responsible for all of the rapid inhibitory transmission in the nervous system. In addition, there are a great many receptors mediating various forms of metabotropic inhibition in the CNS, and some of these receptors and their G-protein-linked pathways are described in Chapters 11–13.

Inhibitory ligand-gated channels are among the most important proteins in the nervous system. GABA receptors in particular are by far the most common sites of action of general anesthetics, including barbiturates and volatile anesthetics like halothane (Franks and Lieb, 1994). These receptors are also important sites of action of many drugs and are promising targets for the treatment of nervous disorders. They produce inhibition in many cases by generating negative-going changes in membrane potential called *inhibitory postsynaptic potentials* (or IPSPs). These sum with EPSPs to reduce excitation and decrease Ca^{2+} influx or action potential generation. GABA and glycine channels are selective for anions, such as Cl^- and HCO_3^- (see Chapter 3). For most neuronal cell bodies, the equilibrium potential for anions is more negative than the resting membrane potential (because Cl^- is pumped out of the cell—see Chapter 4), and an increase in anion permeability produces a hyperpolarization (Eccles, 1964; Nicoll, 1988; Ebihara et al., 1995).

In some muscles (Dudel and Kuffler, 1961) or neurons (Adams and Brown, 1975), the opening of ligand-gated channels for GABA or glycine may produce little or no change in membrane potential. This would occur if anions were passively distributed across the cell membrane. In the absence of a change in membrane potential, inhibition could still occur, since an increase in a conductance whose reversal potential is equal to the resting potential would tend to clamp the membrane potential near the resting potential and prevent EPSPs from depolarizing the cell to the threshold needed to generate an action potential.

At dendrites or axon terminals (Alger and Nicoll, 1982; Nicoll, 1988; Zhang and Jackson, 1993), the equilibrium potential for anions is sometimes more positive than the resting membrane potential (because Cl⁻ was pumped *into* the cell), and the opening of GABA or glycine channels produces a depolarization. In this case the effect could still be inhibitory, since the resulting depolarization might be too small to produce an action potential and the membrane potential would still be held below the spike threshold. Furthermore, if the depolarization were small and slow, it might inactivate Na⁺ channels by a process called *accommodation* (see the summary in Chapter 6). The Na⁺ channels might enter an inactivated state before any action potentials were produced, which could have the effect of preventing excitatory synaptic potentials from stimulating the cell (Zhang and Jackson, 1995; Jackson and Zhang, 1995).

Structure of GABA and Glycine Receptors

GABA and glycine receptors share many similarities with excitatory ACh and 5-HT receptors, and it is possible they evolved from a common ancestor (Ortells and Lunt, 1995). The excitatory ACh and 5-HT receptors are thought to have diverged rather early from the inhibitory GABA and glycine receptors, but these proteins nevertheless all share a common structure. All are thought to contain a large N-terminal region, which is at least partially responsible for ligand (transmitter) binding; all have 4 transmembrane domains, of which the second (M2) is at least partially responsible for forming the ion channel; and all have a large cytoplasmic domain between M3 and M4, which often contains regulatory sites for protein phosphorylation (see Fig. 10.1).

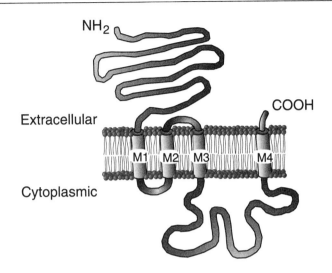

Fig. 10.1 Proposed structure of inhibitory GABA$_A$ and glycine receptors. (After Macdonald and Olsen, 1994.)

GABA receptors are much more widely dispersed than glycine receptors within the central nervous system and are abundantly expressed by cells in cortex, cerebellum, and most major brain nuclei. Glycine receptors are mostly restricted to the spinal cord, brainstem, and retina. GABA receptors seem to occur in much greater variety than glycine receptors, and there is some evidence that glycine receptors may have evolved from GABA receptors (Ortells and Lunt, 1995). For these reasons, I begin with GABA.

GABA Receptors

The first GABA receptors (like the first ACh receptors) were isolated biochemically (from brain), and partial sequences were used to make probes from which receptor clones were pulled out of brain cDNA libraries (Schofield et al., 1987; see Macdonald and Olsen, 1994; Tyndale, Olsen, and Tobin, 1995; Sieghart, 1995; Whiting, McKernan, and Wafford, 1995; for the ε subunit, see Davies et al., 1997). There are of the order of 20 different receptor subunit genes (in rodents), which have been placed into 6 subfamilies on the basis of the similarity of their sequences, called α, β, γ, δ, ε, and ρ. The variety of receptor proteins is further increased by alternative splicing: for example, genes for the γ2 and β2 subunit may be expressed as forms called L and S, and the L form (but not the S) may include an additional sequence that contains a potential site for phosphorylation by protein kinase C (see Chapter 12).

For nicotinic ACh receptors at the electroplax or neuromuscular junction, we know that functional receptors are pentamers with a stoichiometry of either $\alpha_2\beta\gamma\delta$ or $\alpha_2\beta\epsilon\delta$. GABA receptors are also believed to be pentamers, but the stoichiometry of the subunits seems to be quite variable and is still the subject of considerable investigation (see Whiting, McKernan, and Wafford, 1995; McKernan and Whiting, 1996). Although the numerous different receptor genes and their alternatively spliced products would seem to provide for many thousands of possible assembled pentamers, the number of receptors actually found in the CNS is probably much lower than this, perhaps of the order of 20–30.

Many studies using immunoprecipitation and immunolocalization with antibodies specific to different subunits, as well as other evidence from *in vitro* hybridization and Western blot analysis, have shown that most GABA receptors actually found in the CNS are probably constructed from at least one α, at least one β, and at least one γ (or δ or ϵ) subunit. The most common brain receptor (representing nearly half of the GABA receptors in CNS) seems to be constructed from $\alpha 1$, $\beta 2$, and $\gamma 2$, apparently with a stoichiometry of $2\alpha:2\beta:1\gamma$ (Chang et al., 1996; Tretter et al., 1997). Some receptors may contain more than one type of α (e.g., $\alpha 1$ and $\alpha 3$— Verdoorn, 1994) or more than one type of β or γ. In general, receptors with γ subunits do not appear to have δ subunits, but there may be exceptions to this rule (Saxena and Macdonald, 1994).

Ligand-gated GABA receptors constructed from α, β, γ, δ, and ϵ subunits are usually referred to as $GABA_A$ receptors. The many different pentamers constructed from these subunits presumably have different properties (Gingrich, Roberts, and Kass, 1995), and much research is currently directed toward understanding what distinguishes the different subunit combinations. Because of the importance of GABA receptors in neural processing and as sites for drug action, considerable effort is being made to localize specific receptor combinations in different parts of the brain and to characterize their function and pharmacologicy.

Receptors constructed from ρ subunits are sometimes placed in a separate category, since they form GABA-gated channels that are quite insensitive to the drug bicuculline (Shimada, Cutting, and

Uhl, 1992; Wang, Guggino, and Cutting, 1994), which is an effective competitive antagonist for most GABA$_A$ receptors. Bicuculline-insensitive GABA receptors are sometimes called GABA$_C$. Receptors formed from ρ subunits have so far been found only in the retina, where they seem to play an important role in ligand-gated GABA inhibition (Qian and Dowling, 1993; Feigenspan, Wässle, and Bormann, 1993; Lukasiewicz, Maple, and Werblin, 1994). In addition to ligand-gated GABA channels, there are also several different kinds of metabotropic or G-protein-coupled receptors that bind GABA, which are usually referred to as GABA$_B$ receptors (see Chapter 11).

Glycine Receptors

Receptors gated by the amino acid glycine were also identified by a combination of biochemical isolation and cDNA cloning (Grenningloh et al., 1987; see Langosch, 1995; Kuhse, Betz, and Kirsch, 1995). There are at least four genes for glycine receptor subunits, grouped into two families: $\alpha 1$–$\alpha 3$ and β. Both $\alpha 1$ and $\alpha 2$ have been shown to be alternatively spliced. Glycine receptors are probably pentamers (Langosch, Thomas, and Betz, 1988) and can be formed *in vitro* homomerically from α subunits, from combinations of different α subunits, and from mixtures of α and β subunits (Bormann et al., 1993; Kuhse et al., 1993). It is likely that native receptors are formed from α and β subunits assembled together, perhaps with the stoichiometry 3α:2β. The cytoplasmic side of the glycine receptor has a binding site for another protein, called gephyrin, which in turn binds cytoskeletal proteins and probably helps position the glycine receptor in clusters at the postsynaptic membrane (see for example Kirsch et al., 1993).

A vivid demonstration of the close relationship between GABA and glycine receptors has been given by Schmieden, Kuhse, and Betz (1993), who showed that the alteration of only 1 or 2 amino acids in the N-terminal region of the glycine receptor is sufficient to make this receptor responsive to GABA. Since GABA and glycine receptors are so similar in their structure and function, it would be quite interesting to know why two inhibitory receptors have evolved with two different transmitters. The vertebrate retina is a particularly interesting case in point, since for one large class of inhibitory interneurons (called amacrine cells), consisting of perhaps 20–30 different cell subtypes, about half release GABA and the other half glycine at synapses onto other neurons (MacNeil and Masland, 1998). It is possible that for this tissue we may eventually discover why this is so.

Ion Selectivity and the Structure of the Channel

Both GABA and glycine channels are highly selective for anions. Chapter 3 presented a partial description of the careful study of Bormann, Hamill, and Sakmann (1987) of the ion selectivity of inhibitory receptors in mouse spinal neurons. Using both whole-cell and single-channel recordings, they showed that many different anions could permeate both GABA and glycine channels. Neither receptor was measurably permeable to cations. Figure 10.2 plots the relative permeability for each of the anions (A) used in their experiments (P_A/P_{Cl}) against the *Stokes diameter* of the ion. The Stokes diameter is the apparent size of the ion estimated from its mobility in aqueous solution (see MacInnes, 1961). The lines through the points give the permeabilities expected for spherical particles moving through a cylindrical channel of a specified diameter, with no other feature of the channel taken into consideration. With the exception of the thiocyanate ion (SCN^-), the fit is fairly good. The channel diameters assumed for the calculations were 0.52 nm for the glycine receptor (Fig. 10.2A) and 0.56 nm for the GABA receptor (Fig. 10.2B). Thus the pores of both receptors seem to be fairly well described by a cylinder whose diameter is between 0.5 and 0.6 nm (5–6 Å).

The only two anions normally present in sufficient quantity under physiological conditions to make a significant contribution to current through inhibitory channels are Cl^- and HCO_3^-. Although the relative permeability of bicarbonate to chloride is only 0.1–0.2, bicarbonate is still permeable enough to affect both the amplitude of the current and its reversal potential (Kaila and Voipio, 1990). Furthermore, since GABA and glycine can produce a net movement of HCO_3^- across the cell membrane, they can cause both intracellular and extracellular changes in pH (see Chapter 4 and Fig. 4.11).

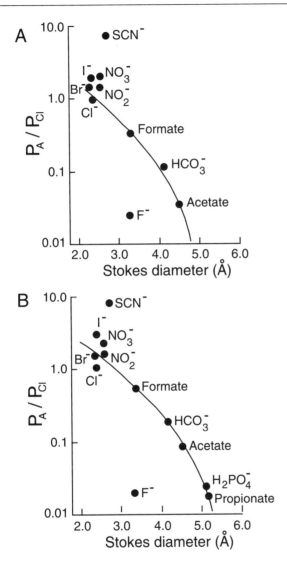

Fig. 10.2 Relative permeabilities of $GABA_A$ and glycine channels to anions. Graphs plot for GABA responses **(A)** and glycine responses **(B)** the relative permeability (P_A/P_{Cl}) as a function of the Stokes diameter of the anion. Permeability measurements were made with the whole-cell patch-clamp method, as described in Chapter 3, from dissociated embryonic spinal cord neurons. The Stokes diameter is the apparent size of the ion, as estimated from its mobility in aqueous solution. Mobility in turn was estimated from Λ_0, the limiting conductivity of the ion at infinite dilution (see MacInnes, 1961). (Reprinted from Bormann, Hamill, and Sakmann, 1987, with permission of the authors and of the Physiological Society.)

M2 Lines the Channel

It is likely that the channels of both GABA and glycine receptors are formed at least in part by the M2 transmembrane domain. Bormann et al. (1993) showed that the glycine single-channel conductance can be altered by mutations in M2. Xu and Akabas (1996) probed the conformation of the GABA channel by mutating amino acids of the GABA M2 domain to cysteines and then exposing the receptors to sulfhydryl-specific reagents, like *p*-chloromercuribenzenesulfonate (pCMBS), placed in the extracellular medium. Since pCMBS is negatively charged and rather bulky, it would not be expected to permeate the lipid bilayer of the plasma membrane and would be expected to react only to amino acids that are somehow accessible to the extracellular space. Sulfhydryl reagents successfully reacted with cysteines on several of the M2 amino acids, producing a change in channel conductance. This would suggest that these amino acids are somehow accessible to the extracellular solution, as would be the case if M2 lined the channel pore. Only a fraction of the M2 amino acids were susceptible to reaction with sulfhydryl reagents, suggesting that only these amino acids were accessible (Fig. 10.3A). On the likely supposition that M2 is α-helical, most of the reacting residues appear to face the same direction (Fig. 10.3B), presumably toward the pore of the channel. Since amino acids that reacted even in closed channels were found almost as far along M2 at the cytoplasmic terminus (Xu, Covey, and Akabas, 1995), it is probable that the channel gate is near the cytoplasmic side of the protein. This appears also to be the case for ACh receptors (see Akabas et al., 1994, and Chapter 9).

What Makes Inhibitory Receptors Permeable to Anions?

ACH and 5-HT receptors are permeable to cations but GABA and glycine receptors are permeable to anions. Since all of these receptors are quite similar in structure, it would be interesting to know what determines the sign of the ions to which the channels are permeable. If the M2 regions of an ACh receptor are compared to those of the subunits of GABA and glycine receptors (Fig. 10.4), several differences are noted. In particular, between positions 236

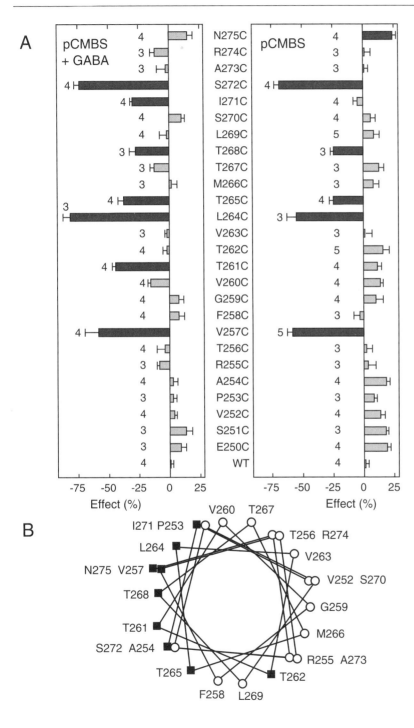

Fig. 10.3 Probing the GABA_A receptor's channel pore with sulfhydryl reagents. The cRNAs from rat wild-type and mutated GABA_A receptor genes were expressed in *Xenopus* oocytes, and recordings were made of responses to perfused GABA with a two-electrode voltage clamp. Amino acid residues of the GABA_A $\alpha 1$ gene near and within the membrane-spanning M2 domain were mutated one at a time to cysteine residues and expressed with wild-type $\beta 1$ and $\lambda 2$. Oocytes were treated with the sulfhydryl reagent pCMBS for 1 min in the presence or absence of 100 μM GABA (with channels open or closed), and GABA responses were subsequently recorded to test for an irreversible change in the properties of the GABA response due to reaction of the reagent with the cysteine. **(A)** Effect of 0.5 mM pCMBS. Black bars indicate statistically significant effects on the GABA response, with a negative change indicating inhibition and a positive change potentiation. Gray bars indicate nonsignificant effects. For both, mean effect and standard error are shown. Number of oocytes tested is indicated to left of bar. Mutations are designated as follows: *L264C* means amino acid 264 of $\alpha 1$, which is leucine (L), was mutated to cysteine (C). **(B)** Positions of affected amino acids. Amino acids near and within M2 have been drawn as an α-helical wheel to depict their approximate positions with respect to the (presumed) helix perimeter of the M2 domain. Black squares are mutated residues that showed a significant response to sulfhydryl reagents (including but not limited to pCMBS), and white squares are nonreactive mutants. (Reprinted from Xu and Akabas, 1996, with permission of the authors and of Rockefeller University Press.)

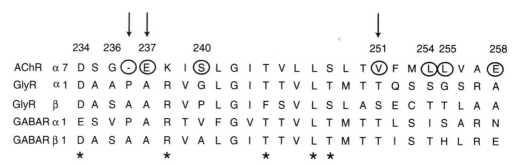

Fig. 10.4 Comparison of sequences of M2 membrane-spanning domains for the neuronal nicotinic ACh $\alpha 7$ gene with genes for subunits from inhibitory GABA$_A$ and glycine receptors. Numbers refer to positions of amino acids in the $\alpha 7$ sequence, and stars indicate highly conserved residues. Circled amino acids were mutated in experiments, as described in the text. The one-letter code for amino acids (see Stryer, 1995) is used here, with dash (negative sign) indicating that no amino acid was present in the corresponding position. (Reprinted from Galzi et al., 1992, with permission of the authors and of Macmillan Magazines Limited.)

and 237 of the ACh receptor, the corresponding locations on GABA and glycine receptors have an additional amino acid, either a proline (P) or an alanine (A). If M2 is an α-helix, the addition of an amino acid just before M2 would have the effect of twisting the helix, so that different amino acids would then be exposed to the channel wall (see Fig. 10.3B).

In an attempt to see which amino acids might be critical in determining the sign of permeable ions, Galzi et al. (1992) mutated the ACh receptor gene $\alpha 7$ to introduce several amino acid changes like those expressed by the glycine receptor gene $\alpha 1$. The changes they made are indicated by the circles in Fig. 10.4: a proline was introduced between positions 236 and 237, and single substitutions were made for each of the circled amino acids from the ACh sequence to mimic the sequence found in GlyR $\alpha 1$. For example, at position 237, glutamate (E) was mutated to alanine (A). A mutant protein containing all of the changes shown in Fig. 10.4 (mutant $\alpha 7$-1) was expressed in *Xenopus* oocytes and responded to ACh to produce an increase in conductance. Remarkably, the current through the channel was no longer cationic like the original $\alpha 7$ ACh receptor but was now carried almost exclusively by anions.

To see which amino acids were critical in producing this change, Galzi and colleagues made successively smaller changes in the $\alpha 7$

ACh receptor gene. An anionic receptor could be produced with only three amino acid alterations (mutant $\alpha7$-2): the insertion of a proline between positions 236 and 237, the substitution of an alanine (A) for a glutamate (E) in position 237, and the substitution of a threonine (T) for a valine (V) in position 251. The most important change seems to have been the insertion of the amino acid between positions 236 and 237. If only this change was made, the RNA unfortunately did not produce a functional protein in *Xenopus* oocytes, for reasons which are unclear. If, however, mutations of the $\alpha7$ receptor gene were made only at the other two loci (237 and 251), the protein was expressed but the channel remained cationic.

These experiments provide additional evidence that M2 is important in forming the channel within the ACh/5-HT/GABA/glycine superfamily of receptors. Furthermore, they show that small changes in the structure of M2 are sufficient to produce a rather dramatic shift in the permeability of the receptor.

Pharmacology

GABA$_A$ responses can be produced by a variety of agonists, including muscimol (from the hallucinogenic mushroom *Amanita muscaria*), 4,5,6,7-tetrahydroisoxazolo-[4,5-*c*]pyridin-3-ol (THIP), and isoguvacine. They can be competitively blocked by several antagonists, of which the most commonly used is bicuculline (see Fig. 10.5A). GABA$_C$ responses, as noted above, have somewhat different pharmacological properties: GABA$_C$ receptors are resistant to bicuculline but in some preparations can be competitively antagonized by imidazole-4-acetic acid (see for example Qian and Dowling, 1994).

Glycine agonists include several compounds similar in structure to glycine, such as β-alanine, taurine, and β-aminoisobutyric acid. Glycine receptors are rather insensitive to bicuculline but can be blocked by the competitive antagonist strychnine and its derivatives (aminostrychnine, methylstrychnine, and isostrychnine), by 1,5-diphenyl-3,7-diaza-adamantan-9-ol, and by the steroid RU 5135. These antagonists are not as a rule terribly selective: RU 5135 and strychnine can both inhibit GABA$_A$ receptors, though the concentration of strychnine required for inhibition is in general higher for GABA$_A$ than for glycine receptors (see for example Fig.

Fig. 10.5 Pharmacology of GABA$_A$ and glycine receptors. **(A)** Effects of common antagonists on inhibitory receptor responses. Whole-cell patch-clamp recordings from dissociated retinal ganglion cells from the goldfish. External and internal (pipette) solutions contained equimolar Cl$^-$ (E_{rev} for Cl$^-$ was 0 mV), and holding potentials for the different experiments were between −70 and −75 mV. Drugs were applied by rapid perfusion. Bars indicate duration of solution application for GABA and glycine (both at 30 μM), with and without co-application of 3 μM bicuculline *(Bi)* and 1 μM strychnine *(S)*. Bicuculline preferentially blocked GABA responses, whereas strychnine blocked glycine responses. (Reprinted from Cohen, Fain, and Fain, 1989, with permission of the authors and of the Physiological Society) **(B)** Effects of barbiturates and benzodiazepines. Whole-cell patch-recordings from embryonic human kidney (293) cells, transfected with DNA for human GABA$_A$ $\alpha 1$, $\beta 1$, and $\lambda 2$ genes. Bars indicate application of 10 μM GABA alone or in the presence of 1 μM of the benzodiazepines diazepam *(DZP)* or flunitrazepam *(FNZM)* or of 50 μM of the barbiturate pentobarbital *(PB)*. Five-minute intervals between records marked by double slashes. (Reprinted from Pritchett et al., 1989, with permission of the authors and of Macmillan Journals, Ltd.) **(C)** The benzodiazepine diazepam increases the single-channel conductance of GABA$_A$ receptors in hippocampal neurons. Recordings from cell-attached patch from hippocampal cell of neonatal rat, perfused through the patch pipette with 5 μM GABA *(left)* or with 5 μM GABA plus 10 μM diazepam. (From Eghbali et al., 1997, with permission of the authors and of Macmillan Magazines Limited.)

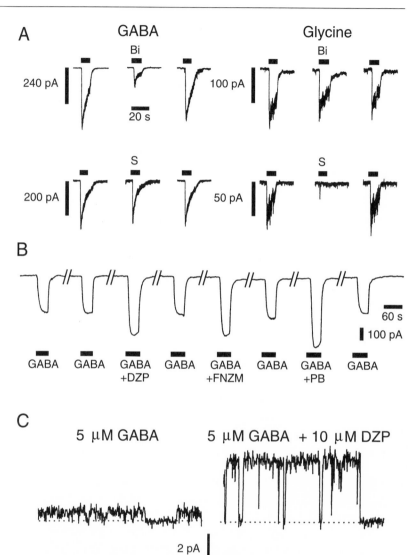

10.5A). Strychnine is also an antagonist for some neuronal nicotinic ACh receptors.

In addition to competitive antagonists, GABA$_A$ responses can be blocked by the noncompetitive antagonist picrotoxin or picrotoxinin, as well as by a variety of other compounds that seem to bind to the picrotoxin binding site, including cyclodiene insecticides and *t*-butyl-bicyclo-phosphorothionate (TBPS). Although the mechanism of action of picrotoxin seems to be complex (see Newland and Cull-Candy, 1992; Yoon, Covey, and Rothman, 1993), two lines of evidence indicate that picrotoxin may inhibit at least in part by binding to a site within the channel. The first is that a point mutation within M2 can greatly reduce the effect of picrotoxin and of the other compounds acting at the picrotoxin binding site (ffrench-Constant, Rocheleau, Steichen, and Chalmers, 1993; Zhang, ffrench-Constant, and Jackson, 1994). The second is that picrotoxin can protect at least one cysteine-mutated residue within M2 from reacting with sulfhydryl reagents (Xu, Covey, and Akabas, 1995). This result seems to suggest that picrotoxin enters the channel and binds, occluding the pore and preventing the passage or binding of sulfhydryl reagents and perhaps also of permeant anions.

Barbiturates and Benzodiazepines

One of the most interesting features of GABA receptors is their sensitivity to barbiturates and benzodiazepines, many of which are widely used as sedatives and relaxants (see Macdonald and Olsen, 1994; Sieghart, 1995; Lüddens, Korpi, and Seeburg, 1995). Barbiturates such as pentobarbitol increase the amplitude of GABA responses (Fig. 10.5B), probably by altering the kinetics of the channels so that the average open time of the channel is increased (Macdonald, Rogers, and Twyman, 1989a). The increase in the size of the GABA response produces an increase in IPSP amplitude, which increases inhibition throughout the nervous system.

Benzodiazepines can have a variety of effects. Benzodiazepine agonists such as flunitrazepam and diazepam facilitate the GABA response, as barbiturates do (see Fig. 10.5B), though by a different mechanism. For some receptor types they probably act by increasing the affinity of GABA for its binding site (Rogers, Twyman, and Macdonald, 1994). For others, they appear to produce an increase in the amplitude of the single-channel conductance (see Fig. 10.5C, from Eghbali et al., 1997). In addition to benzodiazepine agonists, which facilitate GABA$_A$ responses, there are compounds, called *inverse agonists,* that *decrease* the amplitude of responses to GABA, as well as benzodiazepine antagonists, which block the binding of benzodiazepine agonists or of inverse agonists.

Because of the importance of barbiturates and benzodiazepines in clinical medicine, a considerable effort has been made to understand how these compounds act. It seems unlikely that the body contains intrinsic "barbiturate-like" or "benzodiazepine-like" compounds that modulate GABA receptors under physiological conditions (though this possibility cannot as yet be excluded). It is more likely that the effects of these compounds are a consequence of the particular conformation of the receptor proteins. That is, barbiturates and benzodiazepines probably bind to sites that have been formed as a part of the mechanism of receptor function, and the effects of these drugs are probably an accident of receptor evolution.

Since benzodiazepines appear to work by affecting GABA binding, understanding their mechanism of action might provide useful information about the conformation of the binding site (see for example Smith and Olsen, 1995). Unfortunately, the binding site for GABA is complex and probably formed from more than one subunit (α: Smith and Olsen, 1994; β: Amin and Weiss, 1993). Benzodiazepine binding is affected by amino acid substitutions on the α subunit (Pritchett and Seeburg, 1991), and the affinity for benzodiazepines seems to be dramatically influenced by the particular α subunit or subunits contained in the receptor (Lüddens, Korpi, and Seeburg, 1995). Benzodiazepine binding is also critically dependent on the presence and nature of the γ subunit (Pritchett et al., 1989; Lüddens, Korpi, and Seeburg, 1995). Some GABA subunit combinations are much more sensitive to benzodiazepines than others, and different receptors have different sensitivities to different drugs. Other receptors are completely insensitive. These differences may be telling us something important about the geometry of the binding site, but it may be difficult to know what this is until we know how many of each subunit a functioning receptor contains, and how these subunits are arranged in the pentamer.

Receptor Activation and Desensitization

When an action potential invades the axon terminal of an inhibitory (presynaptic) neuron, GABA or glycine is released from the

A

B

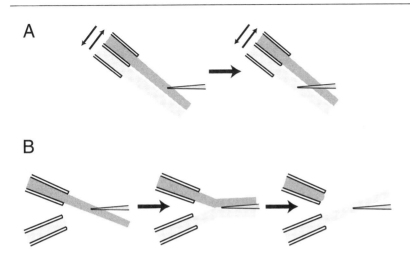

Fig. 10.6 Two methods for making ultra-rapid solution changes to outside-out patches containing ligand-gated channels. **(A)** In the first method, the solutions or patch pipettes are moved. One solution containing Ringer and another containing Ringer with agonist are placed in barrels of a double-barreled piece of "theta" pipette tubing. Solution flows continuously into both barrels, and the position of the pipette or solution tubing is switched rapidly from one place to the next, often with a piezo-electric device. (After Lester and Jahr, 1992.) **(B)** The second method requires no motion of the pipette or solution tubing. Two solution-containing barrels are directed at the pipette containing the outside-out patch. At first only one solution barrel is open *(left)*. To change solutions, a second solution barrel is opened and the first barrel is closed. This initially forms a solution interface *(middle)*, which rapidly displaces across the patch pipette oriface as the flow velocity from the first barrel decreases. After complete closing of first barrel, only solution from second barrel reaches patch pipette *(right)*. (After Maconochie and Knight, 1989.)

terminal and binds to receptors in the membrane of the post-synaptic cell to produce a change in its conductance. The concentration of GABA in the cleft is thought to rise to between 0.5 and 1 mM. This conclusion is based, in part, upon a comparison of the rate of rise of the postsynaptic current with the rate of rise of the GABA response in an isolated outside-out patch (Maconochie, Zempel, and Steinbach, 1994; Jones and Westbrook, 1995).

An outside-out patch (Fig. 1.4) can be rapidly exposed to medium containing GABA, either by moving the pipette containing the membrane patch rapidly back and forth between two streams of solution at the end of a piece of "theta" tubing (Fig. 10.6A, Lester and Jahr, 1992), or by directing two streams of solution toward the patch and rapidly switching them on and off by altering their flow rates (Fig. 10.6B, Maconochie and Knight, 1989). The second of these methods is fast enough to change solutions in less than 100 μs, a speed of the same order as the rate of the delivery of transmitter across the synaptic cleft.

The recordings in Fig. 10.7 show averages of responses to different GABA concentrations for an outside-out patch from a cerebellar granule cell, taken from the study of Maconochie, Zempel, and Steinbach (1994). Notice that the rate of the solution change (bottom two traces) is faster than the rate of any of the GABA responses. This is comforting, since it indicates that the method used to deliver solution to the patch was not rate-limiting.

Fig. 10.7 Rate of activation of $GABA_A$ receptors. Currents recorded from an outside-out patch, excised from a rat cerebellar granule cell in culture. Responses are averages of 6–60 presentations. Bars indicate time course of GABA application at each of the concentrations noted. Traces to right are for applications of 300 µM to 10 mM GABA; they repeat the same responses appearing to the left, at the same concentrations, but on a faster time scale (note timebars). The two lowest traces display the time course of the solution change at slow and fast time scales, measured by exposing an open patch pipette to solutions of different composition and measuring the resulting change in junction current. (Reprinted from Maconochie, Zempel, and Steinbach, 1994, with permission of the authors and of Cell Press.)

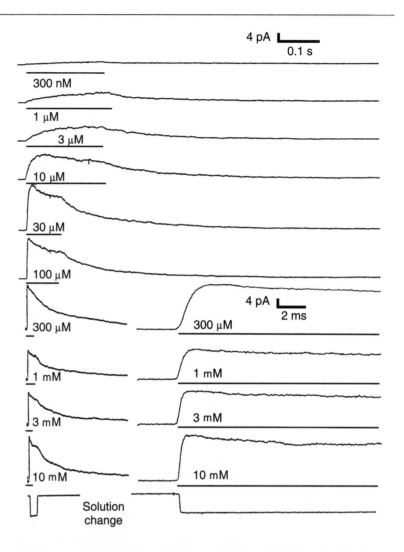

The rate of rise of the inhibitory synaptic current (the IPSC) was then measured, also from an intact granule cell in a cerebellar culture. When this was compared to the rise times of the responses in Fig. 10.7, the concentration of GABA that produced an equivalent rise time for the IPSC could be estimated to be 0.5 to 1 mM. This is the concentration that would be expected to be reached within the synaptic cleft, but it may be a lower limit, since the rate of rise of the IPSC could have been underestimated during the recording, as a result of slowing of the IPSP time course due to electrotonic conduction from synapses to the recording pipette (see Fig. 2.11A).

If the concentration of GABA in the synaptic cleft rises to 0.5–1.0 mM, then the GABA receptors are likely to be saturated (or nearly so) at the peak of the IPSP. As I explained in Chapter 8, the release of a single vesicle at a synapse in the central nervous system is likely to increase the concentration in the synapse cleft by at least 0.5–1 mM (see Clements, 1996). Thus a single vesicle probably is sufficient to saturate the GABA receptors at an inhibitory synapse. The response from each synapse is then equivalent to a miniature IPSP, and many such responses sum from many different points of synaptic contact within the dendritic field of a cell to produce the summed IPSP recorded at the cell body.

The notion that a single vesicle is sufficient to saturate GABA receptors at a CNS synapse is consistent with the observation that benzodiazepines, which for some GABA$_A$ receptors appear to act by increasing GABA binding, do not increase the amplitude of miniature IPSCs (Mody et al., 1994; DeKoninck and Mody, 1994; but see Frerking, Borges, and Wilson, 1995). Benzodiazepines would not increase the amplitude of the response to a single vesicle if the binding of GABA to the receptor were already saturated during synaptic activation.

This observation, however, poses an important question that is still not entirely resolved. If benzodiazepines do not actually increase the amount of binding because the binding sites are saturated, how do they increase the level of inhibition at central synapses? One answer to this question is that there are some CNS synapses for which benzodiazepines increase the single-channel conductance, as in Fig. 10.5C. This would increase the size of the inhibitory current even if no greater binding of GABA were to occur. Another possibility is that benzodiazepines, by increasing GABA binding, increase the *duration* of the IPSP (Mody et al., 1994). The duration is increased because the increased affinity of GABA causes the GABA to be released from the receptor more slowly once GABA has bound. Imagine a neuron receiving inhibitory input at synapses in many different locations. Provided inputs at these synapses are not exactly synchronized in time, miniature IPSPs will arrive from these synapses at the cell body at different moments. If these miniature IPSPs are longer in duration in the presence of benzodiazepines, they would be expected to sum to-gether to produce a larger and longer inhibitory input.

Channel Activation

Once GABA or glycine binds to its receptor, it gates the opening of channels. Since GABA and glycine receptors are structurally so similar to ACh receptors, it is reasonable to suppose that the mechanism of activation is similar. That is, channel gating may occur by a scheme like this,

$$C \underset{k_{-1}}{\overset{k_1}{\rightleftharpoons}} CA \underset{k_{-2}}{\overset{k_2}{\rightleftharpoons}} CA_2 \underset{\beta_2}{\overset{\alpha_2}{\rightleftharpoons}} OA_2$$

much as I described the sequence of changes for ACh receptors at the muscle endplate in Chapter 9.

There are reasons to suppose, however, that GABA channel activation may be more complicated than this. In the first place, several attempts have been made to model the kinetics of activation of GABA receptors from single-channel recordings, and these studies indicate that more closed and open states may be necessary to describe the gating of GABA receptors than were needed to model gating of ACh receptors (Weiss and Magleby, 1989; Macdonald, Rogers, and Twyman, 1989b; Twyman, Rogers, and Macdonald, 1990). Openings seem to occur for both singly and doubly liganded receptors, but there appear to be a total of at least three open states and as many (or more) closed states. It is possible that ACh receptors also enter similar additional open and closed states but much less frequently. The apparent difference between ACh and GABA receptors may be fundamental in nature, or it may reflect a variation on the same basic pattern. The latter seems more likely, but the truth is that we really do not know at present.

In addition to these complexities, both GABA and glycine receptors have numerous subconductance states, which in many recordings are quite commonly observed. The recordings of Bormann, Hamill, and Sakmann (1987) from mouse spinal cord neurons are typical. In outside-out patches with the same (145 mM) concentration of Cl^- on both sides of the membrane, the most frequently observed conductance for GABA receptors was 30 pS, but substates were also frequently observed at 44, 19, and 12 pS. For glycine receptors the most frequently observed conductance was 46 pS, with subconductance states at 30, 20, and 12 pS. Subconductance states were also observed in on-cell recordings and so are unlikely to be an artifact of the excision of the patch. In some recordings, the main conductance represented nearly all of the openings, but in other cases nearly half of the openings were to subconductance levels.

A typical example of data recorded from an outside-out patch containing only a single active glycine receptor is given in Fig. 10.8. Part A shows the receptor's response to 100 μM glycine on a slow time base, and in part B the same response is displayed at a higher temporal resolution. The most frequently observed conductance was near 27 pS, but there were many openings to near 22 pS, and a few to near 10 pS. The 27 and 22 pS conductance states represent conformational changes of the same macromolecule, and this is probably the case for the 10 pS openings as well. The evidence for this claim is given in Fig. 10.8C, which is a histogram of the frequency of appearance of specific current measurements. Zero current is, of course, the baseline. The lines drawn through the frequency data fit Gaussian distributions to the distributions for the different conductance levels, and from these distributions we can calculate the probability of occurrence of the different conductance values. These calculations indicate that for about 47 percent of the time the conductance of the receptor occupied the 27 pS level, and for about 35 percent the 22 pS level. The frequency of occurrence of 10 pS openings was not estimated, but these openings probably accounted for the nonzero value of the opening frequency for current values near -1 pA.

Suppose the 27 and 22 pS openings represented different, independently gated channels. Then there should have been a $(0.47)(0.35) = 16$ percent chance of seeing *both* the 27 and 22 pS channels open simultaneously. However, $27 + 22 = 49$ pS events were never observed. This is rather strong evidence that the 27 and 22 pS events were not different, independently gated channels but

Fig. 10.8 Responses of an outside-out patch excised from cultured retinal ganglion cell containing a single active glycine receptor. Solutions inside and outside the patch contained nearly equal Cl⁻ concentrations ($E_{rev} \sim 0$ mV), and V_H was -94 mV. **(A)** Response to 10 s application of 100 µM glycine. Noise in record just before first channel opening is an artifact produced by motorized switch that changed solutions of microperfusion system. **(B)** Single-channel openings from **(A)** shown on a faster time scale. The most common open state was at a conductance of 27 pS, but openings were also observed at 10 pS and 22 pS. **(C)** Amplitude histogram for segment of record in **(A)** containing channel activity. Histogram was constructed by sampling the value of the current in **(A)** every 115 µs. The current values were then sorted into bins of 0.1 pA, and the number of observations in each bin was plotted against bin value. Dotted and dashed lines are Gaussian fits for currents of -2.6 ± 0.2 pA (corresponding to 27 pS channel openings) and -2.1 ± 0.3 pA (corresponding to 22 pS openings). Solid line is sum of these two Gaussians plus Gaussian at 0 pA for baseline. Note the poor fit of solid line near -1 pA, corresponding to infrequent 10 pA openings illustrated in **(B)**. (Reprinted from Cohen, Fain, and Fain, 1989, with permission of the authors and of the Physiological Society.)

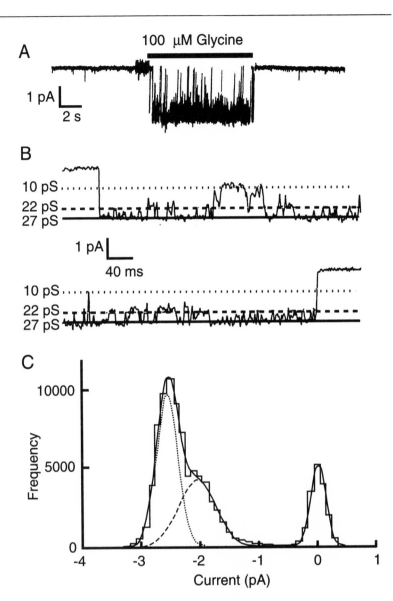

rather different conductance states of the same channel. Presumably the same macromolecule can undergo several different conformational states, each of which may have a pore of a different diameter. The multiplicity of conductance states and their greater frequency of occurrence makes the kinetics of GABA and glycine receptors much more difficult to analyze and understand than for ACh receptors in muscle, where subconductance states are occasionally seen but are by comparison rather rare (see Hamill and Sakmann, 1981).

Desensitization

Although some studies have suggested that the desensitization of GABA or glycine receptors is too slow to contribute to the time course of the IPSP (see for example Borst, Lodder, and Kits, 1994), this may not be true in every case. IPSPs transmitted through GABA receptors seem to occur with a variety of different waveforms, some much faster than others (see for example Puia, Costa, and Vicini, 1994). Rapid desensitization has now been observed in several different preparations and may be characteristic of many inhibitory synapses in the CNS.

It is possible that desensitization may help prolong the duration of inhibitory IPSPs (Jones and Westbrook, 1995). This could happen in the following way. Receptors could bind GABA during the short period of time when the GABA concentration was high in the synaptic cleft, before GABA diffused away. The receptor could open and close, and then desensitize before GABA became unbound. If we can assume that the affinity of the GABA receptor for GABA in the desensitized state is high (this is true for the ACh receptor), the GABA could remain bound to the desensitized form of the receptor for as long as the receptor remained desensitized. The receptor could then reopen from the desensitized state once or even several times. The multiple passage of the receptor from its desensitized state to its open state may prolong the duration of inhibition.

Presynaptic Inhibition

Inhibition produced by synapses directly onto a nerve cell soma or dendrite is called *postsynaptic inhibition* (see Fig. 10.9A). IPSPs produced by postsynaptic inhibition are commonly hyperpolarizing and sum with excitatory EPSPs to modulate the excitability of the postsynaptic cell. Most neurons receive many excitatory and inhibitory synapses, and the output of the cell depends upon the relative number and amplitudes of the postsynaptic potentials. The location of the input can also be important. In a pyramidal cell, for example, inhibition would be most effective when the synapse is positioned between the excitatory input and the site of action potential generation. If, for example, excitation were to occur at synapses onto the spines of distal dendrites, inhibition would be most effective if it were between those spines and the cell body, or at the soma itself.

As a general rule, the closer the inhibitory synapses are to the axon hillock of the postsynaptic cell, the greater is their influence on the probability of spiking. Inhibition directly at the soma, however, suffers from the disadvantage of being rather nonselective: it inhibits excitatory input from any of the main branches of the dendritic tree. Inhibition onto dendrites can be much more discriminating, depressing excitation at only one or a few of the dendritic branches of the cell.

Mechanism of Presynaptic Inhibition

If the inhibitory synapse occurs not on the soma or dendrite of the postsynaptic cell but rather on another synaptic terminal, the inhibition is said to be *presynaptic* (Fig. 10.9A). The mechanism of presynaptic inhibition was first elucidated by Dudel and Kuffler (1961) in recordings from the crayfish neuromuscular junction. The abductor muscles in the walking legs of the crayfish receive input from two kinds of fibers: excitatory fibers, which are glutamatergic, and inhibitory fibers, which are GABAergic. The two kinds of fibers can be separated and separately stimulated. When the excitatory fibers are stimulated, the muscle depolarizes and occasionally generates action potentials, which are Ca^{2+}-dependent (see Chapter 7). Simultaneous stimulation of the inhibitory fibers decreases the amplitude of this excitation, in part through synapses made by the inhibitory fibers directly onto the muscle. Inhibition of this sort is of course postsynaptic (Fig. 10.9A) and can be explained by changes in the conductance of the muscle membrane.

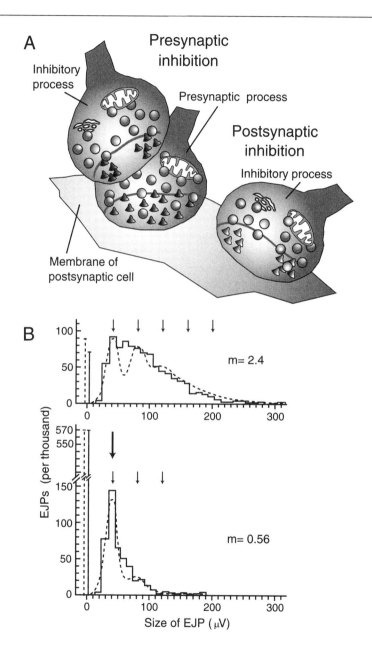

Fig. 10.9 **(A)** Presynaptic and postsynaptic inhibition. For presynaptic inhibition, the inhibitory process terminates on a presynaptic terminal, which in turn forms a synapse with the postsynaptic neuron. The release of inhibitory transmitter alters the probability of release of transmitter from the presynaptic terminal. For postsynaptic inhibition, the inhibitory process terminates directly on the postsynaptic neuron. **(B)** Demonstration of presynaptic inhibition at the crayfish neuromuscular junction. Excitatory junctional potentials (EJPs) were recorded extracellularly (as in Fig. 8.10) after stimulation of presynaptic nerve. Graphs show frequency of EJPs grouped in 10 μV bins with amplitudes indicated on abscissa. Heavy arrow indicates mean amplitude of spontaneous miniature EJPs and smaller arrows point to calculated mean amplitudes of events containing 1–5 quanta. Upper graph is for stimulation of excitatory nerve alone, lower graph for stimulation of both excitatory and inhibitory nerves. Both graphs contain a total of 1,000 recorded EJPs. Dashed line in both figures indicates number of failures and gives fit with Poisson equation for value of mean quantal content (m) given in insert to graph. Note that inhibition decreases m, increases the probability of failures, and shifts the whole probability distribution toward smaller amplitudes. Inhibition at this synapse must therefore be at least in part presynaptic, since postsynaptic inhibition would have simply scaled the distribution to smaller amplitudes without changing its shape or the value of m. (Redrawn from Dudel and Kuffler, 1961.)

Dudel and Kuffler also observed that stimulation of the inhibitory nerve fibers produces another kind of inhibition, which could not be explained by a postsynaptic mechanism. They made extracellular recordings of excitatory synaptic potentials, much as I previously described in Chapter 8 (see Fig. 8.10A). When the excitatory nerve was stimulated, single excitatory junctional potentials (EJPs) could be recorded, whose amplitude was distributed approximately according to a Poisson distribution (Fig. 10.9B). If, however, the inhibitory nerve was stimulated at the same time as the excitatory nerve, the distribution of EJPs changed dramatically. There were many more failures, and the whole distribution was shifted toward smaller amplitudes.

The change in the distribution of amplitudes is not a result that would be expected for postsynaptic inhibition. Postsynaptic inhibition might change the *amplitude* of the junctional potentials, but the shape of the histogram would not be altered, since the probability of release of quanta would not be affected. The change in the shape of the histogram indicates that inhibition produced a change in *quantal content, m*. As described in Chapter 8, the quantal content can be thought of as the mean number of quanta (or vesicles) released by the excitatory nerve, and it is given by the ratio of the mean EJP amplitude to the mean amplitude of the miniature potentials. In addition, quantal content can be calculated from the number of failures, since $p_0 = e^{-m}$ (see Eqn. 10 of Chapter 8). Using either method, Dudel and Kuffler (1961) showed that inhibition produces a decrease in m. Thus inhibition of this sort reduces the *number* of quanta released by the excitatory axon rather than the amplitude of the quantal response.

Presynaptic inhibition is widespread throughout the central and peripheral nervous system, in invertebrates such as crayfish as well as in vertebrates and mammals. Its mechanism is still unclear. Activation of GABA or glycine receptors on the presynaptic membrane may produce a hyperpolarization, which would increase the threshold for action potential propagation into the presynaptic terminal; or it may produce depolarization, which would lead to inactivation of the Na^+ channels of the presynaptic process and block spike propagation in this way (Jackson and Zhang, 1995). Presynaptic inhibition can also be mediated by metabotropic receptors. Certain metabotropic receptors can produce either an increase in K^+ conductance or a reduction in inward Ca^{2+} current in the presynaptic terminal (see Chapter 12). An increase in K^+ conductance would hyperpolarize and prevent depolarization of the presynaptic terminal, whereas a reduction in Ca^{2+} current would reduce Ca^{2+} influx and decrease the probability of transmitter release directly. Metabotropic receptors and neuromodulation are described in the next section of this book.

Summary

Ligand-gated GABA and glycine channels are the most important sources of inhibition in the central nervous system. These channels are similar in structure to ionotropic ACh receptors, but there is one essential difference. Activation of ACh receptors produces a nonselective increase in permeability to cations, which generally depolarizes the postsynaptic neuron. Activation of GABA and glycine receptors, on the other hand, increases permeability to anions and may hyperpolarize or depolarize the postsynaptic neuron, or produce no change in potential whatever. Regardless of the sign of the potential change, the activation of inhibitory receptors decreases the probability of spike production in the postsynaptic cell and modulates the level of neural activity.

GABA receptors are composed of different subunits from at least 6 subfamilies; in spite of considerable progress, the stoichiometry of individual receptors is still not entirely understood. Glycine receptors are far simpler: so far genes for only 4 subunits have been described in 2 subfamilies, though again the stoichiometry remains uncertain. One of the most interesting aspects of GABA receptors is their complicated pharmacology. They can be blocked by many different competitive and noncompetitive antagonists, but in addition they can be modulated by barbiturates and benzodiazepine agonists and antagonists, as well as by neurosteroids. GABA receptors are the principal targets of general anesthetics in the CNS, and the effects of these drugs provide useful clinical applications and may eventually reveal much of interest about the structure of the receptor proteins. Both GABA and glycine receptors probably gate (open and close) in much the same way as do ACh receptors, though the kinetics of channel gating appear to be more complicated for inhibitory receptors.

The pharmacological effects of barbiturates or of the glycine antagonist strychnine provide ample evidence that inhibitory pathways are crucial in determining the level of activity in the brain. In spite of their importance, we know considerably less about inhibitory receptors and the mechanisms of inhibitory transmission than we do for excitatory receptors and excitation. As our understanding of inhibition improves, we are likely to gain a new appreciation for the way GABA and glycine receptors shape patterns of neural processing.

PART FOUR

Metabotropic Transmission and Neuromodulation

11

Receptors and G Proteins

IN ADDITION TO the ligand-gated receptors described in Part Three, neurons and most other cells in the body express a variety of receptors that are not themselves ion channels. These receptors bind transmitter and then produce some alteration in the response of the cell, often by means of a second messenger. Second messengers can gate ion channels directly or regulate the activity of protein kinases and phosphatases, enzymes that phosphorylate proteins and alter their properties. Virtually every protein that plays a role in neuronal signaling can be modulated by phosphorylation: voltage- and ligand-gated channels, enzymes that synthesize or release second messengers, gap-junctional proteins, and proteins that direct the release of synaptic transmitter. Protein phosphorylation is one of the most common mechanisms for altering neural behavior and undoubtedly plays a large role in synaptic plasticity, learning, and memory (see Chapter 14).

The great majority of receptors that are not ligand-gated channels and that contribute to nerve cell signaling belong to a superfamily of *seven transmembrane-spanning* proteins, which are often called *G-protein-coupled receptors* or *metabotropic receptors*. These receptors all work in a similar way: the binding of transmitter to the receptor produces activation of a G protein, which then alters the activity of an effector molecule. The effector may be an ion channel, or it may be an enzyme that synthesizes or hydrolyzes a second messenger, such as *adenylyl cyclase* (which synthesizes cyclic AMP), *phospholipase C* (which hydrolyzes phosphatidyl inositol to produce inositol trisphosphate and diacylglycerol), *phospholipase A$_2$* (which generates arachidonic acid), or *phosphodiesterase* (which hydrolyzes cyclic AMP and cyclic GMP). Effectors can lead to changes in the concentration of *second messengers,* such as cyclic nucleotides or Ca^{2+}, which can themselves modulate the opening or closing of ion channels. Second messengers may also regulate the activity of protein kinases and phosphatases.

Some of the more important signaling pathways used by metabotropic receptors in the nervous system are schematized in Fig. 11.1. As this figure shows, the receptors, G proteins, and effector molecules are for the most part associated with the plasma membrane, as are some second messengers (diacylglycerol and arachidonic acid); other second messengers are soluble and diffuse throughout the cytoplasm (cyclic nucleotides and Ca^{2+}). In many cases, a single receptor can have more than one effect. For example, the binding of acetylcholine to an m_3 muscarinic receptor (one of the subtypes of metabotropic ACh receptors) causes an activation of the membrane-bound enzyme phospholipase $C\beta$ (PLCβ), which hydrolyzes the plasma-membrane lipid *phosphatidyl inositol 4,5-bisphosphate* (PIP$_2$). Hydrolysis of PIP$_2$ produces two second messengers, diacylglycerol (DAG), which activates *protein kinase C* (PKC); and 1,4,5-inositol trisphosphate (IP$_3$—see Fig. 12.11). IP$_3$ diffuses through the cytoplasm and binds to IP$_3$ receptors on calcisomes or smooth endoplasmic reticulum (labeled *Ca²⁺ store* in Fig. 11.1), releasing Ca^{2+} from these vesicles and increasing the cytosolic Ca^{2+} concentration. Ca^{2+} then in turn acts as a messenger, and the effect of the Ca^{2+} increase can vary from one cell type to another. Among the many possibilities are these: (1) the direct gating of ion channels (Ca^{2+}-dependent K^+ or Cl^- channels); (2) the activation of adenylyl cyclase to increase cAMP, which in turn activates cAMP-dependent protein kinase (or protein kinase A—PKA); (3) stimulation (via the Ca^{2+}-binding protein calmodulin) of another protein kinase, called *calcium-calmodulin kinase II* (CaM KII), and/or of a protein phosphatase called *calcineurin;* and (4) the triggering (also via calmodulin) of nitric oxide (NO) synthesis by the enzyme NO synthase (NOS), which in turn activates soluble guanylyl cyclase and results in an increase in the concentration of cGMP. Increased cGMP may then stimulate cGMP-dependent protein kinase (or protein kinase G—PKG).

Because of the great complexity of metabotropic pathways in cells, it is often difficult to determine which pathways are of greatest significance in individual cases. Furthermore, the many effects of receptor stimulation are further confounded by feedback pathways, including phosphorylation of the receptors and the effector

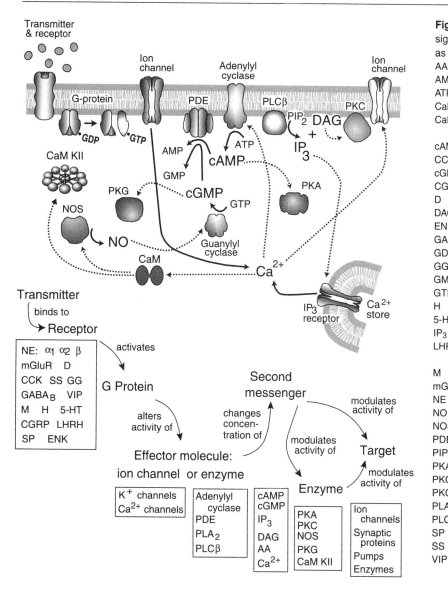

Fig. 11.1 Pathways for G-protein-mediated signal transduction in neurons. Abbreviations as follows:

AA	arachidonic acid
AMP	adenosine monophosphate
ATP	adenosine triphosphate
CaM	calmodulin
CaM KII	Ca^{2+}/calmodulin-dependent protein kinase II
cAMP	adenosine 3′,5′-cyclic monophosphate
CCK	cholecystokinin receptor
cGMP	guanosine 3′,5′-cyclic monophosphate
CGRP	calcitonin gene-related peptide receptor
D	dopamine receptor
DAG	diacylglycerol
ENK	enkephalin receptor
GABA$_B$	GABA$_B$ receptor
GDP	guanosine diphosphate
GG	glucagon receptor
GMP	guanosine monophosphate
GTP	guanosine triphosphate
H	histamine receptor
5-HT	5-hydroxytryptamine (serotonin) receptor
IP$_3$	inositol 1,4,5-trisphosphate
LHRH	luteinizing hormone releasing hormone receptor
M	muscarinic ACh receptor
mGluR	metabotropic glutamate receptor
NE	norepinephrine receptor
NO	nitric oxide
NOS	nitric oxide synthase
PDE	cyclic nucleotide phosphodiesterase
PIP$_2$	phosphatidylinositol 4,5-bisphosphate
PKA	protein kinase A
PKC	protein kinase C
PKG	protein kinase G
PLA$_2$	phospholipase A$_2$
PLCβ	phospholipase Cβ
SP	substance P receptor
SS	somatostatin receptor
VIP	vasoactive intestinal peptide receptor

molecules themselves. Some of these mechanisms are of considerable interest. The kinase CaM KII, for example, can phosphorylate itself, with dramatic effects on its activity (see Chapter 13 and Braun and Schulman, 1995).

This is the first of four chapters that describe the most common pathways of metabotropic transmission in the nervous system and their effects on nerve cell behavior. I shall begin with the receptors themselves and describe a bit of their structure and function, as I did for ionotropic receptors in Chapters 9 and 10. Then I show how these receptors couple to G proteins. In the following two chapters, effector molecules, second messengers, phosphorylation, and the parts they play in metabotropic transmission and neuromodulation are described. Although emphasis will be placed on the role of these processes in the nervous system, many of the mechanisms described in these chapters are quite general and are used (at least in part) by nearly every cell in the body.

The complexity of metabotropic receptor activation is so great that understanding how modulation occurs for particular cell types would seem to be nearly hopeless. Fortunately, this has not proved to be the case, and I shall present several well-studied examples for which the effects of receptor activation seem reasonably well understood. Some metabotropic receptors are present in postsynaptic membrane and function purely and simply as synaptic receptors, much like ligand-gated channels. Other metabotropic receptors generate a more complicated response, with branching pathways of protein phosphorylation, and these responses are more difficult to understand in detail. It is these more complex pathways, however, which may hold the clue to complex behavior (see Chapter 14).

G-Protein-Coupled Receptors

The mammalian genome contains perhaps a thousand or more genes for G-protein-coupled receptors, over 400 of which have been cloned and sequenced (Watson and Arkinstall, 1994; Peroutka, 1994). The proteins in this megafamily all have a common structure consisting of seven transmembrane, probably α-helical domains. For this reason these receptors are sometimes called *heptahelical* receptors. Within this megafamily there are at least three superfamilies of related proteins: the *rhodopsin* family, the *glucagon/secretin* family, and the *Ca/mGluR/GABA$_B$* family. Members of all three of these families are found in the nervous system and together include receptors for many common synaptic transmitters (acetylcholine, GABA, glutamate, adenosine, 5-hydroxytryptamine, epinephrine, dopamine, histamine), Ca^{2+}, neuropeptides (vasoactive intestinal peptide, or VIP, somatostatin, angiotensin, cholecystokinin, tachykinin, opioid peptides), and hormones (luteinizing hormone, follicle-stimulating hormone, thyrotropin, thyrotropin releasing hormone, oxytocin, vasopressin, antidiuretic hormone). Also among these families of proteins are visual pigments for both invertebrate and vertebrate photoreceptors and the receptor proteins of olfactory nerve cells.

All of these proteins are thought to share a similar three-dimensional structure (see Fig. 11.2 and Birnbaumer and Birnbaumer, 1994; Strader et al., 1994; Baldwin, 1994). Each has seven hydrophobic stretches of 20–25 amino acids, which are thought to form the transmembrane α-helices. Structural studies of rhodopsin indicate that the α-helices may be oriented nearly perpendicular or somewhat tilted to the plane of the membrane (see Chapter 16 and Schertler, Villa, and Henderson, 1993; Unger et al., 1997). Most (probably all) receptors are glycosylated, usually at sites near the amino-terminal region of the protein, which is extracellular. There are three extracellular loop domains, and many G-protein-coupled receptors have a disulfide bond between two often-conserved cysteines on the first and second extracellular loops, which may contribute to the stability of the protein. The carboxyl terminus is intracellular and often contains sites for protein phosphorylation. The use of site-directed mutagenesis in many studies has demonstrated that several of the intracellular loop domains contribute to the interaction between the receptors and the G proteins (Strader et al., 1994; Baldwin, 1994).

Adrenergic Receptors

We shall look at two classes of G-protein-coupled receptors as examples. Adrenergic receptors (Fig. 11.2A and C) are members of the rhodopsin superfamily and bind the catecholamines epinephrine and norepinephrine, also called adrenaline and noradrenaline (see Fig. 9.1). There are several different subtypes of adrenergic receptors, each with a distinctive pharmacology (Pepperl and Regan, 1994). The β receptors, for example, are selectively blocked by the drug propranolol and are functionally coupled to adenylyl cyclase to produce an increase in cAMP. In contrast, α_1 receptors are blocked by prazosin and have been shown to produce PIP_2 hydrolysis and Ca^{2+} release; and α_2 receptors are blocked by yohimbine and produce an inhibition of adenylyl cyclase and a decrease in

Fig. 11.2 Structure of G-protein-coupled receptors. **(A)** Hypothesized membrane topology of adrenergic receptor. (After Freedman and Lefkowitz, 1996.) **(B)** Hypothesized membrane topology of metabotropic glutamate receptor. (After Pin and Duvoisin, 1995.) **(C)** Schematic drawing of adrenergic receptor with seven transmembrane domains (labeled *TM1–7*) and hypothesized intramembranous binding site for norepinephrine. **(D)** Schematic drawing of metabotropic glutamate receptor with seven transmembrane domains (labeled *TM1–7*) and hypothesized binding site for glutamate in extracellular amino-terminal domain. (After Pin and Bockaert, 1995.)

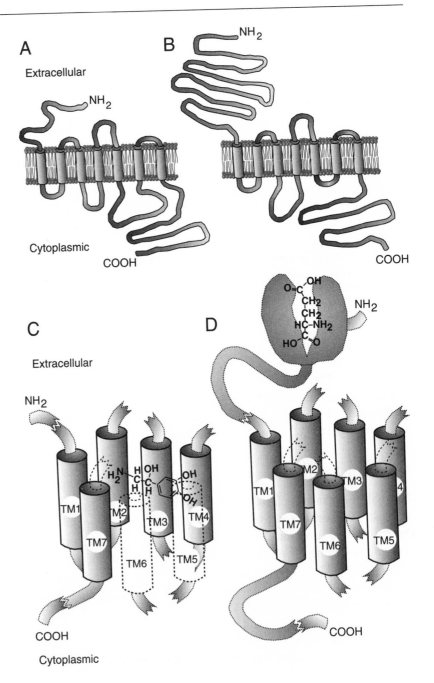

cAMP. Additional functions for several of these receptors have also been suggested, including G-protein-mediated modulation of ion channels.

Adrenergic receptors are representative of a large number of G-protein-coupled receptors that bind relatively small-molecular-weight neurotransmitters, for which the binding site is thought to lie in a pocket formed by the membrane-spanning domains (Kobilka, 1992; Strader et al., 1994). Evidence of the location of the binding site on adrenergic receptors has been obtained primarily by site-directed mutagenesis. All adrenergic receptors, for example, have a negatively charged aspartate in the third transmembrane domain. Norepinephrine has an amino group at one end of its structure (see Fig. 9.1), which is mostly positively charged at neutral pH. Epinephrine is identical in structure to norepinephrine, except that this amine is replaced by a methylamine ($-NHCH_3$), which is also mostly positively charged. The negatively charged aspartate in the third transmembrane domain of the receptor probably serves as a counter-ion for the positively charged nitrogens of the agonists, since substitution of this aspartate with asparagine or serine produces a 10,000-fold decrease in agonist affinity. All muscarinic acetylcholine receptors also have an aspartate in a similar position, which probably serves as a counter-ion for the positively charged amine group of ACh (see Fig. 9.1).

Less dramatic changes in agonist or antagonist affinity can also be produced by substitutions in other transmembrane domains, and residues important for agonist binding probably occur in different places for different receptor types (Baldwin, 1994). The picture that emerges is of rods (formed by the seven α-helices) creating a pocket and providing specific sites of contact; these sites, which are all buried within the membrane-spanning regions of the protein, are somewhat different for different receptors, and this specificity is probably responsible for the receptor's selectivity for agonist binding.

Metabotropic Glutamate Receptors

Metabotropic glutamate receptors (mGluRs) belong to a different subfamily of G-protein-coupled receptors, which also includes GABA$_B$ receptors (Kaupmann et al., 1997) and a Ca^{2+}-sensing receptor isolated from the parathyroid gland (Brown et al., 1993). Glutamate receptors (and $GABA_B$ and Ca^{2+}-sensing receptors) possess a large amino-terminal extracellular loop not present on adrenergic receptors (Fig. 11.2B and D). For the glutamate receptors, these N-terminal peptides are essential for agonist binding. The relative effectiveness of different agonists can be altered, for example, merely by exchanging a portion of the N-terminal region of one glutamate receptor with that of another of different pharmacology (Takahashi et al., 1993). In addition, site-directed mutations within the N-terminal region can alter agonist effectiveness, in a way that suggests that glutamate may bind within a cleft between two globular masses of N-terminal peptides. It has been proposed that these globular masses swing together and close when agonist binds (see Fig. 11.2D), like two halves of a clam shell (O'Hara et al., 1993). This picture of agonist binding is in dramatic contrast to that for the adrenergic receptors, for which the entire amino-terminal region can be removed with little effect on agonist affinity (see Kobilka, 1992).

There are at least eight genes coding for metabotropic glutamate receptors in mammals, and at least some of these can be alternatively spliced to produce different gene products (Nakanishi, 1994; Conn and Patel, 1994; Pin and Duvoisin, 1995; Pin and Bockaert, 1995). Amino acid sequence comparison has been used to classify the receptors into three groups with somewhat different pharmacology. All of the metabotropic glutamate receptors so far studied respond to glutamate but not to the ionotropic glutamate receptor agonists AMPA, NMDA, or kainate (see Fig. 9.11). Group I (mGluR1 and mGluR5) and Group II (mGluR2 and mGluR3) metabotropic glutamate receptors respond to (1S, 3R)-1-aminocyclopentane-1,3-dicarboxylate (ACPD—see Fig. 11.3); Group I receptors are relatively more sensitive than Group II to quisqualate and Group II, relatively more sensitive than Group I to ACPD and to (2S,3S,4S)-α-(carboxycyclopropyl)-glycine (L-CCG-1, see Fig. 11.3). Both Group I and Group II receptors are insensitive to L-2-amino-4-phosphonobutyric acid (L-AP4—see Fig. 11.3), which is an excellent agonist for Group III receptors (mGluRs 4, 6, 7, and 8).

Metabotropic glutamate receptors have been shown to have a

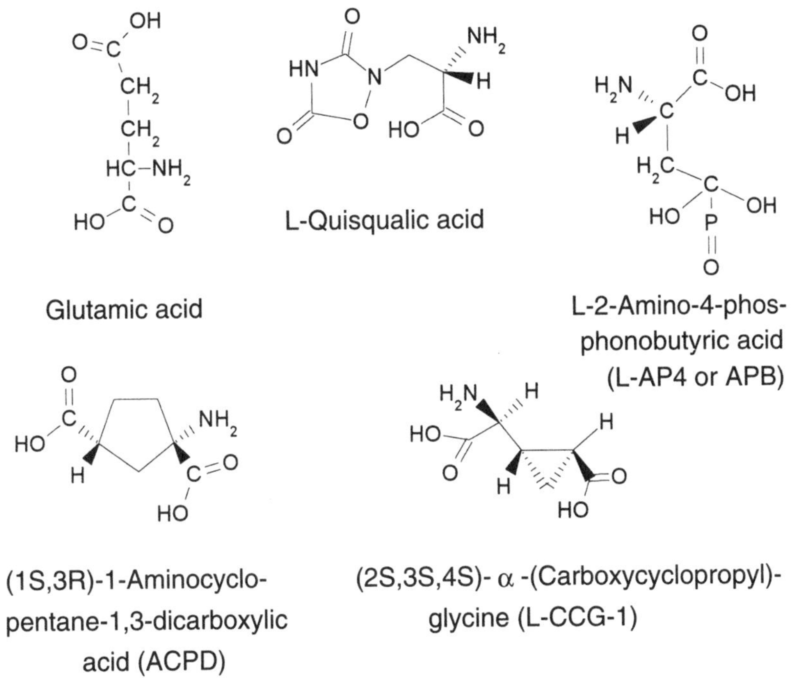

Fig. 11.3 Structures of common agonists for metabotropic glutamate receptors.

Glutamic acid

L-Quisqualic acid

L-2-Amino-4-phosphonobutyric acid (L-AP4 or APB)

(1S,3R)-1-Aminocyclopentane-1,3-dicarboxylic acid (ACPD)

(2S,3S,4S)- α -(Carboxycyclopropyl)-glycine (L-CCG-1)

large number of actions, including direct effects on ion channels, Ca²⁺ release, generation of arachidonic acid, stimulation and inhibition of adenylyl cyclase, and regulation of ligand-gated receptors, perhaps by protein phosphorylation (see Pin and Duvoisin, 1995). In some cases, particularly for mGluR6, the metabotropic receptors are located in the postsynaptic membrane and function as a synaptic transmitter receptor, much like ligand-gated channels. I shall describe the role of mGluR6 in more detail in Chapter 12. Other metabotropic glutamate receptors seem to be localized just to one side of the synapse (Baude et al., 1993; Nusser et al., 1994). This is of particular interest, since metabotropic receptors positioned in this way could use the same transmitter as the ionotropic receptors located in the postsynaptic membrane directly adjacent to release sites (see Fig. 11.4). The function of peripherally placed metabotropic receptors is unknown, but it seems possible that they serve in some way to modulate ionotropic transmission. Metabotropic glutamate receptors have also been proposed to function presynaptically, to modulate release at synaptic terminals (see Sánchez-Prieto et al., 1996).

Activation and Desensitization

The binding of a ligand produces a change in the conformation of the receptor (see Fig. 11.5). Studies on the visual pigment rhodopsin suggest that this change is modest and may be limited to small, "rigid body" motions of the membrane-spanning α-helices (see Chapter 16 and Farahbakhsh, Hideg, and Hubbell, 1993; Farrens et al., 1996). These motions are somehow communicated to the cytosolic loops and carboxyl-terminal peptides of the receptor, where G protein binds. Binding does two things. It increases the

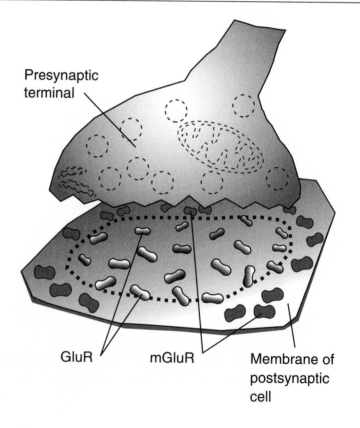

Fig. 11.4 At some synapses in the central nervous system, ligand-gated glutamate receptors are located directly opposite the presynaptic terminal, whereas metabotropic glutamate receptors are placed peripherally, just to the side of the synapse. See for example Baude et al. (1993) and Nusser et al. (1994). Dotted line indicates approximate area of postsynaptic active zone. Receptor densities are much greater than illustrated.

Presynaptic terminal

GluR   mGluR   Membrane of postsynaptic cell

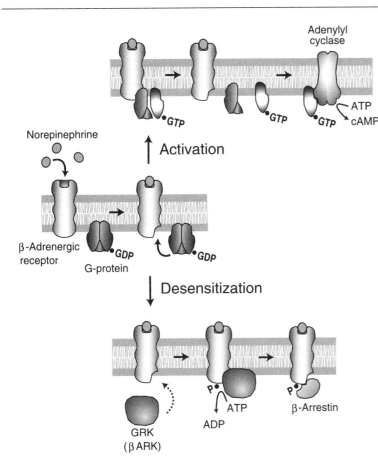

Adenylyl
cyclase

GTP
GTP
GTP
ATP
cAMP

Activation

Norepinephrine

β-Adrenergic
receptor

G-protein

GDP
GDP

Desensitization

P
ATP
ADP

P
β-Arrestin

GRK
(βARK)

Fig. 11.5 Mechanism of activation and desensitization of G-protein-coupled receptors. *GTP*, guanosine triphosphate; *ATP*, adenosine triphosphate; *cAMP*, adenosine 3′,5′-cyclic monophosphate; *GDP*, guanosine diphosphate; *GRK*, G-protein-coupled receptor kinase; *βARK*, β-adrenergic receptor kinase; *P*, phosphate group; *ADP*, adenosine diphosphate. (After Freedman and Lefkowitz, 1996.)

affinity of the receptor for ligand, and it facilitates an exchange of GTP for GDP on the G protein α subunit, activating the G protein. Activated G protein dissociates, and the α subunit and βγ dimer can then diffuse away from the receptor to an effector molecule (for the β-adrenergic receptor in Fig. 11.5, adenylyl cyclase). This leaves the G protein's binding site on the receptor unoccupied, and the receptor may then bind and activate another G protein. Multiple activation of G proteins may be an important source of gain at this first step in signal transduction: for rhodopsin, as many as 500 G proteins can be activated during the lifetime of the activated form of the receptor (Fung and Stryer, 1980).

The activation of G protein ceases either when ligand falls off the receptor or when the receptor desensitizes. Desensitization of G-protein-coupled receptors appears to occur predominantly by phosphorylation (Kobilka, 1992; Premont, Inglese, and Lefkowitz, 1995; Freedman and Lefkowitz, 1996). Kinases called G-protein-coupled receptor kinases (or GRK's) bind specifically to activated receptors and phosphorylate serine and threonine residues on the receptor's carboxyl tail. There are at least 6 members of the GRK gene family but many hundreds of different G-protein receptors, so these kinases are probably rather promiscuous, phosphorylating many different receptor types. The exceptions are rhodopsin kinase (GRK1), which appears to be specific for rod and cone visual pigments (see Chapter 15); and GRK4, which is found mostly in the testis. The other G-protein kinases, including the one that phosphorylates the β-adrenergic receptor (GRK2 or βARK), are widely dispersed throughout the body, including the brain.

G-protein kinases are cytoplasmic proteins that become active when agonist is bound to the receptor, and they then phosphorylate the receptor. Phosphorylation may be sufficient by itself to produce a small degree of desensitization, but substantial desensitization occurs only when a cytoplasmic protein called *arrestin* binds to the phosphorylated receptor (see Fig. 11.5). As for the kinases, several different arrestin genes are expressed by the cells of the body, most with alternatively spliced variants; but there are many fewer types of arrestins than G-protein-coupled receptors. The photoreceptors again have their own arrestins, but other arrestins (including the one for β-adrenergic receptors, called *β-arrestin*) are expressed all throughout the body, including the nervous system, with some differences in expression in different tissues and in different parts of the brain.

The binding of arrestin to phosphorylated receptor sterically hinders the binding of G protein to the receptor, effectively terminating signal transduction. The receptor must then be regenerated by dephosphorylation, but little is known at present about how this occurs. Many receptor types can also be desensitized by phosphorylation by other kinases, such as protein kinase A (see Freedman and Lefkowitz, 1996). They may also be *sequestered*: that is, the receptor may be removed from the plasma membrane and localized within the membranes of intracellular vesicles. The purpose of sequestration is unclear, since desensitization of the receptor can occur even when sequestration is blocked. It is possible that sequestration is a part of the mechanism for dephosphorylating and regenerating the desensitized receptor (see Liggett and Lefkowitz, 1994).

Heterotrimeric G Proteins

Heterotrimeric G proteins are proteins, about 100 kilodaltons in molecular weight, that bind guanosine nucleotides (GDP and GTP). Purified, unactivated proteins consist of three subunits (and so are *trimers*), each with a different composition (and so *hetero*trimers). The subunits are called α (or G_α), β (or G_β), and γ (or G_γ), and the completely assembled protein is called $\alpha\beta\gamma$ or $G_{\alpha\beta\gamma}$.

There are a large number of different α, β, and γ subunits, which in different combinations form a still greater number of differently assembled heterotrimers, and a considerable amount has been learned about the structure and function of these proteins (see Simon, Strathmann, and Gautam, 1991; Conklin and Bourne, 1993; Birnbaumer and Birnbaumer, 1994; Spiegel et al., 1994; Bourne, 1995; Neer, 1995; Hamm and Gilchrist, 1996; Gudermann, Schöneberg, and Schultz, 1997). At latest count there are 23 different α subunits, 5 β's, and 12 γ's (including splice variants). As Fig. 11.5 illustrates, the α subunit can dissociate from β and γ, but β and γ form a functional, noncovalently assembled dimer ($\beta\gamma$) that does not dissociate except after denaturation.

G-protein α Subunits

The α subunits have received more attention than β and γ, since α's appear to be the most diverse and are responsible for the specificity of G-protein/receptor interaction. G-protein α subunits have been divided into four families on the basis of their amino acid identities (see Simon, Strathmann, and Gautam, 1991). These families are delineated in Table 11.1. The α_s family includes α_s itself, a ubiquitous protein that is coupled to adenylyl cyclase and stimulates synthesis of cAMP. Also in this family is α_{olf}, which is found predominantly (though not exclusively) in olfactory receptors, where it too is coupled to adenylyl cyclase; it is an essential component of olfactory transduction (see Chapter 16).

Table 11.1   The Family of G-Protein α Subunits in Mammals

Subfamily	G_α	Typical Receptor	Effectors	Location
α_s	α_s	β-adrenoreceptor	Adenylyl cyclase Ca²⁺ channels	Ubiquitous
	α_{olf}	Odorant receptors	Adenylyl cyclase	Olfactory epithelium
α_i/α_o	$\alpha_{i1}, \alpha_{i2},$ and α_{i3}	Somatostatin receptor	Adenylyl cyclase K⁺ channels	Ubiquitous
	α_o	m2 muscarinic ACh receptor	Ca²⁺ channels	Brain
	α_z	Unknown	Adenylyl cyclase	Brain
	α_{t1}	Rhodopsin	cGMP-PDE	Retinal rods
	α_{t2}	Cone opsins	cGMP-PDE	Retinal cones
	α_{gust}	Taste receptors	Unknown	Taste buds
α_q	α_q, α_{11} α_{14}, α_{15}	m1 muscarinic ACh receptor	PLCβ	Ubiquitous
α_{12}/α_{13}	α_{12}, α_{13}	Unknown	Unknown	Ubiquitous

Modified from Conklin and Bourne (1993) and Birnbaumer and Birnbaumer (1994).

The α_i/α_o family is the most diverse and perhaps most interesting of the α families. The α_i's are ubiquitously distributed throughout the body and are thought again to be coupled to adenylyl cyclase, but instead of stimulating this enzyme, they inhibit it and reduce the synthesis of cAMP. G proteins containing α_i's appear also to be coupled to K⁺ channels (see for example Ito et al., 1992; Schreibmayer et al., 1996). The role of α_o's is still unclear. They are quite abundant in brain tissue, and there is considerable evidence that, at least in some neurons, they are a part of a cascade leading to the inhibition of Ca²⁺ channels (see for example Kleuss et al., 1991; Campbell, Berrow, and Dolphin, 1993). G-protein-mediated increases in K⁺ conductance and decreases in Ca²⁺ conductance seem to be important mechanisms for presynaptic inhibition in the central nervous system, which I shall describe in more detail in Chapter 12.

In addition to α_i and α_o themselves, the α_i/α_o family also contains the α subunits of *transducins,* which are the G proteins of photoreceptors (α_{t1} in rods and α_{t2} in cones). These α subunits are coupled to the enzyme cGMP phosphodiesterase, which hydrolyzes cGMP. The α_i/α_o family also contains α_{gust}, found in certain taste receptors, and α_z, localized primarily within neurons and platelets. Little is known about the function of either of these proteins. Activation of all the members of the α_i/α_o family except α_z can be blocked by pertussis toxin, from the bacterium that causes whooping cough. This toxin catalyzes the transfer of ADP-ribose from NAD^+ to a cysteine residue on the α subunit (see Stryer, 1995), preventing the exchange of GTP for GDP.

The final two α subunit families are α_q and α_{12}/α_{13}. The α_q's are ubiquitous proteins that are coupled to phospholipase Cβ (PLCβ), an enzyme which hydrolyzes PIP_2 to generate IP_3 and diacylglycerol (see Figs. 11.1 and 12.11). The α_{12} and α_{13} proteins are also ubiquitous, but little is known about what they do. A typical cell may have 9–10 different G proteins, some expressed at higher levels than others (see Birnbaumer and Birnbaumer, 1994). The levels of expression of α_s, α_{12}/α_{13}, and α_q are relatively low; in neurons α_o can be quite high, 50–100 times higher than α_s, for example, and as much as 1–2 percent of the total membrane protein.

G-protein β and λ Subunits

The β and γ subunits have been less thoroughly investigated than the α's. For a long time they were thought merely to facilitate the association of the G protein with the receptor but not to contribute much to the rest of the signaling cascade. We now know this is not true. The βγ dimers appear directly to activate many different effector molecules, including ion channels (see Clapham, 1994; Wickman and Clapham, 1995), phospholipase Cβ (see Clapham and Neer, 1993; Sternweis, 1994) and phospholipase A_2 (Jelsema and Axelrod, 1987). Understanding how the β and γ subunits work is now clearly recognized as an essential component of the complete picture of metabotropic signaling.

There are several genes for β and γ subunits, though less is known about their function or distribution than about α's. The different β proteins are rather similar, sharing from 50 to 83 percent identity in amino acid sequence, but the γ subunits are much more diverse, for reasons still poorly understood. There seem to be some rules for specifying which β's can associate with which γ's, and which combinations can modulate the activity of effector molecules. Some of the best evidence for the existence of these rules comes from experiments on GH_3 cells, a cell line derived from the pituitary gland (see Kleuss et al., 1991, 1992, 1993).

GH_3 cells have metabotropic receptors for a variety of transmitters, including acetylcholine and the peptide somatostatin. The application of either the cholinergic agonist carbachol or somatostatin produces a decrease in voltage-gated Ca^{2+} current (see Fig. 11.6), via a G-protein-mediated cascade. Both the carbachol and somatostatin responses can be blocked by pertussis toxin and so are mediated by G proteins from the α_i/α_o family. Other experiments indicate that both responses are produced by G proteins containing α_o, though quite possibly by different splice variants: α_{o1} may produce the cholinergic response and α_{o2} the response to somatostatin (Kleuss et al., 1991).

These different forms of α_o appear to be combined with different forms of β and γ. This was demonstrated by Kleuss and collaborators by injecting the nuclei of GH_3 cells with *antisense DNA* for the different β and γ subunits. Antisense DNA is DNA complementary to mRNA for the particular protein whose function is to be tested. Usually synthesized as an oligomer 20–40 nucleotides long, it is often designed to be complementary to the nucleotide sequence of the protein near the site where translation is initiated. By binding to the mRNA, the antisense DNA can prevent the translation machinery from attaching to the mRNA and so may inhibit the production of protein. Since the sequences of nucleotides of mRNAs even for closely related proteins are often quite different, experimental strategies using antisense DNA (when successful) can be used to block the production of proteins with high specificity.

Figure 11.6 shows that antisense DNA for $\beta 1$ blocks the reduction of the Ca^{2+} current by somatostatin but does not alter the response to carbachol. Since antisense for $\beta 1$ would be expected to stop the synthesis of the $\beta 1$ protein, it would appear that $\beta 1$ is required to produce the somatostatin response. Antisense for $\beta 3$ blocks the response to carbachol but has no effect on that to somatostatin, and antisense for $\beta 2$ and $\beta 4$ have no effect on either

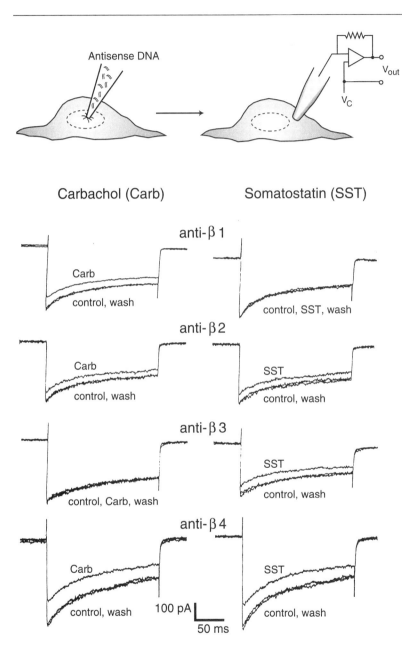

Carbachol (Carb)   Somatostatin (SST)

anti-β 1

Carb

control, wash   control, SST, wash

anti-β 2

Carb   SST

control, wash   control, wash

anti-β 3

                                    SST

control, Carb, wash   control, wash

anti-β 4

Carb   SST

control, wash   100 pA   control, wash
                 50 ms

Fig. 11.6 Specificity of G-protein β subunits for carbachol and somatostatin inhibition of Ca^{2+} currents in rat pituitary (GH_3) cells. Whole-cell patch recordings. Intracellular (pipette) solution contained 120 mM $CsCl_2$ (to block K^+ currents), and the extracellular solution contained 10.8 mM Ba^{2+} as a charge carrier for Ca^{2+} currents. Responses are to voltage pulses from $V_H = -80$ mV to 0 mV. Each panel of figure shows current responses from one cell superimposed for three conditions: control (before drug exposure), in presence of drug (either 10 μM carbachol or 1 μM somatostatin), and wash (after drug exposure). Recordings were made 40 hours after injection with indicated antisense nucleotides. (Records relabeled from Kleuss et al., 1992; used with permission of the authors and of Macmillan Magazines Limited.)

response (Kleuss et al., 1992). Similar experiments with γ's show that γ4 is necessary for the carbachol response and γ3 for the somatostatin response (Kleuss et al., 1993). Thus it would appear that the carbachol response is mediated by $\alpha_{o1}\beta_3\gamma_4$, whereas the somatostatin response is coupled to $\alpha_{o2}\beta_1\gamma_3$. Both G proteins somehow act to reduce Ca^{2+} currents, as I shall describe more fully in the following chapter.

The γ subunits (but not β) are covalently modified by the attachment of lipid to their C-terminus (see Wedegaertner, Wilson, and Bourne, 1995). This lipid appears to be important for the coupling of βγ to α and as a site of interaction with the membrane. Dimers of βγ produced without γ-lipid attachment become localized to the cytosol and do not associate with α subunits to form active heterotrimers. The α subunits can also be lipidated, near the N-terminus, and this association also appears to aid in membrane attachment.

G-protein Activation and Deactivation

The α subunit of the G protein contains a binding site for guanosine nucleotides that, in the inactive form, is occupied by GDP. Inactive α•GDP has a high affinity for βγ, which means that the inactive heterotrimer normally exists as an α•GDP•βγ complex (see Fig. 11.7). When ligand binds to receptor, the conformation of the receptor is subtly altered. The receptor is then able to bind to α•GDP•βγ, and there is some evidence that the C-terminus of α may be an important determinant of the specificity of receptor binding (see for example Conklin et al., 1993). The binding of α•GDP•βγ to the receptor often increases the affinity of the receptor for its ligand and also alters the conformation of the G-protein α subunit, triggering the release of GDP from the nucleotide binding site. The α subunit of the trimer is then free to bind GTP. The binding of GTP produces an α•GTP•βγ complex, which is unstable and rapidly dissociates to α•GTP and βγ. As Fig. 11.7 shows, both α•GTP and βγ can diffuse, for the most part near or within the membrane, and independently bind to effector molecules to alter their behavior.

The α subunits of heterotrimeric G proteins are actually GTPases: that is, they have intrinsic enzymatic activity and catalyze the hydrolysis of GTP to GDP. As soon as GTP binds to G protein

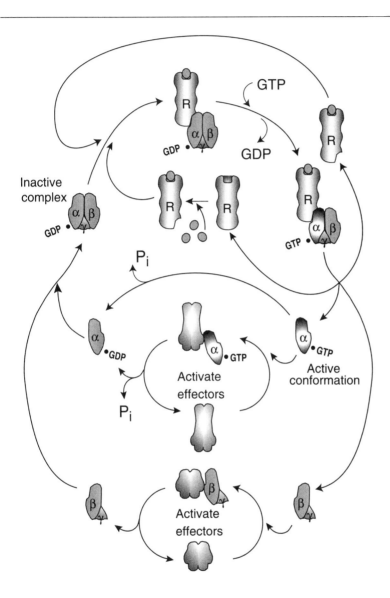

Fig. 11.7 Heterotrimeric G-protein activation. *GDP,* guanosine diphosphate; *R,* receptor; *GTP,* guanosine triphosphate; *P$_i$,* inorganic phosphate.

and $\alpha \cdot$GTP is formed, the α subunit begins hydrolyzing the terminal phosphate of the bound nucleotide to $\alpha \cdot$GDP. Since $\alpha \cdot$GTP can activate effector molecules but $\alpha \cdot$GDP cannot, the lifetime of active G$_\alpha$ is determined by the rate of hydrolysis of GTP. The rate of hydrolysis also determines the lifetime of $\beta\gamma$, since once GTP is hydrolyzed, $\alpha \cdot$GDP recombines with $\beta\gamma$ to form the inactive $\alpha \cdot$GDP$\cdot \beta\gamma$ complex.

For most α subunits the intrinsic rate of hydrolysis of GTP is rather slow, with a half-time of the order of several seconds to a minute, but there is increasing evidence that many if not all cells contain *GTPase-activating proteins,* or *GAPs,* which speed up the rate of GTP hydrolysis. A group of GAPs called *RGS proteins* have been shown to accelerate the rate of GTP hydrolysis at least for some α subunits of trimeric G proteins by 40-fold or more (see for example Berman, Wilkie, and Gilman, 1996; Berman, Kozasa, and Gilman, 1996). There is also evidence that the association of some G proteins with their effector molecules produces an acceleration in the rate of GTP hydrolysis (see for example Biddlecome, Berstein, and Ross, 1996). I shall describe the interactions of G proteins with effectors in the next chapter.

Summary

In addition to ionotropic, ligand-gated channels, nerve cells also contain metabotropic receptors, most of which belong to a large family of proteins containing seven transmembrane-spanning domains. The many different proteins in this family have common structural features but also exhibit interesting differences. For adrenergic and muscarinic ACh receptors, for example, ligand appears to bind within a pocket formed by the membrane-spanning domains. For other receptors, including those binding glutamate and GABA, ligand appears to bind to a large extracellular domain near the amino terminus. The binding of ligand appears to trigger subtle changes in the conformation of the membrane-spanning domains, which are communicated to the cytoplasmic loops and the cytoplasmic carboxyl terminus.

The change in conformation of these cytoplasmically exposed regions of the receptor causes them to bind heterotrimeric G proteins. Heterotrimeric G proteins are composed of three subunits, called α, β, and γ. Each of these subunits is coded by a number of different genes, which can be alternatively spliced, resulting in great variety in trimeric composition. The α subunits can be divided into four families, which appear to interact with different effector molecules, and the β and γ subunits are also quite variable. Certain combinations of α, β, and γ seem to be specified for particular metabotropic responses. The β and γ subunits are tightly bound to one another and function as a single unit, called the βγ dimer.

The binding of G protein to activated receptor catalyzes the exchange of GTP for GDP on a guanosine nucleotide binding site on the α subunit. The α•GTP•βγ complex then dissociates to form α•GTP and βγ, both of which can interact with effectors and modulate their activity. The α subunit has intrinsic GTPase activity and hydrolyzes bound GTP to GDP, in a reaction that may be accelerated by GAPs or RGS proteins. The lifetime of both activated α and βγ is determined by the rate of GTP hydrolysis, since once α•GTP is changed to α•GDP, the α•GDP recombines with β and γ to reconstitute the inactive G-protein trimer.

The receptors and G proteins described here are the major components of metabotropic transmission in the nervous system. Recently, however, other receptor and G-protein types have been receiving increasing attention. Ionotropic glutamate receptors in cortex have been reported to act in some cells as metabotropic receptors, directly stimulating G proteins (Wang et al., 1997). Most cells in the body contain *receptor tyrosine kinases,* membrane proteins that have extracellular binding domains for peptide growth factors or hormones, including insulin, and intracellular catalytic domains that phosphorylate target proteins on specific tyrosine residues. Receptor tyrosine kinases have been implicated in cell proliferation, differentiation, and migration, but they may also play a role in modulating neuronal behavior (Wang and Salter, 1994; Holmes, Fadool, and Levitan, 1996; Jonas et al., 1996; Llinás et al., 1997). Recent experiments suggest that certain tyrosine kinases may even be associated with ionotropic receptors and stimulated by receptor binding (Hayashi et al., 1999). Another receptor type can act as protein tyrosine phosphatases removing tyrosine phosphates (see Streuli, 1996), though a function of these receptors in nerve cell signaling has not yet been described. Finally, there are membrane protein receptors that function as guanylyl cyclases, catalyzing the synthesis of cGMP (see Yuen and Garbers, 1992; Garbers and Lowe, 1994).

The cells of the body contain many different kinds of G proteins in addition to the heterotrimeric G proteins described in this chapter. Especially interesting are the small-molecular-weight G proteins known as *ras,* which are highly expressed in the nervous system and have an essential function in growth and development (Finkbeiner and Greenberg, 1996). As we learn more about neuronal signaling, we may discover that electrical impulse propagation, synaptic transmission, and cell growth and differentiation are intimately linked through the same group of effectors and second messengers. It is these effectors and second messengers that will be described in the next two chapters.

12

Effector Molecules

Aᴄᴛɪᴠᴀᴛᴇᴅ ɢ ᴘʀᴏᴛᴇɪɴ, either as $G_\alpha \cdot GTP$ or as $G_{\beta\gamma}$, dissociates from a liganded receptor and diffuses near or within the membrane to reach target proteins called *effectors*. Several effectors have been discovered, including ion channels and enzymes that synthesize or degrade second messengers. The $\alpha \cdot GTP$ and $\beta\gamma$ molecules are thought to bind directly to the effectors to regulate their activity. For some effectors the evidence for direct binding is now rather strong (see for example Hargrave and Hamm, 1994; Huang et al., 1995; Inanobe et al., 1995; Krapivinsky et al., 1995). In many cases $\alpha \cdot GTP$'s and $\beta\gamma$'s are thought to act independently of one another to trigger a change in effector activity, but in other cases there is evidence that both subunit moieties may bind to the same molecule, each inhibiting the effects of the other (Schreibmayer et al., 1996) or together synergistically stimulating the effector (Tang and Gilman, 1991).

A single G-protein $\alpha \cdot GTP$ or $\beta\gamma$ can influence more than one effector (see Gudermann, Schöneberg, and Schultz, 1997). For example, α_{i1} can inhibit adenylyl cyclase, as well as decrease the probability that K^+ channels will open (Schreibmayer et al., 1996). Whether certain G-protein subunits do one thing rather than another may be determined by their location within the cell. It seems quite likely (though as yet unproved) that receptors are placed in the membrane in close proximity to specific G-protein types and selected effectors and target molecules. There is considerable evidence, for example, that some protein kinases are localized to specific sites within cells by anchoring proteins (Mochly-Rosen, 1995). A large fraction of the protein kinase A (PKA) in the CNS seems to be localized at postsynaptic densities, probably by *A kinase anchoring proteins* (or AKAPs), which anchor PKA, perhaps selectively, near to the proteins it normally phosphorylates (Rosenmund et al., 1994; Cooper, Mons, and Karpen, 1995). The localization of components of signaling cascades to specific parts of the nerve cell may play an important role in determining how particular receptors, G proteins, and effectors function in concert.

In this chapter, I describe the properties of several well-characterized effector molecules and the consequences of effector activation, including the ways second messengers, protein kinases, and kinase target molecules act together to produce alterations in signaling. The literature on metabotropic transmission is vast, and I make no attempt to be exhaustive. I hope instead to give a representative sample of the variety of effects produced by metabotropic signaling cascades.

Adenylyl Cyclase, cAMP, and Protein Kinase A

One of the principal functions of trimeric G proteins containing α_s subunits is the regulation of adenylyl cyclase. The binding of norepinephrine to the β-adrenergic receptor, for example, produces activated $\alpha_s \bullet GTP$, which can bind to any of the many forms of adenylyl cyclase. Adenylyl cyclase catalyzes the reaction

$$ATP \rightarrow cAMP$$

converting ATP to adenosine 3′,5′-cyclic monophosphate, or cAMP, the first second messenger to be discovered (Sutherland, 1972).

G-protein-regulated adenylyl cyclase is a membrane-bound protein composed of two similarly constructed halves, probably arising from gene duplication (see Tang and Gilman, 1992; Birnbaumer and Birnbaumer, 1994; Cooper, Mons, and Karpen, 1995; Sunahara, Dessauer, and Gilman, 1996). Each "half" consists of a series of six membrane-spanning domains, superficially resembling a K^+ channel or a membrane transporter but with no significant sequence homology to these proteins (see Fig. 12.1A). The membrane-spanning domains are then followed by large cytosolic regions, which contain catalytic domains required for cAMP synthesis.

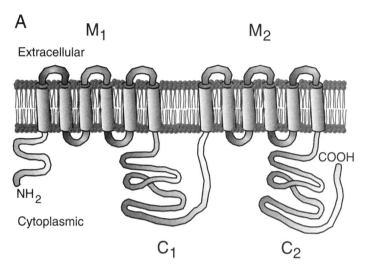

A

M$_1$ M$_2$

Extracellular

COOH

NH$_2$

Cytoplasmic

C$_1$ C$_2$

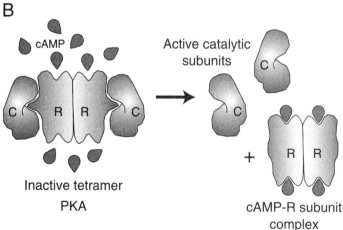

B

cAMP

Active catalytic
subunits

C   C

C   R   R   C   C

+   R   R

Inactive tetramer
PKA

cAMP-R subunit
complex

Fig. 12.1 Adenylyl cyclase and protein kinase A. **(A)** Hypothesized membrane topology of adenylyl cyclase. M_1 and M_2 are two membrane-spanning regions, each containing 6 membrane-spanning domains; C_1 and C_2 are the two catalytic segments of the protein, which together catalyze cAMP synthesis. (After Birnbaumer and Birnbaumer, 1994.) **(B)** Struture and mechanism of activation of protein kinase A (PKA). Inactive tetramer (*left*) is composed of two catalytic subunits (labeled *C*) and two regulatory subunits (labeled *R*). Each regulatory subunit has two binding sites for cAMP, and the binding of cAMP to these sites causes the catalytic subunits to dissociate from the regulatory subunits, leaving the catalytic subunits free to phosphorylate protein.

There are at least ten different genes for G-protein-regulated adenylyl cyclases, each coding for proteins with somewhat different properties (Birnbaumer and Birnbaumer, 1994; Cooper, Mons, and Karpen, 1995; Sunahara, Dessauer, and Gilman, 1996). All adenylyl cyclases can be stimulated by α_s, as well as by the drug forskolin; they differ in almost every other respect. Some can be stimulated or inhibited by Ca^{2+} or Ca^{2+}-calmodulin, some are inhibited by α_i or by other G-protein α subunits, some are regulated by βγ with little apparent specificity for different βγ isoforms, and some can be stimulated by phosphorylation from protein kinase C (I shall have more to say about this protein later in the chapter). The many opportunities for regulation of adenylyl cyclase activity make this family of enzymes an important target for interacting signaling pathways, whose common output is reflected in the rate of synthesis of cAMP.

Cyclic AMP was first discovered as a regulator of carbohydrate metabolism (Robison, Butcher, and Sutherland, 1968, 1971) but is now recognized to be involved in many important cellular functions, including neuronal signaling. It diffuses readily throughout the cytoplasm and can even diffuse between cells through gap junctions. Although in olfactory receptors cAMP can directly gate the opening of ion channels (see Chapter 16), in most neurons the predominant effect of cAMP is to stimulate the phosphorylation of proteins. It does this via activation of cAMP-dependent protein kinase (protein kinase A, or PKA), which then phosphorylates target proteins, including both voltage-gated and ligand-gated ion channels.

Protein kinase A is a tetramer (see Walaas and Greengard, 1991; Francis and Corbin, 1994), consisting of two regulatory and two catalytic subunits (see Fig. 12.1B). In its inactive form, the regulatory and catalytic subunits are bound to one another, and the regulatory subunits inhibit the catalytic subunits. Each regulatory subunit has two binding sites for cAMP, and binding of cAMP causes the catalytic subunits to dissociate from the regulatory subunits, releasing the catalytic subunits as active monomers. There are several different isoforms of both regulatory and catalytic subunits—all with different patterns of expression in different tissues, including brain—but the significance of this diversity is presently unknown.

Phosphorylation of Ion Channels

Since the initial demonstration of cAMP's effect on the action potential waveform in heart cells (Tsien, 1973), many studies have shown that PKA can and does phosphorylate and modulate the activity of channels of physiological interest, including Na^+, K^+, and Ca^{2+} channels, as well as ACh, GABA, and glutamate receptors of the AMPA, kainate, and NMDA classes (see Raymond, Blackstone, and Huganir, 1993; Roche, Tingley, and Huganir, 1994; Levitan, 1994; Browning and Rogers, 1994; Catterall, 1994; Jonas and Kaczmarek, 1996). It does this by catalyzing the transfer of the terminal (γ) phosphate of ATP to specific serines or threonines on target proteins.

I shall give just one example. When RNA for rat brain Na^+ channels is injected into *Xenopus* oocytes and the oocytes are voltage-clamped, a large inward current is produced in response to depolarizing voltage steps. If the oocyte is now penetrated with an injection pipette containing cAMP and the cAMP is introduced into the cell (Gershon et al., 1992), the Na^+ current decreases (Fig. 12.2A). A similar effect occurs when oocytes are injected with the catalytic subunit of protein kinase A (Fig. 12.2B).

A more direct demonstration of the effect of PKA is given in Fig. 12.2C–E (Li et al., 1992). Here rat brain Na^+ channel DNA was expressed at high density in Chinese hamster ovary fibroblasts (a cell line). Inside-out patches from these cells contained large numbers of Na^+ channels, from which an inward current could be recorded in response to a depolarizing voltage step. Direct perfusion of the inside surface of the membrane with the catalytic subunit of PKA together with ATP produced a decrease in the Na^+ current (Fig. 12.2C) but little or no change in the voltage dependence either of activation (Fig. 12.2D) or of steady-state inactivation (Fig. 12.2E). A similar effect was observed with inside-out patches pulled from actual rat brain cells, indicating that brain Na^+ channels *in situ* can also be regulated by cAMP and PKA.

The phosphorylation of brain Na^+ channels by PKA probably occurs at sites within the domain linking repeat units I and II of the α subunit. Some of the evidence for this conclusion is given in Fig. 12.3. In these experiments (Smith and Goldin, 1996), chimeras were made between RIIA Na^+ channels from rat brain (which show PKA modulation) and skeletal muscle SkM1 channels (which do not—see Fig. 12.3A). Brain RIIA α subunits have five putative sites for PKA phosphorylation distributed throughout the I–II linker (Fig. 12.3A, arrow), but these sites are not present in the skeletal muscle protein. To prepare the chimeras, the I–II linkers were exchanged between the brain and muscle proteins. Samples of RNA for the normal brain and muscle channels as well as for the chimeric proteins were injected in separate experiments into

Fig. 12.2 Protein kinase A reduces voltage-gated Na^+ current. *Top:* Xenopus oocytes were injected with cRNA for the α subunit of a voltage-gated Na^+ channel from rat brain, and currents were recorded with a two-electrode voltage clamp in response to voltage steps from -100 mV to $+10$ mV. Responses were recorded before and after injection of 10 pmol of cAMP **(A),** or 0.2 to 0.3 units of purified PKA catalytic subunit **(B).** Injections were performed by applying pressure to a microneedle inserted into the oocyte. (From Gershon et al., 1992, reprinted with permission of the authors and of the Society for Neuroscience.) *Bottom:* Inside-out recordings made from plasma membrane excised from Chinese hamster ovary fibroblasts (a cell line), transfected with DNA for rat brain IIA Na^+ channels. **(C)** Currents in response to test pulses from $V_H = -110$ mV to -20 mV, before and 2 min after exposure of the cytoplasmic surface of the patch to 2 µM of the catalytic subunit of PKA plus 1 mM ATP. **(D)** Comparison of current-voltage curve for peak amplitude of Na^+ currents to test pulses from $V_H = -110$ mV, before and after exposure to catalytic subunit of PKA and ATP. **(E)** Normalized steady-state inactivation of Na^+ currents (h_∞) measured as in Fig. 5.15A. Inactivation was produced by a 250 ms prepulse to the potential plotted on the abscissa. Inactivation was then measured with a subsequent voltage pulse to -20 mV, and the current with prepulse was normalized to the current without and plotted on the ordinate (as in Fig. 5.15B and 5.17B). (Reprinted with minor modification from Li et al., 1992, with permission of the authors and of Cell Press.)

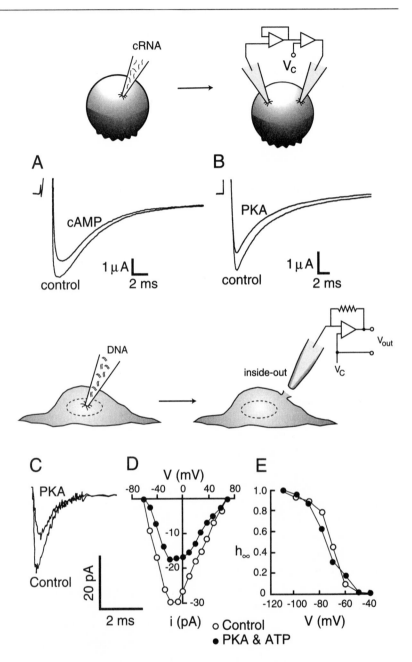

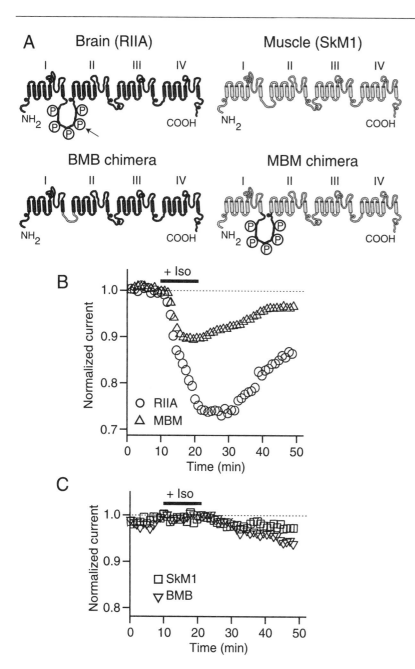

Fig. 12.3 The presence of the I–II linker is required for PKA-dependent modulation of rat brain Na$^+$ channels. **(A)** Formation of chimeras. The P's surrounded by circles indicate putative phosphorylation sites *(arrow)*. **(B)** and **(C)** Na$^+$ currents recorded from *Xenopus* oocytes after expression of RNA for the proteins in **(A)**, together with RNA for the β-adrenergic receptor. Currents were recorded with a two-electrode voltage clamp in response to voltage pulses from $V_H = -100$ mV to -10 mV, and peak current amplitudes for each cell were normalized to the response recorded from that cell for the first voltage pulse in the series (at $t = 0$). Bars indicate period of 10 min application of 4 μM isoproterenol. (Modified from Smith and Goldin, 1996.)

Xenopus oocytes, along with RNA for the β-adrenergic receptor. Since the β-adrenergic receptor is normally coupled to adenylyl cyclase, the β-adrenergic agonist isoproterenol could be used to test for PKA modulation of the Na^+ current.

There was a large decrease in peak current for the Na^+ channels from the rat brain when the oocyte was exposed to isoproterenol. This occurred because activation of expressed β-adrenergic receptors produced $\alpha_s \cdot GTP$ from G_s endogenous to the oocyte. The $\alpha_s \cdot GTP$ then activated adenylyl cyclase, which increased the cAMP concentration, and cAMP stimulated PKA to phosphorylate the Na^+ channels. A somewhat smaller decrease was also seen for the current of chimeric muscle Na^+ channels containing the brain I–II linker (Fig. 12.3B, *MBM*). No effect of isoproterenol was seen for either the skeletal muscle channel or the brain chimera containing the muscle I–II linker (Fig. 12.3C, *BMB*). These results indicate that the I–II linker is necessary for PKA-dependent modulation of the Na^+ channel current.

Phosphorylation does not appear to affect the single-channel conductance of the Na^+ channel (Li et al., 1992), and so it probably does not interfere with ion permeation. Since the voltage dependence of activation is unaltered (Fig. 12.2D), it seems unlikely that phosphorylation produces a change in the movement of the gating charges. One possible explanation for the effect of phosphorylation is that the negative charge of the phosphate in some way interferes with the transitions in conformation that occur during gating, so that the movement of gating charge is less likely to result in channel opening. The exact location of the negative charge within the structure of the channel is probably critical for producing this effect, since phosphorylation of *cardiac* Na^+ channels by PKA produces an *increase* in Na^+ current rather than a decrease (Schreibmayer et al., 1994).

Protein Phosphatases

In the experiments just described, the diffusion of cAMP to binding sites on the regulatory subunits of protein kinase A causes the release of active catalytic subunits, which appear directly to phosphorylate the Na^+ channels. One implication of this mechanism is that the effect of a single application of isoproterenol would remain indefinitely unless some process existed for subsequently removing these phosphates. The removal of phosphates from proteins is performed by enzymes called *protein phosphatases,* which are probably just as important in the modulation of nerve cell activity as are the kinases; but our understanding of the role of phosphatases is at present rather primitive. It has been estimated that the mammalian genome may contain a large number of genes for protein phosphatases (Hunter, 1995), but only a small number of phosphatase genes have so far been discovered (see for example Walaas and Greengard, 1991; Wera and Hemmings, 1995; Villafranca, Kissinger, and Parge, 1996).

There are several indications that phosphatases may be sites of neuromodulation. Phosphatases that are likely to be directly regulated by second-messenger pathways include protein phosphatase 2B, or *calcineurin.* This enzyme has the interesting property that it is activated by an increase in intracellular Ca^{2+}, either by entry through Ca^{2+} channels or by the release of Ca^{2+} from internal stores (Chapter 13). Another phosphatase, *protein phosphatase 1,* is inhibited by a regulatory protein called *dopamine and cAMP-regulated phosphoprotein* (DARPP-32). The activity of DARPP-32 is in turn controlled by phosphorylation, presumably as a result of receptor activation (Walaas and Greengard, 1991). DARPP-32 is expressed in regions of the brain (or other parts of the body) where dopamine receptors are present. Exactly what this protein does is still not clear, but it is reasonable to suppose that it serves some regulatory role in dopamine transmission.

Na^+ channels and other proteins seem to be present in cells at some basal level of phosphorylation determined by the activity of kinases like PKA, which are constantly adding phosphates, and phosphatases, which are constantly removing them (Hunter, 1995). The extent of phosphorylation could then be modulated upward by kinase activation or downward by stimulation of a phosphatase. Some evidence that phosphatases are involved in neuromodulation has been obtained, for example for NMDA receptors, by observing the effects on channel activity of exogenously applied phosphatases or of phosphatase inhibitors like okadaic acid or calyculin A (Wang et al., 1994; Lieberman and Mody, 1994). One possible role of phosphatases in regulating neural activity will be described in Chapter 14.

Phosphodiesterase and cGMP

Certain G-protein α subunits of the α_i/α_o subclass, and in particular the transducins of rod and cone photoreceptors, are known to be coupled to an enzyme called *cGMP phosphodiesterase* (or PDE), which catalyzes the hydrolysis of cyclic GMP to GMP:

$$cGMP \rightarrow GMP$$

In photoreceptors, the PDE exists as an inactive tetramer, much like protein kinase A. There are two catalytic subunits (called α and β), which are each bound to identical regulatory subunits (called γ). The direct binding of the activated G_α of the photoreceptor G-protein *transducin* to PDE γ subunits relieves the inhibition of γ on either the α or β PDE catalytic subunits (or both), activating PDE (see Chapter 16 and Fig. 16.4A).

PDE activation leads to increased hydrolysis of cGMP and a decrease in cGMP concentration. Although we have only a limited notion of what cGMP does in neurons, we do know that it can bind to and regulate specific cGMP-gated ion channels (Finn, Grunwald, and Yau, 1996; Zagotta and Siegelbaum, 1996), and it can activate cGMP-dependent protein kinase (PKG). PKG is less widely distributed than PKA, but different isoforms of PKG are present throughout the body, including in the CNS, as soluble or membrane-bound proteins (Francis and Corbin, 1994). Very little is known about the function of cGMP-dependent phosphorylation, and few target proteins have been identified. I shall return to cGMP and PKG in the next chapter, when I describe the role of nitric oxide (NO) and carbon monoxide (CO) as second messengers.

mGluR6 and ON Bipolar Cells

One of the most interesting examples of PDE as an effector in metabotropic signaling is found in the transduction cascade for the mGluR6 receptor, which is located in the postsynaptic membranes of *ON bipolar cells* in the retina and probably nowhere else in the nervous system. Bipolar cells are retinal interneurons that receive synaptic input predominantly from photoreceptors and that synapse in turn onto amacrine and ganglion cells. There are two classes of bipolar cells: the ON cells, which depolarize when the photoreceptors respond to a light stimulus, and the OFF cells, which hyperpolarize. These two cells together enable the visual system to respond to both light increments and light decrements.

The evidence is rather strong that photoreceptors use glutamate as their transmitter (see for example Copenhagen and Jahr, 1989). There is, however, one peculiar feature of this glutamate release. As I shall describe in Chapter 16, photoreceptors are depolarized in darkness by a resting conductance to cations. Light reduces this conductance, and the photoreceptor membrane potential *hyperpolarizes*. As a result, glutamate is released from photoreceptors continuously in darkness, and light *reduces* the release of glutamate. If, therefore, light depolarizes ON bipolar cells, glutamate must hyperpolarize these cells; and if light hyperpolarizes OFF bipolar cells, glutamate must depolarize them (see Dowling, 1987).

This may become clearer when we examine in detail the effects of transmitters on the bipolar cells. In the experiments of Fig. 12.4, (from de la Villa, Kurahashi, and Kaneko, 1995), a cat ON bipolar cell was exposed to glutamate and the mGluR6 agonist L-AP4 (see Fig. 11.3). In the absence of glutamate (marked *control*), there is a large resting conductance, which has its reversal potential near zero. This conductance is produced by channels nonselectively permeable to cations (Na$^+$, K$^+$—see Nawy and Copenhagen, 1987; Shiells and Falk, 1990; Nawy and Jahr, 1991). The effect of glutamate or L-AP4 is to decrease this conductance by closing these channels, as summarized in the inset to the figure. Glutamate, which is released by the photoreceptor in darkness, closes channels whose reversal potential is near zero. In light, the glutamate release is decreased, these channels open, and the cell depolarizes.

For the OFF bipolar cells (Fig. 12.4B), glutamate has just the opposite effect: it increases membrane conductance, again to channels nonselectively permeable to cations. Notice, however, that these channels are not activated by L-AP4. The reason for this is that the postsynaptic receptors of OFF bipolar cells are not mGluR6 receptors but rather ionotropic glutamate receptors, probably of the kainate type (DeVries and Schwartz, 1999). Glutamate, which is released by the photoreceptor in darkness, opens these channels, and the bipolar cell's membrane potential is kept at a depolarized value. In light, the glutamate release is decreased, these channels close, and the cell hyperpolarizes.

Fig. 12.4 Whole-cell recordings made with patch electrodes from dissociated cat retinal bipolar cells. Pipette solution contained mostly (120 mM) $CsCl_2$ and included also 1 mM cGMP and GTP. Extracellular solution was mostly (135 mM) NaCl. Current-voltage curves were recorded under voltage clamp with voltage ramps (from −40 mV to +40 mV) as command voltages. **(A)** Recording from ON bipolar cell, identified by positive immunoreactivity to an antibody against PKC (see Negishi, Kato, and Teranishi, 1988). **(B)** Recording from OFF bipolar cell, which did not react to PKC antibody. Transduction mechanisms for channel activation in the two cell types are illustrated at right. (Data redrawn from de la Villa, Kurahashi, and Kaneko, 1995.)

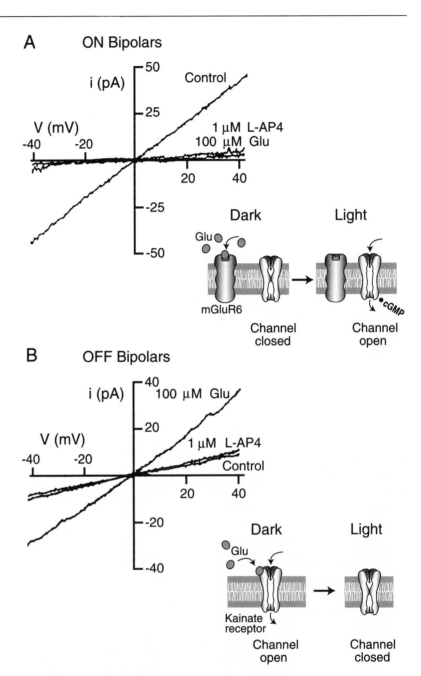

The ON bipolar cells are, at present, the only example we have of a cell for which a metabotropic receptor is present at the synapse as the primary receptor in the postsynaptic membrane. Antibodies specific to mGluR6 have been used to localize these receptors to the postsynaptic membranes of ON bipolar cells (Nomura et al., 1994), and transgenic mice lacking mGluR6 receptors exhibit a specific disruption of ON bipolar cell responses and no other known deficit (Masu et al., 1995). There seems now little doubt that mGluR6 receptors, and only these receptors, mediate transmission from the photoreceptors to the ON bipolar cells. This is at present the only example we have of a metabotropic receptor serving as the principal postsynaptic receptor at a synapse.

Signal Cascade of ON Bipolar Cells

When a patch-clamp whole-cell recording is made from an ON bipolar cell, either in a retinal slice or from a dissociated cell, there is initially a small, resting inward current which often disappears with time ("washes out"). This current can be maintained or even increased if the whole-cell pipette contains exogenous cGMP or GTP (Nawy and Jahr, 1990, 1991; Shiells and Falk, 1990). The ON bipolar cell in Fig. 12.5A, for example, was internally dialyzed with a patch-pipette solution containing 1 mM cGMP. A resting inward current developed and grew with increasing time, but it could be suppressed by application of 1 μM L-AP4 (bars). If, however, the bipolar cell was dialyzed with cGMP as well as the PDE inhibitor dipyridamole, an inward current developed as the cGMP opened channels in the bipolar cell membrane, but this current could not be suppressed with L-AP4. A likely explanation for these results is that cGMP is gating a channel in the bipolar cell, probably a cGMP-gated channel similar though apparently not identical to that of photoreceptors. Activation of glutamate receptors then stimulates a PDE, which hydrolyzes cGMP and transiently lowers the intracellular cGMP concentration, closing the channels (see Fig. 12.6A). This response to glutamate can be eliminated by blocking the PDE.

The mGluR6 receptors at the ON bipolar cell synapse are coupled to PDE activation via a G protein. One way to show this is to internally dialyze bipolar cells with the compound guanosine-5′-O-

Fig. 12.5 Whole-cell recordings made with patch pipettes from bipolar cells in thin slices of salamander retina. At bars above traces, 1 μM of the mGluR6 agonist L-AP4 was microperfused onto the bipolar cell from a multibarrel pipette assembly, positioned near the bipolar cell. Recordings were made from light-adapted slices, superfused with 1 mM Co^{2+} to block synaptic transmission. $V_H = -70$ mV. **(A)** Whole-cell recording pipette contained 1 mM cGMP. Gradual increase in current produced by opening of channels by cGMP is blocked by application of L-AP4. **(B)** Recording pipette contained 1 mM cGMP plus 200 μM of the PDE inhibitor dipyridamole. Effect of L-AP4 is abolished. (Reprinted from Nawy and Jahr, 1991, with permission of the authors and of Cell Press.)

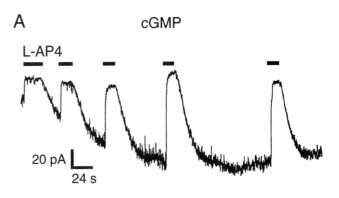

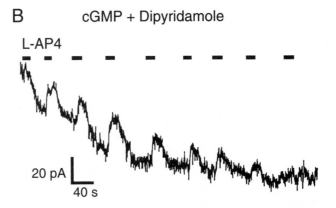

(3-thiotriphosphate), or GTPγS. GTPγS is identical in structure to GTP except for the presence of one sulphur atom replacing an oxygen bonded to the terminal (γ) phosphate. GTPγS has been shown in many experiments to bind to G proteins in exchange for GDP and to activate them almost irreversibly, since the rate of hydrolysis of GTPγS is much slower than that of GTP as a result of the presence of the sulphur atom. Since α•GTPγS is only very slowly converted to α•GDP, effector activation by G proteins is quite prolonged. When an ON bipolar cell is dialyzed with GTPγS, stimulation of the cell with glutamate or L-AP4 produces a nearly irreversible decrease in the cGMP-gated conductance (Shiells and Falk, 1990; Nawy and Jahr, 1991).

Rate of Activation of Cascade

The mGluR6-containing synapse between photoreceptors and ON bipolar cells is crucially important for the proper functioning of the visual system. If this synapse is blocked (by injecting L-AP4 into the vitreous in the middle of the eye), there are marked effects on visual behavior (Schiller, Sandell, and Maunsell, 1986). Why is a metabotropic receptor used at this synapse rather than an ionotropic receptor? The explanation may reside in the higher gain that metabotropic transmission provides. As explained in the previous chapter, one activated receptor can produce the activation of many G proteins, which in turn can cause a large change in the concentration of a second messenger like cGMP. One disadvantage of metabotropic transmission, however, would be a slower rate of activation than for ionotropic transmission (Hille, 1992), particularly in situations (like the one of the ON bipolar cell) where a diffusible intracellular messenger seems to be a necessary part of the transduction pathway.

The notion that transmission at the ON bipolar cell synapse should be much slower than at a synapse using ionotropic receptors was tested by Shiells and Falk (1994), in a clever way. These investigators first recorded from bipolar cells in functioning slices of retina, since they could then use the polarity of the light response of the cell to distinguish ON cells from OFF cells. After recording the polarity of the light response, the patch pipette was pulled away from the slice, and on some occasions the cell from which they were recording remained attached to the pipette and could be pulled entirely out of the retina. Fast solution-change methods (as in Fig. 10.6A) were then used to make "solution jumps"—that is, to place the whole of the bipolar cell into a glutamate-containing solution as fast as possible.

The results of these experiments are shown in Fig. 12.6B and C, on the left from an ON bipolar cell and on the right from an OFF cell. In both series of experiments, the bipolar cells were first jumped into a solution with an altered K^+ concentration. The point of doing this was to measure the rate of the solution change, since a change in the K^+ concentration should change the membrane potential of the cell very rapidly. The cell was then exposed to glu-

Fig. 12.6 Comparison of speed of activation for mGluR6 receptors at ON bipolar cells, and for ionotropic glutamate receptors at OFF bipolar cells. Recordings were made initially from intact cells in slices of dogfish retina, and cells were identified from their light responses as ON or OFF. The patch pipette was then carefully pulled away from the slice, in some cases yielding cells with dendrites isolated from the retina. These cells were then rapidly stepped across the interface between two solutions emerging from the end of theta tubing (as in Fig. 10.6A). **(A)** Postulated scheme for signal transduction at postsynaptic membrane for two bipolar cell types. Below is a comparison of averaged responses to steps from 160 μM glutamate into Ringer with responses to steps into altered K^+ for **(B)**, ON bipolar and **(C)** OFF bipolar cells. Duration of solution step was 1–3 ms, estimated from the time course of change of junction currents with an open patch pipette. Upper traces show solution step from 3 mM K^+ to 23 mM K^+ (in B), or from 23 mM K^+ to 3 mM K^+ (in C); middle traces show steps from 160 μM glutamate into Ringer solution. In the lower traces, the two responses have been superimposed after normalization to the same peak amplitude. (Traces relabeled from Shiells and Falk, 1994, reprinted with permission of the authors and of Cambridge University Press.)

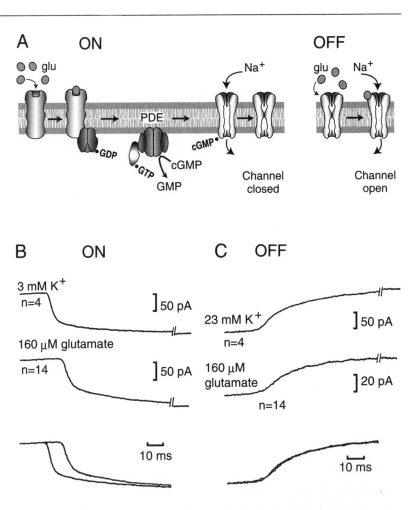

tamate, and the responses were compared (the lowermost trace superimposes the responses to glutamate and K^+). For the OFF bipolar cell, these traces are indistinguishable, indicating that glutamate opens OFF cell glutamate receptors as fast as the solution can be changed. This is not unexpected, since non-NMDA glutamate channel opening is normally quite rapid and would not be distinguishable from the rate of solution change unless the solution change were made very rapidly to a small area of membrane, such as a membrane patch (as in Fig. 10.7). For the ON bipolar cell, on the other hand, the response to glutamate is significantly slower;

there is an additional delay of about 10 ms. The surprise here is not that metabotropic transmission is slower than ionotropic, but rather how small the difference is. Clearly the rate of activation of mGluR6 at the bipolar cell is sufficiently rapid to mediate signal transmission at this important synapse, and it will be interesting to see whether metabotropic receptors also serve as the primary postsynaptic receptors at other synapses in the CNS.

Membrane-Delimited Modulation of Ion Channels

Activated G-protein α and $\beta\gamma$ subunits appear to be able to bind directly to ion channels to alter their probability of opening. Thus ion channels can be thought of as effector molecules, which catalyze the passage of ions through the plasma membrane. Although G proteins may modulate many different channel types (Brown et al., 1988; Clapham, 1994; Wickman and Clapham, 1995), the best evidence is for the modulation of certain inwardly rectifying K^+ channels and of Ca^{2+} channels.

G-protein Modulation of K+ Channels

The very first demonstration that a chemical released by a nerve can alter the behavior of another cell was Otto Loewi's discovery that acetylcholine, released by the vagus nerve, causes a slowing of the rate of the heart beat (Loewi, 1921). ACh binds to muscarinic cholinergic receptors to produce an increase in an inwardly rectifying K^+ conductance, which causes membrane hyperpolarization and a decrease in both the frequency and duration of cardiac action potentials.

The way acetylcholine regulates the K^+ conductance is unlike anything I have so far described. A first indication of the mechanism emerged from experiments by Soejima and Noma (1984) on single atrial cells isolated from the rabbit heart. They made on-cell patch recordings and tested the effects of ACh in two ways. In the first, the more traditional approach, they added the ACh to the bathing solution. In the second, they perfused the external membrane of the on-cell patch with ACh by replacing the solution *inside of the patch pipette*. They did this by inserting a fine polyethylene tube into the patch pipette, one end of which was heated and pulled to a diameter of 70 μm. This was fine enough so that the end of the tubing could be placed relatively near the pipette tip. The other end of the tubing was inserted into one of several reservoirs filled with test solutions. Gentle suction was applied not to the tube but rather to the back of the patch pipette. This had the effect of pulling solution from one of the reservoirs down into the tubing and into the region near the pipette tip (see Fig. 12.7A).

In the absence of ACh, occasional openings were observed in on-cell patches of a 45–50 pS, inwardly rectifying K^+ channel (Fig. 12.7B). When ACh was added to the bath, there was little or no change in channel activity; but when ACh was perfused into the patch pipette, there was a large increase in opening frequency. This can be seen even more clearly in Fig. 12.7C, which shows the effect of introducing ACh into the patch pipette on a slower time base.

The results in Fig. 12.7 are just those expected if ACh were activating an ionotropic (nicotinic) receptor. ACh would be expected to activate receptors in an on-cell patch only if it were applied directly to the membrane containing the channels. Considerable pharmacological evidence, however, indicates that the cholinergic receptors of atrial cells are *not* ionotropic but rather metabotropic. Additional evidence is given in Fig. 12.8 (from Kurachi, Nakajima, and Sugimoto, 1986). In recordings from on-cell patches again from atrial cells with ACh in the pipette, frequent K^+ channel openings can be observed, but these disappear when the patch is pulled away from the cell to form an inside-out patch (Fig. 12.8A). This experiment alone would seem to suggest that the receptors may not be ionotropic, since nicotinic ACh channels are generally quite stable in isolated membrane patches.

Stronger evidence comes from the demonstration that addition of GTP to the medium bathing the inside surface of the membrane causes the channels to reappear (Fig. 12.8A, at right). This effect of GTP is reversible (see Fig. 12.8C, at left) but becomes irreversible if the poorly hydrolyzable analogue GTPγS is used instead of GTP. If in the presence of GTP or GTPγS, pertussis toxin (which blocks G proteins of the α_i/α_o family—see Chapter 11) is added together with NAD^+, the channel activity slowly disappears (Fig. 12.8B). Finally, channel activity can be restored even in the absence of GTP and even in the presence of pertussis toxin if the inside surface of the patch is perfused with G-protein βγ subunits (Fig. 12.8C).

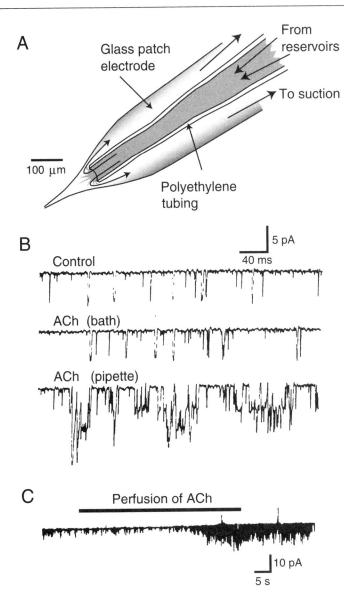

A

Glass patch
electrode

From
reservoirs

To suction

100 μm

Polyethylene
tubing

B

5 pA

40 ms

Control

ACh (bath)

ACh (pipette)

C

Perfusion of ACh

10 pA

5 s

Fig. 12.7 Membrane-delimited gating of cardiac K^+ channels by ACh. **(A)** Method for perfusing inside of patch pipette. A piece of 1 mm polyethylene tubing was heated with a tungsten wire and pulled to a tip diameter of 70 μm. The tube was then inserted into the pipette with its tip as close as possible to the pipette tip. The other end of the tube was connected to open reservoirs filled with test solutions, and solution was pulled into the pipette from these reservoirs by applying suction at the back of the patch pipette, as illustrated. **(B)** Single-channel on-cell recordings from atrial cells dissociated from the rabbit heart. Holding potential was set by applying a potential of +20 mV to the pipette. Since the resting potential of the cell was not affected by this procedure (the patch of membrane clamped by the pipette was a small fraction of the total membrane area), an increased positivity applied to the pipette had the result of increasing the potential drop across the membrane patch and therefore *hyperpolarized* the patch by 20 mV negative of V_{rest}. Channels were recorded at this potential in absence of ACh (*Control*), with ACh in the bath, and with ACh in the pipette (0.1 μM). **(C)** Response to application of 0.1 μM ACh to pipette, recorded on slower time scale. In **(B)** and **(C)**, inward currents are shown as downward deflections. Two upward deflections in **(C)** are perfusion drip artifacts. (Traces relabeled and figure redrawn from Soejima and Noma, 1984.)

Fig. 12.8 Activation of cardiac K^+ channels by ACh requires GTP or $G_{\beta\gamma}$ and is blocked by pertussis toxin. Single-channel recordings were made with patch electrodes from atrial cells dissociated from the guinea pig heart. **(A)** Beginning of recording shows inward single-channel openings on slow time scale in cell-attatched (on-cell) recording with 1.1 μM ACh in the recording pipette. At arrow, the patch was pulled away from the cell to form an inside-out patch, and channel activity gradually disappeared. The cytoplasmic surface of the patch was then perfused with 100 μM GTP, and channel activity reappeared. **(B)** Same patch as in **(A)**. Pipette contained 1.1 μM ACh, and bathing solution perfusing cytosolic side of inside-out patch contained 100 μM GTP. At bar, pertussis toxin and NAD^+ were added at the indicated concentrations, and channel activity was slowly blocked. (For **(A)** and **(B)**, traces relabeled and figures redrawn from Kurachi, Nakajima, and Sugimoto, 1986.) **(C)** Inside-out patch recording, with 0.3 μM ACh in pipette. At beginning of recording, bathing solution facing cytosolic side of patch contained 100 μM GTP. Removal of GTP caused dramatic decrease in channel activity. Activity was then restored by adding 10 nM of $G_{\beta\gamma}$ purified from bovine brain. (Traces relabeled and figures redrawn from Ito et al., 1992.)

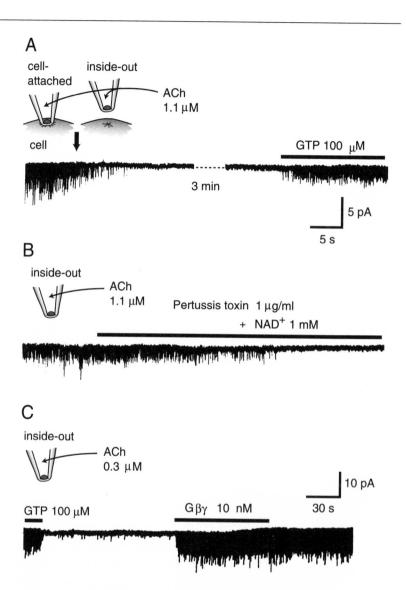

These experiments provide strong evidence that the opening of K^+ channels is somehow mediated by a G protein, which would be unlikely if the receptor were ionotropic but obligatory if it were G-protein regulated.

Since during on-cell recording ACh produces channel activation only when it is applied to the inside of the patch pipette, the ACh is unlikely to be acting via a diffusable second messenger such as cAMP or cGMP. Suppose for example that ACh were acting by way of α_s to produce an increase in the activity of an adenylyl cyclase. The adenylyl cyclase would synthesize cAMP, which would spread within the cytoplasm, and it should then make no difference whether ACh was added to the bath or to the solution within the patch pipette. The effect of the ACh seems to be localized to a very small region less than or equal to the diameter of a patch pipette (about 1 μm), close to the K^+ channels within the on-cell patch from which recordings are made. For this reason, the mechanism of channel activation is often referred to as *membrane-delimited* (Brown et al., 1988). The metabotropic receptor activates a G protein, and the G protein is then somehow coupled to K^+ channels, all within the restricted space of the patch of membrane directly beneath the orifice of the pipette.

Although membrane-delimited channel activation was a topic of considerable controversy for many years, there is now excellent evidence, at least for the cholinergic response of atrial cells, that the K^+ channels are directly activated by G-protein βγ subunits (see for example Logothetis et al., 1987; Ito et al., 1992; Wickman et al., 1994; Reuveny et al., 1994; Kofuji, Davidson, and Lester, 1995). Our understanding of the mechanism was greatly advanced by the cloning (from the heart of the rat) of the first of the inwardly rectifying K^+ channels modulated by G proteins, called GIRK1 or Kir3.1 (Kubo et al., 1993; Dascal et al., 1993). This was soon followed by the isolation of several other members of this family (see Doupnik, Davidson, and Lester, 1995; Jan and Jan, 1997), which together with GIRK1 are widely expressed throughout the brain (see for example Karschin et al., 1996; Navarro et al., 1996; Liao, Jan, and Jan, 1996). These channels show considerable homology to other inward rectifiers, with a structure consisting of cytosolic amino and carboxyl termini and two membrane-spanning domains (see Chapter 7 and Fig. 7.12). The expression of these channels made possible not only the demonstration that purified βγ subunits activate the channels but also that the βγ subunits physically bind directly to the channels (Huang et al., 1995; Inanobe et al., 1995; Krapivinsky et al., 1995), probably at regions near the amino and carboxyl termini (Slesinger et al., 1995).

Direct G-protein modulation of inwardly rectifying K^+ channels

Fig. 12.9 Membrane-delimited receptor activation in the CNS. **(A)** Intracellular recordings of membrane potential of locus ceruleus neurons in slices of rat brain. Bars indicate application of [Met[5]]enkephalin (an opioid receptor agonist) at the indicated concentrations, which produced a dose-dependent hyperpolarization. (Reprinted from North and Williams, 1985, with permission of the authors and of the Physiological Society.) **(B)** Single K^+ channels recorded from neurons of the locus ceruleus. Recordings were made on-cell with agonists included in the pipette solutions at the indicated concentrations: *Enk-ol,* Tyr-D-Ala-Gly-MePhe-Gly-ol; *SST,* somatostatin; *UK 14304,* an α_2-adrenoreceptor agonist. (Reprinted from Miyake, Christie, and North, 1989, with permission of the authors.)

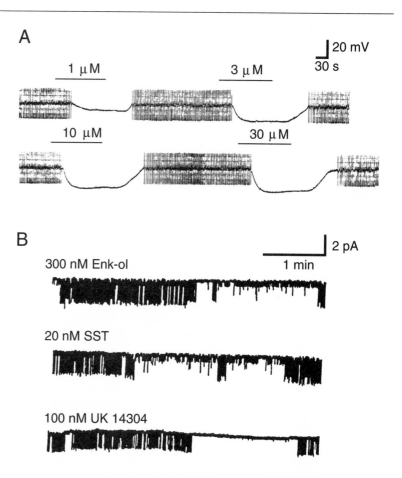

is thought to occur widely throughout the brain for a variety of different transmitter substances, including acetylcholine, GABA, adenosine, glutamate, dopamine, 5-hydroxytryptamine, and the opioid peptides (see North, 1989). The responses in Fig. 12.9 are typical (North and Williams, 1985; Miyake, Christie, and North, 1989). When [Met[5]]enkephalin or Enk-ol, an agonist for μ opioid receptors, is perfused across a brain slice, neurons from the locus ceruleus in the hindbrain are hyperpolarized (Fig. 12.9A). This hyperpolarization is caused by an increase in an inwardly rectifying K^+ conductance, produced by the opening of 45–50 pS channels (Fig. 12.9B). These same channels appear to be also activated in these cells by somatostatin and by the α_2 adrenergic receptor agonist UK 14304.

The mechanism of K$^+$ channel activation in the brain seems to be quite similar to that in the heart. Activation has been shown in some cases to be blocked by pertussis toxin and to become irreversible in the presence of GTPγS. For the neurons of the locus ceruleus, the probability of channel opening is increased in on-cell patches only when the agonist is placed inside the pipette, and not when the agonist is placed in the bath. Thus activation is membrane delimited, just as for atrial cells, and is probably also produced by direct modulation of the channels by G proteins.

K$^+$ channels modulated by G proteins are found postsynaptically (Ponce et al., 1996), although it is not yet known whether they are coupled to postsynaptic receptors directly opposite release sites or to receptors which, like some metabotropic glutamate receptors (see Chapter 11), are located at the periphery of the synapse and somehow modulate the principal pathway of transmission. It is of considerable interest that these K$^+$ channels seem also to be located presynaptically (Ponce et al., 1996). Since many of the transmitters that activate inwardly rectifying K$^+$ channels have been shown to function in presynaptic inhibition (see Dunwiddie and Lovinger, 1993), it is quite possible that membrane-delimited activation of a K$^+$ conductance may hyperpolarize presynaptic terminals and serve as an important mechanism for regulating synaptic transmitter release.

G-protein Modulation of Ca^{2+} Channels

Another important mechanism of presynaptic regulation is the modulation of Ca^{2+} channels. If activation of a metabotropic receptor were to produce an increase in the probability of opening of Ca^{2+} channels, synaptic transmitter release would be enhanced; a decrease in the probability of opening could, on the other hand, cause presynaptic inhibition (see for example Takahashi et al., 1996).

There is now considerable evidence for Ca^{2+} channel regulation by a metabotropic pathway, and in at least some cases the mechanism appears to be membrane-delimited (see Hille, 1994; Dolphin,

1995). One particularly interesting form of Ca^{2+} channel regulation has been called *voltage-sensitive modulation*, since it is nearly abolished by large depolarizations. Voltage-sensitive modulation has been demonstrated for a variety of different Ca^{2+} channel types, including proteins expressed from the genes α_{1A} (P/Q) and α_{1B} (N—see for example Bourinet et al., 1996), both of which are known to be present at presynaptic terminals and to trigger the release of neurotransmitter.

Fig. 12.10A illustrates voltage-sensitive modulation of Ca^{2+} currents in bullfrog dorsal root ganglion cells (Bean, 1989). Most of the Ca^{2+} current in these cells can be blocked by ω-conotoxin and seems therefore to be N-type (α_{1B}). Administration of norepinephrine or a number of other transmitters (5-HT, GABA) produces a prominent decrease in the amplitude of the Ca^{2+} current, which is largest near −10 mV, the voltage at which the Ca^{2+} current is maximal, but it is much smaller and nearly absent at depolarizing voltages (+110 mV—see current-voltage curve to right in Fig. 12.10A).

Some of the characteristics of this sort of inhibition are illustrated in Fig. 12.10B for rat sympathetic neurons (Ikeda, 1996), for which the Ca^{2+} current is also primarily N-type. The inhibition is accompanied by a characteristic slow phase of activation of the Ca^{2+} current, which seems to occur because voltage-sensitive modulation produces an alteration in Ca^{2+} channel gating. Exposure to an agonist like norepinephrine causes the channels to move from a mode in which they are "willing" to open to a mode in which they are "reluctant" (Bean, 1989—see also Delcour and Tsien, 1993; Patil et al., 1996), but the equilibrium between "reluctant" and "willing" seems to be voltage-dependent, with depolarization favoring the "willing" mode. This is probably the reason for the slow increase in channel current in the left panel of Fig. 12.10B: the norepinephrine moves the channels into a "reluctant" mode, but the depolarization used to evoke the current then produces a slow conversion of some of the channels from "reluctant" to "willing," and as more channels occupy the "willing" mode, the channel current slowly increases. The voltage dependence of channel gating is apparently also the reason for the difference in channel modulation at −10 mV and +110 mV in Fig. 12.10A. At +110 mV, most of the channels occupy the "willing" mode even in the presence of agonist.

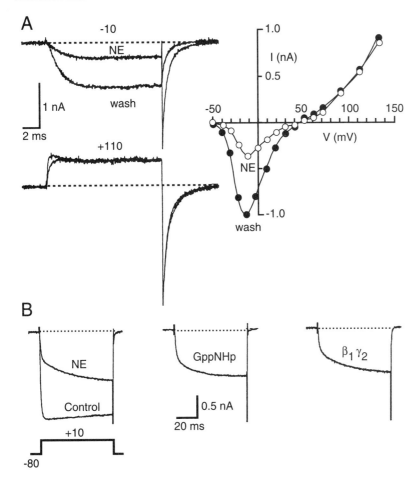

Fig. 12.10 Voltage-dependent modulation of Ca^{2+} channels by G-protein $\beta\gamma$. **(A)** Voltage-dependent inhibition of Ca^{2+} currents by norepinephrine. Traces show whole-cell patch recordings from freshly dissociated dorsal root ganglion (DRG) neurons from the frog. Responses are superimposed to voltage steps in medium containing 30 μM norepinephrine (*NE*) and in control medium 1–2 min after exposure to drug (*wash*), for two voltage protocols: *above*, from $V_H = -60$ mV to -10 mV; *below*, $V_H = -60$ mV to $+110$ mV. Current-voltage curve to right plots steady-state current as a function of voltage in medium containing 30 μM norepinephrine (*NE*) and in control medium 1–2 min after drug exposure (*wash*). Note that inhibition is voltage-dependent and virtually disappears at large positive voltages. (Reprinted from Bean, 1989, with permission of the author and of Macmillan Magazines, Ltd.) **(B)** Ca^{2+} channel modulation by G proteins. Whole-cell patch recordings from rat sympathetic neurons, dissociated from the superior cervical ganglion. *Left:* Ca^{2+} currents recorded in normal medium (*Control*) and in 10 μM norepinephrine (*NE*). Note the slow increase in current amplitude in the presence of norepinephrine, due to voltage-dependent shift of Ca^{2+} channels from "reluctant" to "willing." See text. *Middle:* Recording pipette contained 500 μM 5'-guanylyl-imidodiphosphate (GppNHp). *Right:* Neurons previously transfected by injection into cell nucleus with plasmids containing DNA for bovine G protein β_1 and γ_2. (Reprinted from Ikeda, 1996, with permission of the author and of Macmillan Magazines Limited.)

Voltage-sensitive modulation is produced by G-protein activation. As the middle panel in Fig. 12.10B illustrates, intracellular dialysis of a rat sympathetic neuron with 5'guanylyl-imidodiphosphate (GppNHp), a poorly hydrolyzable GTP analogue like GTPγS, produces a voltage-sensitive inhibition of the Ca^{2+} current even in the absence of transmitter. GppNHp, like GTPγS, produces an irreversible activation of G proteins, and this is apparently sufficient to produce a maintained Ca^{2+} current inhibition. Inhibition has been shown in many systems to be blocked by pertussis toxin and to be mediated by receptors linked primarily to G_o (see for example Kleuss et al., 1991 and Fig. 11.6).

This particular form of Ca^{2+} channel inhibition seems not to be produced by a diffusable second messenger but rather by a membrane-delimited system, probably by G proteins interacting directly with the Ca^{2+} channels (see Hille, 1994; Dolphin, 1995). There is evidence that inhibition can be produced by G-protein $\beta\gamma$ (see for example Fig. 12.10B, right panel) but not G_α (Ikeda, 1996; Herlitze et al., 1996). This suggests that $\beta\gamma$ may mediate at least some forms of voltage-sensitive modulation, just as it does for inwardly rectifying K^+ channels. Furthermore, $\beta\gamma$ has been shown to bind directly to Ca^{2+} channel α subunits. At least one binding site seems to occur on the domain I–II linker (Zamponi et al., 1997; Waard et al., 1997; Herlitze et al., 1997), but the C-terminus of the α subunit appears to contain an additional site of interaction (Qin et al., 1997).

Phospholipases and Protein Kinase C

Phospholipases are enzymes that hydrolyze membrane phospholipids (see Stryer, 1995). At least two families of phospholipases appear to act as effectors after activation by G proteins: phospholipase A_2 and phospholipase C. Phospholipase A_2 (PLA_2) occurs in several different forms, but the one most commonly studied binds to the plasma membrane and generates the lipophilic second messenger *arachidonic acid*. Arachidonic acid is commonly found as one of the long-chained fatty acids esterified to the phospholipid headgroup of a variety of phospholipids, including phosphatidyl choline, phosphatidyl ethanolamine, and phosphatidyl inositol (see Fig. 12.11). PLA_2 can be activated by increases in intracellular Ca^{2+}, and it has been reported also to be stimulated by G-protein $\beta\gamma$ (Jelsema and Axelrod, 1987); it then hydrolyzes the bond between the arachidonic acid and the rest of the lipid (dotted arrow, Fig. 12.11; see Exton, 1994a; Nishizuka, 1995).

Arachidonic acid is highly hydrophobic and would be expected to diffuse in the membrane, where it may modulate the activity of ion channels and other proteins (see for example Kim and Clapham, 1989). In addition, arachidonic acid is an important intermediate in lipid metabolism and is readily converted to biologically active compounds called *eicosanoids*. These have been shown to have many different effects on cells in a multiplicity of tissues (see Piomelli, 1993), but little is known about their physiological importance in neuronal signaling.

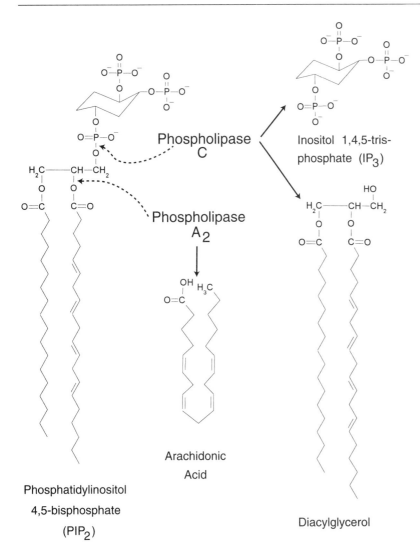

Fig. 12.11 Phospholipases as effectors: structures and mechanism of generation of the second messengers IP₃, diacylglycerol, and arachidonic acid.

Phospholipase C

Inositol 1,4,5-tris-phosphate (IP₃)

Phospholipase A₂

Arachidonic Acid

Phosphatidylinositol 4,5-bisphosphate (PIP₂)

Diacylglycerol

Considerably more is known about the functional importance of another lipase effector, phosphoinositide-specific phospholipase C (PLC—see Meldrum, Parker, and Carozzi, 1991; Rhee and Choi, 1992; Birnbaumer and Birnbaumer, 1994; Exton, 1994b, 1996; Divecha and Irvine, 1995). Phosphoinositides are a relatively minor component (<10 percent) of membrane lipids, which contain as a part of their head group an inositol ring that can be multiply phosphorylated. The phosphoinositide thought to be of greatest importance in metabotropic transmission is triply phosphorylated and is called phosphatidylinositol 4,5-bisphosphate, or PIP_2 (see Figure 12.11). Phosphoinositide-specific PLC hydrolyzes the phosphate bond connecting the inositol ring to the lipid head group, releasing two important second messengers, inositol 1,4,5-trisphosphate (IP_3) and diacylglycerol (DAG).

There are several different types of phosphoinositide-specific PLCs (Birnbaumer and Birnbaumer, 1994; Exton, 1994b, 1996), but only one family, the β family, can be activated by G proteins and is known to be involved in metabotropic signal cascades. There are at least four varieties of PLCβ proteins, each of which has different specificities for G-protein subunits and is probably linked to different receptor types. Some of the PLCβ isoforms can be activated by G-protein α subunits, particularly of the α_q class (α_q, α_{11}, α_{14}, α_{15}). G proteins in this class are insensitive to pertussis toxin and probably mediate the most common form of PLCβ activation. However, some PLCβs can be activated by pertussis-toxin-sensitive G proteins (G_i and G_o), and there is increasing evidence that much of this activation may be due to G-protein $\beta\gamma$ subunits rather than to α_i or α_o.

Of the two second messengers produced by PLC activation, IP_3 is soluble and diffuses from the membrane through the cytosol to specific receptors in the smooth endoplasmic reticulum. There, the binding of IP_3 causes an ion channel within the IP_3 receptor to open, releasing Ca^{2+} into the cytoplasm (see Fig. 11.1). I shall describe IP_3-gated Ca^{2+} release in considerable detail in the following chapter. Diacylglycerol, the other second messenger produced by PLCβ, is highly lipophilic and remains in the membrane. Its most important known function is to activate a protein called *C kinase*, which is here referred to by the name *protein kinase C*.

Protein Kinase C

Protein kinase C *(PKC)*, like PKA, transfers the terminal phosphate of ATP to specific serines or threonines on target proteins and is present in high concentrations in the central nervous system. There are a large number of different forms of PKC, which seem not to differ greatly in their specificity for different substrate proteins but *do* differ in their mode of activation and location in the cell (see

Tanaka and Nishizuka, 1994; Nishizuka, 1995). Most forms of PKC are strongly stimulated by diacylglycerol, but some show in addition a dependence upon other lipids and on Ca^{2+}. It is of considerable interest that different forms of PKC are found in different parts of the brain, and that more than one type may be found in the same cell but differentially localized, for example to the cell body or to the dendrites.

Many studies have shown that PKC phosphorylates and modulates the activity of channels of physiological interest, including Na^+, K^+, and Ca^{2+} channels, as well as ACh, GABA, and glutamate receptors (see Raymond, Blackstone, and Huganir, 1993; Roche, Tingley, and Huganir, 1994; Levitan, 1994; Browning and Rogers, 1994; Catterall, 1994; Jonas and Kaczmarek, 1996). PKC activation has also been found to augment synaptic transmitter release (see Tanaka and Nishizuka, 1994). One way to study the effects of protein phosphorylation by PKC is to treat isolated cells or tissues with diacylglycerol analogues (for example 1,2-oleoylacetylglycerol, or OAG) or with compounds called *phorbol esters,* highly lipophilic molecules that bind to the DAG-binding site and activate the enzyme. Two phorbol esters in particular, phorbol 12-myristate-13-acetate (PMA) and phorbol 12,13-dibutyrate (PDBu), enhance transmitter release from nerve terminals in many parts of the brain. An important control in such experiments is to show that the effect of the phorbol esters can be blocked with PKC inhibitors, since phorbol esters may also have direct effects on ion channels independent of PKC activation (see for example Hockberger et al., 1989). The most commonly used inhibitor is the antibiotic *staurosporine,* but a more specific inhibitor is *PKC 19–36,* constructed from amino acids 19–36 of some isoforms of the PKC protein. This sequence is apparently a regulatory sequence that binds specifically to the active site of PKC and prevents protein phosphorylation (House and Kemp, 1987).

PKC Modulation of Ca^{2+} Currents

The enhancement of transmitter release mediated by PKC is thought to be caused at least in part by modulation of presynaptic Ca^{2+} currents. Fig. 12.12A, from Swartz, Merritt, Bean, and Lovinger (1993), shows the effect of the phorbol ester PMA on the

Fig. 12.12 PKC modulation of Ca^{2+} currents. **(A)** The phorbol ester phorbol-12-myristate-13-acetate (*PMA*) was perfused onto a pyramidal neuron dissociated from the CA3 region of rat hippocampus. Currents through Ca^{2+} channels were measured with a whole-cell patch clamp in an external medium containing 25 mM $BaCl_2$, by stepping from $V_H = -80$ to -10 mV and then back to -60 mV. Sample recordings before (*control*) and 2 min after application of 500 nM PMA are shown in inset. Graph plots peak amplitude of inward current carried by Ba^{2+} as a function of time. Duration of PMA exposure indicated by bar. **(B)** Recordings as in **(A)**. Effect of 200 μM of the metabotropic glutamate agonist (1S,3R)-1-aminocyclopentane-1,3-dicarboxylic acid (ACPD) before (*control*) and 1 min after application of PMA (*post-PMA*). (From Swartz et al., 1993, reprinted with the permission of the authors and of Macmillan Magazines Limited.) **(C)** Formation of chimera between gene for α_{1A}, which is not modulated by PKC, and gene for α_{1B}, which is. The complete I–II linker from α_{1B} was inserted into α_{1A}, and the proteins for these genes were expressed in *Xenopus* oocytes together with that for the β_{1b} auxiliary subunit. **(D)** Comparison of effect of PMA on currents recorded from oocytes after expression of α_{1A}, α_{1B}, and the chimera $\alpha_{1A/B}$, each together with β_{1b}. Data are shown as means ± S.E.s, as a percentage of current amplitudes before PMA exposure, for the number of experiments shown above each bar. (Redrawn from Stea, Soong, and Snutch, 1995 and used with the permission of the authors and of Cell Press.)

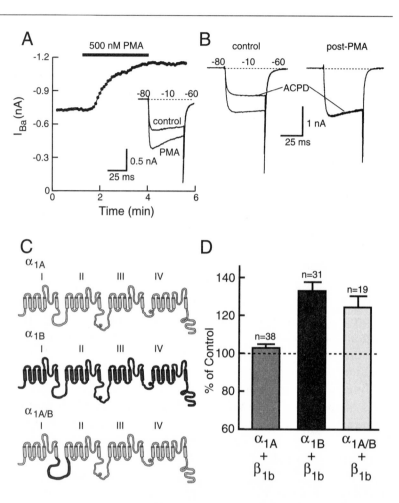

Ca^{2+} current of a dissociated pyramidal cell from the rat hippocampus. The current has been labeled I_{Ba} in this figure because the external medium contained 25 mM $BaCl_2$ and no $CaCl_2$. Recall that, for most voltage-gated Ca^{2+} channels, Ba^{2+} permeates more readily than Ca^{2+}, which means that currents in Ba^{2+} are larger (see Chapter 7). This makes the effect of the phorbol ester on the Ca^{2+} channels easier to detect.

PMA produced a sizable increase in the current, which can be blocked when the inhibitor PKC 19–36 is included in the pipette solution. The effect of PKC activation is opposite in sign to the voltage-sensitive modulation previously described, which *decreases* the amplitude of the Ca^{2+} current (see Fig. 12.10). The voltage-sensitive and PKC-mediated pathways seem to interact in some way, as can be seen in Fig. 12.12B. In this experiment, the metabotropic glutamate agonist ACPD was first perfused onto the pyramidal cell. Other experiments had previously shown that ACPD produces a voltage-sensitive decrease in the Ca^{2+} current (Swartz and Bean, 1992), and a decrease in current is observed in the left panel of Fig. 12.12B (labeled *control*). Notice, however, that if ACPD is added 1 min after treatment with PMA, no effect of the glutamate agonist can be detected (Fig. 12.12B, right panel, labeled *Post-PMA*).

The mechanism of PKC modulation is still unclear, but there are indications that PKC may directly phosphorylate the Ca^{2+} channels and increase their probability of opening (Yang and Tsien, 1993; Zamponi et al., 1997; but see also Swartz, 1993). When Ca^{2+} channels are expressed in oocytes, the phorbol ester PMA augments the currents of channel types α_{1B} and α_{1E} (Stea, Soong, and Snutch, 1995). Since there are PKC phosphorylation sites on the domain I–II linker of these channels, in the same general region as the PKA sites of Na^+ channels described earlier in the chapter (see Fig. 12.3A), this linker may be exchanged between channels that show PKC modulation and those that don't. For example (see Fig. 12.12C), the I–II linker of α_{1B} (which shows the modulation) can be moved to α_{1A} (which doesn't), much as in the experiment for PKA modulation of Na^+ channels (Fig. 12.3). In this hybrid channel the effect of PKC activation is nearly as large as it is for α_{1B} (Fig. 12.12D). Although this experiment doesn't show that the Ca^{2+} channel is itself directly phosphorylated by the PKC, other results indicate that direct phosphorylation probably does occur (Zamponi et al., 1997).

PKC modulation of Ca^{2+} currents is a subject of considerable interest, since it may provide a general mechanism for the enhancement of synaptic transmission. There is still much we don't understand about this phenomenon, but many of the tools needed to study it are now available. The modulation of synaptic transmission by metabotropic transmitters is an important mechanism for the regulation of integration in the brain and will continue to be an active area of investigation.

Summary

When metabotropic receptors bind agonist, they initiate a signaling cascade by stimulating guanosine nucleotide exchange on the G_α subunit, releasing $\alpha \bullet GTP$ and G-protein $\beta\gamma$. There is considerable evidence that different receptors bind to different G proteins, so that, for example, activated β-adrenergic receptor binds G_s and generates $\alpha_s \bullet GTP$, which stimulates adenylyl cyclase; whereas the m_1 muscarinic ACh receptor stimulates G_q and/or G_{11}, which activates PLC. This specificity is not absolute: muscarinic m_3 receptors, for example, may interact with G_o but also with G_i. This seems to have the consequence, at least in some cells, that m_3 receptors can both inhibit Ca^{2+} currents (through G_o) and activate inwardly rectifying K^+ currents (through G_i), both of which could act presynaptically to reduce transmitter release. We are just beginning to understand the multiplicity of metabotropic pathways that act together to alter cell signaling (see Gudermann, Schöneberg, and Schultz, 1997).

Many of the effectors described in this chapter act by altering the concentration of second messengers: adenylyl cyclase synthesizes cAMP, cGMP phosphodiesterase hydrolyzes cGMP, phosphoinositide-specific PLC liberates both IP_3 and DAG. Alternatively, signal transduction may occur via a membrane-delimited cascade, for which a G-protein subunit seems to bind directly to an ion channel to change its probability of opening. There is now strong evidence that G-protein subunits bind directly to certain inwardly rectifying K^+ channels and may also directly regulate presynaptic Ca^{2+} channels. In the next chapter, I describe some additional second messengers (Ca^{2+} and NO), which have also been shown to participate in metabotropic signaling. Yet another second messenger, ceramide, has received increasing attention in the regulation of cell growth, differentiation, and cell death (see Liscovitch and Cantley, 1994; Divecha and Irvine, 1995; Hannun, 1994, 1996), but we still know too little to know if it plays a significant role in neural function.

Metabotropic transmission is often called *neuromodulation*. Since many metabotropic receptors produce second messengers that ultimately activate protein kinases and produce protein phosphorylation, it used to be thought that the only role of metabotropic receptors was to produce a modification of the basic pathways of synaptic transmission, which in turn were mediated exclusively by ionotropic mechanisms. It should now be clear that this is an oversimplification. Metabotropic and ionotropic transmission often use the same transmitters, released presynaptically in the same way. Both can produce changes in membrane potential by altering the probability of opening of ion channels. It is difficult to see why one of these mechanisms should be graced with the name "neurotransmission" and the other labeled "neuromodulation." Furthermore, at least for ON bipolar cells in the retina, a metabotropic receptor *is* the postsynaptic receptor at the synapse, and so far as we know the *only* postsynaptic receptor. Although it is sometimes supposed that ON bipolar cells are an exception, we really do not know how often metabotropic transmission functions purely and simply as *synaptic* transmission.

We used to think of metabotropic receptors as mediating long-term changes in neural activity, and they *do* do this. Neuromodulation is likely to be of considerable importance, for example in learning and memory (see Chapter 14). It is, however, now clear that neuromodulation produced by long-acting modulation of protein function is only one of the functions mediated by metabotropic receptors. Many studies now suggest that a large part of G-protein-mediated transmission in the nervous system uses quite short-acting mechanisms of presynaptic excitation or inhibition.

In this chapter I have emphasized the effects of metabotropic activation on ion channel activity, since these often have been best characterized. It is possible and even likely that many of the most interesting actions of second messengers are those that act on other aspects of cell behavior, for example on the proteins involved in vesicle exocytosis (see for example Trudeau, Emery, and Haydon, 1996). Effects of this kind are receiving increasing attention, since they have the potential to have very wide-spread influence on brain function (see Chapter 14).

13

Calcium and Nitric Oxide

CALCIUM IS ONE of the most important second messengers in the nervous system (Berridge, 1993; Clapham, 1995). It enters through voltage-gated Ca^{2+} channels and regulates the release of synaptic transmitter (see Chapter 8). It can also be released from intracellular stores through IP_3-gated channels in the membrane of endoplasmic reticulum (or calcisomes—see Chapter 4). Ca^{2+} can alter the activity of many proteins in nerve cells, often by binding first to small-molecular-weight proteins such as *calmodulin* (see Fig. 11.1). The Ca^{2+}/calmodulin complex then activates other proteins, including Ca^{2+}/calmodulin-dependent protein kinase (CaM kinase) II, which is present at high concentration throughout the central nervous system. This protein by itself accounts for 1–2 percent of the total protein of the hippocampus and is particularly enriched in synaptic terminals. Like PKA and PKC, it is a serine/threonine kinase that specifically phosphorylates membrane channels and synaptic proteins such as synaptophysin and synaptotagmin. CaM kinase may be an important modulator of synaptic transmission and, as such, make an essential contribution to learning and memory.

Ca^{2+} can also stimulate the enzyme nitric oxide synthase (NOS) which synthesizes nitric oxide (see Fig. 11.1). Since NO is a gas, it can readily diffuse across cell membranes and so can spread not only within a single cell but also from one cell to another. This may give NO a special ability to regulate the activity of many cells simultaneously. NO can bind to a soluble form of guanylyl cyclase and so produce an increase in cGMP concentration. It is therefore entirely conceivable that binding of agonist to receptor could activate PLCβ, generate IP_3, cause intracellular Ca^{2+} to rise, increase the concentration of NO, and elevate cGMP. I shall refer to all of these substances as "second messengers," though in some cases it would appear that they may actually function as third, fourth, or even fifth messengers in some signal cascades.

Tools for Studying Ca²⁺

Ca²⁺ Buffers

Ca²⁺ buffers function like pH buffers, but they bind Ca^{2+} instead of H^+. Ca²⁺ buffers are used to decrease the rate of change of the intracellular free-Ca²⁺ concentration. An effect of a buffer is often an important indication that Ca²⁺ is playing some role in a physiological response. Highly selective Ca²⁺ buffers are also essential as experimental tools to reduce the level of intracellular free-Ca²⁺ concentration, in order to study the Ca²⁺ dependence of transmitter release or synaptic modulation. Ca²⁺ impurities in salts, such as NaCl and KCl, and leaching from ordinary laboratory glassware can produce Ca²⁺ concentrations of 1–10 μM even in solutions to which no Ca²⁺ has been specifically added. A buffer can bind this Ca²⁺, remove it from solution, and decrease the Ca²⁺ concentration to much lower values.

The choice of Ca²⁺ buffer, like the choice of a pH buffer, if often dictated by the range of concentrations for which the buffer is intended to be used. Since the resting Ca²⁺ concentration in most cells is of the order of 100 nM (see Chapter 4), appropriate buffers in many experiments are those with a dissociation constant (K_d) near 10^{-7} M. Buffers with lower dissociation constants would seldom be useful, since they would be saturated with bound Ca²⁺ at the normal free-Ca²⁺ concentration and would not be able to bind additional Ca²⁺; buffers with higher dissociation constants would be useful only in experiments for which the intracellular free-Ca²⁺ level would be expected to increase to a very high level (above 1 μM).

The most commonly used Ca²⁺ buffers are EGTA and BAPTA (see Fig. 13.1). EGTA is ethylene glycol bis(β-aminoethyl ether)-N,N,N′,N′-tetraacetic acid. The Ca²⁺ binding site is formed by four negatively charged acetic acid groups that make a cage around the bound ion. The affinity of EGTA for Ca²⁺ is very high (the K_d at neutral pH is between 10^{-6} and 10^{-7} M). EGTA has little affinity for common monovalent cations like Na$^+$ and K$^+$, and the affinity of EGTA for Ca^{2+} is over 10^5 times greater than for Mg^{2+}, the only other divalent ion found in abundance in cells or extracellular media.

The principal difficulty with EGTA is that, at physiological pH, the acetocarboxyl groups of the molecule also bind H$^+$, and the binding of H$^+$ competes with the binding of Ca^{2+}. As a consequence Ca^{2+} binds relatively slowly, since it must effectively compete with H$^+$ to enter the coordination site of the buffer. It also means that the K_d of Ca^{2+} binding is dependent on pH. Finally, the binding of Ca^{2+} by EGTA can produce the *release* of H$^+$, making it difficult to distinguish experimentally between a decrease in Ca^{2+} concentration produced by injection of EGTA into a cell and an increase in the concentration of protons.

A more useful buffer in many experiments is BAPTA (1,2-bis(*o*-aminophenoxy)ethane-*N,N,N',N'*-tetraacetic acid), which has a Ca^{2+} affinity and divalent ion selectivity similar to that of EGTA but is nearly unaffected by pH within the physiological range (Tsien, 1980). The benzene rings of the BAPTA molecule decrease the H$^+$ affinity of the carboxyl groups in the Ca^{2+} binding site (see Fig. 13.1), so these groups are largely unprotonated at neutral pH. Because of its diminished proton binding, BAPTA is a much faster buffer than EGTA. At neutral pH and a buffer concentration of 10 mM, the binding of Ca^{2+} approaches equilibrium with a time constant of 50–100 µs for EGTA, whereas the equivalent time constant for BAPTA is several hundred times shorter (0.1–0.2 µs—see Tsien,

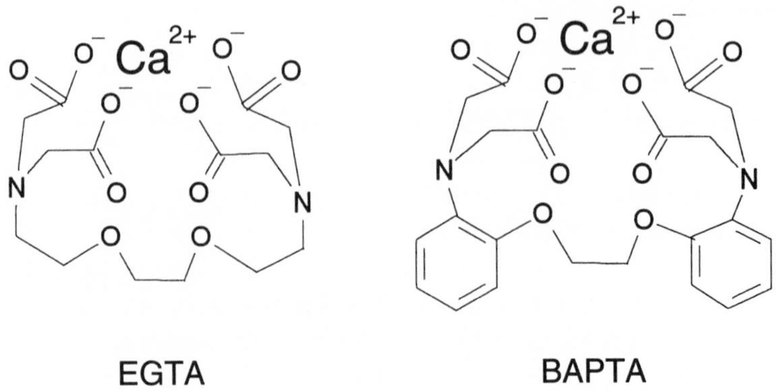

Fig. 13.1 Chemical structures of the Ca^{2+} buffers EGTA and BAPTA, shown with a Ca^{2+} ion adjacent to the negatively charged carboxyl groups that form the binding sites of these two molecules.

EGTA   BAPTA

1980; Adler et al., 1991). This is a critical advantage in many experiments, as we have already seen for studies of the Ca^{2+} dependence of transmitter release (see Chapter 8).

Ca^{2+} Indicators

To monitor the release of Ca^{2+} from internal stores, it would be useful to measure the increase in free-Ca^{2+} concentration within the cell, and even better to visualize the part of the cell within which the Ca^{2+} concentration is changing. In Chapter 8 I described several experiments that made use of luminescent proteins or indicator dyes to measure $[Ca^{2+}]_i$. I now describe these methods in more detail (see Thomas, 1982; McCormack and Cobbold, 1991).

The first technique widely used to measure the free-Ca^{2+} concentration in a living cell employed the luminescent protein *aequorin* (see Shimomura and Johnson, 1976; Cobbold and Lee, 1991). This is a 21 kDa protein extracted from *Aequora,* a luminescent jellyfish which can be found in abundance in late summer in the coastal waters of Puget Sound in the Pacific Northwest. When aequorin binds Ca^{2+}, the protein luminesces (emits) a blue light. Aequorin has many favorable properties. It responds to Ca^{2+} within the physiological range, it is unaffected by monovalent cations or Mg^{2+}, it can be injected into cells and is nontoxic, and the emitted luminescence is relatively easy to measure with a photodetecting device, such as a photomultiplier tube.

Unfortunately, aequorin also has several serious limitations. The amount of luminescence depends nonlinearly on the Ca^{2+} concentration, the aequorin molecule has multiple Ca^{2+} binding sites, and the activity of the protein declines during luminescence (which means that no baseline can be measured). This makes the aequorin signal difficult (perhaps impossible) to calibrate and therefore to use to measure the absolute concentration of free Ca^{2+}. Aequorin is also rather slow, responding to changes in Ca^{2+} with a time constant of the order of 10 ms (Hastings et al., 1969). Aequorin is therefore a poor choice for measuring rapid changes in Ca^{2+}.

More satisfactory results in many experiments have been obtained with the dye Arsenazo III, which is not luminescent but rather changes absorbance when it binds Ca^{2+} (Thomas, 1991). Arsenazo III responds to changes in Ca^{2+} much more rapidly than aequorin, but it too has multiple binding sites for Ca^{2+} and is difficult to use quantitatively. In spite of these limitations, Arsenazo III has proved useful in many investigations, as we have already seen in Chapter 8.

Methods for measuring Ca^{2+} were revolutionized by the synthesis of the dyes indo, fura-2, and their relatives, which have a single binding site for Ca^{2+} and simple stoichiometry (Grynkiewicz, Poenie, and Tsien, 1985). These properties make these dyes much easier to calibrate and use quantitatively. The structure of fura-2 (Fig. 13.2A) is similar to that of BAPTA, with one difference. At one of the benzene rings, an additional group has been added, which causes the compound to fluoresce. Fura-2, like BAPTA, is selective for Ca^{2+} and has an affinity between 10^{-6} and 10^{-7} M. It can be easily injected into a cell with a patch-pipette, or it can be loaded into the cell by means of a form of fura-2 called fura-2-AM, to which acetoxymethyl esters have been attached at one or more of the four acetic acid carboxyl groups. The technique of attaching acetoxymethyl esters, first developed by Tsien (1981) for BAPTA, is widely used. The acetyoxymethyl ester groups are hydrophobic and neutralize the charge of the acetic acid carboxyl groups; this has the effect of greatly increasing the membrane permeability of the esterified compound. Once within the cell, native cytosolic enzymes called acetylesterases cleave the ester groups away from the rest of the dye, trapping the dye within the cell. The AM forms of BAPTA and the Ca^{2+} fluorescent indicator dyes must be used with some care, however, since the ability of these molecules to cross lipid membranes means that the dyes can become internalized inside the organelles and vesicles of the cytoplasm.

One particularly useful feature of fura-2 is that changes in Ca^{2+} concentration produce a change not simply in the magnitude of the fluorescence, but in the spectrum of light that excites the molecule to produce the fluorescence. These differences are graphed in Fig. 13.2B, where the ordinate gives (in arbitrary units) the intensity of the *emitted* fluorescence, measured in the green (at 510 nm), and the abscissa gives the wavelength of the *exciting* light. The amplitude of the emitted fluorescence changes when the wavelength of the exciting light is changed, producing an *excitation spectrum*. The shape of this spectrum varies at different concentrations of Ca^{2+} and so changes as Ca^{2+} binds to the fura-2 dye.

A

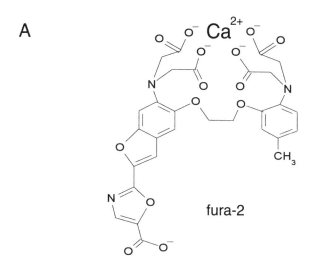

fura-2

B

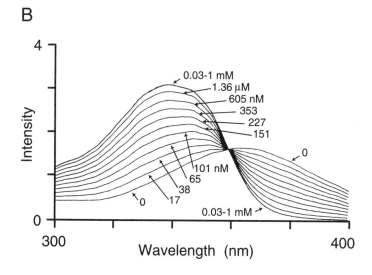

Fig. 13.2 The Ca^{2+} fluorescent indicator dye fura-2. **(A)** Chemical structure of fura-2, shown with a Ca^{2+} ion adjacent to the negatively charged carboxyl groups that form the binding site. **(B)** Excitation spectrum for fura-2 as a function of Ca^{2+} concentration. Dye in solution was excited by light at the wavelength shown on the abscissa. The ordinate gives the intensity of emitted light as a function of the wavelength of the excitation illumination for each of the indicated Ca^{2+} concentrations. Emitted light was collected over a fixed region of the spectrum (510 ± 5 nm) in the green. Notice that as the Ca^{2+} concentration increases, the intensity of fluorescence emitted by the dye increases for excitation wavelengths less than about 360 nm but *decreases* for wavelengths greater than this. (Data relabeled from Grynkiewicz, Poenie, and Tsien, 1985, and used with the permission of the authors and of the American Society for Biochemistry and Molecular Biology.)

In many experiments, particularly those which follow changes in Ca^{2+} over long periods of time, the constant exposure of the dye to ultraviolet excitation light causes the dye to bleach and the dye concentration to decrease. Measurements of Ca^{2+} with fura-2 are relatively insensitive to dye bleaching, since it is possible to excite the dye alternately at two wavelengths, say 340 nm and 380 nm (see Fig. 13.2B). By measuring the ratio of the emitted light for these two excitation wavelengths, it is possible to measure the change in Ca^{2+} in a way that is relatively insensitive to changes in dye concentration, since bleaching reduces the signals for both excitation wavelengths, and the ratio of these signals remains relatively constant. Provided bleaching is not too great, the method of comparing ratios for alternating excitation wavelengths can often be quite helpful. "Ratioing" can also be used for the related dye indo, but for indo it is the emission spectrum, not the excitation spectrum, that changes when Ca^{2+} binds.

In addition to indo and fura-2, there are now many other Ca^{2+}-sensitive fluorescent dyes, most notably the rhod and fluo families (Minta, Kao, and Tsien, 1989) and Calcium Green™ and its relatives (Haugland, 1996). Several of these dyes have affinities similar to fura-2 but produce larger changes in fluorescence and can be excited by light in the visible part of the spectrum (fura-2 requires light in the ultraviolet—see Fig. 13.2B). For these dyes, the binding of Ca^{2+} changes the magnitude of the fluorescence but does not alter either the excitation or emission spectrum. However, the much larger increase in the intensity of the fluorescence produced by Ca^{2+} binding has the advantage that rather dim excitation intensities can be used to measure changes in Ca^{2+} concentrations so that bleaching of the dye can be minimized. Furthermore, in many experiments changes in Ca^{2+} are measured for a brief period (for example during synaptic transmission). Provided conditions can be found that keep dye bleaching small, accurate measurements can be made at a single excitation wavelength, without ratioing (Neher and Augustine, 1992). Other dyes, for example Furaptra, Calcium Green–5N™, and Calcium Orange–5N™, have dissociation constants in the micromolar and so are less sensitive to changes in calcium concentration. They are particularly useful in experiments for which very large changes in Ca^{2+} occur (as at the presynaptic terminal—see Chapter 8) or for very rapid measurements of Ca^{2+} (Escobar, Cifuentes, and Vergara, 1995).

The use of Ca^{2+} fluorescent indicators together with video microscopy has made possible the imaging of changes in Ca^{2+} throughout a cell and the detection of the distribution of Ca^{2+} changes, for example in different parts of a dendritic tree. An example is shown in Fig. 13.3 (from Eilers, Augustine, and Konnerth, 1995).

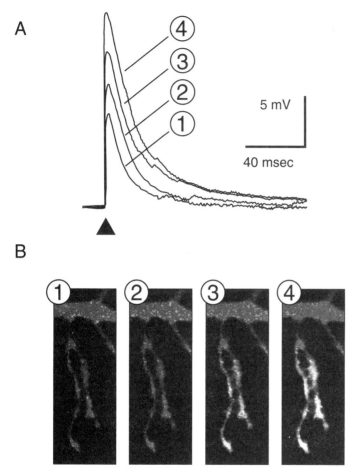

A

B

Fig. 13.3 Dependence of postsynaptic Ca^{2+} increase on EPSP amplitude in the fine dendrites of a rat cerebellar Purkinje neuron. **(A)** Voltage recordings of EPSPs from Purkinje cell in slice. Presynaptic input was stimulated at arrow with an extracellular electrode, placed in the vicinity of parallel fibers (which provide a major pathway for excitatory synapses onto Purkinje cells). For records marked *1–4,* the amplitude of the stimulation voltage was progressively increased, increasing the number of parallel fibers excited by the extracellular electrode. Since these fibers then synapse onto the Purkinje cell, the increase in their stimulation produces an increase in the size of the postsynaptic response. **(B)** Images of a Purkinje cell's fine dendrite, showing the change in intracellular free Ca^{2+}. The Ca^{2+} was measured from the ratio of the brightness of the fluorescence of the Ca^{2+} indicator dye Calcium Green™, before and after stimulation. Increases in Ca^{2+} are indicated by an increase in the lightness of the image. The records *1–4* in **(A)** correspond to the images numbered *1–4* in **(B)**. Notice that increasing the amplitude of stimulation increases the free Ca^{2+} concentration in the dendrite, but the change in free Ca^{2+} remains confined to a small dendritic area and does not spread to the larger dendrite at the top of the images or to adjacent dendrites. (From Eilers, Augustine, and Konnerth, 1995, reprinted with permission of the authors and of Macmillan Magazines Limited.)

5 mV

40 msec

A whole-cell patch recording was made from a Purkinje cell in a slice of cerebellum from rat brain, with a pipette containing the Ca^{2+} fluorescent indicator Calcium Green™. After the Calcium Green™ diffused into the cell, the pipette was used to record EPSPs produced in the Purkinje cell dendrites by stimulation of presynaptic inputs, and a confocal microscope simultaneously recorded the distribution of the Ca^{2+} change in the dendrites, as a function of the size of the EPSP. Such experiments indicate that changes in free-Ca^{2+} concentration can sometimes be localized to a very small region of the dendritic tree, even to a single spine (Yuste and Denk, 1995). The technology for imaging changes in Ca^{2+} is evolving rapidly, as a result of recent developments in confocal microscopy (Eilers, Schneggenburger, and Konnerth, 1995) and two-photon fluorescence microscopy (Yuste and Denk, 1995; Svoboda et al., 1997). The further refinement of these techniques should provide enormous power for investigating the role of Ca^{2+} in nerve cell behavior.

Caged Ca^{2+}

Caged compounds are molecules whose structure and biological activity can be altered by intense, usually ultraviolet illumination. The first molecule of this type shown to be useful in functional studies was caged ATP (Kaplan, Forbush, and Hoffman, 1978), but many similar molecules have now been synthesized to control the release of a variety of metabolites, including Ca^{2+} (Adams and Tsien, 1993; Wang and Augustine, 1995; Nerbonne, 1996). The name *caged* would seem to imply that the compound encloses something which is then somehow released by illumination, and this is approximately true for caged-Ca^{2+} compounds, as we shall see. It is *not* true for most other caged molecules. In most cases, a molecule such as glutamate (Wieboldt, Gee, et al., 1994) or GABA (Wiebolt et al., 1994) is simply attached to a photosensitive group, which makes the glutamate or GABA inactive. This group then undergoes a photochemical reaction during illumination and releases active glutamate or GABA rapidly and with high yield. "Caged" nitric oxide compounds are even simpler (Makings and Tsien, 1994): they are nontoxic organic molecules which undergo a photochemical reaction that produces NO.

Caged compounds are useful in many kinds of experiments. Caged glutamate, for example, can be placed in the extracellular medium and then illuminated with a scanning laser spot in different locations, in order to map the locations of glutamate receptors within the dendritic fields of single neurons (Dalva and Katz, 1994). It can also be used to deliver glutamate very rapidly without rapid perfusion, a technique used to study the kinetics of transmitter activation and desensitization (see for example Otis, Zhang, and Trussell, 1996).

Caged Ca^{2+} compounds are modified Ca^{2+} buffers, whose affinity is altered by light. The most commonly used are DM-nitrophen

A

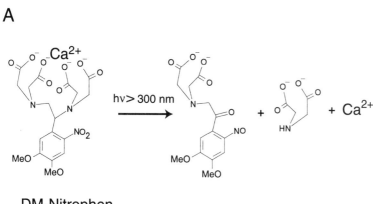

DM-Nitrophen

B

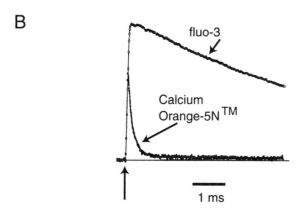

fluo-3

Calcium
Orange-5N™

1 ms

Fig. 13.4 The caged-Ca^{2+} compound DM-nitrophen: structure and kinetics of Ca^{2+} release. **(A)** Chemical structure of DM-nitrophen, with Ca^{2+} bound in unexcited state *(left)* and after excitation with ultraviolet light *(right)*. The molecule undergoes a photochemical reaction that severs a part of the Ca^{2+} binding site from the rest of the compound and releases the bound Ca^{2+}. *Me,* methyl group; *hν,* light exposure (photon). **(B)** Kinetics of Ca^{2+} release. DM-nitrophen was mixed in solution with either of the Ca^{2+} indicator dyes fluo-3 or Calcium Orange–5N™. A brief (30 ns) flash of light from an ultraviolet laser was used to excite the DM-nitrophen and release Ca^{2+}, and the fluorescence emitted for a fixed excitation wavelength was then measured with a photodiode. The diode current is plotted in arbitrary units on the ordinate as a function of time on the abscissa (note calibration bar). The much faster decay of signal measured with Calcium Orange–5N™ is a result of the much lower affinity of this dye for Ca^{2+} due to the much larger rate constant for unbinding (k_{off}). This dye consequently gives a more accurate indication of the time dependence of change in free-Ca^{2+} concentration. (Data relabeled from Escobar, Cifuentes, and Vergara, 1995.)

(Kaplan and Ellis-Davies, 1988); the *nitr* compounds, particularly nitr-5 and nitr-7 (Adams et al., 1988); and nitrophenyl-EGTA (Ellis-Davies and Kaplan, 1994). All bind Ca^{2+} with high affinity but can undergo a photochemical reaction that decreases the affinity of the buffer and releases bound Ca^{2+} to the solution.

As an example, the structure and photochemical transformation of DM-nitrophen are given in Fig. 13.4A. Light exposure produces a very large change in Ca^{2+} affinity, since the DM-nitrophen actually falls apart during the photochemical reaction. The release of Ca^{2+} is quite rapid. This can be shown by measuring the change in Ca^{2+} after brief, intense illumination (delivered with a laser). If the released Ca^{2+} is measured with the Ca^{2+} indicator dye Calcium Orange–5N™(Escobar, Cifuentes, and Vergara, 1995), the increase in Ca^{2+} under favorable conditions rises and decays in less than a millisecond (Fig. 13.4B). Calcium Orange–5N™is a useful indicator for these experiments, since, as I have previously mentioned, it has a low affinity for Ca^{2+} (Escobar et al., 1997). Ca^{2+} therefore binds and unbinds rapidly, and the dye responds very quickly to changes in free Ca^{2+}. Notice that *the very same Ca^{2+} increase* produced by the caged-Ca^{2+} compound and the laser flash appears to be much slower when measured with the higher-affinity dye fluo-3, since Ca^{2+} dissociates from fluo-3 much more slowly than from Calcium Orange–5N™. This result emphasizes the importance of selecting Ca^{2+} indicator dyes carefully and understanding their limitations. In particular, when the change in free Ca^{2+} is large enough to permit them to be used, low-affinity dyes will always provide a more accurate indication of the magnitude and kinetics of the Ca^{2+} concentration change.

Caged-Ca^{2+} compounds are useful for producing localized increases in Ca^{2+} concentration but, like the indicator dyes, they have important limitations. DM-nitrophen, for example, binds Mg^{2+} as well as Ca^{2+}. Nitrophenyl-EGTA has a lower affinity for Mg^{2+} but, like EGTA, binds H^+; this means that the association constant for Ca^{2+} binding depends upon pH. The *nitr* compounds have little affinity for either Mg^{2+} or H^+ but undergo a relatively small change in Ca^{2+} affinity upon illumination. For all of these compounds, the increase in Ca^{2+} must be carefully quantitated with an indicator dye. Even given the difficulties, however, Ca^{2+} compounds have been useful in many experiments—for example, for studying the role of Ca^{2+} in synaptic transmission (Chapter 8) and in long-term potentiation (Chapter 14).

Intracellular Ca^{2+} Release

When a cerebellar Purkinje cell is exposed to glutamate or to the metabotropic glutamate agonists quisqualate or ACPD, the calcium concentration in the dendrites of the cell increases dramatically (Llano et al., 1991; Yuzaki and Mikoshiba, 1992; Linden, Smeyne, and Connor, 1994). This increase can be observed even when calcium is removed from the extracellular bathing medium. It must therefore be produced by a release of calcium from within the cell.

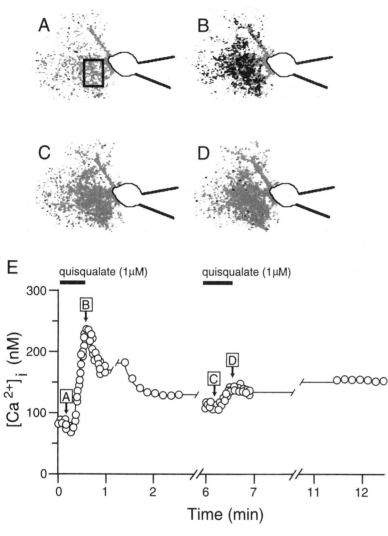

Fig. 13.5 Glutamate agonists produce a release of Ca^{2+} from internal stores in cerebellar Purkinje cells. Whole-cell patch recordings were made from a Purkinje cell in a rat brain slice with an electrode containing 200 μM of the Ca^{2+} indicator dye fura-2. Ca^{2+} measurements were then made from the dendrites of the cell. Bathing medium contained 20 μM EGTA and no added Ca^{2+}. **(A)** Resting Ca^{2+} level in dendrites was about 80 nM (gray shading). Cell body and recording pipette are outlined to right. Box indicates region of dendrites averaged for part E (see below). **(B)** Change in Ca^{2+} 30 s after bath perfusion of 1 μM of the metabotropic glutamate agonist L-quisqualic acid (quisqualate). Black shading indicates region of the dendritic field for which a Ca^{2+} increase was detected. **(C)** Recovery of resting Ca^{2+} concentration. **(D)** Second application of quisqualate elicits much smaller response. **(E)** Mean Ca^{2+} level in dendrites in region shown by box in **(A)** as function of time. Letters correspond to schedule of events displayed above. Bars indicate duration of exposure to 1 μM L-quisqualic acid. (Modified from Llano et al., 1991, and used with the permission of the authors and of Cell Press.)

In the experiment illustrated in Fig. 13.5 (from Llano et al., 1991), a Purkinje cell in a slice from rat brain was whole-cell patch-clamped with an electrode containing the Ca^{2+} indicator dye fura-2. After allowing sufficient time for the fura-2 to enter the cell, calcium measurements were made by recording video images of the dye emission alternately for two excitation wavelengths (see Fig. 13.2). The intensity of the images produced by the two excitation wavelengths was collected for each of the points *(pixels)* of the video image, digitized, and stored in the memory of a computer. The ratio of the intensities was then calculated pixel by pixel, and from this ratio the Ca^{2+} concentration was calculated and displayed as an image, much as in Fig. 13.3B. In this case, however, an increase in Ca^{2+} is represented by an increase in the darkness of the image, and the position of the cell body and the patch pipette are shown to the right of the dendrites, in white.

The solution used for this experiment contained no added calcium and 20 μM of the calcium buffer EGTA. Perfusion of the slice with 1 μM of the glutamate agonist L-quisqualic acid produced a large increase in intracellular free Ca^{2+}, which was localized to the dendrites of the Purkinje cell (Fig. 13.5B). When the same cell was exposed to quisqualate a second time, little or no release of Ca^{2+} occurred (Fig. 13.5D). The reason for this was probably that the first exposure to quisqualate depleted the intracellular Ca^{2+} stores, and in the absence of extracellular Ca^{2+}, these stores could not be replenished.

The time course of the Ca^{2+} increase for the cell in parts A–D of Fig. 13.5 is graphed in part E. The amplitude of the calcium change plotted in this figure was determined from the area of dendrites shown by the black box in Fig. 13.5A, just to the left of the cell soma. Fig. 13.5E confirms the impression of A–D: quisqualate increases the intracellular Ca^{2+} concentration even in the absence of extracellular Ca^{2+}, and only the first exposure produced a significant release of Ca^{2+}.

The increase in calcium produced by quisqualate in the Purkinje cell is probably a consequence of the activation of phospholipase C by a metabotropic glutamate receptor (see Fig. 11.1). Glutamate and quisqualate have been shown to produce an increase in IP_3 turnover in cerebellum, probably in the Purkinje cells (Blackstone, Supattapone, and Snyder, 1989). There are high concentrations of IP_3 receptors in Purkinje cells, among the highest anywhere in the brain (Nakanishi, Maeda, and Mikoshiba, 1991; Sharp et al., 1993). Blockers of IP_3-mediated Ca^{2+} release block the Ca^{2+} increase produced by metabotropic glutamate agonists in these cells (Yuzaki and Mikoshiba, 1992). Finally, an increase in IP_3 concentration in the Purkinje cells produced by illumination of caged IP_3 has been shown to lead to an increase in intracellular Ca^{2+} concentration (Khodakhah and Ogden, 1993, 1995).

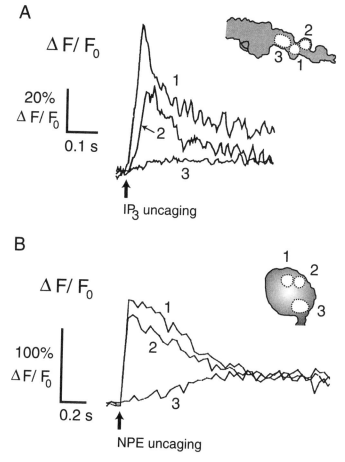

A

$\Delta F/ F_0$

20%
$\Delta F/ F_0$

0.1 s

1

2

3

↑
IP$_3$ uncaging

B

$\Delta F/ F_0$

100%
$\Delta F/ F_0$

0.2 s

1

2

3

↑
NPE uncaging

Fig. 13.6 Focal release of Ca^{2+} in a Purkinje cell dendrite. Whole-cell patch recordings were made from Purkinje cells in rat brain slices. The pipette solution contained the calcium indicator dye Calcium Green™ as well as either caged IP$_3$ or caged Ca^{2+}. The change in Ca^{2+} concentration was estimated from $\Delta F/F_0$, i.e., the change in the fluorescence of the dye divided by the initial (resting) fluorescence, measured with a confocal microscope. An argon ion laser was used to focus a spot 3–5 μm in diameter of high-intensity ultraviolet illumination onto the specimen, and the duration of laser exposure was controlled with an electronic shutter. **(A)** Recording pipette contained 150 μM caged IP$_3$. Inset shows a portion of the dendritic arbor of the Purkinje cell used for the experiment. Graph plots relative change in Ca^{2+} concentration as a function of time at three regions of the dendritic tree (indicated by numbers in inset). Position of spot generated by the uncaging laser is labeled as *1*. **(B)** Experiment similar to that in **(A)**, but recording pipette contained the caged-Ca^{2+} compound nitrophenyl-EGTA (*NPE*), and measurements were made from Purkinje cell soma instead of dendrite. Position of spot generated by the uncaging laser is again labeled as *1*. (Reprinted from Wang and Augustine, 1995, with permission of the authors and of Cell Press.)

One way to investigate IP$_3$-dependent Ca^{2+} release is to use confocal microscopy to image a Purkinje cell from a cerebellar slice, and to make simultaneous whole-cell recordings from this cell with a patch-clamp electrode containing caged IP$_3$ and a Ca^{2+} indicator dye. In an experiment of this kind (Wang and Augustine, 1995), ultraviolet light from a laser was focused to a spot 3–5 μm in diameter, which was positioned within one of the dendrites of the cell, and a 4 ms pulse from the laser was used to uncage the IP$_3$. The confocal microscope was then employed to detect the spatial distribution and relative amplitude of the increase in calcium concentration, determined from the fluorescence of the dye Calcium Green™.

A sizable increase in Ca^{2+} can be observed at the position of the laser spot (Fig. 13.6A), but the amplitude of the Ca^{2+} concentration increase is smaller at some distance away from the site of IP_3 uncaging. A similar experiment with the caged Ca^{2+} compound nitrophenol-EGTA found a similar localized increase in Ca^{2+} concentration in the cell soma (Fig. 13.6B). The Ca^{2+} increase is local, probably the result of buffering and sequestration of Ca^{2+} within the cytoplasm (Chapter 4).

IP_3 and Ryanodine Receptors

IP_3 produces Ca^{2+} release by binding to specialized membrane proteins called *IP_3 receptors*, which are located within vesicles of the smooth endoplasmic reticulum and in the sarcoplasmic reticulum of muscle, perhaps in a special group of vesicles called calcisomes. As previously described (see Chapter 4), these vesicles have a Ca^{2+} ATPase (or SERCA) that pumps Ca^{2+} into the vesicle, and the Ca^{2+} inside the vesicle is buffered by Ca^{2+}-binding proteins. The binding of IP_3 to its receptor causes the opening of a channel and the efflux of Ca^{2+} out of the vesicle into the cytosol (see Fig. 13.8B).

Structure and Function of IP_3 Receptors

Functional IP_3 receptors are tetramers with an apparent molecular mass of over one million Daltons (see Berridge, 1993; Mikoshiba et al., 1993; Bezprozvanny and Ehrlich, 1995; Bezprozvanny, 1996). Each of the four monomers has a binding site for IP_3 and six transmembrane domains, which are thought to form the channel for Ca^{2+}, with both carboxyl- and amino-terminal ends of the protein located cytoplasmically (see Fig. 13.7A). Much of the mass of the protein lies within the cytoplasmic amino terminus, which contains the binding site for IP_3 and a large sequence usually referred to as the *regulatory* or *coupling domain*. The coupling domain is thought to coordinate the binding of IP_3 with the opening of the channel, which is nearly nonselective for divalent cations and can also be permeated by monovalent cations. Since there is probably no difference in the K^+, Na^+, or Mg^{2+} concentration across the vesicle membrane, most of the current through the IP_3 receptor chan-

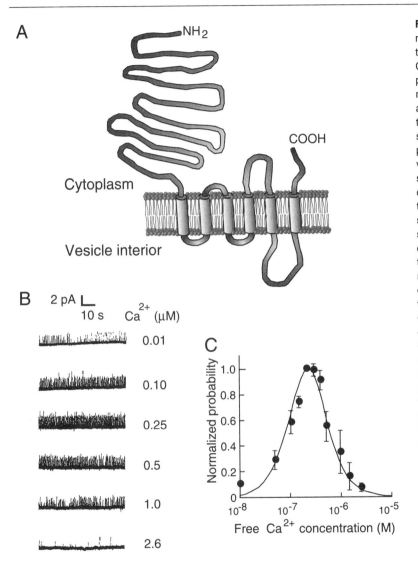

Fig. 13.7 IP$_3$ receptors. **(A)** Hypothesized membrane topology of monomer of IP$_3$ receptor. (After Mikoshiba et al., 1993.) **(B)** and **(C)** Ca^{2+} dependence of IP$_3$ receptor opening probability. IP$_3$ receptors were isolated from canine cerebellum and incorporated into an artificial lipid bilayer, formed by painting a solution of lipid across a 100 μm hole in a Teflon sheet. The Teflon sheet was supported in a plastic chamber, and the lipid membrane was voltage-clamped by placing electrodes in the solutions on the two sides of the lipid. Vesicles containing IP$_3$ receptor protein were added only to one side of the lipid bilayer, called the *cis* side, and IP$_3$ receptor was incorporated by fusion of the vesicles with the bilayer. This occurred in such a way that the cytosolic side of the protein faced the *cis* side of the bilayer. Current recordings in **(B)** show sample channel openings as a function of the Ca^{2+} concentration on the *cis* or cytosolic side of the bilayer. Graph in **(C)** plots the probability a channel is open as a function of cytosolic (i.e., *cis*) free Ca^{2+} concentration. Data, from four experiments, are means ± standard errors. Probabilities have been normalized to maximum channel activity observed in each experiment, which was always less than 0.15. See Bezprozvanny, Watras, and Ehrlich (1991) for details. (After Bezprozvanny, Watras, and Ehrlich, 1991, and Bezprozvanny, 1996.)

nel under physiological conditions is carried by Ca^{2+} leaving the vesicle interior.

There are at least three (and probably more) different genes for IP$_3$ receptors, with several splice variants, which are differently expressed in different parts of the nervous system and other parts of the body. All have a similar structure and probably function in a similar fashion. A large fraction of the sequence differences between the different forms of receptors occurs within the coupling domain, which is an indication that regulation of IP_3-gated Ca^{2+} release may differ in different cells or even different parts of the same cell. The coupling domain appears to have binding sites for Ca^{2+} (or for an unidentified Ca^{2+}-binding protein) and for ATP. This part of the protein can also be phosphorylated by protein kinases.

The regulation of the IP_3 receptor could be very important in the life of the cell, since changes in the response of this receptor to IP_3 could alter the effect of activation of metabotropic receptors that act through $PLC\beta$. In particular, suppose Ca^{2+} itself were to modulate the receptor and increase its probability of opening. An initial efflux of Ca^{2+} from the Ca^{2+} store would facilitate further efflux, and the Ca^{2+} release would then become regenerative, like an action potential. If Ca^{2+} were to inhibit the release, this would produce a kind of negative feedback, which could limit the increase in free-Ca^{2+} concentration.

Several studies have addressed the possible effect of Ca^{2+} on IP_3 receptors. The data in Fig. 13.7B and C are from the paper of Bezprozvanny, Watras, and Ehrlich (1991), who incorporated cerebellar endoplasmic reticulum into an artificial lipid membrane and measured the activity of the IP_3 receptor at a fixed IP_3 concentration but a varying concentration of Ca^{2+}. The probability that the receptor would open in the presence of IP_3 was increased by small increases in Ca^{2+} but inhibited by large ones, with most of the modulation occurring within the physiological range of Ca^{2+} concentrations. Thus, release of Ca^{2+} from intracellular vesicles is likely *both* to stimulate *and* inhibit further Ca^{2+} release, depending upon the total Ca^{2+} concentration present in the vicinity of the vesicle.

Structure and Function of Ryanodine Receptors

In addition to IP_3 receptors, other Ca^{2+} channel proteins, called *ryanodine receptors,* are also present in the vesicles of the endoplasmic reticulum (Meissner, 1994; Berridge et al., 1996; Verkhratsky and Shmigol, 1996). These proteins were first discovered in skeletal and cardiac muscle, where they are known to be responsible for the Ca^{2+} release which facilitates muscle contraction. They are called ryanodine receptors because they bind the plant alkaloid ryanodine, which was used for the first biochemical isolation and subsequent cloning of the DNA encoding these proteins.

There are at least three ryanodine receptor genes, with several splice variants (Sorrentino, 1996). Like IP_3 receptors, the ryanodine receptor monomers have several (perhaps also 6) membrane-spanning domains near the carboxyl terminus, and these domains show significant sequence homology to the carboxyl-terminal membrane-spanning domains of the IP_3 receptor. When 4 ryanodine receptor monomers assemble into a tetramer, the Ca^{2+} channel formed is also similar to that of IP_3 receptors: the relative selectivity of the receptors for divalent and monovalent cations is nearly identical, though the unitary conductance of the ryanodine channel is approximately a factor of 4 larger (see Bezprozvanny and Ehrlich, 1995). One difference between the two receptor families is that the molecular weight of ryanodine receptor monomers is nearly twice that of IP_3 receptors, with most of the additional amino acids occurring within the coupling domain.

Ryanodine receptors are expressed in many parts of the brain, with different isoforms localized to different regions of the CNS (Nori, Gorza, and Volpe, 1996; Berridge et al., 1996). The function of these receptors in neurons seems to be to mediate Ca^{2+}-induced Ca^{2+} release. That is, Ca^{2+} entering the cell (or released from IP_3 receptors) appears to be able to gate the release of further Ca^{2+} from vesicles containing ryanodine receptors (see Fig. 13.8B). In voltage-clamped Purkinje cells, for example, Ca^{2+} entering through voltage-gated Ca^{2+} channels produces an increase in intracellular free Ca^{2+}, which rises more than linearly with pulse duration: doubling the pulse duration can produce a fivefold increase in free Ca^{2+} (Llano, DiPolo, and Marty, 1994). Similar effects have been observed in sensory neurons (Shmigol, Verkhratsky, and Isenberg, 1995). The Ca^{2+} increase can be nearly completely blocked by exposing the cells to ruthenium red, which inhibits Ca^{2+}-induced Ca^{2+} release in skeletal muscle (see Ehrlich et al., 1994) and blocks the opening of ryanodine receptor channels from cerebellum (Bezprozvanny, Watras, and Ehrlich, 1991). Furthermore, caffeine, which activates Ca^{2+} release from vesicles containing ryanodine receptors (see Ehrlich et al., 1994), has been shown to produce increases in Ca^{2+} in many types of neurons (see Verkhratsky and Shmigol, 1996).

Since ryanodine receptors have even larger cytoplasmic domains than IP$_3$ receptors, it would not be surprising if these proteins were regulated in a variety of ways. As already mentioned, Ca^{2+} stimulates release of more calcium, and very high concentrations of Ca^{2+} (>100 μM) can also inhibit further release, though it is not clear whether this inhibition occurs under physiological conditions. Release is also modulated by ATP, by calmodulin, and by phosphorylation by serine/threonine protein kinases. Perhaps the most interesting of the ryanodine receptor modulators is cyclic ADP-ribose, which has been postulated to act as a second messenger in some cells (Dousa, Chini, and Beers, 1996; Lee, 1996; Galione and Summerhill, 1996). There is evidence in several tissues, including the nervous system (Hua et al., 1994), that cyclic ADP-ribose can facilitate Ca^{2+} release from ryanodine-receptor-containing vesicles, perhaps by directly binding to the receptor. Cyclic ADP-ribose is synthesized by ADP-ribosyl cyclase, which in sea urchin eggs has been reported to be activated by cGMP (Galione et al., 1993). Thus it is conceivable that second messenger cascades that produce an increase in cGMP lead to an increase in cyclic ADP-ribose, which then alters the intracellular Ca^{2+} concentration.

Ca^{2+} Oscillations and Ca^{2+} Waves

Results from many experiments suggest that for the most part IP$_3$ and ryanodine receptors are located on different vesicle populations; that is, Ca^{2+} can be released from two mostly separate groups of vesicles containing different kinds of Ca^{2+} channels. The receptor-mediated activation of PLCβ generates the diffusible messenger IP$_3$, which binds to IP$_3$ receptors and produces an efflux of Ca^{2+} from one sort of vesicle. This Ca^{2+} could then act on the IP$_3$ receptors themselves, to stimulate further release. The Ca^{2+} could also bind to ryanodine receptors, producing additional release from a second population of vesicles. Provided the two vesicle populations were located in the same region of the cell, which seems to be the case in some cells (though not in others), release from one population could have a dramatic effect on release from the other.

In many cell types metabotropic agonists and IP$_3$ have been shown to trigger regenerative oscillations of intracellular Ca^{2+}, as well as Ca^{2+} waves that can travel in complicated patterns across the cytoplasm (Meyer and Stryer, 1991; Berridge and Dupont, 1994; Petersen, Petersen, and Kasai, 1994; Bootman and Berridge, 1995; Clapham, 1995; Clapham and Sneyd, 1995). The origin of these waves is unknown. Although it is possible to imagine complex interactions between vesicles containing IP$_3$ and ryanodine receptors, spectacular waves have been observed in *Xenopus* oocytes (Lechleiter et al., 1991) that appear to lack ryanodine receptors completely. Other proposed mechanisms for the waves include Ca^{2+}-dependent regulation of IP$_3$ synthesis (Harootunian et al., 1991) and stimulatory and inhibitory Ca^{2+} feedback of release by binding of Ca^{2+} to IP$_3$ receptors (see Clapham and Sneyd, 1995; Bezprozvanny, 1996).

The role of Ca^{2+} oscillations and waves in the nervous system is not at present understood. It is intriguing to speculate that Ca^{2+} entry through voltage- or receptor-gated channels may trigger waves of Ca^{2+} that propagate throughout the dendritic tree. Ryanodine receptors, for example, seem to be located in the spines of hippocampal pyramidal cells (and IP$_3$ receptors in the spines of Purkinje cells). It is possible that Ca^{2+} stores in spines participate in boosting Ca^{2+} entry or Ca^{2+} release. Since Ca^{2+} seems to play such an important role in synaptic modulation in the nervous system (Chapter 14), the spread of Ca^{2+} in dendrites may have important implications for signal processing.

Refilling the Stores: I$_{CRAC}$

The intracellular free-Ca^{2+} increase produced by a metabotropic agonist in many cells has two phases: an initial transient response, which is often relatively independent of external Ca^{2+} and seems to represent release from internal stores; and a sustained response, which disappears when external Ca^{2+} is removed and seems to be caused by the opening of Ca^{2+} channels in the plasma membrane (see Fig. 13.8A). When cells are bathed in zero-Ca^{2+} solution, the stores are rapidly depleted, often after the very first exposure to a metabotropic agonist (see Fig. 13.5). When Ca^{2+} is present in the bathing solution, Ca^{2+} can enter the cell, and the stores can be rapidly refilled.

Putney (1986, 1990) suggested that the depletion of Ca^{2+} from the vesicle produces a signal that gates Ca^{2+} entry into the cell,

Fig. 13.8 **(A)** Calcium influx measured in rat basophilic leukemia cells (RBL-2H3) stably transfected with m1 muscarinic receptors (RBL-m1 cells; from Dr. O. Choi, NIH). RBL-m1 cells were loaded with fura-2-AM. Intracellular Ca^{2+} concentration was monitored in single cells with a photomultiplier-based system and calculated from the fluorescence ratio for excitation at 360 and 390 nm by standard methods (Neher, 1989). The cholinergic agonist carbachol (100 μM) was introduced by local pressure application from a wide-tipped micropipette placed within 20 μM of the cell and was applied *(solid bar)* in the presence ($+Ca^{2+}$ = 10 mM) or absence of external Ca^{+2} ($-Ca^{2+}$ = no added Ca). The figure shows averages from 17 ($+Ca^{2+}$) and 5 cells ($-Ca^{2+}$). In both cases 10 mM Cs was included in the bath solution to block endogenous inward-rectifier K^+ channels, thus preventing changes in membrane potential during carbachol application. (Modified in part from Mathes, Fleig, and Penner, 1997, and from data provided by the authors of this paper.) **(B)** Schema for the major mechanisms for Ca^{2+} release from internal stores. Vesicle to left contains IP_3 receptor, whereas that to right contains ryanodine receptor. Both also contain Ca^{2+}-ATPase (SERCA) to pump Ca^{2+} into the vesicles (not shown) and have high concentrations of Ca^{2+} (Ca^{2+} store). Plasma membrane contains two kinds of entry pathways for Ca^{2+}: the release-activated channels (I_{CRAC}) and voltage-gated channels.

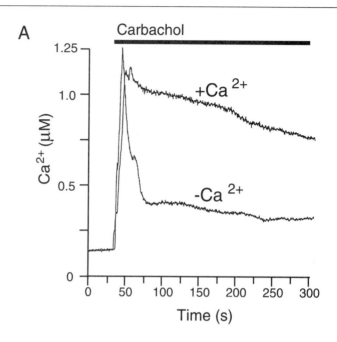

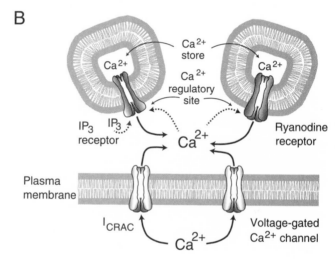

which he termed *capacitative calcium entry*. He first envisaged a pathway directly from the extracellular space into the vesicle, but later he proposed that something in the vesicle senses the decrease in vesicular Ca^{2+}, and this is then communicated to a plasma membrane Ca^{2+} channel, either via some direct physical connection between the vesicle and the membrane (Berridge, 1995) or, as now seems more likely, via the diffusion of some intracellular messenger (Randriamampita and Tsien, 1993; Thomas and Hanley, 1995; for reviews, see Fasolato, Innocenti, and Pozzan, 1994; Clapham, 1996).

The nature of the Ca^{2+} entry pathway is still unclear, but in several cell types a novel Ca^{2+} current has been observed that is gated by vesicle depletion. This current has been called the *Ca^{2+}-release activated Ca^{2+} current,* or I_{CRAC} (see Penner, Fasolato, and Hoth, 1993; Parekh and Penner, 1996; Lewis, Dolmetsch, and Zweifach, 1996). I_{CRAC} was first observed in blood cells (Hoth and Penner, 1992; Zweifach and Lewis, 1993) but has now been found in many other cell types, including neurons (Mathes and Thompson, 1994). Fig. 13.9 (from Parekh and Penner, 1996) shows the development of I_{CRAC} in a mast cell, a blood-derived cell that has also been useful for studying the mechanism of vesicle exocytosis (Chapter 8). The mast cell was approached with a patch electrode containing IP_3 and 10 mM EGTA. After a seal was formed, additional suction was applied to the pipette to produce a whole-cell recording, and the IP_3 and EGTA diffused from the pipette into the cell. The upper part of the figure shows the response of the cell to a series of voltage ramps from -100 mV to $+100$ mV. The current of the cell was recorded as the voltage was systematically changed by the ramp, automatically generating a current-voltage curve for the cell. The amplitude of the peak current at three different voltages is plotted in the lower graph, as a function of time after formation of the whole-cell recording.

At the beginning of the recording, there was little current. As the IP_3 and EGTA diffused into the cell, the IP_3 presumably released Ca^{2+} from vesicles and depleted the vesicle's Ca^{2+} store, and EGTA kept the cytosolic Ca^{2+} concentration at a low value. As this occurred, a membrane conductance gradually increased with time. This conductance was probably gated by depletion of Ca^{2+} from

Fig. 13.9 Activation of I_{CRAC}. Whole-cell patch recordings were made from isolated rat basophilic leukemia (RBL-2H3) cells. Depletion of Ca^{2+} stores was initiated by including 20 μM IP_3 in the patch pipette. Formation of whole-cell recording (at $t = 0$) caused the slow dialysis of IP_3 into the cell, which gated IP_3 receptors, depleted Ca^{2+} from intracellular vesicles, and gated the opening of a plasma membrane Ca^{2+} conductance. Extracellular medium contained 10 mM Ca^{2+}, and Ca^{2+} in pipette solution was buffered to very low levels with 10 mM EGTA. **(A)** Membrane conductance was measured with voltage ramps from −100 mV to +100 mV *(upper traces)*. Lower traces show current responses to voltage ramps at times indicated by filled circles in **(B)**. Arrows (for fourth record) indicate currents at three potentials, whose values are plotted in **(B)**. **(B)** Current as a function of time measured from voltage ramps at 2 s intervals at 0 mV, −40 mV, and −80 mV. (Reprinted with minor modification from Parekh and Penner, 1996, with permission of the authors and of Rockefeller University Press.)

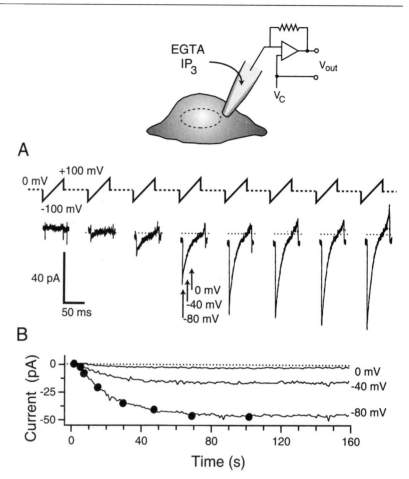

the vesicle, since it could also be produced by agonists that produce vesicular Ca^{2+} release.

I_{CRAC} channels have now been studied in some detail and have the following properties: (1) they are highly selective for Ca^{2+} and are normally much less permeable to monovalent cations and even to Ba^{2+} or Sr^{2+}, which readily permeate voltage-gated Ca^{2+} channels; (2) they are inwardly rectifying, probably as the result of Goldman rectification (because the Ca^{2+} concentration inside the cell is so low) and not as the result of any intrinsic voltage dependence of the current; and (3) they can be blocked by La^{3+} and by a host of divalent cations, including Zn^{2+}, Cd^{2+}, and Co^{2+}. I_{CRAC} appears to inactivate, apparently by a Ca^{2+}-dependent mechanism (Hoth and Penner, 1993; Zweifach and Lewis, 1995).

The molecular structure of the molecule responsible for I_{CRAC} is still unclear. Attention has focused on a protein called trp (see Clapham, 1996; Minke and Selinger, 1996), which is a Ca^{2+}-permeable channel protein that plays an essential role in phototransduction in the eye of *Drosophila*. When this protein is expressed in insect cells (Vaca et al., 1994) or in oocytes (Petersen et al., 1995; Gillo et al., 1996), it produces a current activated by store depletion. The structure of trp is similar to one of the repeat domains of a voltage-sensitive Ca^{2+} channel, and its putative membrane-spanning domains show some sequence homologies to these channels (Phillips, Bull, and Kelly, 1992). Mammalian analogues of trp seem also to form depletion-activated channels (Zhu et al., 1996; Zitt et al., 1996), and it is possible (though as yet unproved) that these channels produce currents similar to I_{CRAC} currents.

CaM Kinase II

Ca^{2+} entering the cytoplasm through plasma membrane channels or from internal stores can act as a second messenger to alter the activity of enzymes and other proteins within the cell. Many of the effects of Ca^{2+} are mediated by small-molecular-weight Ca^{2+}-binding proteins. That is, the Ca^{2+} binds to a soluble and diffusible binding protein, and this protein then binds to some other protein to alter its activity. The best characterized of the Ca^{2+}-binding proteins is *calmodulin* (see Fig. 11.1), which has a molecular weight of about 17 kDa and four Ca^{2+}-binding sites, each with a dissociation constant of about 1 μM (Cohen and Klee, 1988; Gnegy, 1993). When Ca^{2+} binds to calmodulin, the protein undergoes a change in conformation, which increases its affinity for binding at sites on effector proteins (Weinstein and Mehler, 1994). Ca^{2+}/calmodulin has been shown to activate the plasma-membrane form of Ca^{2+} ATPase (Chapter 4), some isoforms of adenylyl cyclase (Chapter 12), protein phosphatase 2B (calcineurin—Chapter 12), Ca^{2+}/calmodulin-dependent cyclic nucleotide phosphodiesterase, and several types of Ca^{2+}/calmodulin-dependent protein kinases, called *CaM kinases* (Gnegy, 1993).

Of the many different kinds of CaM kinase, the most thoroughly studied and best understood is undoubtedly CaM kinase II (see Hanson and Schulman, 1992; Schulman, 1995; Ghosh and Greenberg, 1995; Braun and Schulman, 1995; Soderling, 1996). This protein is 20–50 times more abundant in the CNS than in most nonneuronal tissues. It has been shown to phosphorylate a variety of targets, including Ca^{2+} channels, IP_3 receptors, GABA receptors, and nitric oxide synthase. It can also phosphorylate many of the proteins that have been postulated to mediate synaptic vesicle mobilization and release.

CaM kinase II, like PKA, PKG, and PKC, is a serine/threonine protein kinase, but it has some peculiar and interesting properties. It is a large, heteromeric protein containing from 8 to 12 homologous subunits. The subunits are encoded by at least four genes, whose gene products (called α, β, γ, and δ) have all been reported to be expressed in the CNS. Messages for these proteins have been identified in a total of at least 17 different splice variants. The sequence of each of the homomers can be divided into three domains (see Fig. 13.10A): a catalytic domain, a regulatory domain containing partially overlapping inhibitory and calmodulin-binding regions, and an association domain. The catalytic domain contains sites for the binding of ATP and the substrate protein, and it is this part of the protein that catalyzes protein phosphorylation. The inhibitory region of the regulatory domain seems to be able to fold over a portion of the catalytic domain, rendering the enzyme inactive. When Ca^{2+}/calmodulin binds to the adjacent CaM-binding region, the inhibitory sequence is lifted away from the catalytic domain, and the enzyme then becomes active to phosphorylate proteins. The association domain is required for the assembly of monomers into the holoenzyme. If this domain is removed from the protein, the monomers retain activity but do not co-assemble.

The monomers of the holoenzyme are distributed in a hub-and-spoke arrangement (see Fig. 13.10B), which has been directly observed in the electron microscope (Kanaseki et al., 1991). This configuration may have evolved to facilitate one of the most remarkable features of CaM kinase II: its ability to regulate its own activity by autophosphorylation. All of the different monomer isoforms contain an important threonine residue within the regulatory domain, which is normally buried inside the structure of the pro-

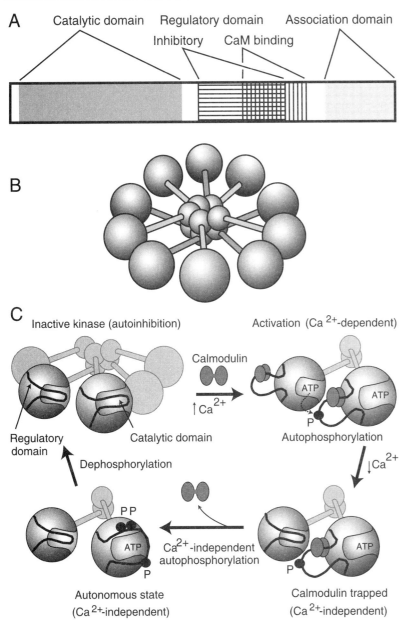

A Catalytic domain   Regulatory domain   Association domain

Inhibitory   CaM binding

B

C

Inactive kinase (autoinhibition)   Activation (Ca²⁺-dependent)

Calmodulin

↑Ca²⁺

ATP

ATP

Regulatory
domain   Catalytic domain   Autophosphorylation

P

Dephosphorylation   ↓Ca²⁺

P P   ATP

ATP   Ca²⁺-independent
autophosphorylation   P

P

Autonomous state   Calmodulin trapped
(Ca²⁺-independent)   (Ca²⁺-independent)

Fig. 13.10   Structure and function of CaM kinase II. **(A)** Each monomer of CaM kinase II (amino terminus at left) consists of three major domains: a catalytic domain, which mediates actual protein phosphorylation; a regulatory domain, with partially overlapping inhibitory and calmodulin-binding sites; and an association domain, which mediates association of monomers into holoenzyme. **(B)** "Hub-and-spoke" structure of CaM kinase II. Hub in center is composed of association domains, and spokes with terminal knobs are composed of regulatory and catalytic domains. **(C)** Autophosphorylation. Increase in Ca^{2+} causes binding of Ca^{2+}/calmodulin to regulatory domain of enzyme, removing enzyme inhibition. Adjacent activated monomers can phosphorylate substrate proteins as well as one another, and autophosphorylation greatly increases calmodulin affinity of the calmodulin-binding site, effectively trapping calmodulin on the enzyme for up to several minutes. Even after calmodulin falls off the enzyme, the presence of phosphate produces an *autonomous* state, which is Ca^{2+}-independent and has partial activity. Removal of the phosphate returns the enzyme to its resting state. (After Braun and Schulman, 1995.)

tein but which becomes exposed after the binding of calmodulin. This threonine is apparently autophosphorylated *by an adjacent monomer on the same holoenzyme* (Hanson et al., 1994). The attachment of a phosphate group at this site has two very important consequences: first, the affinity for calmodulin binding to the protein is increased as much as 1000-fold (Meyer et al., 1992), so calmodulin remains bound for as long as several minutes even after the free-Ca^{2+} concentration in the cell has fallen; and second, the enzyme retains some activity even after calmodulin has dissociated from the protein. This Ca^{2+}-independent activity is stable until the threonine is dephosphorylated by protein phosphatases (Miller and Kennedy, 1986; Lai, Nairn, and Greengard, 1986). Thus a cytoplasmic increase in free Ca^{2+}, provided it is sufficiently large and prolonged to produce autophosphorylation of a substantial fraction of the enzyme monomers, can produce a prolonged activation of CaM kinase and an extended physiological effect.

CaM Kinase Modulation of Glutamate Responses

Because glutamate AMPA receptors are probably the most common excitatory receptors in the brain, the phosphorylation of these receptors by protein kinases could provide an important mechanism for synaptic modulation. Since the first discovery of AMPA receptor modulation by PKA at the photoreceptor synapse in the retina (Knapp and Dowling, 1987), the role of phosphorylation in the modulation of glutamate receptor responses has been studied with keen interest (see Roche, Tingley, and Huganir, 1994; Levitan, 1994). The great abundance of CaM kinase II in the CNS would seem to indicate that this protein may play a major role in receptor modulation, and several groups have investigated possible effects of this kinase on glutamate receptor function.

One approach has been to introduce CaM kinase into cells expressing AMPA receptors (Yakel et al., 1995) or into dissociated neurons or cells in brain slices (McGlade-McCulloh et al., 1993; Kolaj et al., 1994; Lledo et al., 1995). This experiment is usually done with a form of the enzyme made nearly irreversibly active by incubation with ATPγS, a form of ATP for which one of the oxygens in the terminal phosphate is replaced with a sulphur atom (like GTPγS—see Chapter 12). This substitution has the conse-

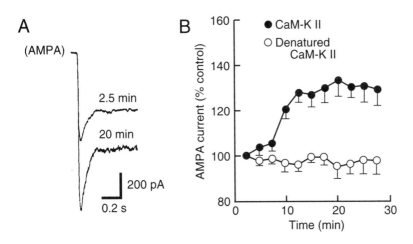

A (AMPA)

2.5 min

20 min

200 pA

0.2 s

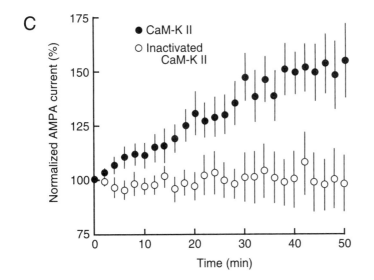

Fig. 13.11 CaM kinase II enhances glutamate currents. **(A)** and **(B)** Whole-cell recordings from dissociated neurons of the dorsal horn of the spinal cord. **(A)** Recording pipette contained 200 nM of CaM kinase II stably activated by thiophosphorylation with ATPγS. Superimposed responses, at indicated times (given as time after forming whole-cell recording), to applications of 30 μM AMPA by rapid perfusion. **(B)** Peak AMPA-induced current as a function of time after forming whole-cell recording for pipettes containing stably activated and heat-denatured CaM kinase II. Data points show means and one standard error. AMPA current is given as a percentage of the first response recorded after going whole-cell. $V_H = -60$ mV. (Reprinted from Kolaj et al., 1994, with permission of the authors and of the American Physiological Society.) **(C)** Experiments similar to those in **(A)** and **(B)** but from CA1 pyramidal cells recorded in slices of guinea pig hippocampus. Whole-cell recording, $V_H = -75$ mV. Pipettes contained 200 nM either of heat-inactivated or thiophosphorylated CaM kinase II. Responses to AMPA were evoked *iontophoretically,* with a pipette (placed close to the cell) containing 10 mM AMPA at pH 8. At this pH, AMPA has a net negative charge, and negative current passed from the pipette into the bathing solution caused AMPA to be delivered to the vicinity of the cell. Data show means ± standard errors as percentage of response recorded just after formation of whole-cell recording. (Reprinted from Lledo et al., 1995, with permission of the authors and of the National Academy of Sciences.)

quence of making this terminal phosphate group more resistant to dephosphorylation by phosphatases, and autothiophosphorylated CaM kinase II remains active almost indefinitely.

These experiments all appear to give a similar result (see Fig. 13.11). The responses in Figs. 13.11A and B were recorded from dissociated neurons from the dorsal horn of the spinal cord (from

Kolaj et al., 1994). Application of AMPA 2.5 and 20 minutes after establishing a whole-cell recording with a pipette containing auto-thiophosphorylated CaM kinase II resulted in a consistent increase in the size of the AMPA response (Fig. 13.11A). A summary of many such experiments is given in Fig. 13.11B, for activated CaM kinase II and for a similar series of experiments in which the enzyme was heat-denatured. Similar recordings (Fib. 13.11C) were obtained from a different series of experiments from hippocampal slices (Lledo et al., 1995). Activated CaM kinase II was again introduced by dialysis during whole-cell recording, this time into CA1 pyramidal cells. The effect of the kinase on AMPA currents was similar.

Numerous experiments demonstrate that CaM kinase II can become activated during normal neuronal activity (see Hanson and Schulman, 1992; Braun and Schulman, 1995). The results in Fig. 13.11 show that activated CaM kinase II can increase the amplitude of AMPA responses, and other evidence indicates that this may occur by direct phosphorylation of the glutamate receptors (McGlade-McCulloh et al., 1993; Tan, Wenthold, and Soderling, 1994; Yakel et al., 1995). Effects of CaM kinase on glutamate receptors could have dramatic effects on excitatory synapses in the central nervous system, perhaps contributing to the mechanism for long-term changes in synaptic efficacy (Barria et al., 1997—see Chapter 14).

NO

The gas nitric oxide (NO) was first identified as a second messenger in studies of the smooth muscle fibers surrounding the blood vessels of the circulatory system (see Ignarro, 1990; Umans and Levi, 1995). When vascular smooth muscle is contracted by exposure, say, to norepinephrine, it can be relaxed again by exposure to, for example, the peptide bradykinin. The signal cascade responsible for this relaxation is, however, not initiated within the smooth muscle cells themselves but rather within the endothelial cells surrounding the muscle cells (Furchgott and Zawadzki, 1980). The endothelial cells release a factor with the following properties: (1) it is unstable, with a half-life of the order of several seconds; (2) it can diffuse freely between cells; (3) its effects can be blocked by extracellular hemoglobin (hemoglobin binds NO with an affinity even higher than it binds O_2); and (4) its effects can be mimicked by compounds called S-nitrosothiols and by sodium nitroprusside (SNP), which undergo spontaneous decomposition in aqueous solution to release NO. Nitroglycerin, which is used clinically as a vasodilator of coronary blood vessels, reacts with the amino acid cysteine to produce S-nitrosocysteine, which generates liberated NO. Finally, (5) the endothelium-derived releasing factor produces an increase in muscle cGMP by stimulating soluble guanylyl cyclase.

Three groups showed at about the same time that the endothelial cells surrounding blood vessels can release chemically identifiable NO (Palmer, Ferrige, and Moncada, 1987; Ignarro et al., 1987; Furchgott, 1988). Subsequently, NO was shown to participate in a variety of functions mediated by the autonomic nervous system (see Schmidt and Walter, 1994; Hobbs and Ignarro, 1997), including, for example, penile erection (see Furchgott, 1988; Burnett et al., 1992). NO is probably also an important mediator of synaptic function in the central nervous system, since the enzyme responsible for synthesizing NO (called nitric oxide synthase, or NOS) is present in many areas of the brain (Schuman and Madison, 1994; Garthwaite and Boulton, 1995; Zhang and Snyder, 1995). Furthermore, male mice lacking brain NOS exhibit increased aggressive and sexual behavior (Nelson et al., 1995), suggesting that NO serves some important neurological function.

Nitric oxide synthase has been isolated, and its genes have been cloned and sequenced from several different tissues in the body. These genes direct the synthesis of a family of related proteins with similar properties (Marietta, 1994; Griffith and Stuehr, 1995; Hobbs and Ignarro, 1997). All are large, heme-containing proteins with binding sites for the electron donors FMN, FAD, and FADPH, and all catalyze a redox reaction that oxidizes the amino acid L-arginine to L-citrulline, releasing NO (Crane et al., 1997). The forms of NOS found in endothelial cells and in the brain also contain a binding site for Ca^{2+}/calmodulin and are activated by an increase in the intracellular free-Ca^{2+} concentration. Thus Ca^{2+}, released from internal stores or entering the cell through ion channels, can bind to calmodulin and activate the synthesis of NO.

Although the role of NO in the peripheral nervous system is well established, we have little idea what it does in the CNS. This molecule is an unusual second messenger, since as a gas it is able to diffuse freely across cell membranes and so can travel both within and between cells over long distances before it is inactivated. The lifetime of NO is probably limited mostly by its instability in solution and is likely to be of the order of several seconds. Within this time NO would be able to diffuse many micrometers away from the cell that produced it and, in the dense plexiform layers of the central nervous system, potentially affect millions of synaptic terminals (Garthwaite and Boulton, 1995).

NO has been shown to bind to and stimulate the soluble form of the enzyme guanylyl cyclase (see Hobbs and Ignarro, 1997). Like NOS, soluble guanylyl cyclase is a heme-containing protein, and NO binds to the heme and produces a change in conformation that activates the synthesis of cGMP (see Schmidt, Lohmann, and Walter, 1993; Garthwaite and Boulton, 1995). In smooth muscle, NO has long been known to produce an increase in cGMP concentration (see Ignarro, 1990), which is thought to be responsible for the relaxation of the muscle. In the CNS, glutamate has been shown to produce large increases in cGMP, particularly in the cerebellum (see Garthwaite, 1991; Schuman and Madison, 1994; Zhang and Snyder, 1995). The cerebellum contains a high concentration of the brain form of NOS—it is from the cerebellum that brain NOS was first biochemically isolated (Bredt and Snyder, 1990). The cerebellum also has relatively high concentrations of soluble guanylyl cyclase.

When cerebellar slices or cell suspensions are exposed to glutamate or to NMDA, the cGMP increases, and this effect is selectively blocked by NMDA receptor antagonists like AP5. It is also blocked by inhibitors of NOS (like N^{ω}-monomethyl-L-arginine) or by hemoglobin, and it therefore seems likely that the increase in cGMP is mediated by NO. Bredt and Snyder (1989) measured the rate of NOS activity in the cerebellum by incubating cerebellar slices in tritiated arginine and measuring the production of tritiated citrulline. They discovered that the increase in cGMP concentration and the production of tritiated citrulline had an almost identical dependence on NMDA concentration (Fig. 13.12A). NMDA seemed to be stimulating NOS, and the NO produced then appeared to be activating guanylyl cyclase to produce cGMP.

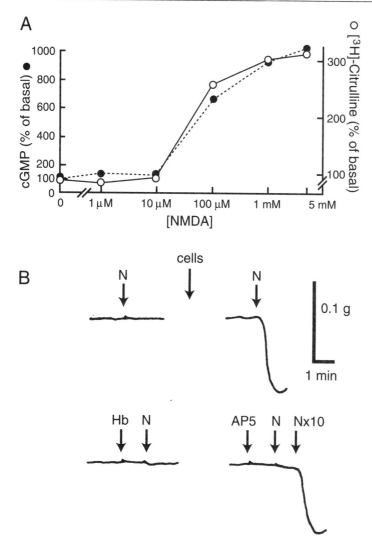

A

B

Fig. 13.12 NMDA receptor activation produces NO evolution in the cerebellum. **(A)** Cerebellar slices, pooled from several rats, were stimulated by incubation with NMDA at the concentration given on the abscissa. The cGMP levels were determined biochemically by standard procedures (radioimmunoassay), and the activity of NO synthase was determined by incubating the tissue in radioactive [³H]-arginine and measuring the production of [³H]-citrulline. Other experiments (not shown) indicate that citrulline production is stoichiometric with NO formation. Formation of NO and cGMP show an almost identical dependence on NMDA concentration. (From Bredt and Snyder, 1989, with permission of the authors.) **(B)** NO evolution was assayed by measuring contraction of smooth muscle stripped of endothelial cells from rat aorta. Traces show tension of aorta smooth muscle after addition of 100 µM NMDA (*N*), first in the absence of cerebellar cells (*top, left*) and then after their addition (*top, right*). The muscle was then washed to remove cells, and fresh cells were added in the presence of hemoglobin *(Hb)*, which binds NO. Now NMDA *(N)* has no effect (*bottom, left*). After washing and further addition of fresh cells, 50 µM AP5 inhibited the response to 100 µM NMDA but not to 1 mM NMDA (*bottom, right*). (Reprinted from Garthwaite, Charles, and Chess-Williams, 1988, with permission of the authors and of Macmillan Magazine Limited.)

Direct evidence for the production of NO by the cells of the cerebellum was obtained by Garthwaite, Charles, and Chess-Williams (1988), who substituted suspensions of cerebellar cells for endothelial cells in preparations of vascular smooth muscle. When the muscle was incubated in the presence of cerebellar cells, NMDA produced a large relaxation of muscle tension, which could be blocked by hemoglobin or by AP5 (Fig. 13.12B).

Fig. 13.13 Mechanism of activation of NOS and guanylyl cyclase in the central nervous system. *GTP,* guanosine triphosphate; *cGMP,* guanosine 3′,5′-cyclic monophosphate; *GC,* guanylyl cyclase; *CaM,* calmodulin; NOS, NO synthase.

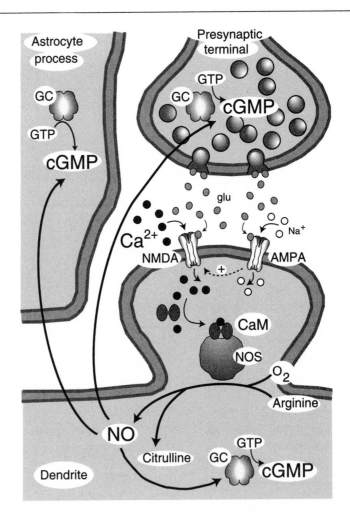

How is NMDA activating NOS? Since increases in cGMP do not occur in the cerebellum in the absence of extracellular Ca^{2+} (Garthwaite, Charles, and Chess-Williams, 1988), the most likely explanation is that Ca^{2+}, entering through open NMDA receptors, binds to calmodulin and stimulates NOS. Although the facts of this scheme, depicted in Fig. 13.13, seem well established, we still do not know for certain which cells in the cerebellum produce the NO and which the cGMP. Similar uncertainties exist for other areas of the CNS (e.g., the cortex), where glutamate-induced NO production and cGMP increases have also been observed.

Even more puzzling is the question of what the cGMP actually does. In photoreceptors (Chapter 16) and retinal bipolar cells (Chapter 12), cGMP acts directly on specialized ion channels to alter their probability of opening. Many cell populations within the central nervous system and elsewhere in the body contain a cGMP-dependent protein kinase (PKG), and it is conceivable that the increase in cGMP activates this protein, which then phosphorylates specific protein targets (see Francis and Corbin, 1994; Hobbs and Ignarro, 1997). In the substantia nigra, an NO-stimulated increase in cGMP produces phosphorylation of DARPP-32 (Tsou, Snyder, and Greengard, 1993), a protein inhibitor of protein phosphatase 1 (see Chapter 12). Other targets probably exist but have not yet been identified, and we still have little notion of the physiological significance of the cGMP increase.

Summary

Important molecular tools have revolutionized the study of Ca^{2+} in cells. These include buffers like BAPTA, which can be used to retard changes in intracellular Ca^{2+} concentration; fluorescent Ca^{2+} indicator molecules, like fura-2 and fluo-3, which make possible the measurement of the free-Ca^{2+} concentration; and caged compounds, which permit the rapid release of Ca^{2+} and other substances at specific locations inside or outside of cells. Methods for studying Ca^{2+} have become almost as powerful as techniques for measuring electrical activity, and together they have established Ca^{2+} as one of the best-characterized messenger substances in the CNS.

These tools have been used to show that neurotransmitters can produce increases in intracellular free Ca^{2+} concentration, often by release from internal stores. Ca^{2+} is contained in cellular vesicles whose membranes have large tetrameric receptors belonging to two related families, the IP$_3$ receptors and the ryanodine receptors. Both are Ca^{2+} channels gated by the binding either of the second messenger IP$_3$ or of Ca^{2+} itself. The opening of the Ca^{2+} channel permits the efflux of Ca^{2+} from the vesicle into the cytoplasm. In many cells, the Ca^{2+} increase can take the form of slow oscillations in Ca^{2+} concentration or of waves spreading across the cell. The depletion of Ca^{2+} from the vesicles somehow triggers the opening of Ca^{2+} channels in the plasma membrane, called *Ca^{2+}-release-*

activated Ca²⁺ channels. The influx of Ca^{2+} through these channels produces a further increase in intracellular Ca^{2+} and causes the depleted vesicles to be refilled.

All this is important because of what increases in Ca^{2+} do in neurons. Of the many proteins and enzymes shown to be regulated by Ca^{2+} or by Ca^{2+} bound to calmodulin, this chapter focused on just two: CaM kinase II and nitric oxide synthase. CaM kinase II is a serine/threonine protein kinase activated by the binding of Ca^{2+}/calmodulin. It has peculiar properties: an unusual hub-and-spoke arrangement of the protein monomers forming the holoenzyme facilitates its autophosphorylation by adjacent monomers, which greatly prolongs the activation of the enzyme to increases in intracellular Ca^{2+}. Experiments suggest that CaM kinase II may play an important role in the modulation of AMPA receptors.

The other enzyme described, nitric oxide synthase (or NOS), synthesizes the unconventional second messenger NO. Like CaM kinase II, NOS is activated by Ca^{2+}/calmodulin, and there is now excellent evidence that brain NOS is widely distributed and can be stimulated, for example, by the opening of NMDA-type glutamate receptors. Since NO is highly reactive, it may have many different effects on neurons (Schuman and Madison, 1994) and may be an important cause of nerve cell death following stroke (Iadecola, 1997). NO can also bind to the heme group of soluble guanylyl cyclase and stimulate the synthesis of cGMP. These pathways are likely to be of considerable importance, but our understanding of NO in the brain is probably in its infancy.

Why would the central nervous system use a gas as a second messenger? Wouldn't the spread of a gas be too large? If millions of presynaptic terminals are exposed to NO, what are the rules that determine which cells respond and which do not? Does the increase in cGMP caused by NO produce nonselective systemic effects, or are the increases in cyclic nucleotide actually carefully localized to produce specific results? We do not know the answers to these questions, but we do know that answering them will probably reveal important new aspects of CNS function. The mechanism of action of NO may be of rather general significance, since NO may not be the only gas used by the brain as a second messenger. Neurons also contain the enzyme heme oxygenase, which synthesizes carbon monoxide (CO). CO can also bind to soluble guanylyl cyclase, and there is evidence that CO can regulate brain cGMP (Verma et al., 1993; Dawson and Snyder, 1994). Metabotropic transmission in the nervous system probably has many more surprises in store for us; the more we understand, the richer and more varied this mode of communication seems to become.

14

Long-Term Potentiation

THOMAS O'DELL

THE STRENGTH or efficacy of synaptic transmission at many excitatory synapses in the brain is not fixed but instead is modulated, over a time scale of seconds to minutes, by neurotransmitters acting through many of the G-protein-mediated second-messenger signaling pathways described in Chapters 11–13. In addition to these relatively short-lived modulatory influences, synaptic transmission at many excitatory synapses can also be modified on a much longer time scale, ranging from many hours to several weeks or more. These longer-lasting changes in synaptic strength are induced by certain patterns of synaptic activity and are thought to have important roles in long-term changes in synaptic function, such as the refinement of synaptic connections during development and the storage of new information during learning.

Although many synapses in the brain are capable of activity-dependent changes in strength, much of what we know about the cellular and molecular processes that underlie these changes comes from studies of synaptic transmission in a region of the brain known as the hippocampus. Why has there been such a strong focus on the plasticity of hippocampal synapses? Part of the answer to this question is simply convenience—compared with many other brain regions, the relatively simple anatomy of the hippocampus makes it amenable to both *in vivo* and *in vitro* electrophysiological studies of synaptic transmission. In addition, neuropsychological studies in humans as well as behavioral studies in animals indicate that the hippocampus has a crucial role in some forms of learning and memory (Squire and Zola-Morgan, 1991). The hippocampus has thus become a major region of focus for investigators interested in understanding the molecular events responsible for activity-dependent changes in synaptic strength and the way these changes may be used by neurons to store new information during memory formation. As we will see in this chapter, although multiple cellular mechanisms (involving many of the signaling molecules discussed in Chapters 11–13) control the strength of excitatory synaptic transmission in the hippocampus, all of these processes share a common dependence on Ca^{2+} as a second messenger.

Synaptic Circuitry of the Hippocampus

The hippocampal formation consists of three major regions—the dentate gyrus and the CA3 and CA1 regions of the hippocampus proper. In a general sense these three regions can be thought of as forming a "trisynaptic circuit" through which information flows into, through, and then out of the hippocampus (Fig. 14.1A). A major anatomical pathway through which information flows into this circuit is the perforant pathway, a collection of axons from neurons in nearby cortical regions that make excitatory synaptic connections onto the granule cells of the dentate gyrus. The dentate gyrus granule cells in turn send axonal projections, known as the mossy fibers, to the CA3 region of the hippocampus, where they make excitatory synapses onto the large CA3 pyramidal cells. Finally, CA3 pyramidal cell axons, known as the Schaffer collaterals, project to the CA1 region of the hippocampus and form excitatory synaptic contacts onto the dendrites of the CA1 pyramidal cells. From here, information leaves the hippocampus through CA1 pyramidal cell projections to neurons in other regions of the brain.

Although the trisynaptic circuit shown in Fig. 14.1A ignores the presence of numerous types of interneurons, as well as other types of synaptic connections onto the principal cells in the three regions of the hippocampal formation, it helps to emphasize an important point. At each of the three major synapses in the circuit a brief period of high-frequency synaptic stimulation (also called *tetanic* stimulation) induces a persistent increase in the strength of synaptic transmission known as *long-term potentiation* (LTP) (Bliss and Lømo, 1973; Bliss and Collingridge, 1993; Nicoll and Malenka, 1995).

Studies of the mechanisms responsible for LTP at hippocampal synapses suggest that there are at least two different types of LTP. One type requires activation of *N*-methyl-D-aspartate (NMDA) re-

Fig. 14.1 **(A)** The three major excitatory synaptic connections of the trisynaptic circuit as seen in a slice of the hippocampus cut perpendicular to its long axis. Arrows indicate some of the major pathways into and between the subdivisions of the hippocampal formation. **(B)** Coincident pre- and postsynaptic activity is required for the induction of LTP. The graph plots the mean size of the EPSPs (estimated from the initial slope) in CA1 pyramidal cells elicited by repetitive, low-frequency stimulation of the Schaffer collateral fibers. After a recording was made of a baseline period of evoked EPSPs for approximately 15 minutes, presynaptic fiber stimulation *(STIM)* was stopped and current was injected through an intracellular microelectrode to strongly depolarize the postsynaptic membrane potential *(MP)*. EPSPs were unchanged when the postsynaptic membrane potential was returned to resting levels and presynaptic fiber stimulation was resumed, indicating that strong postsynaptic depolarization alone is not sufficient for the induction of LTP. As can be seen in the second part of the experiment, synaptic transmission does undergo LTP if presynaptic stimulation is continued during depolarization of the postsynaptic cell. The traces above the graph show EPSPs evoked at the time points indicated by the circled numbers. (Adapted from Malenka, Kauer, Perkel, and Nicoll, 1989, with permission of the authors and of Elsevier Science Ltd.)

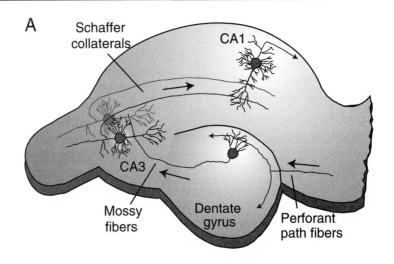

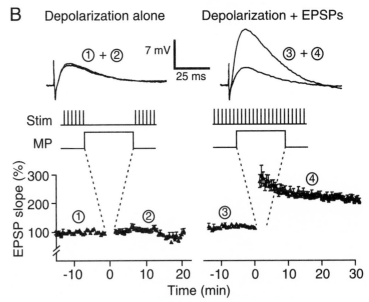

ceptors and is seen at both the perforant pathway synapses onto dentate gyrus granule cells and at the Schaffer collateral synapses onto CA1 pyramidal cells. The second type of LTP, seen at mossy fiber synapses onto the CA3 pyramidal cells, does not require NMDA receptor action and is often referred to as mossy fiber LTP (or more generally as NMDA receptor–independent LTP). Below I consider what is known about the cellular and molecular processes responsible for these two forms of LTP, emphasizing studies on CA1 and CA3 pyramidal cells. I also consider mechanisms that may be responsible for a third type of synaptic plasticity, long-term depression (LTD).

NMDA Receptor–Dependent LTP

If the Schaffer collateral fibers are electrically stimulated at a low rate (once every minute or so), the average amplitude of postsynaptic potentials recorded either from individual CA1 pyramidal cells using intracellular recording techniques or from populations of pyramidal cells using extracellular methods is relatively stable. Following a brief, high-frequency burst of Schaffer collateral fiber stimulation, however, synaptic transmission undergoes a dramatic and persistent potentiation (see Fig. 14.2A). This enhancement of synaptic transmission can persist for several hours and, when studied *in vivo,* even for as long as several weeks—hence the name *long-term* potentiation. The long-lasting nature of LTP was one of the characteristics that first suggested that it might be an important synaptic mechanism involved in memory formation.

Early studies revealed that LTP had several characteristics that provided important insights into the synaptic processes involved in inducing LTP (Nicoll, Kauer, and Malenka, 1988). First, LTP was found to be *synapse-specific.* This characteristic of LTP was seen in experiments where synaptic responses evoked by two independent groups of presynaptic afferents were monitored before and after tetanic stimulation of only one group of afferents. In these experiments only those synapses that had been activated by the tetanus underwent LTP; other synapses that were not active during the tetanus did not potentiate (Fig. 14.2A). Although more recent experiments suggest that LTP induced at one synapse may result in potentiation of nearby inactive synapses, this "spreading" LTP is anatomically discrete, ocurring over a distance of less than 70 μm from the activated synapses (Engert and Bonhoeffer, 1997). The restriction of LTP to only those synapses directly activated during the tetanus, or ones located close to the activated synapses, suggests that the strength of small groups of synapses onto a neuron can be potentiated independently, providing a powerful mechanism whereby neuronal circuits could store large amounts of information through a process like LTP.

A second characteristic of LTP became evident when investigators began to examine the effects of presynaptic stimulation intensity on the induction of LTP. These studies showed that tetanic stimulation easily induced LTP when strong-intensity presynaptic stimulation was used to activate a large number of presynaptic fibers. However, the same high-frequency stimulation protocols fail to induce LTP at weak-intensity presynaptic stimulation strengths, which activate only a small number of fibers (Fig. 14.2B) (McNaughton, Douglas, and Goddard, 1978). There thus appears to be a threshold number of synaptic inputs that must be coactivated for LTP to occur, and presynaptic fibers interact to reach this threshold, a property known as *cooperativity*.

Cooperativity gives rise to a third, related property of LTP, *associativity*. High-frequency activation of a small number of presynaptic inputs typically fails to induce LTP (because of the lack of cooperativity). If this small group of fibers is activated at the same time a separate, larger group of Schaffer collateral fibers is activated, however, then the small group of fibers (as well as the larger group) will undergo LTP (Fig. 14.2C). Thus by virtue of being active when a larger group of fibers is activated, synapses can associate with one another and undergo LTP (Barrionuevo and Brown, 1983; Levy and Steward, 1979).

The key to understanding the initial events responsible for the induction of LTP, and how these processes account for the synapse-specific, cooperative, and associative properties of LTP, lies in thinking about what happens on both the pre- and postsynaptic sides of the synapse during the high-frequency synaptic stimulation. The tetanic stimulation of presynaptic fibers induces glutamate release from the presynaptic terminals and depolarization of the postsynaptic cell via activation of postsynaptic AMPA-type glutamate receptors. The size of the postsynaptic depolarization will be directly related to the number of presynaptic fibers activated. From the properties of LTP discussed above, it seems that the size of the postsynaptic depolarization during a tetanus is crucial for the induction of LTP. Thus, if a synapse is inactive (no depolarization) or if only a few presynaptic fibers are tetanically stimulated

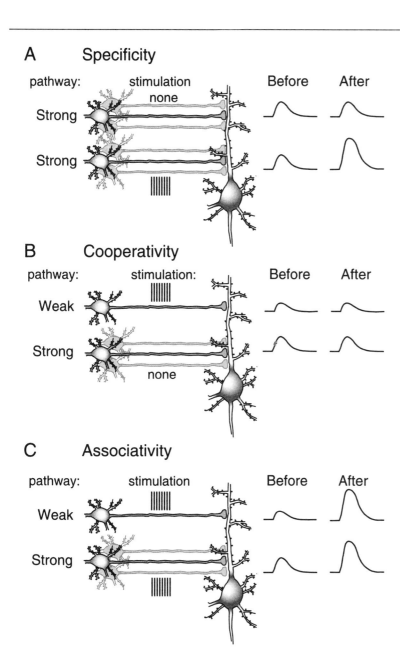

A Specificity

pathway: stimulation
                 none   Before   After

Strong

Strong

B Cooperativity

pathway: stimulation: Before   After

Weak

Strong
                 none

C Associativity

pathway: stimulation   Before   After

Weak

Strong

Fig. 14.2 Synapse-specific, cooperative, and associative properties of NMDA receptor–dependent LTP in the CA1 region of the hippocampus. **(A)** The induction of LTP is restricted to only those synapses that undergo high-frequency stimulation. As indicated by the lines near the axons, following high-frequency stimulation of a group of presynaptic fibers (strong pathway), EPSPs (shown on the right) are increased. Other synaptic inputs that were not active at the same time do not undergo LTP. **(B)** Although high-frequency stimulation of a large group of axons can induce LTP, the same stimulation delivered to one or only a few axons (weak pathway) fails to induce LTP. This indicates that a minimum number of presynaptic fibers must be co-activated to induce LTP with high-frequency synaptic stimulation. **(C)** Although the weak pathway fails to undergo LTP when activated alone, the synapses formed by these axons will potentiate if they are activated at the same time as the strong pathway. In this case, LTP of the weak pathway occurs because activity in this pathway was associated in time with activity in another group of fibers. (Adapted from Nicoll, Kauer, and Malenka, 1988.)

(producing a small postsynaptic depolarization), no LTP is induced. If a larger group of fibers are activated, either alone or in combination with a smaller collection of afferents, then a large postsynaptic depolarization will be elicited, and under these conditions LTP will be induced. Strong postsynaptic depolarization thus seems to be required for the induction of LTP. Consistent with this notion, if the postsynaptic depolarization produced by tetanic stimulation of a large group of presynaptic fibers is prevented by injection of a hyperpolarizing current through an intracellular recording electrode, the induction of LTP is blocked (Malinow and Miller, 1986).

In the absence of synaptic stimulation, no LTP is seen when a CA1 pyramidal cell is depolarized with a strong depolarizing current pulse delivered to the cell through an intracellular recording electrode (Fig. 14.1B). Thus, while postsynaptic depolarization is necessary for the induction of LTP, it is not sufficient. LTP is induced, however, if this postsynaptic membrane depolarization is paired with low-frequency presynaptic fiber stimulation (Fig. 14.1B—see Kelso, Ganong, and Brown, 1986; Sastry, Goh, and Auyeung, 1986; Gustafsson, Wigström, and Abraham, 1987). This suggests that two conditions, strong postsynaptic depolarization along with presynaptic activity, are both necessary for inducing LTP.

Activation of NMDA-type Glutamate Receptors Is Required for the Induction of LTP

As progress was made in understanding the properties of the glutamate receptor subtypes involved in fast excitatory synaptic transmission in the central nervous system, it became clear that the NMDA receptor had properties that could enable it to detect the coincident presynaptic activity and postsynaptic depolarization required for the induction of LTP. As discussed in Chapters 1 and 9, in addition to glycine binding to the NMDA receptor, activation requires two signals: glutamate binding must occur, as must sufficient membrane depolarization to relieve the voltage-dependent Mg^{2+} ion block of the NMDA receptor ion channel (see Fig. 1.9). Synaptic NMDA receptors will thus be activated only during periods of coincident pre- and postsynaptic activity, just the conditions required for the induction of LTP. Indeed, selective NMDA receptor antagonists like AP5 (see Chapter 9) have little effect on synaptic transmission during low-frequency Schaffer collateral fiber stimulation, but they potently block the induction of LTP (Collingridge, Kehl, and McLennan, 1983).

Ca²⁺ Influx Through the NMDA Receptor Ion Channel Triggers the Induction of LTP

If the NMDA receptor detects the coincidence of pre- and postsynaptic activity required for inducing LTP, how does it signal the occurrence of this coincidence to the cell? Since the NMDA receptor ion channel is highly permeable to Ca^{2+}, patterns of synaptic activity that induce LTP should produce a large influx of Ca^{2+} into the cell. This increase in intracellular Ca^{2+} could thus serve as the trigger that activates postsynaptic mechanisms responsible for increasing synaptic strength. Direct evidence for this hypothesis first came from experiments showing that Ca^{2+} chelators, like EGTA or BAPTA (Fig. 13.1), block the induction of LTP when they are injected into CA1 pyramidal cells (Lynch et al., 1983; Malenka et al., 1988).

Additional support for the idea that Ca^{2+} has an essential role in the induction of LTP was obtained from studies examining changes in intracellular Ca^{2+} in CA1 pyramidal cells, loaded with the Ca^{2+} indicator dye fura-2 (see Fig. 13.2). In these experiments pyramidal cells in a hippocampal slice (as in Fig. 14.1) were loaded with fura-2, and an array of photodiodes was positioned along the length of the pyramidal cells to measure changes in dye fluorescence during trains of synaptic stimulation. Weak trains of synaptic activation that did not induce LTP produced changes in dye fluorescence throughout the cells, presumably via influx of Ca^{2+} through voltage-gated calcium channels. In contrast, patterns of synaptic stimulation that induced LTP elicited an additional, AP5-sensitive increase in intracellular Ca^{2+} that was specifically localized to the dendritic region containing the activated synapses (Regehr and Tank, 1990; see Fig. 14.3). These experiments show that patterns of synaptic stimulation that induce LTP produce an NMDA receptor–mediated increase in intracellular Ca^{2+}. Along with previous experiments showing that Ca^{2+} chelators block LTP, they provide

Fig. 14.3 High-frequency synaptic stimulation induces NMDA receptor–dependent increases in intracellular calcium. **(A)** In these experiments an intracellular electrode was used to introduce the calcium-sensitive dye fura-2 into individual CA1 pyramidal cells, and an array of photodiodes was used to measure fura-2 fluorescence at the cell body and at several points along the apical dendrite of a CA1 pyramidal cell *(boxes)*. **(B)** Increases in intracellular calcium concentration measured from fura-2 fluorescence when high-frequency (100 Hz) synaptic stimulation was delivered either in the presence or absence of the NMDA receptor blocker AP5. **(C)** The change in intracellular calcium that occurred during high-frequency stimulation in AP5 was subtracted from the change occurring in the absence of AP5 to give the component of the calcium increase due to activation of NMDA receptors. Note that this component is greatest near the site of the activated synapses. (Adapted from Regehr and Tank, 1990, and used with the permission of the authors and of Macmillan Magazines Limited.)

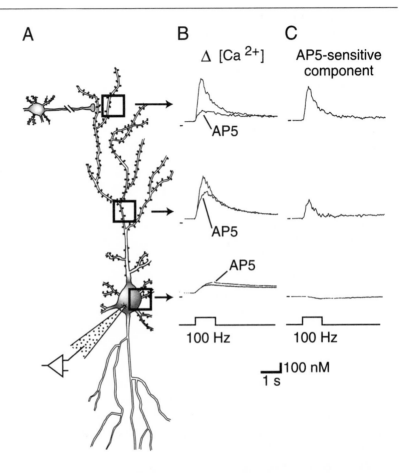

strong evidence that Ca^{2+} influx through NMDA receptors is required for the induction of LTP.

Although many experiments now indicate that Ca^{2+} serves as a crucial trigger for the cellular mechanisms responsible for LTP, it is not clear from these results whether this increase in intracellular Ca^{2+} is sufficient for the induction of LTP, or if other factors are also necessary. Evidence addressing this point has come from experiments using the photolabile caged-Ca^{2+} compound nitr-5. As discussed in Chapter 13, the affinity of nitr-5 for Ca^{2+} (like that of DM-nitrophen—see Fig. 13.4) is markedly reduced by exposure to UV light. Thus, nitr-5 can be preloaded with Ca^{2+} (by mixing it with a Ca^{2+}-containing solution) and then injected into cells from an intracellular microelectrode. Following a flash of UV light, intracellular levels of Ca^{2+} increase as nitr-5 is rapidly converted to its low-Ca^{2+}-affinity form and Ca^{2+} is released into the cytoplasm. When this experiment was done for hippocampal CA1 pyramidal cells, flashes of UV light produced a large and lasting potentiation of synaptic transmission (Malenka et al., 1988; see Fig. 14.4B). If pyramidal cells were filled with nitr-5 that had not been loaded with Ca^{2+}, flashes of UV light had no effect on synaptic strength. Indeed, in other experiments the induction of LTP by high-frequency stimulation was blocked when cells were injected with nitr-5 that had not been Ca^{2+} loaded and was not exposed to UV illumination (Fig. 14.4C). This is as expected, since unloaded, unilluminated Nitr-5 is a potent Ca^{2+} chelator like EGTA or BAPTA. Thus it appears that an increase in intracellular Ca^{2+} is not only necessary but also sufficient for the induction of LTP.

Ca^{2+} as a Second Messenger in LTP: The CaM Kinase II Hypothesis

Although it is now clear that the induction of LTP in CA1 pyramidal cells critically depends on NMDA receptor activation and subsequent increases in intracellular Ca^{2+}, less is known about the Ca^{2+}-activated processes actually responsible for potentiating synaptic transmission. It is known, however, that the induction of LTP requires the activity of a number of different protein kinases. The list of kinases that may be involved in LTP is long; just a few examples are PKC (Reymann et al., 1988; Malinow, Schulman, and Tsien, 1989), PKA (Frey, Huang, and Kandel, 1993), PKG (Zhuo et al., 1994), and one or more types of tyrosine kinases (O'Dell et al., 1991). However, one protein kinase, the multifunctional, Ca^{2+}/calmodulin-dependent protein kinase CaM kinase II, has a central role in the induction of LTP (Malinow, Schulman and Tsien, 1989; Malenka et al., 1989).

CaM kinase II has a number of properties that make it an attractive candidate to be a "downstream" target for Ca^{2+} in the signaling pathway responsible for LTP (see Chapter 13). First, as its name implies, CaM kinase II is activated by the Ca^{2+}-binding protein calmodulin following increases in intracellular Ca^{2+} (see Fig. 11.1). Second, CaM kinase II is an extremely abundant protein in

Fig. 14.4 Increases in postsynaptic calcium are sufficient for the induction of LTP. **(A)** In hippocampal slices maintained *in vitro,* an intracellular microelectrode was used both to introduce the photolabile Ca^{2+} chelator nitr-5 into individual CA1 pyramidal cells and to make intracellular recordings of EPSPs evoked by Schaffer collateral fiber stimulation. An extracellular electrode was used to monitor EPSPs elicited in other nearby cells. **(B)** EPSPs intracellularly recorded before and after photolysis of nitr-5 by a flash of UV light. When the intracellular electrode contained Ca^{2+}-loaded nitr-5, increases in intracellular Ca^{2+} following the UV light flash induced a large potentiation of synaptic transmission *(solid circles).* In contrast, flashes of UV light had no persistent effect on synaptic transmission in cells injected with unloaded Nitr-5 *(open circles).* **(C)** Tetanic stimulation fails to induce LTP in cells injected with unloaded, unilluminated nitr-5, which is a potent Ca^{2+} chelator *(bottom graph).* Extracellular recordings of EPSPs in other cells indicate that the tetanus does induce LTP at synapses onto other cells in slice *(top graph).* Examples of both intracellularly and extracellularly recorded EPSPs evoked at times indicated by the circled numbers are shown to the right. (Adapted from Malenka et al., 1988.)

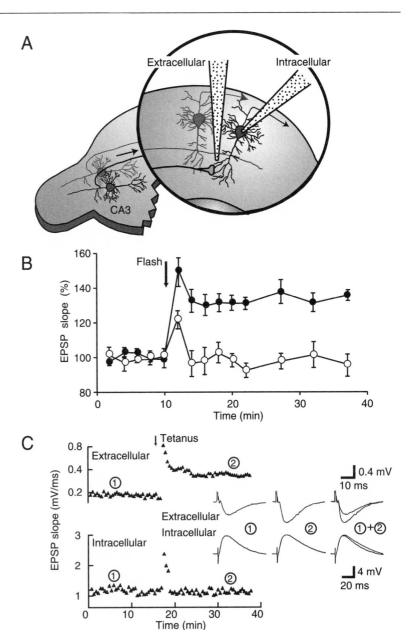

the nervous system and is highly localized to the postsynaptic density at excitatory synapses in the hippocampus. Thus CaM kinase II is localized in a manner consistent with its having an important role in synaptic transmission. Third, CaM kinase II activity is regulated by autophosphorylation, an intermolecular enzymatic event whereby one CaM kinase II monomer phosphorylates other activated CaM kinase II monomers on a threonine residue that resides within the regulatory domain of the enzyme (see Fig. 13.10). Because the autophosphorylated form of CaM kinase II remains active long after Ca^{2+} levels have returned to basal levels, the holoenzyme is able to act as sort of a molecular switch that is persistently activated by a transient increase in intracellular Ca^{2+} (Miller and Kennedy, 1986). The prolonged activation of CaM kinase II that results from autophosphorylation thus provides a mechanism whereby a transient increase in intracellular Ca^{2+} during high-frequency synaptic activity can induce a persistent biochemical change that could, at least in part, underlie the persistent potentiation of synaptic transmission seen in LTP (Lisman, 1989, 1994).

Numerous experiments suggest that CaM kinase II is an important component of the signaling pathway responsible for LTP. For instance, a selective peptide inhibitor of CaM kinase II derived from the inhibitory domain of the enzyme, CaMKII(273–302), blocks LTP when injected into CA1 pyramidal cells (Malinow, Schulman, and Tsien, 1989). In these experiments, synaptic transmission is only transiently potentiated; it returns to baseline levels 50 minutes or so after high-frequency stimulation (Fig. 14.5A). When pyramidal cells were injected with similar amounts of a truncated peptide that does not block CaM kinase II activity, CaMKII(284–302), normal LTP could be induced by high-frequency stimulation (Fig. 14.5B).

Molecular genetic approaches have also been used to inhibit CaM kinase II by introducing a null mutation in the mouse αCaM *kinase II* gene (Silva et al., 1992). In these "knock-out" animals, levels of αCaM kinase II protein are undetectable biochemically (the α isoform of CaM kinase II is normally highly expressed by hippocampal neurons), and high-frequency stimulation protocols that induce strong LTP in hippocampal slices from wild-type animals (Fig. 14.5C) fail to induce LTP in slices from αCaM kinase II

Fig. 14.5 Both pharmacological and molecular genetic inhibition of CaM kinase II blocks the induction of LTP in the CA1 region of the hippocampus. **(A)** An intracellular microelectrode was used both to record EPSPs and to inject an inhibitory peptide derived from the autoinhibitory domain of CaM kinase II into individual pyramidal cells. In these experiments, high-frequency synaptic stimulation (delivered at the arrow) induced only a transient, short-term potentiation of synaptic transmission. The traces marked *1* and *2* are EPSPs evoked during the times indicated on the graph. **(B)** LTP is not inhibited in cells injected with a related peptide, CaMKII (284–302), that does not block CaM kinase II activity. (Adapted from Malinow, Schulman, and Tsien, 1989.) At bottom are the results of experiments investigating the induction of LTP by high-frequency stimulation in hippocampal slices from wild-type **(C)** and transgenic mice with a null mutation in the α *CaM kinase II* gene **(D)**. Each point plots the slope of field EPSPs *(f-EPSP)* evoked by presynaptic fiber stimulation delivered once every 30 seconds. The arrows indicate when synapses were stimulated with a high-frequency (100 Hz) tetanus. Note that while robust LTP is induced in slices from wild-type animals, only a very short lasting potentiation (probably corresponding to posttetanic potentiation) is seen in slices from the CaM kinase II mutant animals. (Adapted from Silva et al., 1992.)

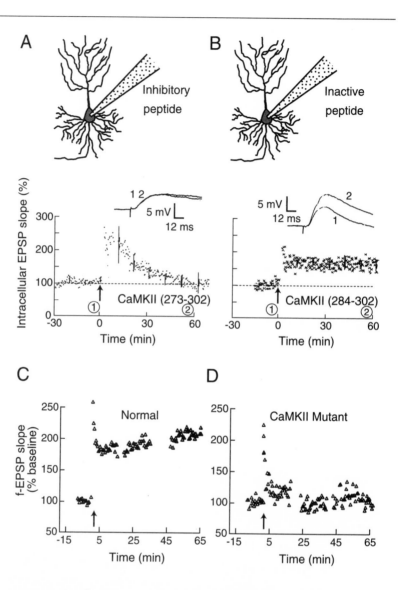

mutant animals (Fig. 14.5D). Thus when the activity of CaM kinase II is inhibited with either pharmacological or molecular genetic approaches, LTP is greatly diminished.

While these experiments are consistent with the notion that CaM kinase II has an important role in LTP, they suffer from experimental disadvantages that make it difficult to conclude definitively that

CaM kinase II has a *central* role in LTP. First, pharmacological inhibitors of protein kinases can be nonselective, and it is often difficult to rule out the possibility that the block of LTP actually occurs via effects of the inhibitor on some unknown molecule. Second, while molecular genetic approaches are exquisitely selective, they suffer from a different disadvantage. The presence of a null mutation means that these animals grow and develop in the complete absence of a gene and the protein it encodes. Thus, the absence of LTP in the αCaM kinase II mutant mice might not be due to the absence of αCaM kinase II per se but rather to a developmental abnormality that altered synaptic transmission in a way that precluded the induction of LTP.

Fortunately, there are additional pieces of evidence from other experimental approaches that strengthen the identification of CaM kinase II as a key molecule in LTP. For instance, biochemical studies have shown that the induction of LTP in hippocampal slices produces an increase in the amount of CaM kinase II in the Ca^{2+}-independent, autophosphorylated state (Fukunaga et al., 1993). This change in CaM kinase II does not occur when the induction of LTP by high-frequency synaptic stimulation is blocked by AP5, indicating that the induction of LTP is specifically associated with CaM kinase II activation. Moreover, as shown in Fig. 14.6, CaM kinase II activation can mimic the induction of LTP. In these experiments, preactivated CaM kinase II was introduced into CA1 pyramidal cells via a patch-clamp electrode and synaptic transmission was gradually potentiated as activated CaM kinase II diffused out of the recording electrode and into the cell (Lledo et al., 1995). No increase in synaptic transmission was observed in control experiments where inactivated (denatured) CaM kinase II was present in the electrode.

Does LTP Arise from Pre- or Postsynaptic Changes in Synaptic Transmission?

Although there is now considerable evidence that the induction of LTP in CA1 pyramidal cells depends on NMDA receptor activation, followed by increases in intracellular Ca^{2+} and CaM kinase II activation, the next steps in the signaling pathway are less well understood. One possibility is that CaM kinase II–mediated phos-

Fig. 14.6 Activated CaM kinase II enhances synaptic transmission in CA1 pyramidal cells. In these experiments patch-clamp electrodes were used to introduce αCaM kinase II monomers into CA1 pyramidal cells and to measure synaptic currents **(A)** evoked by presynaptic fiber stimulation. When CaM kinase II monomers that were preactivated by autophosphorylation were introduced into the cells, the excitatory postsynaptic currents, or EPSCs, gradually increased as CaM kinase II diffused out of the recording electrode into the cell; see the top set of EPSC recordings in **(A)** and filled symbols in **(B)**. Time zero corresponds to the time of "break-in," when the whole-cell recording configuration was first achieved and CaM kinase II was able to diffuse into the cell. No enhancement of synaptic currents occurred when the recording electrode contained CaM kinase II that was inactivated (denatured) by heating to 100 °C for 10 minutes; see the open circles in **(B)** and bottom set of traces in **(A)**. This suggests that the increase in EPSCs produced by active CaM kinase II was produced by phosphorylation rather than by some nonspecific effect of the protein. (Adapted from Lledo et al., 1995, and used with the permission of the authors and of the National Academy of Sciences, U.S.A.)

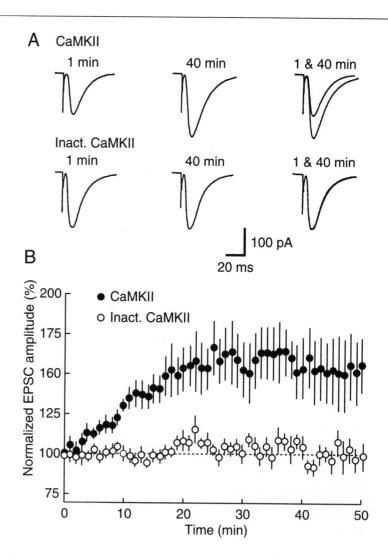

phorylation of the postsynaptic AMPA receptors enhances their activity and thus potentiates synaptic transmission (see Chapter 13 and Fig. 13.11). Indeed, it has been shown that AMPA receptors are phosphorylated by CaM kinase II following the induction of LTP (Barria et al., 1997), and that AMPA receptor–mediated responses are enhanced by CaM kinase II activation (McGlade-McCulloh et al., 1993; Lledo et al., 1995). In some ways, this hypothetical mechanism is appealing in its simplicity, and it is supported by a number of experimental observations; however, it fails to incorporate several details of what is known about the mechanisms involved in LTP, particularly the potential involvement of PKC and PKA (Reymann et al., 1988; Malinow, Schulman, and Tsien, 1989; Frey, Huang, and Kandel, 1993; Blitzer et al., 1995; Thomas et al., 1996).

Our understanding of the mechanism of LTP becomes even less clear when we consider the results of a number of investigations that have attempted to answer what would seem to be a simple question: Does the increase in synaptic strength that occurs with the induction of LTP involve presynaptic or postsynaptic changes? That is, is LTP caused, for example, by an increased glutamate receptor sensitivity or increased activity of the glutamate receptor ion channels in the postsynaptic cell, or is it caused instead by presynaptic changes resulting in enhanced transmitter release? We know that the induction of LTP requires postsynaptic increases in intracellular Ca^{2+} and the activation of postsynaptic NMDA receptors and protein kinases. It would therefore seem reasonable to assume that postsynaptic changes would underlie the enhancement of synaptic strength. Just the opposite conclusion, however, was drawn when investigators examined the statistics of transmitter release with quantal analysis techniques, which suggested that *presynaptic* changes in transmitter release were responsible for LTP, perhaps through increases in the probability of transmitter exocytosis.

One approach in these studies has been to measure the synaptic responses evoked by "minimal stimulation" of the Schaffer collateral pathway in the CA1 region of the hippocampus. The technique of minimal stimulation involves adjusting the intensity of extracellular stimulation delivered to the presynaptic fibers in a hippocampal slice to a level just slightly stronger than that which produces no response in a postsynaptic pyramidal cell. By this means the experimenters hope to activate only a single presynaptic fiber. When this sort of stimulation protocol is used along with whole-cell voltage-clamp techniques to record synaptic currents from CA1 pyramidal cells, clear failures of synaptic transmission occur for some stimulation pulses, while synaptic currents ranging in size from about 1 to 20 pA are elicited by other pulses (Fig. 14.7A). Because synaptic currents are recorded over a large number of stimulation trials before and after the induction of LTP, this approach should make it possible to examine how the quantal parameters of synaptic transmission may change after LTP.

Recall from Chapter 8 that quantal analysis permits the evaluation of two aspects of synaptic transmission: the average number of synaptic vesicles released by a presynaptic action potential, known as the quantal content of the EPSP *(m)*; and the mean amplitude of the postsynaptic response produced by a single quantum of transmitter, known as the quantal size (*<mepsp>*—see Chapter 8, Eqns. 8–10). Quantal size can be estimated from the amplitude of single miniature synaptic events or from the response size corresponding to the first, nonzero peak of the amplitude distribution of postsynaptic responses (see Fig. 8.15). Quantal content can be estimated with either the direct method, where the average amplitude of the evoked EPSP is divided by the quantal size to give the mean number of quanta that make up the evoked response (*m* = *<epsp>/<mepsp>*). Alternatively, when release probability is low and Poission statistics are appropriate, quantal content can be estimated from the number of failures of synaptic transmission according to the equation: $m = \ln(1/p_0)$, where p_0 is the probability of observing a failure.

A third way that quantal content of the synaptic response can be estimated is by calculating the *coefficient of variation (CV)*. In statistical terms the CV is the standard deviation divided by the mean. If the EPSPs recorded from a pyramidal cell are infrequent (as, for example, during minimal stimulation), then the probability *(p$_i$)* of observing *i* quanta is distributed according to the Poisson distribution, where

$$p_i = \frac{m^i}{i!} e^{-m}$$

This was previously given as Eqn. (10) in Chapter 8. It is a property of this distribution that the variance and mean are both equal to *m*, the quantal content. Therefore the coefficient of variation is given by CV = $\sqrt{m}/m$, since the standard deviation is the square root of the variance; and $1/(CV)^2 = m$.

At high levels of synaptic activity, a binomial distribution would have to be used instead of a Poisson distribution, since release probability cannot be assumed to be low. The mean number of quanta observed will still be given by m, since m is equal to the probability of release at any release site multiplied by the number of release sites (see Chapter 8, Eqn. 9). The product of the probability of release and the number of release sites must clearly give the mean number of quanta observed, and this is the definition of the quantal content. The variance of the binomial distribution is, however, not m but rather $m(1 - p)$. Hence

$$\frac{1}{(\mathrm{CV})^2} = \frac{m}{(1 - p)}$$

Note that when binomial statistics apply we cannot directly estimate quantal content from $1/(\mathrm{CV})^2$ without an independent measure of either n or p. Regardless of whether we use the binomial or Poisson distribution, however, this equation has some experimental advantages for the study of LTP. First, one doesn't have to measure n, p, or quantal size directly to calculate $1/(\mathrm{CV})^2$ but can instead simply measure the mean and variance of the synaptic responses evoked following numerous presynaptic fiber stimulations. Second, and more important, there are no postsynaptic variables in the equation for CV. Thus if LTP causes postsynaptic changes in synaptic transmission, then $1/(\mathrm{CV})^2$ should remain unchanged following the induction of LTP, even though mean synaptic response is potentiated. If LTP involves presynaptic changes that increase either n or p, however, then $1/(\mathrm{CV})^2$ should increase as synaptic transmission is potentiated. Using this sort of analysis, it has been shown that $1/(\mathrm{CV})^2$ increases following the induction of LTP (Fig. 14.7B), suggesting that the potentiation of synaptic transmission that occurs in LTP is due to presynaptic changes in transmitter release (Malinow and Tsien, 1990; Bekkers and Stevens, 1990). Moreover, a fairly common finding observed in these sorts of experiments is that the induction of LTP is accompanied by a decrease in the number of failures in synaptic transmission, a result consistent with the notion that LTP arises from an increased probability of transmitter release (Fig. 14.7C).

Fig. 14.7 Minimal stimulation experiments measuring $1/(CV)^2$ and synaptic failures suggest that LTP is due to presynaptic changes in transmitter release. **(A)** A patch-clamp electrode is used for whole-cell voltage-clamping and an extracellular stimulating electrode is used to activate presynaptic fibers. At low stimulation strengths only a single presynaptic fiber will be activated, producing small EPSCs and numerous failures of synaptic transmission, as illustrated by the superimposed current traces. (From Issac, Nicoll, and Malenka, 1995, with permission of the authors and of Cell Press.) **(B)** Two separate inputs onto a CA1 pyramidal cell were alternately activated with two stimulating electrodes. After a short period of baseline recording, LTP was induced *(arrows)* by pairing postsynaptic depolarization with activation of only one of the presynaptic inputs *(solid symbols)*. The mean synaptic current evoked by this input increase to about 4 × the baseline mean after pairing, whereas the currents evoked following stimulation of the second pathway *(open symbols)* remained unchanged. Furthermore, $1/(CV)^2$ increased only for the synapses that underwent LTP *(bottom)*. **(C)** Data from several individual experiments compiled to graph the number of failures of synaptic transmission (as a percentage of total stimulation pulses) before *(Control)* and after the induction of LTP. Note the large decrease in failure rate that occurs with the induction of LTP. Each symbol represents a different cell, with bars giving the mean percentage of failures. (Adapted from Malinow and Tsien, 1990, with permission of the authors and of Macmillan Magazines Limited.)

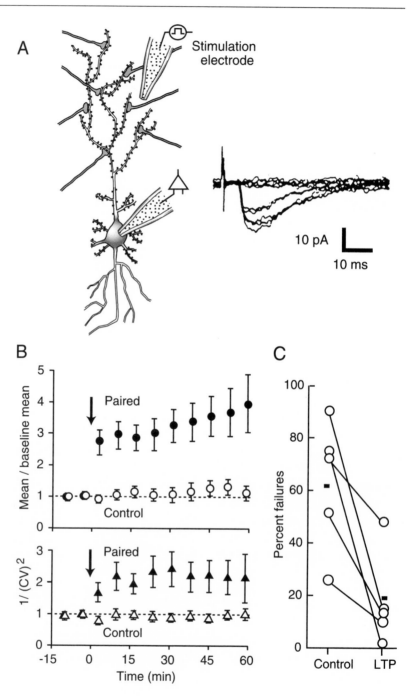

The possibility that LTP involves presynaptic changes in transmitter release while the induction of LTP depends on activation of postsynaptic processes suggests that there must be some form of communication from the postsynaptic to the presynaptic side of the synapse. One possibility that has attracted considerable attention is that the postsynaptic processes involved in LTP include the generation of signaling molecules that diffuse out of the postsynaptic cell and travel across the synapse in a retrograde manner to modulate the presynaptic release machinery. In addition, the induction of LTP may also produce structural changes at synapses, perhaps by means of a retrograde messenger that produces a structurally coordinated presynaptic and postsynaptic increase in synaptic size (Lisman and Harris, 1993). Although there are several candidate retrograde messengers, such as nitric oxide (Schuman and Madison, 1991; O'Dell, Grant, and Kandel, 1991), carbon dioxide (Stevens and Wang, 1993), arachidonic acid (Williams et al., 1989), and platelet activating factor (Arai and Lynch, 1992; Kato et al., 1994), none has yet been convincingly identified as carrying the retrograde signal in LTP (Williams et al., 1993; Bear and Malenka, 1994).

The notion that LTP involves a presynaptic change in transmitter release is not universally accepted. Numerous investigators have applied the techniques of quantal analysis (and other approaches) to examine this question and, while the results of some experiments support a presynaptic locus for LTP (Stevens and Wang, 1994; Malgaroli and Tsien, 1992; Bolshakov and Siegelbaum, 1995), other experimental results are most consistent with a predominately postsynaptic change (Manabe, Renner, and Nicoll, 1992; Manabe and Nicoll, 1994; Oliet, Malenka, and Nicoll, 1996). Some experiments even indicate that LTP involves both pre- and postsynaptic modifications of synaptic transmission (Kullmann and Nicoll, 1992). This confusion probably partly arises from the fact that we currently know very little about even basic aspects of excitatory synaptic transmission in the mammalian central nervous system. Thus it is not clear whether many of the assumptions underlying quantal analysis as developed from studies of the neuromuscular junction are equally valid for CNS synapses (see Chapter 8). For instance, failures of synaptic transmission during minimal stimulation are typically interpreted as failures of transmitter release. Thus, if the failure rate decreases, as it does following the induction of LTP, then there must have been a presynaptic change in release probability. The results of recent studies suggest, however, that the interpretation of the decrease in the failure rate of synaptic transmission following the induction of LTP may not be so straightforward.

This need for reinterpretreation has arisen from new findings about the distribution of glutamate receptors at synapses in the CNS. Although it is often assumed that NMDA and AMPA glutamate receptors are always co-localized postsynaptically (as in Fig. 9.17), recent evidence suggests that at some (and perhaps many) synapses onto CA1 pyramidal cells, only NMDA-type receptors are present postsynaptically (Kullman, 1994; Liao, Hessler, and Malinow, 1995). At the normal resting membrane potential of these cells, release of glutamate from the presynaptic terminal at one of these pure NMDA receptor synapses would produce no postsynaptic response, because of the voltage-dependent Mg^{2+} block of the NMDA receptor ion channel. In other words, at the normal resting membrane potential these synapses would be essentially silent or nonfunctional.

An example of the behavior of a pure NMDA receptor or "silent" synapse can be seen in Fig. 14.8A. At a holding potential of -60 mV, no excitatory postsynaptic currents (EPSCs) are evoked over many stimulation pulses. However, when the postsynaptic membrane potential is changed to $+30$ mV (thus relieving the Mg^{+2} ion block of the NMDA receptor ion channels), clear EPSCs now appear. The synaptic currents seen at $+30$ mV are the result of activation of NMDA-type glutamate receptors, since they are completely blocked by AP5. Note that in these experiments the failure rate was dramatically affected by a *postsynaptic* change (a change in membrane potential).

Suppose that AMPA-type receptors are inserted or converted to a functional form after LTP induction at these silent synapses (Fig. 14.8B). Then synapses that produced few postsynaptic responses before LTP with a high rate of failure would be converted to synapses producing frequent responses, with a low failure rate. Fig. 14.8C shows just such an effect. Here a silent synapse was repeatedly activated with the postsynaptic cell voltage-clamped at its resting membrane portential, and no synaptic responses were observed

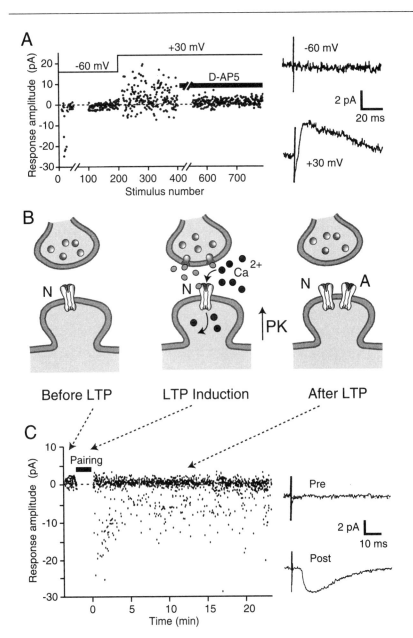

Fig. 14.8 Activation of AMPA-type glutamate receptors at "silent synapses" may provide a postsynaptic explanation for decreases in failure rate following the induction of LTP. **(A)** The behavior of a silent synapse onto a CA1 pyramidal cell. When the postsynaptic cell is voltage-clamped near the resting membrane potential, presynaptic stimulation appears to produce only failures of synaptic transmission, as there are no detectable postsynaptic responses over many presynaptic stimulation pulses. Following depolarization of the postsynaptic membrane potential to +30 mV, clear postsynaptic currents can be detected on some stimulation pulses. The NMDA receptor antagonist D-AP5 (applied for the duration indicated by the bar) blocked these EPSCs, indicating that they are mediated by NMDA receptors. The current traces on the right show the average of 100 consecutive responses to presynaptic stimulations when the postsynaptic cell was held at −60 mV or +30 mV. **(B)** Possible mechanism for LTP-dependent insertion or activation of previously nonfunctional AMPA receptors, perhaps by phosphorylation by protein kinases triggered by the entry of Ca^{2+} through NMDA channels. *N,* NMDA receptor; *A,* AMPA receptor; *PK,* protein kinase (adapted from Liao et al., 1995). **(C)** When LTP is induced by pairing presynaptic stimulation with postsynaptic depolarization, previously silent synapses can become functional, giving clear synaptic responses even at the resting membrane potential. The traces shown at bottom right are the averages of 100 EPSCs recorded before *(Pre)* and 1 minute after pairing postsynaptic depolarization with presynaptic stimulation *(Post)*. (Adapted from Issac, Nicoll, and Malenka, 1995, with permission of the authors and of Cell Press.)

over many stimulation pulses. The postynaptic membrane potential was then depolarized and synaptic stimulation was continued in an attempt to induce LTP of the silent synapse. Following this pairing of depolarization and synaptic stimulation, clear EPSCs are now evoked at the negative holding potential, just as expected if new AMPA receptors had been activated or inserted into the postsynaptic membrane (Liao, Hessler, and Malinow, 1995; Issac, Nicoll, and Malenka, 1995). This finding indicates that the decrease in synaptic failures observed in quantal analysis studies of LTP may not represent a presynaptic change in release probability but may instead reflect postsynaptic changes that unmask previously silent synapses.

Clearly, until we have a better understanding of the behavior of excitatory synapses in the CA1 region of the hippocampus (as well as elsewhere in the brain), there will probably be no definitive answer to what initially appeared to be a rather simple question—does LTP arise from pre- or postsynaptic changes in synaptic transmission, or both?

Long-Term Depression

Synaptic transmission at Schaffer collateral inputs onto CA1 pyramidal cells is not only capable of undergoing LTP but can also be persistently depressed by certain patterns of synaptic stimulation, a phenomenon known as long-term depression (LTD). Unlike LTP, which is typically induced by brief periods of high-frequency stimulation, LTD occurs when synapses are repeatedly stimulated at relatively low rates (1 to 5 Hz) for several minutes (Dudek and Bear, 1992). Although LTP and LTD are induced by very different patterns of synaptic activity, the initial events involved in the induction of LTD are surprisingly similar to those involved in LTP. For instance, the induction of LTD, like LTP, requires NMDA receptor activation (Fig. 14.9A), since it is blocked by AP5 (Dudek and Bear, 1992). This suggests that the cellular mechanisms responsible for LTD may also be Ca^{2+}-dependent. Indeed, loading cells with Ca^{2+} chelators, such as BAPTA, blocks the induction of LTD just as it blocks the induction of LTP (Mulkey and Malenka, 1992). Beyond this common dependence on NMDA receptor activation and subsequent increases in intracellular Ca^{2+}, however, the molecular processes responsible for LTD diverge from those responsible for LTP.

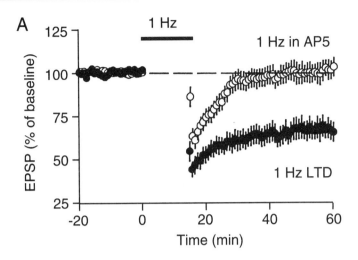

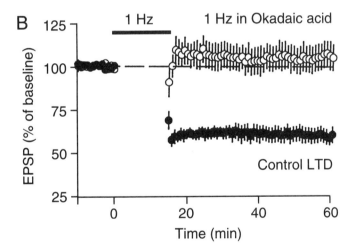

Fig. 14.9 LTD of synaptic transmission requires an NMDA receptor–dependent activation of protein phosphatases. **(A)** After monitoring the amplitude of EPSPs evoked by 0.02 Hz presynaptic stimulation for 20 minutes, LTD was induced by increasing the presynaptic stimulation rate to 1 Hz for 15 minutes. The amplitude of EPSPs evoked during 1 Hz stimulation is not shown. In control experiments *(solid symbols)* a long-lasting depression of synaptic transmission is evident when the stimulation rate is returned to 0.02 Hz. When NMDA receptors are blocked with AP5, however, the induction of LTD is inhibited and only a transient depression of synaptic transmission follows 1 Hz stimulation *(open symbols).* **(B)** The protein phosphatase type 1 and 2A inhibitor okadaic acid (1.0 μM) also blocks the induction of LTD *(open symbols),* suggesting that the induction of LTD requires the activity of one or more types of protein phosphatases.

One important distinction between the mechanisms of LTP and LTD is that the induction of LTD requires activation of protein phosphatases (see Chapter 12). For instance, LTD is blocked when hippocampal slices are exposed to okadaic acid, a potent, membrane-permeable inhibitor of protein phosphatases 1 (PP1) and 2A (Fig. 14.9B) (Mulkey, Herron, and Malenka, 1993). PP1, which is the major protein phosphatase present in the postsynaptic density (Shields, Ingebritsen, and Kelly, 1985), is not directly activated by calcium but instead by dephosphorylation of an associated, regulatory phosphoprotein called inhibitor 1 (inhibitor 1 behaves in a manner very similar to the protein DARPP-32 described in Chapter 12). PP1 thus cannot serve as an immediate downstream target for Ca^{2+} in the signaling pathway responsible for LTD. Instead, Ca^{2+} influx through the NMDA receptor ion channels during the induction of LTP is thought to activate the Ca^{2+}-activated phosphatase calcineurin. When activated by Ca^{2+}, calcineurin dephosphorylates inhibitor 1, which in its dephosphorylated state no longer associates with and inhibits PP1.

Calcineurin-mediated dephosphorylation of inhibitor 1 thus provides a possible mechanism for Ca^{2+}-dependent activation of PP1. Two experimental observations suggest that this multistep pathway leading to PP1 activation is actually involved in the induction of LTD. First, experiments have shown that the immunosuppressant compounds cyclosporin A and FK506, which are potent calcineurin inhibitors, block LTD (Mulkey et al., 1994). Second, these same investigators have found that thio-phosphorylated inhibitor 1, which blocks PP1 but is resistant to dephosphorylation by calcineurin, blocks LTD when it is injected into CA1 pyramidal cells.

In some ways the mechanisms responsible for LTD seem to complement those responsible for LTP. Namely, the increase in synaptic strength in LTP appears to require protein kinase activation and subsequent substrate phosphorylation, while the decrease in synaptic strength seen in LTD apparently depends on protein phosphatase activation and substrate dephosphorylation. As with LTP, however, little is known about the substrates that, when dephosphorylated, give rise to a depression of synaptic transmission. Likely candidates include the postsynaptic AMPA-type glutamate receptors or CaM kinase II (PP1 dephosphorylates autophosphorylated CaM kinase II and turns it off).

Our understanding of the synaptic mechanisms underlying LTP and LTD has led to an apparent paradox regarding the induction of these two forms of synaptic plasticity. The induction of LTP and LTD at CA1 pyramidal cells both depend on the same synaptic event, Ca^{2+} influx through NMDA receptor ion channels. What, then, determines whether this Ca^{2+} influx activates the protein kinase–dependent steps responsible for LTP or the protein phosphatase–dependent processes responsible for LTD? One possibility is that the amount and/or duration of Ca^{2+} influx is important. Here, the idea is that high-frequency stimulation produces strong NMDA receptor activation and a large increase in intracellular Ca^{2+} that preferentially activates the protein kinases responsible for LTP. On the other hand, lower-frequency synaptic stimulation should produce weaker NMDA receptor activation and smaller increases in intracellular Ca^{2+} that may preferentially activate the protein phosphatase cascade responsible for LTD (Lisman, 1989; Cummings et al., 1996). Consistent with this notion, calcineurin has a much higher affinity for Ca^{2+}/calmodulin than CaM kinase II has (Klee, 1991) and thus would be expected to be activated by smaller increases in intracellular Ca^{2+}.

One problem with this model is that the large increase in intracellular Ca^{2+} that occurs during LTP-inducing high-frequency stimulation should activate both protein kinases and protein phosphatases, a situation in which no net change in kinase and phosphatase activity might occur. One possibility is that high levels of intracellular Ca^{2+} not only activate the CaM kinase II–dependent steps responsible for LTP but also activate a second signaling pathway that prevents PP1 activation (see Fig. 14.10A). Some evidence suggests that this inhibitory pathway involves Ca^{2+}-sensitive isoforms of adenylyl cyclase, such as ACI or ACVIII (Lisman, 1994). The increase in cAMP generated in response to increases in intracellular Ca^{2+} may activate PKA and lead to phosphorylation of inhibitor 1. This would effectively oppose inhibitor 1 dephosphorylation by calcineurin and thus prevent PP1 activation. Consistent with this notion, PKA activators like 8-Br-cAMP block LTD (see Fig. 14.10B, from Mulkey et al., 1994). As research on the mechanisms of LTP progresses, a clearer picture of the mechanisms responsible for LTD may also emerge.

NMDA Receptor–Independent LTP

NMDA receptor–dependent LTP and LTD can be seen at many excitatory synapses, both within the hippocampus as well as in other regions of the brain, such as the neocortex. But these are not the only types of synaptic plasticity capable of persistently altering the strength of excitatory synaptic transmission in the brain. Indeed, even within the hippocampus some synapses undergo LTP through

Fig. 14.10 Calcium-sensitive isoforms of adenylyl cyclase may provide a mechanism for inhibiting protein phosphatases during the induction of LTP. **(A)** Ca^{2+} influx through NMDA receptor ion channels is hypothesized to activate the CaM kinase II–dependent pathway underlying LTP and also a cascade of protein phosphatase activation. The phosphatase cascade is shown as follows: Ca^{2+} binds to calmodulin *(CaM)* and activates the phosphatase calcineurin. Calcineurin then converts the phosphorylated form of inhibitor 1 *(I-1-P)* to a dephosphorylated form *(I-1)*, releasing inhibitor 1 from protein phosphatase 1 *(PP1)* and activating this phosphatase. PP1 then is hypothesized both to induce LTD and to inhibit the induction of LTP. During high-frequency synaptic stimulation, the consequent large increase in intracellular Ca^{2+} may not only activate CaM kinase but may produce a Ca^{2+}/calmodulin-dependent activation of adenylyl cyclase, thus generating cAMP and activating PKA. PKA phosphorylation of inhibitor 1 *(I-1)* would keep the inhibitor in its phosphorylated form *(I-1-P)*, opposing the effects of calcineurin and preventing activation of PP1. Circled plus signs indicate stimulation and circled minus signs indicate inhibition. (Adapted from Lisman, 1994, and Blitzer et al., 1995.) **(B)** Pharmacological activation of PKA does seem to block LTD, since the cAMP analogue 8-Br-cAMP inhibits the induction of LTD by 1 Hz stimulation. The traces shown above the graph are field EPSPs recorded during baseline and 30 minutes after 1 Hz stimulation. The effects of PKA activation are reversible, since after 8-Br-cAMP is removed from the solution bathing the slices (break in the graph), 1 Hz stimulation can now induce LTD. (Reprinted from Mulkey et al., 1994, with permission of the authors and of Macmillan Magazines Limited.)

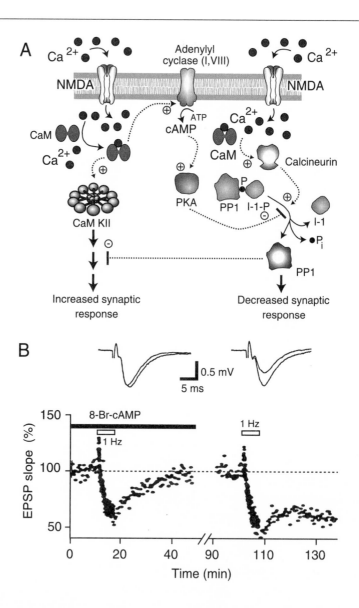

molecular processes that are quite distinct from the NMDA receptor–dependent mechanisms responsible for LTP in the hippocampal CA1 region.

When dentate gyrus granule cell axons (the mossy fibers) are activated at a high frequency, transmission at the mossy fiber synapses onto the pyramidal cells in the CA3 region of the hippocampus undergoes LTP (Fig. 14.11A). The first indication that LTP at the mossy fiber synapse is mechanistically distinct from LTP at the Schaffer collateral synapses onto CA1 pyramidal cells came from studies showing that LTP could still be induced when high-frequency mossy fiber stimulation was delivered in the presence of the NMDA receptor antagonist AP5 (Harris and Cotman, 1986). Thus mossy fiber LTP is often referred to as NMDA receptor–independent LTP. Moreover, mossy fiber LTP differs from LTP in the CA1 region of the hippocampus in that it still occurs when the Ca^{2+} chelator BAPTA is injected into individual postsynaptic CA3 pyramidal cells (Zalutsky and Nicoll, 1990). These results suggest that neither postsynaptic NMDA receptor activation nor increases in postsynaptic Ca^{2+} are required for the induction of mossy fiber LTP. In fact, when high-frequency mossy fiber stimulation is delivered in the presence of the AMPA receptor antagonist kynurenate, so that no postsynaptic excitatory response occurs during LTP induction, synaptic transmission still shows a large potentiation when the blocker is washed away (Castillo, Weisskopf, and Nicoll, 1994; see Fig. 14.11B). Because LTP can still be induced when the postsynaptic response to high-frequency synaptic stimulation is totally blocked, there seems to be little involvement of the postsynaptic cell in the induction of mossy fiber LTP. Instead, this form of LTP may depend solely on processes within the presynaptic mossy fiber terminals.

What is the signal generated during high-frequency mossy fiber stimulation that initiates the induction of LTP at these synapses? If extracellular Ca^{2+} is removed during high-frequency mossy fiber stimulation, no potentiation of synaptic transmission is observed when normal levels of Ca^{2+} are restored (Fig. 14.11C; Castillo, Weisskopf, and Nicoll, 1994). This suggests that, as in LTP in the CA1 region of the hippocampus, Ca^{2+} serves as an essential trigger for the induction of mossy fiber LTP; but it is Ca^{2+} influx into the presynaptic terminal, rather than into the postsynaptic dendritic spine, that triggers the induction of mossy fiber LTP.

Important findings that provided key insights into the nature of the Ca^{2+}-activated signal responsible for mossy fiber LTP came from studies that examined the potential role of PKA (Weisskopf et al., 1994). First it was observed that PKA inhibitors such as Rp-

Fig. 14.11 LTP of mossy fiber synapses in the CA3 region of the hippocampus requires presynaptic calcium influx. **(A)** In these experiments an intracellular microelectrode was used to record EPSPs evoked by mossy fiber stimulation in CA3 pyramidal cells. Mossy fibers were stimulated extracellularly with an electrode in the dentate gyrus. **(B)** Under normal conditions, high-frequency stimulation *(HFS)* of the mossy fibers induces a nearly twofold increase in the strength of synaptic transmission *(open symbols)*. High-frequency stimulation can also induce mossy fiber LTP *(solid symbols)*, even when the tetanus is delivered during a complete blockade of synaptic transmission by the general glutamate receptor antagonist kynurenate (application as indicated by bar). In these experiments, EPSPs blocked by kynurenate recover as kynurenate washes out of the slice, and they eventually reach a potentiated level similar to that produced by high-frequency stimulation in the control experiments. Since LTP can still be induced when the postsynaptic effects of the tetanus are completely blocked, the postsynaptic cell probably has little role in the mechanisms responsible for mossy fiber LTP. **(C)** EPSPs do not recover to a potentiated level following high-frequency stimulation delivered when synaptic transmission is blocked by removing extracellular calcium. The block of LTP in these experiments suggests that the induction of mossy fiber LTP requires increases in intracellular calcium, probably via influx through presynaptic voltage-sensitive calcium channels. (Parts **(B)** and **(C)** adapted from Castillo, Weisskopf, and Nicoll, 1994, with permission of the authors and of Cell Press.)

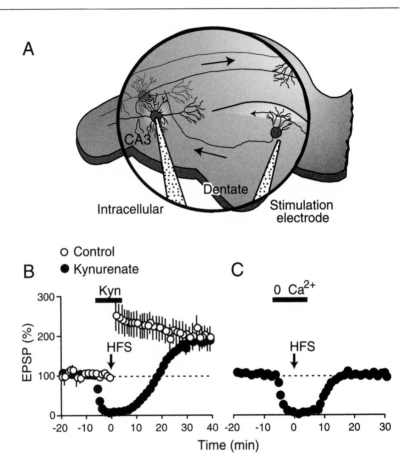

cAMPs and H89 block the induction of mossy fiber LTP. Second, a PKA activator, such as forskolin, which increases levels of cAMP by directly stimulating adenylyl cyclase, induces a potentiation of mossy fiber synaptic transmission with properties similar to mossy fiber LTP induced with high-frequency synaptic stimulation. Thus it seems likely that during high-frequency stimulation, large increases in intracellular Ca²⁺ in the mossy fiber terminal activate Ca²⁺-sensitive isoforms of adenylyl cyclase (like ACI or ACVIII). The resulting increase in cAMP, PKA activation, and substrate phosphorylation then lead to increased transmitter release. As with LTP in the CA1 region of the hippocampus, little is known about the PKA substrates that may participate in this enhancement of transmitter release, although modulation of K⁺ and/or Ca²⁺ channel function, as well as phosphorylation-dependent changes in the molecules involved in the transmitter release machinery, are obvious candidates.

Summary

In many ways this chapter, like the one that preceded it, is about Ca²⁺. As we've seen, all of the cellular mechanisms responsible for activity-dependent, persistent changes in synaptic strength in the hippocampus are activated by increases in intracellular Ca²⁺. There are important differences, however, in the Ca²⁺-activated signaling pathways responsible for different forms of synaptic plasticity. In the CA1 region of the hippocampus, Ca²⁺ influx through postsynaptic NMDA receptors and activation of CaM kinase II are thought to be key components of the molecular mechanism responsible for LTP at the Schaffer collateral synapses (Fig. 14.12A). Although CaM kinase II apparently has a central role in LTP at these synapses, other Ca²⁺-activated signaling pathways are also important. For instance, Ca²⁺ may activate enzymes that generate retrograde messengers, such as NO, that diffuse back across the synapse and enhance transmitter release. In addition, activation of Ca²⁺-sensitive forms of adenylyl cyclase and subsequent PKA activation seem to be important parts of a mechanism for suppressing protein phosphatases, which if left uninhibited could oppose the protein kinase activity needed for LTP (Fig. 14.10).

Ca²⁺ also serves as an essential trigger for the induction of mossy fiber LTP in the CA3 region of the hippocampus. In contrast to CA1 LTP, mossy fiber LTP requires Ca²⁺ influx through presynaptic voltage-sensitive Ca²⁺ channels rather than postsynaptic NMDA receptors. Mossy fiber LTP also differs from LTP in the CA1 region of the hippocampus in that PKA, rather than CaM kinase II, has a central role in the enhancement of synaptic transmission (Fig. 14.12B).

Lastly, in addition to LTP, many synapses can also be persistently depressed by certain patterns of synaptic activity. It seems likely that, at least in some regions of the brain, these patterns of synaptic stimulation induce LTD by producing low levels of NMDA receptor activation that elicit modest increases in intracellular Ca²⁺.

Fig. 14.12 Summary of hypothesized cellular mechanisms responsible for LTP of Schaffer collateral synapses in the CA1 region of the hippocampus *(top)* and for mossy fiber LTP in the CA3 region *(bottom)*. At the Schaffer collateral synapses in the CA1 region, LTP is thought to be primarily the result of a postsynaptic, CaM kinase II–dependent process activated by NMDA receptor–mediated increases in intracellular Ca^{2+}. At the mossy fiber synapses in the CA3 region of the hippocampus, the induction of LTP is also dependent on increases in intracellular Ca^{2+}, but here influx through presynaptic voltage-sensitive calcium channels *(VSCC)* and activation of PKA appear to play pivotal roles.

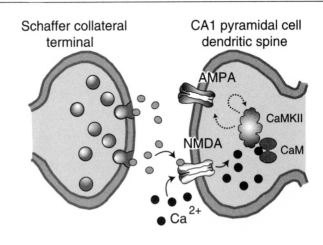

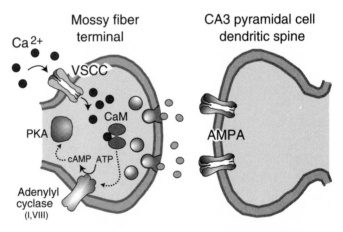

While unable to activate the protein kinase–dependent mechanisms responsible for LTP, these levels of Ca^{2+} may trigger a cascade of protein phosphatase activation that persistently depresses synaptic transmission (Fig. 14.10).

Although many of the essential components of the signaling pathways responsible for LTP and LTD seem to have been identified, we are far from completely understanding the cellular mechanisms responsible for different forms of synaptic plasticity. Many important questions remain. For instance, it is still not clear whether the enhancement of synaptic transmission in CA1 LTP arises from either presynaptic or postsynaptic changes (or both).

Moreover, the protein kinase substrates responsible for LTP, as well as those dephosphorylated by calcineurin and PP1 in LTD, remain to be identified. Clearly, a complete understanding of the mechanisms responsible for LTP and LTD must await answers to these fundamental questions.

Finally, most of what we know about the mechanisms underlying activity-dependent forms of synaptic plasticity applies to events that occur within the first hour or so after the induction of LTP or LTD. It seems quite likely that at later times very different signaling pathways and cellular processes may be required to maintain the changes in synaptic strength that have taken place (Matthies, 1989), and structural changes in the size of the synapses may also be important (Lisman and Harris, 1993). The persistence of LTP beyond 2 to 3 hours after tetanic stimulation is dependent on both mRNA and protein synthesis (Huang, Li, and Kandel, 1994; Nguyen, Abel, and Kandel, 1994). The identity of these proteins and their role in synaptic plasticity are important questions for the future.

PART FIVE

Sensory Transduction

15

Mechanoreceptors

SENSORY RECEPTORS are cells singularly sensitive to external stimuli, such as electromagnetic or acoustical radiation, and are usually found in specialized organs like the eye or ear. Sensory receptor cells contain molecules that convert external stimuli into electrical signals, by a process known as *sensory transduction*. The mechanism of transduction in different receptor cells provides a convenient means for dividing them into two classes, which we shall call *ionotropic* and *metabotropic,* by analogy to the mechanism of signal transduction in postsynaptic membrane. For some sensory receptors, external stimuli act directly on ion channels to alter their probability of opening. The most extensively studied examples of such ionotropic sensory receptors are the mechanoreceptors, which are the subject of this chapter. For metabotropic sensory receptor cells, the external stimulus acts on one of a family of seven-transmembrane α-helical receptor proteins. This protein then activates a G protein and triggers a metabotropic cascade leading to a change in the concentration of a second messenger, which may alter the probability of opening of an ion channel. Metabotropic sensory receptor cells, and in particular photoreceptors and olfactory receptors, will be the subject of the chapter to follow.

Mechanosensitive Channels

Channels gated directly by membrane stretch or tension were first discovered in skeletal muscle. Two examples of recordings from this preparation are given in Fig. 15.1: the first (in part A) from a cell-attached (on-cell) patch (from Brehm, Kullberg, and Moody-Corbett, 1984), and the second (in part B) from an excised, inside-

Fig. 15.1 Patch recordings from mechanosensitive channels. **(A)** On-cell recording from intact skeletal muscle from tail of *Xenopus* tadpole. Negative pressure applied to the patch pipette *(arrow)* produced an increase in the frequency of channel opening. (Reprinted from Brehm, Kullberg, and Moody-Corbett, 1984, with permission of the authors and the Physiological Society.) **(B)** Excised, inside-out patch from embryonic chick skeletal muscle. Numbers above traces give value of suction applied to patch pipette. Note that increased suction produces an increase in the frequency of bursts of openings. (Reprinted from Guharay and Sachs, 1984, with permission of the authors and the Physiological Society.)

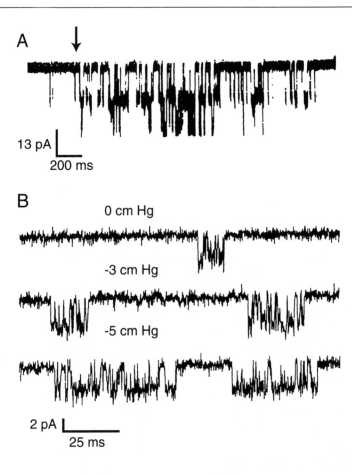

out patch (from Guharay and Sachs, 1984). In both experiments, gentle suction delivered by the patch pipette on the membrane containing the channels elicited an increase in channel opening. Since stretch-induced channel activity can be observed in cell-attached patches, mechanosensitivity is unlikely to be an artifact of patch isolation. Since channel opening can also be observed in excised patches (Fig. 15.1B), a mechanical disturbance seems capable of gating channel opening directly, in the absence of a second messenger or protein kinase.

Following these original reports, many recordings have been made of channels that are either activated or inactivated by mechanical stimulation (see Sachs, 1992; Sackin, 1995). These channels come in a variety of types. The most common may be channels that are selective for cations but permeable to Na^+ as well as to K^+ and even to Ca^{2+}. There are also K^+-selective channels sensitive to stretch, as well as anion-selective channels and (in bacteria) large, nonselective channels. The unitary conductance of mechanosensitive channels varies widely, from 10 to 3,000 pS.

Since mechanosensitive channels have been recorded in so many different cell types, it is perhaps surprising that so little progress has been made isolating and cloning these channels (see García-Añoveros and Corey, 1997). The one exception is a 17 kDa channel, the *mechanosensitive nonselective large* (or MscL), whose gene has been cloned from bacteria. In a cell-free system, this protein has been shown to form a 2,500–3,000 pS channel in lipid membranes that is activated by suction (Sukharev et al., 1994). This is so far the only report of a cloned protein demonstrated to produce a mechanosensitive channel, but it is probably used by bacteria not for sensing mechanical stimuli but rather for responding to osmotic stress. A protein with such a large unitary conductance would seem unsuitable for sensing mechanical disturbances, since the opening of even one channel in a cell as small as a bacterium would have dramatic consequences for the cell membrane potential and intracellular ion concentrations. No homologues of MscL have been detected in eukaryotes, and it remains unclear whether proteins related to MscL serve any role in mechanoreception.

Some of the most interesting experiments attempting to isolate mechanoreceptive proteins have used the nematode *Caenorhabditis elegans* (see Hamill and McBride, 1996; Corey and García-Añoveros, 1996; García-Añoveros and Corey, 1997). *C. elegans* responds to light body touch by moving away, and this reaction appears to be mediated by only 6 touch-sensitive neurons. At least 15 genes have been isolated whose gene products appear to be required for the production of the mechanosensitive response. Although several of these genes encode proteins necessary for the development and differentiation of the touch-sensitive cells, or proteins that form components of the extracellular matrix, at least 2 proteins (called MEC-4 and MEC-10) have sequences resembling those of ion channel subunits. Since these proteins have not as yet been successfully expressed, it is still unclear whether MEC-4 or MEC-10 (or a combination of these and other proteins) forms a channel that mediates touch sensitivity.

Crayfish Stretch Receptor

Channels directly gated by mechanical stimuli seem likely to mediate the touch sensitivity of mechanoreceptors in the skin and in more specialized structures, such as the ear. A direct demonstration of a role for these channels in sensing mechanical disturbances has been difficult to obtain, however (see for example Morris and Horn, 1991). Perhaps the best evidence comes from two particularly well-studied sensory receptors: crayfish stretch receptors and hair cells of the auditory and vestibular system.

The thorax and abdomen of many crustaceans contain specialized cells whose fine processes are closely apposed to accessory muscle cells (Fig. 15.2A). These processes do not innervate the muscle cells but instead form numerous sites of attachment with the muscle cell membrane or adjacent extracellular matrix. The muscle cells are attached to the wall of the exoskeleton and span adjacent segments, so that when the abdomen or thorax of the animal is stretched, the muscle cells are also stretched. Stretching of the muscle causes the dendrites of the stretch receptors to be distended, and this produces a change in the receptor membrane potential, called a *generator potential*.

Responses from crayfish stretch receptors were first recorded by Eyzaguirre and Kuffler (1955), and an example of their recordings is given in Fig. 15.2B. Intracellular responses were detected with fine microelectrodes while stretches were applied to the accessory muscle of the receptor by holding the ends of the muscle with tweezers and gently pulling the ends of the muscle apart. Beginning at the first arrow below the recording in Fig. 15.2B, a stretch was delivered to the muscle and then continuously increased up to the straight line. From this point on, the stretch was maintained at a constant length and then released at the second arrow. The stretch depolarized the cell from its resting potential, typically -70 to -80 mV, and the depolarization caused the generation of action potentials.

In a later study (Nakajima and Onodera, 1969), the muscle was

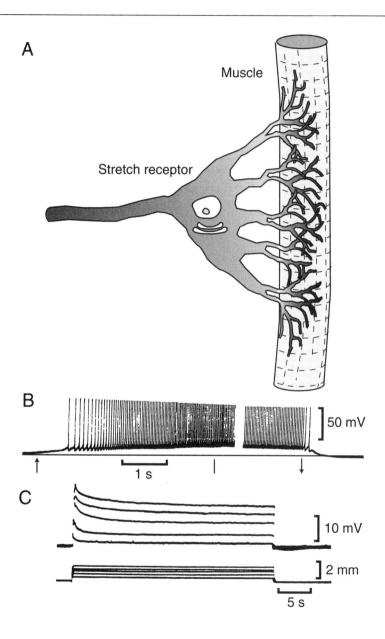

Fig. 15.2 Mechanosensory response of crayfish stretch receptor. **(A)** Anatomy of stretch receptor. (Simplified from Wiersma, 1967.) **(B)** Intracellular recording from crayfish stretch receptor. Resting membrane potential was between −70 and −80 mV. Stretches were applied by clamping the ends of the accessory muscle with tweezers attached to sliding supports, and then gently moving these supports with micrometer screws so as to pull the ends of the muscle apart. At first arrow, a stretch was applied and then gradually increased up to the line. Stretch was then maintained until the downward arrow. Gap in record contained several seconds of rhythmic spiking, not shown. (Data from Eyzaguirre and Kuffler, 1955, relabeled and displayed with contrast reversed.) **(C)** Generator potentials, recorded with intracellular microelectrode from a crayfish stretch receptor bathed in solution containing 2×10^{-7} g/ml TTX. Lower traces show duration and magnitude of stretches of constant length applied to the accessory muscle, and upper traces are superimposed voltage responses from the same receptor. Stretches were applied by a method similar to that in **(B)**. (From Nakajima and Onodera, 1969, with permission of the authors and of the Physiological Society.)

stretched in a preparation bathed in TTX, to block action potentials and reveal the isolated generator potential. For each trace (Fig. 15.2C), a stretch of constant length was given for the duration of the stimulus (indicated by the lowermost traces), and the magnitude of the stretch was varied, producing each of the superimposed responses. Larger stretches produced larger depolarizations, and each response showed a sag in membrane potential, called *adaptation,* probably a result of mechanical relaxation in the tension produced by the muscle during a stretch of constant length. The channel gated by stretch is permeable to a wide variety of monovalent cations, including Tris+ and arginine+ (Brown, Ottoson, and Rydqvist, 1978). The channel also is permeable to divalent cations, including Ca^{2+}, Mg^{2+}, Sr^{2+}, and Ba^{2+} (Edwards et al., 1981).

Since the depolarization of the stretch receptor is produced by a distension of the membrane of the fine dendrites, it seems possible that these dendrites may contain some form of stretch-sensitive channels. This notion was tested by Erxleben (1989), who made on-cell and isolated patch recordings from the cell body and primary dendrites of the crayfish stretch receptors. Erxleben was unable to make recordings from the fine dendritic processes which were directly apposed to the muscle cells, but he supposed that the population of channels in the larger primary dendrites might reflect the population in the finer processes.

He found two kinds of stretch-sensitive channels (see Fig. 15.3), which he called *stretch-activated* (SA) channels and *rectifying stretch-activated* (RSA) channels. Both types were nonselective for cations and permeable to Ca^{2+}, but they differed in single-channel conductance and in voltage dependence. For SA channels, the probability of opening *(p_o)* was largely independent of voltage, whereas for the RSA channels, p_o was very small at the resting membrane potential and increased dramatically as the membrane potential hyperpolarized. The channels also differed in their distribution. RSA channels were more often observed in patches from the cell body or axon hillock, and channel density was usually small. SA channels, on the other hand, were commonly observed in patches from the primary dendrites, and there were usually a large number of channels in each patch.

These results suggest that the mechanosensitivity of the crayfish stretch receptor may be mediated by SA channels. The contribution

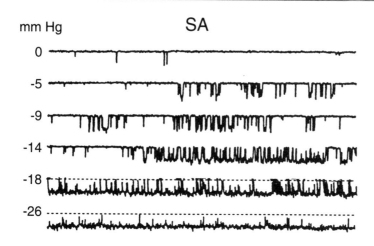

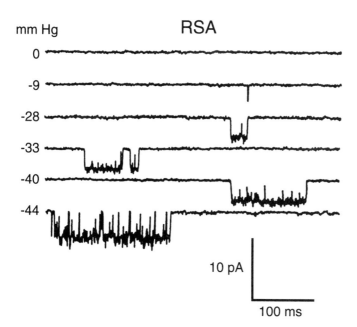

Fig. 15.3 On-cell patch recording of single stretch-sensitive channels from crayfish stretch receptors. Numbers to left give suction applied to patch pipette from a calibrated pressure transducer. Pressure was applied continuously for the length of each record. Recordings were from *SA*, stretch-activated channels; and *RSA*, rectifying stretch-activated channels. Holding potentials were at the cell's resting membrane potential (for *SA*) and 50 mV hyperpolarized from resting membrane potential (for *RSA*). (From Erxleben, 1989, reprinted with permission of the author and of Rockefeller University Press.)

of RSA channels to the mechanosensitive current is unlikely to be large, since the p_o of these channels either at the resting membrane potential or at depolarized potentials is low, and since the density of these channels on the dendrites seems also to be low. Since Erxleben did not make recordings from the finest dendrites actually in contact with the muscle cells, it remains possible that neither the SA nor the RSA channels actually contribute to mechanoreception but that the finest dendrites contain yet another kind of channel which actually mediates the response to stretch.

Hair Cells

An even more convincing case for direct activation of mechano-receptive channels can be made for hair cells. Hair cells are the sensory receptor cells of the vertebrate inner ear and of the semicircular canals of the vestibular system. They are also the sensory cells of lateral line organs, which fish and aquatic amphibians use to detect water movements. Hair cells in all of these tissues have a similar morphology (see Hudspeth, 1985, 1989; Pickles, 1988; Corey and Assad, 1992; Hackney and Furness, 1995). They are modified epithelial cells that appear cylindrical in cross-section or as isolated cells (see Figs. 15.4A and B). They lack axons but contact nerve fibers at afferent synapses along the basal surface of the cell (see Chapter 8 and Fig. 8.8C), which may be glutamatergic (Kataoka and Ohmori, 1994). The most striking morphological feature of these cells is their apical hair bundle, formed from a cluster of 20–300 microvilli-like structures called *stereocilia* (or *stereovilli*) and, in some cases, a single true cilium called a *kinocilium*. These can be seen in cross section in Fig. 15.4A and B but can be more clearly visualized in Fig. 15.4C, a scanning electron micrograph of a portion of the apical surface of the bullfrog sacculus. The round balls in this picture are the bulbous terminations of the lone kinocilium of each hair cell bundle. The stereocilia are generally arranged in order of height, in round, square, or oval bundles or (in higher vertebrate cochlea) in the shape of a *V* or *W*, with the apex of the bundle containing the kinocilium and the tallest stereocilia, behind which stereocilia of progressively shorter height are placed.

Mechanotransduction occurs when the stereocilia are moved either directly by surrounding fluid or by some specialized structure, such as the otolithic membrane of the sacculus and utriculus or the gelatinous cupula of the semicircular canals and lateral line organs. The stereocilia are rigid rods full of actin filaments crosslinked by another protein, fimbrin. They are inserted into the hair cell at the cuticular plate, which is also rigid and is composed of actin as well

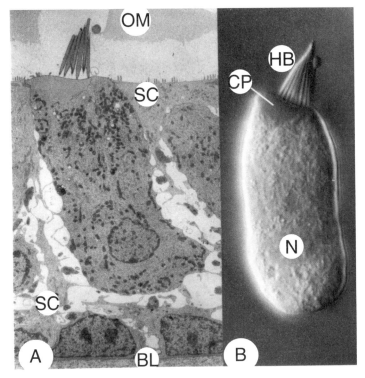

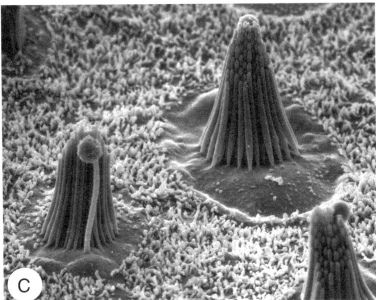

Fig. 15.4 Anatomy of a hair cell. **(A)** Transmission electron micrograph of intact hair cell from bullfrog sacculus. Hair cell and adjacent supporting cells (*SC*) form an epithelial sheet, resting on the basolaminar membrane (*BL,* bottom). The hair bundle of a hair cell is shown at the top of the figure, in contact with the otolithic membrane (*OM*), whose movement conveys the sensory stimulus to the cell (see also Fig. 15.5). **(B)** Light micrograph of single hair cell, enzymatically dissociated from bullfrog sacculus. *HB,* hair bundle; *CP,* cuticular plate; and *N,* cell nucleus. Knob to right of hair bundle is bulbous termination of kinocilium. (Parts **(A)** and **(B)** from Hudspeth, 1985, reprinted with permission of the author and of the American Association for the Advancement of Science.) **(C)** Scanning electron micrograph of sensory epithelium of bullfrog sacculus with otolithic membrane removed. Note organization of hair bundle, with tallest stereocilia placed adjacent to kinocilium (with knob), and stereocilia of progressively smaller length behind. Hair bundles arise from cuticular plates of hair cells, which are surrounded by a sea of shorter microvilli, mostly from supporting cells. (Reprinted with the permission of John A. Assad and David P. Corey.)

as several other cytoskeletal proteins. At the point of insertion the stereocilia narrow, so that only a small fraction of the actin filaments of the stereocilium terminate within the cuticular plate. This anchoring mechanism has the effect that, when the stereocilia are deflected, they remain rigid and pivot at their point of insertion.

The role of the stereocilia in mechanotransduction was first investigated by Åke Flock and his collaborators, who showed that the stereocilial bundle is directionally sensitive: stimuli in the direction of the tallest stereocilium (or the kinocilium) are excitatory, and stimuli in the opposite direction are inhibitory (Flock, 1965). This property of the hair cell was investigated in detail with intracellular recording by Hudspeth and Corey (1977), who stripped the otolithic membrane away from the sacculus of a bullfrog with fine forceps and recorded from hair cells with intracellular electrodes (Fig. 15.5A). Another coarse, stimulating pipette (labeled *Stimulus probe* in Fig. 15.5A) was slipped over the tips of the hair bundles and moved by an electromechanical transducer (a piezoelectric element), which in turn was controlled by a waveform generator.

When the stimulus probe was moved toward the largest stereocilia and the kinocilium, the hair cell membrane potential depolarized (Fig. 15.5B). Movement in the opposite direction produced a hyperpolarization, and movement perpendicular to this axis produced little or no response. The amplitude of the response increased with increasing deflection of the bundle but was asymmetric: depolarizations were larger than hyperpolarizations, and at rest about 15 percent of the mechanoreceptive channels were open and available to be closed (Fig. 15.5C).

The Mechanism of Mechanotransduction

The changes in voltage produced by deflection of the hair bundle are produced by the gating of mechanosensitive channels. Preliminary measurements by Hudspeth and Corey (1977) suggested that depolarization was accompanied by an increase in conductance (that is, the opening of channels) and hyperpolarization by a conductance decrease (channel closing). Conclusive evidence for this hypothesis was later provided by voltage-clamp recordings from hair cells, either with a two-electrode method (Corey and

A

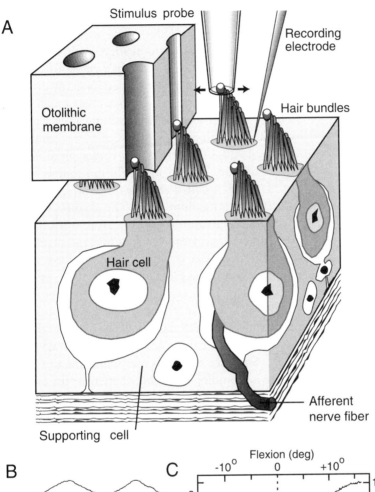

Stimulus probe

Recording electrode

Otolithic membrane

Hair bundles

Hair cell

Afferent nerve fiber

Supporting cell

B

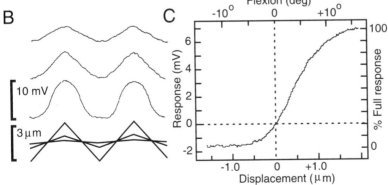

10 mV

3 μm

C

Flexion (deg)

-10° 0 +10°

Response (mV)

% Full response

Displacement (μm)

Fig. 15.5 Intracellular recordings from bullfrog saccular cells. **(A)** Experimental preparation. Otolithic membrane was partially stripped from saccular epithelium, revealing apical ends of hair cells and hair bundles. A stimulus probe was slipped over the top of the hair bundle of a single cell and moved laterally, to produce mechanical movement. Intracellular recording was made with a microelectrode inserted into the hair cell. **(B)** Change in membrane potential of hair cell during mechanical stimulation. Stimulus probe was coupled to a piezo-electric device, which in turn was controlled by a waveform generator. *Lower traces:* Superimposed triangle waves (10 Hz), used as the electrical signal to move the stimulus probe toward the kinocilium and then back again. Three waveforms are shown, corresponding to displacements of the probe with amplitudes as indicated by the scale bar at left. *Upper traces:* Voltage responses of hair cell to these three stimuli. Each trace is the average of 32 responses. **(C)** Curve showing potential change as a function of displacement. Ordinate gives (*left*) change in potential from V_{rest} of −58 mV or (*right*) response as a percentage of maximum response. Abscissa shows magnitude of displacement in μm (*below*) or in degrees of angular flexion of the hair bundle (*above*). Zero displacement is resting position of hair bundle, positive displacements are toward the kinocilium, and negative are away from kinocilium. Note asymmetry in curve. (From Hudspeth and Corey, 1977, reprinted with permission of the authors.)

Hudspeth, 1979; Howard and Hudspeth, 1987) or with patch-clamp recording (Ohmori, 1985; Holton and Hudspeth, 1986; Crawford, Evans, and Fettiplace, 1989). The mechanosensitive current has a reversal potential at or somewhat positive to zero, and the channels are nonselective cationic, like those of crayfish stretch receptors. The channels can be permeated by many different monovalent cations, including Na^+ and K^+, as well as much larger ions, such as choline$^+$ and tetramethylammonium; they can also be permeated by divalent cations, including Ca^{2+}, Sr^{2+}, and Ba^{2+} (Corey and Hudspeth, 1979; Ohmori, 1985). Under physiological conditions, the stereocilia are bathed in a solution that is low in Na^+ and Ca^{2+} but high in K^+, called *endolymph,* and inward current is carried mostly by potassium ions. The channels can be blocked by positively charged aminoglycoside antibiotics, such as streptomycin and neomycin, and the block is voltage-dependent, decreasing with membrane depolarization (Ohmori, 1985).

The channels appear also to be blocked by Ca^{2+}. The evidence for this is that increases in the extracellular Ca^{2+} concentration cause a decrease in the size of the mechanosensitive current (see for example Crawford, Evans, and Fettiplace, 1991), such that the amplitude of the current is several times larger in 50–500 μM Ca^{2+} than in 2.8 mM Ca^{2+}. Since the channels are permeable to Ca^{2+}, it seems likely that there is a binding site somewhere near the channel mouth to which Ca^{2+} binds during its passage through the channel, much as for voltage-dependent Ca^{2+} channels (see Chapter 7).

If the Ca^{2+} concentration is made very low (of the order of 1–10 μM or below), a peculiar thing happens. The mechanoreceptive current is entirely abolished (Sand, 1975; Corey and Hudspeth, 1979; Crawford, Evans, and Fettiplace, 1991). If exposure to such low-Ca^{2+} solutions is prolonged for more than a few seconds, the current disappears and does not come back for many hours. It is as if low-Ca^{2+} solution somehow destroys the sensitivity of the channels to mechanical stimuli.

This effect was exploited by Crawford, Evans, and Fettiplace (1991) to record single-channel currents from hair cells. They exposed dissociated hair cells from the turtle cochlea to 1 μM Ca^{2+} for just long enough to abolish the mechanosensitive current, and they then returned the cell to normal saline solution. In some ex-

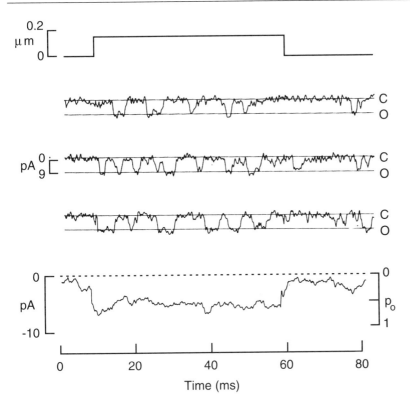

Fig. 15.6 Whole-cell recording of currents from a single mechanosensitive channel from a hair cell isolated from the cochlea of the turtle *Pseudemys scripta elegans*. Hair cell was treated with 1 μM Ca^{2+} solution for a brief period and then restored to normal saline. Upper trace shows stimulus protocol: hair bundle was deflected 0.15 μm toward the kinocilium for 50 ms. Method of stimulation similar to the one illustrated in Fig. 15.5. Middle three traces are representative responses. The cell appeared to have only a single active channel (*C*, closed; *O*, open) with a unitary current of about 9 pA. Lower trace, an average of 55 responses from this cell, indicates that stimulation increased the probability of opening of the channel (p_o) from 0.15 at rest to 0.5 for the 0.15 μm stimulus. (Reprinted from Crawford, Evans, and Fettiplace, 1991, with permission of the authors and of the Physiological Society.)

periments, just one or a few channels survived this treatment, and the opening and closing of the channels could be recorded with a whole-cell voltage clamp. An example is given in Fig. 15.6. The first trace in this figure shows the time course of deflection of the hair bundle, and the three traces below give typical responses from the cell. The records are a bit noisy, since they are whole-cell recordings and not isolated patch recordings, and the recording therefore exhibits the background noise of the whole cell rather than of a small piece of membrane. Nevertheless, the recordings clearly show channel openings with a unitary conductance of about 100 pS (see also Ohmori, 1985). The lowermost trace is an average of many single-channel recordings from this same cell and more clearly demonstrates that the probability of opening of the channels is increased by bundle deflection.

The Tip-Link Hypothesis

The gating of the mechanosensitive channels of hair cells appears to be the result of direct application of a mechanical force on the channel or surrounding membrane, in the absence of any second messenger or metabotropic cascade. The best evidence for this is the short latency of the response, which in submammalian vertebrates is no larger than 100 μs (Corey and Hudspeth, 1983; Crawford, Evans, and Fettiplace, 1989). In Fig. 15.7A, the mechanosensitive current from a single voltage-clamped hair cell from the turtle cochlea is shown as a function of time for a rapid displacement of the hair bundle (uppermost trace). The current responses are given for displacements of different amplitude (measured in μm). They show that the time course of the response was slowest near the resting position of the bundle but became more rapid with increasing bundle displacement. For the largest displacements, the time constant of current increase was about 100 μs. In mammals, the hair cell response is probably even faster than this, since in bats and in aquatic animals, like whales and seals, sounds can be detected at frequencies above 100 kHz. Hair cells in these animals appear to have latencies less than 10 μs, which is far too fast to be produced by even the most rapid metabotropic cascade (Corey and Hudspeth, 1983).

If deflection of the bundle directly gates the mechanosensitive channels, it is clearly of interest to understand the physical mechanism of channel opening. One hypothesis, for which there is now considerable evidence, is that gating is due at least in part to forces produced by structures called *tip links*. Tip links are proteinaceous fibers that connect adjacent stereocilia at their tips (Pickles, Comis, and Osborne, 1984). Pickles and collaborators suggested that the stretching and slackening of the tip links may somehow gate channel opening and closing (Pickles, Comis, and Osborne, 1984; Pickles, 1988); that is, movement of the bundle in the direction of the kinocilium and/or the largest stereocilia may stretch the tip links and somehow pull the channels open, whereas movement in the opposite direction may relax the tip links, allowing the channels to close (see Fig. 15.7B).

If forces produced by the tip links are somehow responsible for gating the channels, then the channels should be located some-

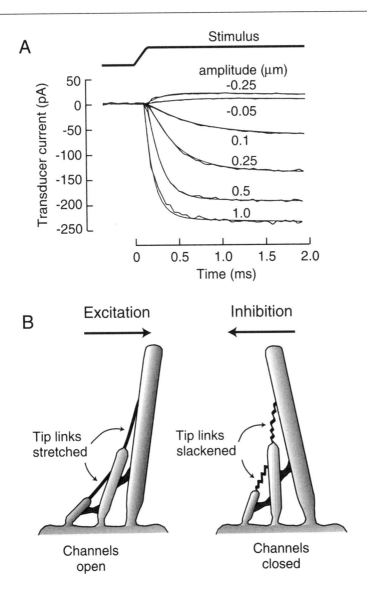

Fig. 15.7 Latency of hair cell response. **(A)** Whole-cell patch recordings from hair cells isolated from the turtle cochlea. Cells were stimulated by rapid displacement of a glass probe glued to a piezo-electric device. Upper trace shows time course of movement of probe, measured optically. Lower traces are current responses at 23°C from voltage-clamped hair cell for hair bundle deflections whose amplitudes are given next to traces. Positive amplitudes are for deflections toward the kinocilium (which produce inward currents), negative amplitudes for deflections away from kinocilium (which produce smaller outward currents). Smooth curves overlaying current responses are fits of currents to two time constants, one of about 50 μs and the other about 400 μs near the resting position of the bundle, but decreasing for either positive or negative displacements. (Reprinted with minor modification from Crawford, Evans, and Fettiplace, 1989, with permission of the authors and of the Physiological Society.) **(B)** Tip-link hypothesis. (After Pickles, Comis, and Osborne, 1984.)

where in the vicinity of the tip links, rather than, for example, at the base of the hair cell bundle near its pivot point. Although this matter was initially controversial (see Ohmori, 1988), there is now nearly universal agreement that the mechanosensitive channels are indeed at the tips. The evidence for this is, first, that the inward current entering the mechanosensitive channels is largest near the tips of the stereocilia (Hudspeth, 1982); and second, that the upper region of the hair cell bundle shows the greatest sensitivity to block by aminoglycoside antibiotics (Jaramillo and Hudspeth, 1991).

In addition to these observations, the location of the channels has been determined by measuring the distribution of Ca^{2+} increase with Ca^{2+}-sensitive fluorescent dyes during displacement of the hair bundle. Recall that the channels are permeable to Ca^{2+}, which means that the opening of the channels should produce a local increase in Ca^{2+} concentration in the vicinity of the channel. Denk, Holt, Shepherd, and Corey (1995) used two-photon microscopy (Denk and Svoboda, 1997) and the fluorometric dye Calcium Green-1™(see Chapter 13) to study the change in Ca^{2+} concentration during bundle deflection. The Ca^{2+} increase was clearly largest and fastest near the top of the hair bundle (see Fig. 15.8B), as would be expected if the channels were also located in this part of the cell (see also Lumpkin and Hudspeth, 1995).

More direct evidence that the tip links are needed for the hair cell's current response comes from the remarkable observations of Assad, Shepherd, and Corey (1991), who showed that exposure to low-Ca^{2+} solution, which abolishes the response of hair cells to mechanical stimuli, also breaks the tip links. The breaking of the tip links causes a sudden movement of the hair bundle, as if the tip links held the bundle under tension (see also Jaramillo and Hudspeth, 1993). After breakage, the tip links regenerate over a period of about 24 hours, and as the tip links return, so do the responses of the hair cells (Zhao, Yamoah, and Gillespie, 1996).

Since the tip lengths exert tension on the hair cell bundle, they may act as *gating springs*, transmitting mechanical force directly to the molecular structure of the channel (see Corey and Hudspeth, 1983; Hudspeth, 1989; Markin and Hudspeth, 1995). If this is so, then the stiffness of the hair cell bundle should be affected by the opening and closing of the channels. To paraphrase Hudspeth (1989), imagine tying an elastic cord to the knob of a door and then measuring the stiffness of the cord by pulling and measuring the distance the cord can be extended. The cord would seem equally stiff if the door were closed or wide open, but a very different result would be obtained if the door were initially closed but

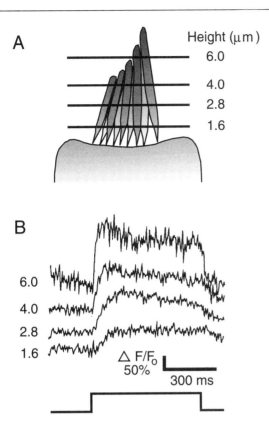

A

Height (μm)

6.0

4.0

2.8

1.6

B

6.0

4.0

2.8

1.6

$\triangle F/F_0$
50%

300 ms

Fig. 15.8 Ca^{2+} measurements from hair bundles. Two-photon confocal microscopy (Denk and Svoboda, 1997) and the fluorescent indicator dye Calcium Green-1™ were used to measure changes in Ca^{2+} as a function of time and distance from the cuticular plate in hair bundles of bullfrog saccular cells. Cells were whole-cell patch-clamped in the intact epithelium with pipettes containing 105 mM Cs^+ to block K^+ currents and 125 μM Calcium Green-1™. Bathing solution contained elevated (4 mM) Ca^{2+} to increase size of Ca^{2+} influx through mechanosensitive channels. **(A)** Schema of hair cell with focal planes from which measurement of Ca^{2+} was made. **(B)** Change in fluorescence as a function of time at indicated focal planes. Fluorescence change normalized to resting fluorescence ($\Delta F/F_0$—see scale bar). Lowermost trace gives waveform of mechanical stimulation, produced by an electronically controlled fluid jet directed at hair bundle. Bundle deflection was ~0.5 μm. (Replotted from Denk et al., 1995, and used with the permission of the authors and of Cell Press.)

free to open. As the cord was pulled, it would initially be stiff but then would relax as the door opened. This would have the effect of making the cord seem less stiff if the door were free to open than if the door were already open or firmly closed. For the hair cell, this would mean that the stiffness of the hair bundle would be greatest when the channels were either all open or all closed, and stiffness should decrease and be at a minimum when the probability of channel opening is near 0.5.

Howard and Hudspeth (1987) tested this notion by measuring the stiffness of the hair bundle during channel gating. They did this by moving the hair bundle of bullfrog saccular cells with a short, flexible fiber (see Fig. 15.9A). The stiffness (or spring constant) of the fiber was measured from its Brownian motion or by attaching weights to the end of the fiber and observing the distance of fiber deflection under the microscope. The fiber was then mounted on the end of a piezo-electric device and attached to the top of a hair cell bundle at the bulbous end of the kinocilium. Since the fiber and the hair bundle had about the same stiffness, movement of the piezo-electric device caused both a bending of the hair bundle and a bending of the fiber (see Fig. 15.9A). From the amplitude of the bending of the fiber and the previously measured spring constant of the fiber, it was possible to calculate the force *(F)* exerted by the fiber, since from Hooke's law

$$F = -kx$$

where k is the spring constant and x is the distance of bending of the fiber. Once this force was known, it was then possible to calculate the stiffness or spring constant of the *hair cell bundle* from the measured distance of *bundle* displacement. Since, as we shall see, the stiffness of the bundle was not a constant but depended upon the amplitude of bundle deflection, it was necessary to express Hooke's law in the form

$$k(x) \approx -\frac{\Delta F}{\Delta x}$$

The results of these experiments are shown in Fig. 15.9B. The bundle stiffness was indeed at its maximal value when the channels were either all open or all closed, and stiffness was a minimum at a bundle deflection of about 30 nm. This happened also to be the value of the deflection for which the receptor potential was about half its maximal value, that is, when p_o was about 0.5. This striking result demonstrates that there is probably some more or less direct connection between a gating spring and the channels. If the gating springs are indeed the tip links, one possibility is that the tip links are connected to the channels by some direct physical attachment. It remains possible, however, that the tip links are inserted in the membrane or cytoskeleton in the vicinity of the channels, and that the tip links and channels are not directly attached though still somehow mechanically coupled to one another.

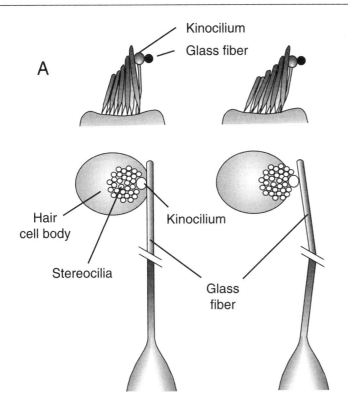

A

Kinocilium

Glass fiber

Hair cell body

Kinocilium

Stereocilia

Glass fiber

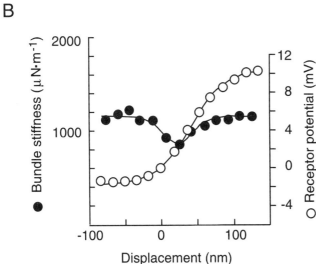

B

Fig. 15.9 Measurement of gating spring. (A) Technique for measuring spring constant of hair cell bundle. A fine glass fiber was pushed up against the end of the hair cell bundle at the kinocilium and spontaneously attached to the bundle. The glass fiber was mounted on a piezo-electric device and could be moved, as shown in side view (upper drawings) and from the top of cell (lower drawings). From the calibration of the spring constant of the fiber, it was possible to calculate the force exerted by the fiber on the bundle, from Hooke's law. From this force and the degree of the movement of the bundle (measured optically), it was possible to calculate the spring constant of the bundle. Fiber was longer than shown (indicated by break). (B) Hair bundle spring constant (bundle stiffness, *solid symbols*) and receptor potential *(open symbols)* measured with an intracellular microelectrode, plotted for the same hair cell against displacement of the hair bundle. Bundle stiffness is at a minimum when the receptor potential is at about half its maximum value. (From Howard and Hudspeth, 1987, reprinted with permission of the authors and of Cell Press.)

Adaptation

One of the most interesting features of the hair cell response is the shift in the dynamic range that occurs in the presence of a steady bundle deflection (see Fettiplace, 1992; Hudspeth and Gillespie, 1994). This readjustment of the dynamic range of the cell is called *adaptation.* It is an important feature of most if not all sensory cells, including photoreceptors and olfactory receptors, as we shall see in Chapter 16. For hair cells in the ear, adaptation has the important role of altering the sensitivity of the cell in the presence of a steady background stimulation, for example the steady sound of a room fan or car motor. As the level of the steady noise changes, the hair cell adjusts its dynamic range to softer or louder sounds so as to retain as large as possible a sensitivity to changes in sound level.

Adaptation can occur within at least some types of hair cells, as can be seen in Fig. 15.10 (from Assad and Corey, 1992). A single saccular hair cell was dissociated from bullfrog for this experiment and then whole-cell voltage-clamped. For each stimulus presentation, the hair cell was first deflected for a short time from its resting position with test displacements of variable amplitude, and changes in current were recorded (see Fig. 15.10A). From these recordings, a stimulus-response curve was determined from the resting position (dashed line in Fig. 15.10B). The hair cell bundle was then deflected 450 nm and held in this position. The hair cell responded with a large inward current (see Fig. 15.10A), which declined with time. Superimposed on top of this declining response are incremental responses to test displacements *from this steady deflected position,* measured at two times after the beginning of the steady deflection. When the values of the peak amplitudes of these responses were plotted as a function of hair bundle position, the resulting curves were shifted along the displacement axis (solid curves in Fig. 15.10B), as if the steady deflection had reset the dynamic range of the cell. Fig. 15.10C shows that this is a fairly rapid effect, requiring less than 5 ms for half completion (see also Eatock, Corey, and Hudspeth, 1987; Crawford, Evans, and Fettiplace, 1989; Shepherd and Corey, 1994; Ricci and Fettiplace, 1997).

The shifting of the positions of the stimulus-response curves in Fig. 15.10B has the effect of changing the region of displacements for which the cell is most sensitive. At the resting bundle posi-

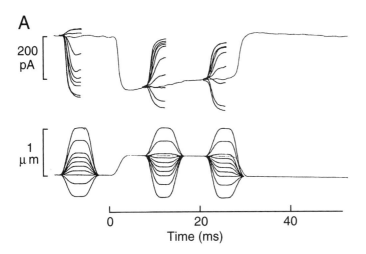

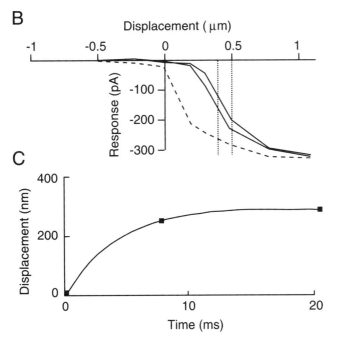

Fig. 15.10 Adaptation in isolated bullfrog saccular cell. Recordings made with whole-cell patch-clamp. Hair cell was stimulated with glass probe attached to kinocilium and displaced with a piezo-electric device. **(A)** Upper traces are superimposed current responses to the stimulation protocol given below. Cell was given a 5 ms test displacement from the resting position, or a steady adapting displacement during which the cell was stimulated with a test displacement at one of two time points during the steady displacement. Only one test displacement was given per experimental run, and this protocol was repeated for each of the three stimulus conditions (with and without the steady displacement) and for each of the 10 test stimulus amplitudes. **(B)** Plot of peak current response amplitude as a function of displacement from the data in **(A)**. Responses to test stimuli from resting position are given as dashed curve, and responses to test stimuli in presence of steady displacement are given as solid curves. Dotted lines are drawn at 0.4 and 0.5 μm (400 and 500 nm), to aid in comparing response amplitudes for these two deflections at rest or in the presence of the adapting stimulus. **(C)** Magnitude of shift of curves in **(B)** along displacement axis as function of time. The displacement of the curves was measured by translating the curve in the resting position in B (the dashed curve) along the displacement axis, and fitting this curve by eye to the two solid curves. The extent of the displacement was then plotted as a function of the time after the beginning of the steady adapting step when the measurements for the two solid curves were made. (Data replotted from Assad and Corey, 1992.)

tion (Fig. 15.10B, dashed curve) deflections to 400 nm and 500 nm produce responses which differ in amplitude by only 10–20 pA (note intersections of dotted and dashed lines). The resting stimulus-response curve is rather shallow for deflections in this range of hair bundle positions, with the consequence that the hair cell would have difficulty distinguishing movements to these two positions. In the presence of the steady displacement, the stimulus-response curve shifts to the right along the displacement axis (Fig. 10B). As a result, there is now a much larger difference in the response to deflections to 400nm and 500nm, and the cell is now better able to distinguish deflections to these two positions.

The shifting of the dynamic range of the hair cell in response to a steady displacement is probably mechanical, as would occur if there were some adjustment in the position or tension of the gating springs. We could imagine, for example, that a steady stretching of the tip links causes the proteins of these fibers to pull on the channels, but that this pull relaxes with time. The machinery for tension adjustment seems to lie within the cytoplasm of the hair cell. The best evidence for this is that adaptation depends critically on a change in intracellular Ca^{2+}. When, for example, the hair cell is dialyzed in a whole-cell patch-clamp with a pipette solution containing 10 mM of the Ca^{2+} buffer BAPTA (see Chapter 13), adaptation is abolished (Crawford, Evans, and Fettiplace, 1989). Adaptation can also be altered by changes in extracellular Ca^{2+} (see for example Hacohen et al., 1989; Crawford, Evans, and Fettiplace, 1989), by ultraviolet irradiation of a hair cell containing the caged-Ca^{2+} compound nitr-5 (Kimitsuki and Ohmori, 1992), and by changes in membrane potential that change the driving force for Ca^{2+} entry (Assad, Hacohen, and Corey, 1989; Crawford, Evans, and Fettiplace, 1989). Finally, adaptation can be abolished by whole-cell dialysis with solutions containing calmodulin inhibitors (Walker and Hudspeth, 1996). These findings suggest that Ca^{2+}, entering the mechanosensitive channels, may somehow alter the dynamic range of channel gating.

One model for adaptation supposes that the tension of the gating springs is adjusted inside the hair cell during a maintained bundle displacement by an active force produced by myosin motors running along the actin fibrils of the stereocilia (see Gillespie, 1995). The sacculus contains myosin (Solc et al., 1994), and immunohistochemistry with myosin monoclonal antibodies suggests that at least one of the isoforms of this protein may be positioned at the tips of the stereocilia, perhaps in the vicinity of the channels (Gillespie, Wagner, and Hudspeth, 1993; see also Hasson et al., 1997). Whole-cell dialysis with agents that inhibit protein ATPases, including myosin, have been shown to abolish adaptation (Gillespie and Hudspeth, 1993; Yamoah and Gillespie, 1996). It seems possible that the entry of Ca^{2+} into the hair cell cytoplasm could trigger the movement of myosin, which then produces an adjustment of the tension of the tip links on the channels. This process would have to be quite rapid, since adaptation in some hair cells can occur in less than 1 ms (see Ricci and Fettiplace, 1997). The rapidity of adaptation (Fig. 15.10C) indicates that there would have to be some highly organized structure within the stereocilia close to the channels, or within the channels themselves, modulating the working range of the mechanoreceptive mechanism.

Hair Cells and the Physiology of Hearing

In the mammalian ear, hair cells are located within a spiral organ called the cochlea (see Pickles, 1988). Changes in air pressure at the tympanic membrane (ear drum) are coupled by the bones of the middle ear (malleus, incus, and stapes) to the oval window of the cochlea (Fig. 15.11A). Vibrations of the oval window are communicated to fluid within the chambers of the cochlea (Fig. 15.11B), and the movement of this fluid initiates a displacement of the basilar membrane just below the hair cells (Fig. 15.12). As the basilar membrane moves, the stereocilia of the hair cells are deflected, and this displacement produces an electrical response.

The response of individual hair cells depends upon the frequency of the sound, and different cells have different *characteristic* or *best* frequencies to which they are most sensitive. In mammals, the characteristic frequency of hair cells varies systematically from one end of the cochlea to the other. In lower vertebrates, such as reptiles and birds, and in particular in the turtle, the frequency tuning of the hair cell may be largely a result of an electrical resonance in the hair cell membrane (Crawford and Fettiplace, 1981), produced by interaction between a voltage-dependent Ca^{2+} conductance and a Ca^{2+}-activated K^+ conductance (Art and Fettiplace, 1987; Art, Wu,

Fig. 15.11   Anatomy of the ear. **(A)** Sound impinges upon tympanic membrane, whose vibrations are communicated by three small bones (malleus, incus, and stapes), known as the *ossicles,* to the oval window of the cochlea. Vibrations in the oval window produce fluid displacements within the spiral cochlea, which are communicated to the hair cells. **(B)** Magnified view of cross-section of cochlea. The oval window pushes against the fluid in the scala vestibuli, which is continuous at the apex of the cochlea with the scala tympani. The motion of fluid produces an undulating displacement of the basilar membrane, which lies at the base of the organ of Corti. (After Pickles, 1988.)

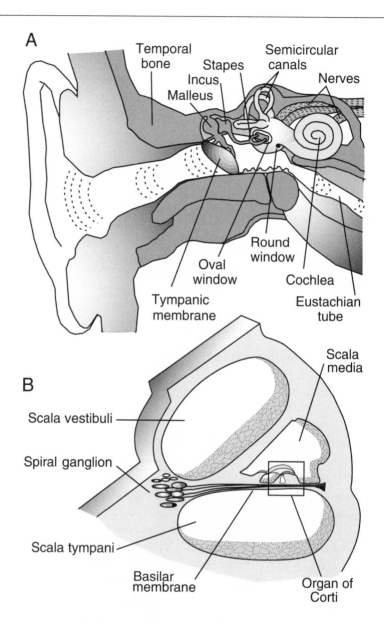

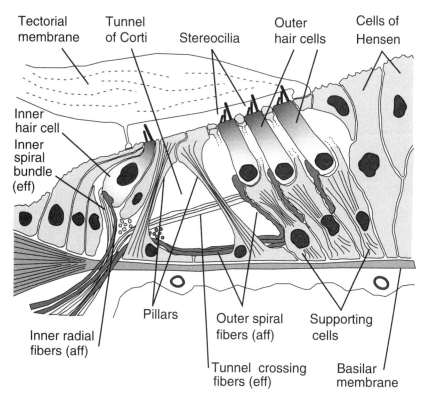

Tectorial membrane

Tunnel of Corti

Stereocilia

Outer hair cells

Cells of Hensen

Inner hair cell

Inner spiral bundle (eff)

Pillars

Inner radial fibers (aff)

Outer spiral fibers (aff)

Supporting cells

Tunnel crossing fibers (eff)

Basilar membrane

Fig. 15.12 The organ of Corti: *eff,* efferent nerve fibers making synapses onto hair cells; *aff,* afferent (sensory) nerve fibers receiving synaptic input from hair cells. (After Pickles, 1988, modified from Ryan and Dallos, 1984.)

and Fettiplace, 1995; Ramanathan et al., 1999). In mammals, however, the frequency selectivity seems to be largely if not entirely produced by mechanical tuning, through a frequency-dependent vibration of the basilar membrane.

The studies of von Békésy (1960) showed that the basilar membrane vibrates passively with a traveling wave initiated near the oval window. This wave reaches a peak amplitude at a characteristic position along the length of the cochlea (see also Pickles, 1988; Ashmore, 1994). High frequencies produce waves that peak near the base of the cochlea, where the basilar membrane is narrowest and least compliant. Low frequencies, on the other hand, peak at the opposite or apical end of the cochlea, within the innermost recesses of its spirals, where the basilar membrane is broadest and vibrates most easily. The stereocilia of the hair cells are close to or actually inserted into a flap of tissue called the tectorial membrane (see Fig. 15.12), and when the basilar membrane moves up and down, the tectorial membrane and surrounding fluid produce a shearing of the hair cell stereocilia and a change in hair cell conductance, just as for the hair cells of the sacculus.

The human ear contains about 15,000 hair cells: a single row of *inner hair cells* and 3–5 rows of *outer hair cells* (see Fig. 15.12). As in the sacculus, the hair cells of the cochlea do not have axons but synapse onto the terminals of the sensory or afferent fibers of the eighth cranial nerve. Although the inner hair cells are much less numerous than the outer hair cells, nearly all of the afferent sensory fibers terminate on these cells rather than on the outer hair cells. Both inner and outer hair cells show responses to auditory stimuli (see for example Cody and Russell, 1987; Dallos, 1985), but it is apparently the single row of inner hair cells that is primarily responsible for auditory perception.

The responses of an inner hair cell to a series of pure tones of variable frequency are illustrated for a cell from the guinea pig ear in Fig. 15.13 (from Russell and Sellick, 1983). As for saccular hair cells (Fig. 15.5), the responses are asymmetric, showing much larger depolarizations than hyperpolarizations. At low frequencies, the hair cell is able to follow the sinusoidal waveform of the sound stimulus, but at high frequencies this is no longer the case. The capacitance of the cell limits its frequency response, and the time constant of the cell (0.2–1 ms) is not sufficiently low to permit the cell to change membrane potential in phase with the stimulating tone. Thus at higher frequencies, the sinusoidal waveform is lost and is replaced by a steady depolarization (called the *D.C. component*).

The responses in Fig. 15.13 are probably produced in much the same way that responses for amphibian saccular hair cells are, by the opening of nonselective cationic channels gated by the movement of the stereocilia. As for the sacculus, the current is carried largely by K^+, since the apical end of the hair cell is bathed in a K^+-rich *endolymph,* contained within the scala media (see Fig. 15.11B). As a result, when the hair cells are stimulated, they are not loaded with Na^+ entering the cell through the mechanosensitive channels, and this may reduce the labor of the Na^+/K^+ ATPase and

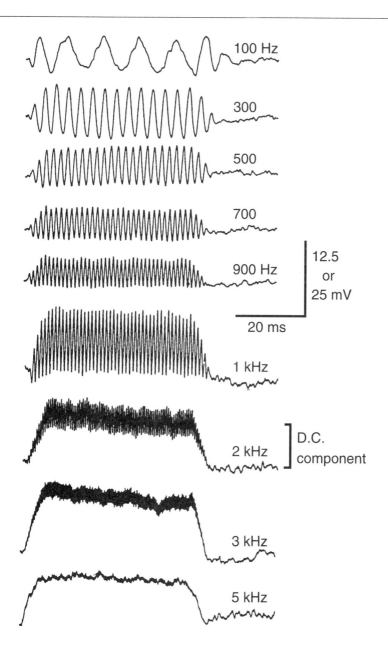

100 Hz

300

500

700

900 Hz

12.5
or
25 mV

20 ms

1 kHz

2 kHz

D.C.
component

3 kHz

5 kHz

Fig. 15.13 Intracellular recordings from hair cells in the intact cochlea of the guinea pig. Animals were stimulated with pure tones at the frequency given adjacent to each response. Responses in this figure were all recorded from the same cell. Amplitude calibration is 25 mV for tones from 100 to 900 Hz, and 12.5 mV for tones from 1 to 5 kHz. Note that responses above 1 kHz do not follow oscillations of tone and are dominated by a steady depolarization called the D.C. component, produced by an asymmetry in the response to positive and negative deflections of the hair bundle (see Fig. 15.5C). (From Russell and Sellick, 1983, reprinted with permission of the authors and of the Physiological Society.)

so decrease the metabolic load of hair cell transduction. The scala vestibuli and scala tympani both contain a Na^+-rich fluid similar in composition to cerebrospinal fluid, called the *perilymph*.

If the inner hair cells are primarily responsible for auditory perception, what do the much more numerous outer hair cells do? Increasing evidence favors the view that these cells are motile and respond to sound by producing an active displacement of the basilar membrane, which greatly enhances the localization and peak amplitude of its passive vibrations (Pickles, 1988; Dallos and Cheatham, 1992; Ashmore, 1994; Ashmore and Kolston, 1994). It has long been recognized that the passive motion of the basilar membrane first described by von Békésy is too small and too broadly tuned to explain the ability of human observers (or of single hair cells) to distinguish sounds of different frequencies. Outer hair cells have been shown to respond to changes in membrane voltage with rapid increases or decreases in cell length (Brownell et al., 1985; Kachar et al., 1986; Ashmore, 1987), and these mechanical motions seem to have a physiological role since they can be produced by deflection of the outer hair cell stereocilia (Evans and Dallos, 1993). Furthermore, stimulation of the outer hair cells has been shown to be sufficient to produce a measurable motion of the basilar membrane (Mammano and Ashmore, 1993). These observations suggest that the outer hair cells may produce a mechanical feedback large enough to produce a local amplification of von Békésy's traveling wave, and this may be an essential step in enabling the ear to detect and distinguish incoming sounds of different frequency.

Summary

Mechanoreceptors are ionotropic sensory receptors: specialized cells sensitive to external stimuli for which the stimulus appears to alter directly the probability of opening of ion channels. Many cell types have been shown to have mechanosensitive channels, which respond to a deformation of the cell membrane by either an increase or a decrease in opening probability. These channels are often nonselective cationic, but channels have also been reported that are selective to K^+ or to anions. In most cells, the function of mechanosensitive channels is still unclear, and it has even been suggested that the mechanosensitivity of these proteins is an artifact of patch-clamp recording. Although this possibility should be given serious consideration, there are at least two examples of mechano-receptors for which mechanosensitive channels are probably responsible for sensory transduction.

The stretch receptors that sense movement of adjacent segments of the exoskeleton in the abdomen and thorax of crustaceans have fine dendritic processes closely apposed to accessory muscle fibers. As the muscle fibers are stretched, the dendrites of the receptors are also stretched, and this produces an increase in a nonselective cationic conductance that depolarizes the receptor and leads to the generation of action potentials. Although recordings have not been made from the finest dendrites of these cells, recordings from larger dendrites reveal an abundant population of mechanosensitive channels with many of the physiological properties of the mechanosensitive current. These channels seem likely to be responsible for mechanotransduction in these receptors.

Hair cells are specialized cells of the auditory and vestibular systems and of lateral line organs. They sense movement by detecting the deflection of hair bundles, formed by clusters of microvilli called stereocilia. The motion of the hair bundle gates the opening and closing of 100 pS, nonselective cationic channels, which are located at the distal ends of the stereocilia. The gating of the channels is too rapid to be produced by a biochemical reaction and seems instead to be generated directly by the mechanical stimulus. Considerable evidence indicates that the channels may be gated by fine fibrous connections between adjacent stereocilia, called tip links, which are stretched or slackened by hair bundle movement. It is likely that the tip links are mechanically coupled to the channels, perhaps even by direct physical connection.

Hair cells in the mammalian ear are located in a spiral structure called the cochlea and are supported at their base by a flexible structure called the basilar membrane. Changes in sound pressure produce vibrations of the basilar membrane, which lead to bending of the hair cell stereocilia. There are two kinds of hair cells, called inner and outer. The inner hair cells respond to vibrations of the basilar membrane with changes in membrane potential, which they communicate at synapses to afferent nerve fibers. The outer hair cells also sense movements of the basilar membrane and may also communicate these responses to higher centers; however, their primary role seems to be to respond to auditory stimuli by generating active extensions and contractions of cell length. These movements are communicated to the basilar membrane and seem to accentuate and sharpen the form of the basilar membrane traveling wave. The outer hair cells appear to provide an active mechanical feedback making an essential contribution to the sensitivity of the ear to differences in pitch.

16

Photoreceptors and Olfactory Receptors

FOR THE SECOND CLASS of sensory receptors, a sensory stimulus does not activate a channel directly, but instead it stimulates a G protein and initiates a transduction cascade. The two most thoroughly studied metabotropic sensory receptors are vertebrate photoreceptors and olfactory receptor neurons, which work in a similar way. For both, the sensory signal (light or odor) is detected by one of a specialized group of heptahelical receptor proteins, similar in design to the β-adrenergic receptor (see Chapter 11 and Fig. 11.2A and C). This receptor protein then interacts with a G protein and an effector molecule to produce a change in the concentration of a second messenger. It is this second messenger that alters the probability of opening of ion channels to change the membrane potential of the cell.

The detection of light by the eye has fascinated scientists, philosophers, and poets since the time of the ancient Greeks. The discovery of even the basic outline of this mechanism is one of the most remarkable achievements of modern neuroscience. As a result of a large body of investigation, most of it within the last 25 years, we now know more about sensory transduction in vertebrate photoreceptors than for any other sensory receptor cell. The generation and modulation of the light responses of rods and cones will be the subject of the first part of this chapter. Transduction in olfactory receptor neurons, similar in many respects to that in photoreceptors, will be summarized in the second part.

I: PHOTORECEPTORS

Phototransduction begins with the absorption of light by a photopigment, called rhodopsin (see Hargrave and Hamm, 1994;

Fig. 16.1 Morphology of vertebrate photoreceptors. The outer segment, the part of the cell where transduction occurs, contains the photopigment, mostly on the disks of rods **(A)** or in the infolded plasma membrane of cones **(B)**. The inner segment is the metabolic part of the cell, containing mitochondria and endoplasmic reticulum for ATP generation and protein synthesis. The most proximal part of the cell is the synaptic terminal, which releases synaptic transmitter (probably glutamate) onto second-order bipolar and horizontal cells in specialized invaginating synapses.

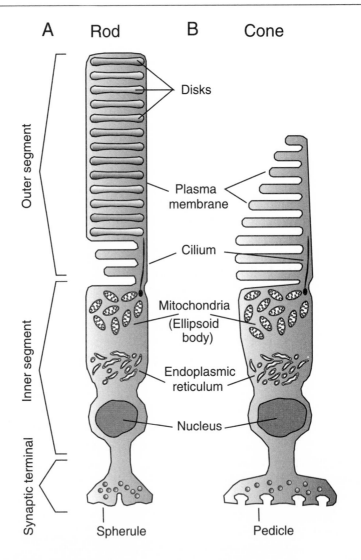

Hargrave, 1995; Rao and Oprian, 1996; Palczewski and Saari, 1997). This pigment is a typical member of the G-protein-coupled receptor family, having seven mostly α-helical transmembrane domains (Schertler and Hargrave, 1995; Sheikh et al., 1996; Unger et al., 1997). In rods, which are the photoreceptors used for dim-light vision, most of the rhodopsin is contained on disks within the outer segment of the cell (see Fig. 16.1A). The disks are formed by membrane infolding at the base of the outer segment. An amphibian rod has 1,000–2,000 of these membrane inclusions, firmly attached to the plasma membrane and to one another by fibrous proteins. In cones, the photoreceptors used for bright-light vision and for color vision, there are no disks (see Fig. 16.1B). The visual pigment is located on the plasma membrane, which is highly infolded.

Rhodopsin is an integral membrane protein (see Fig. 16.2), with about half its mass spanning the disk membrane, about a quarter (including the glycosylated N-terminus) facing the space within the disk (in rods) or the extracellular space (in cones), and about a quarter (including the C-terminus) facing the cytoplasm. The part of the protein facing the cytoplasm contains sites for interaction with G protein and with other proteins in the transduction cascade, as I shall describe in more detail below. Near the C-terminus, two highly conserved cysteines are covalently bound to lipid; they may function to anchor this part of the protein to the lipid bilayer of the membrane. The C-terminal region also contains numerous serines and threonines, which are sites for protein phosphorylation.

Rhodopsin is a peculiar sort of metabotropic receptor, since it is bound to its "agonist" when it is unstimulated (that is, in darkness) and the bond is covalent. Unstimulated rhodopsin can be thought of as consisting of two parts: the protein (called *opsin*) and the molecule bound to the protein (called the *chromophore*), which is analogous to a receptor agonist. The chromophore in most species is *11-cis retinal,* a lipophilic molecule consisting of a ring with a long aliphatic tail of carbon atoms connected by a series of conjugated double bonds (see Fig. 16.3A). At the end of the tail there is an aldehyde group (at C15), which reacts to form a covalent bond with the terminal amino group of a lysine, located about half-way down the seventh α-helix of the opsin protein. The retinal is thus buried within the protein (see Fig. 16.2B), in a pocket enclosed within the boundaries of the lipid bilayer, much as norepinephrine is when it is bound within the β-adrenergic receptor (see Fig. 11.2C).

The chromophore is directly responsible for the absorption of light. Although some insects and even some vertebrates can see in the ultraviolet, in mammals vision is mostly produced by light of wavelengths between about 400 nm (in the violet) and 700 nm (in the deep red). Mammalian visual pigments all absorb best when the stimulus is in this wavelength region: for example, the wavelength of maximal absorption (or λ_{max}) for the primate rod pigment is at about 500 nm (in the green), and for primate cone pigments at

Fig. 16.2 **(A)** Hypothesized membrane topology of rhodopsin. (After Hargrave and Hamm, 1994.) **(B)** Orientation of α-helices in structure of rhodopsin. (Modified from Schertler and Hargrave, 1995; Sheikh et al., 1996; and Unger et al., 1997.)

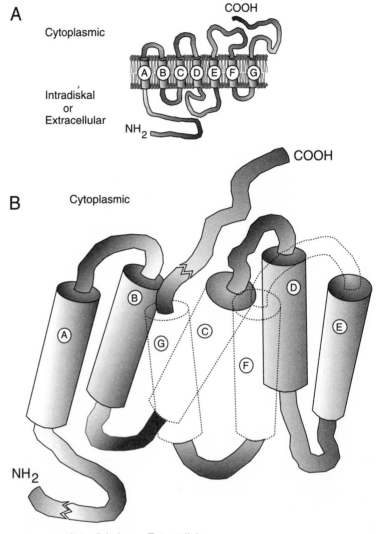

about 415–420 nm (in the blue), 535–540 nm (in the green), and 560–570 (in the yellow—see Bowmaker, Dartnall, and Mollon, 1980; Nunn, Schnapf, and Baylor, 1984).

The absorption of light by most visual pigments occurs at much longer wavelengths than absorption by either the opsin or the chromophore by themselves. In the absence of 11-*cis* retinal, rod and cone opsins absorb in the ultraviolet, like other proteins (see Tanford, 1961). In the absence of opsin, the 11-*cis* retinal also absorbs in the ultraviolet (its λ_{max} is at about 380 nm). When the aldehyde of 11-*cis* retinal reacts with opsin at the terminal amino group of the lysine residue (lys296 in bovine opsin), a double bond is formed between the aldehyde carbon and the lysine nitrogen called a *Schiff base.*

Considerable evidence indicates that the Schiff base at the chromophore-binding site is protonated (see Rao and Oprian, 1996), and protonation is largely responsible for shifting the absorption of the chromophore from 380 nm into the visible part of the spectrum. The positive charge of the proton is balanced by a negative charge from a glutamic acid in the third transmembrane domain of opsin (glu113 in bovine opsin). This glutamate is within the same transmembrane domain and only one helical turn away from the location of an aspartate residue in both adrenergic receptors and muscarinic cholinergic receptors, which is important in agonist binding (see Chapter 11).

The protonated Schiff base and the carboxyl group of glu113 together form an ion pair called a *salt bridge* (see Fig. 16.3B), which is essential for maintaining the conformation of the unstimulated receptor in a quiescent or inactive state. A single rod may contain as many as 10^9 rhodopsin molecules. These molecules are so stable that their half-life for spontaneous (thermal) activation can be measured in the hundreds or even thousands of years (Yau, Matthews, and Baylor, 1979; Baylor, Matthews, and Yau, 1980). Since spontaneous activation is so rare, the rod is exceptionally quiet. This essential feature of phototransduction makes possible the detection of a single photon of light (see Box 16.1).

The absorption of light by the covalently bound chromophore produces a chemical reaction called a *photo-isomerization,* which twists the chromophore tail around the 11–12 bond and converts 11-*cis* retinal to *all-trans* retinal (Fig. 16.3C). The twisting of the chromophore happens very rapidly and then initiates a slower series of transitions of protein structure through several intermediates, eventually removing the Schiff base's nitrogen from the vicinity of the glu113 and breaking the salt bridge. The breaking of the salt bridge is accompanied by small changes in the conformation of the protein (Farahbakhsh, Hideg, and Hubbell, 1993; Farrens et al., 1996; Sheikh et al., 1996), producing an activated conforma-

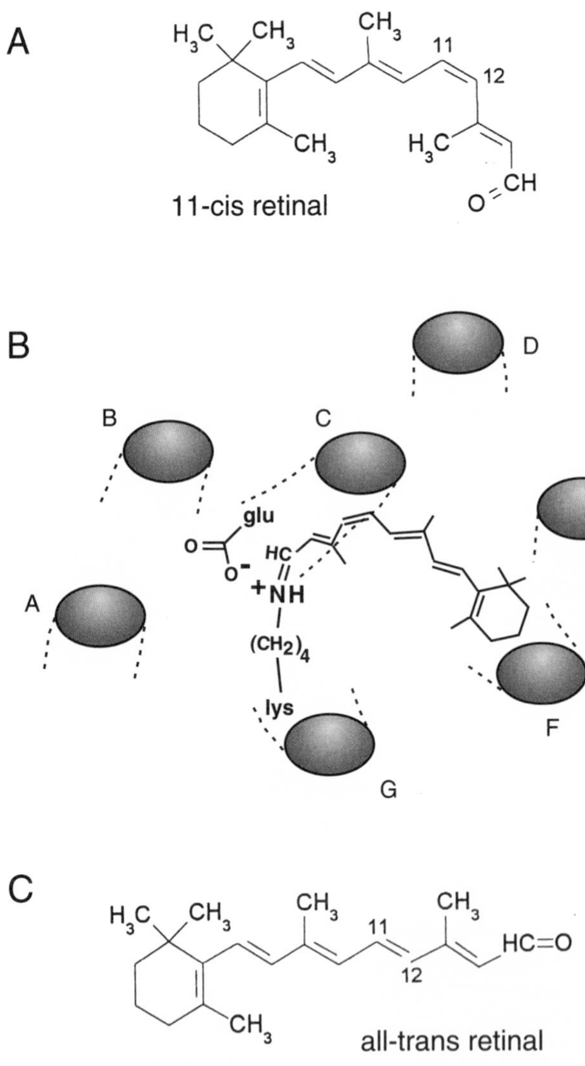

Fig. 16.3 **(A)** Chemical structure of 11-*cis* retinal₁ (often just called 11-*cis* retinal). This chromophore is most commonly found in both vertebrates and invertebrates. Certain aquatic vertebrates, such as freshwater fish, salamanders, and aquatic reptiles, contain a modified chromophore, called 11-*cis* retinal₂, or 3-dehydroretinal. This differs from retinal₁ only by the presence of an extra double bond in the ionone ring, which lengthens the chain of conjugated double bonds by one extra member and shifts the spectra of visual pigments containing retinal₂ to somewhat longer wavelengths. **(B)** Hypothesized position of chromophore within the binding site of rhodopsin. (See Rao and Oprian, 1996, and Sheikh et al., 1996.) **(C)** All-*trans* retinal₁ (often just called all-*trans* retinal).

tion (known as metarhodopsin II, or Rh*), which binds G protein and initiates the transduction cascade.

Mechanism of Transduction

Photoreceptors contain specific heterotrimeric G proteins, called *transducins*. Transducin alpha subunits (T_α's) are members of the

α_i/α_o subfamily (see Table 11.1); they are different for rods and cones, though the different kinds share an 80 percent sequence identity. The mechanism of interaction between Rh* and transducin appears to be very similar to that for other G-protein-mediated cascades (see Figs. 11.5 and 11.7). The binding of transducin to Rh* produces a change in the conformation of the guanosine nucleotide binding site on the transducin α subunit, which decreases the affinity of T_α for GDP. GDP falls off the binding site, and GTP then binds to the α subunit; this greatly decreases the affinity of T_α for both Rh* and $T_{\beta\gamma}$. Although there is some evidence that $T_{\beta\gamma}$ may play a role in photoreceptor function (see for example Jelsema and Axelrod, 1987), the major pathway of the phototransduction cascade is thought to be through $T_\alpha \cdot$ GTP (see Fig. 16.4A).

The lifetime of a photo-activated rhodopsin molecule is likely to be a few tens of milliseconds in a mammalian cone but of the order of a second or two in an amphibian rod. During its lifetime, a single Rh* may activate many transducin molecules, producing (in rods) perhaps as many as 500 to 1,000 $T_\alpha \cdot$ GTP molecules (Fung and Stryer, 1980; Vuong, Chabre, and Stryer, 1984). The activated state of rhodopsin is terminated as other metabotropic receptors are (see Figs. 11.5 and 16.4A). Rhodopsin kinase (GRK1), a G-protein receptor kinase specific for photoreceptors, phosphorylates one or more serines and theonines on the C-terminal tail of rhodopsin. Phosphorylation of this part of the protein is necessary for rhodopsin turnoff: if the C-terminal region of rhodopsin is genetically removed, the decline of the receptor light response is dramatically prolonged (Chen et al., 1995). Phosphorylation is followed by binding of an arrestin protein, and both phosphorylation and arrestin binding are thought to be necessary to deactivate rhodopsin completely.

Activation of Phosphodiesterase

The $T_\alpha \cdot$ GTP generated by photo-activated rhodopsin directly binds to and activates its effector molecule, which for both rods and cones is a cyclic GMP phosphodiesterase (PDE—see Chapter 12). Photoreceptor PDE is a membrane-associated protein consisting of two large (80–90 kDa) subunits, called α and β, which are catalytic; and two much smaller (<10 kDa) inhibitory subunits,

Fig. 16.4 **(A)** Mechanism of activation and in-activation of rhodopsin. The absorption of a photon *(hν)* by rhodopsin generates a conformational state of the molecule called metarhodopsin II or Rh*. This then binds to the G-protein transducin and catalyzes the exchange of GTP for GDP on the transducin α subunit. $T_\alpha \bullet$GTP then binds to the γ subunit of the effector molecule, phosphodiesterase *(PDE),* removing the inhibition of its activity. The PDE then hydrolyzes cGMP to GMP. Inactivation or turnoff of rhodopsin is caused by phosphorylation of rhodopsin from the terminal phosphate of ATP by rhodopsin kinase *(GRK1)* and the binding of arrestin. Transducin is inactivated (not shown) by the dephosphorylation of T_αGTP to T_αGDP, probably facilitated by PDE γ and GAPs or RGS proteins; this step is followed by the recombination of T_α with $T_{\beta\gamma}$. (Adapted in part from Pugh and Lamb, 1993.) **(B)** Relative abundance of molecules of transduction cascade on rod disk membrane. Small dots represent rhodopsin, larger grey dots transducin, and large black dots PDE. A patch of membrane this size would be associated with only one single free cGMP molecule. (Modified from Bownds and Arshavsky, 1995.)

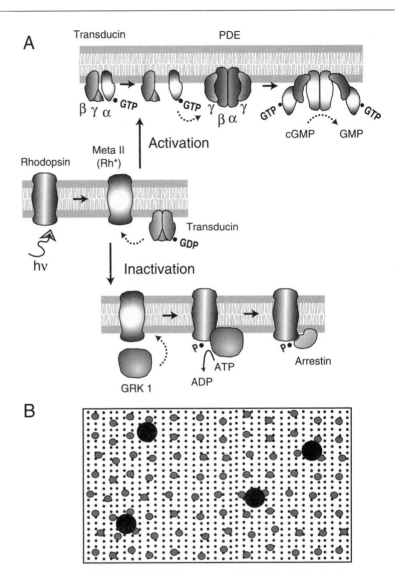

called γ (see Fig. 16.4A). Each of the catalytic subunits has approximately the same enzymatic activity, and each is associated in darkness with an inhibitory γ. $T_\alpha \bullet$GTP generated in the light binds to PDE γ subunits and alters their conformation, with the result that the inhibition of the PDE catalytic subunits is removed. The binding of a $T_\alpha \bullet$GTP to both of the γ subunits is required to produce maximal PDE activity, and the PDE remains activated for as long as $T_\alpha \cdot$GTP remains bound to γ.

PDE activation is terminated by hydrolysis of GTP to GDP by the T_α molecule. As for other heterotrimeric α subunits, T_α has intrinsic GTPase activity and will hydrolyze bound GTP. GTP hydrolysis by transducin is probably accelerated by GTPase-activating proteins, or GAPs, perhaps by PDE itself (Arshavsky and Bownds, 1992) and/or by retinal-specific RGS proteins (see Chapter 11). Hydrolysis of GTP generates $T_\alpha \cdot$GDP, which recombines with $\beta\gamma$ to regenerate inactive transducin.

Rhodopsin molecules in rods have long been known to float freely within the membrane of the disk, as within a sea of olive oil (Poo and Cone, 1974). It is presumed that the other molecules of the transduction cascade behave similarly, and that the reactions leading to the activation of PDE occur largely on the cytoplasmic surface of the disk membrane. Figure 16.4B is a model of a small piece of a disk surface, with each of the transduction proteins represented at approximately their natural abundance. There are 1,000 small dots in this drawing, which represent the rhodopsin molecules; 100 grey dots, which represent $T_{\alpha\beta\gamma}$; and 4 large black dots, which represent PDE molecules. For each piece of disk surface of this size, there would be only a single free cGMP molecule. Activation of rhodopsin produces $T_\alpha \cdot$GTP, which activates PDE, which in turn hydrolyzes cGMP. As Poo and Cone (1974) first observed, the placement of rhodopsin on the surface of the disk greatly increases its effective concentration and collision rates with the other molecules of the cascade. In spite of the many steps of the phototransduction cascade, the change in cGMP concentration occurs rapidly, and the minimum latency of the rod response between the stimulation of rhodopsin and the closing of the first channels in the plasma membrane is only 7 ms (Cobbs and Pugh, 1987).

Cyclic-Nucleotide-Gated Channels

There is now strong evidence that cGMP acts as a second messenger in rods and cones and is directly responsible for regulating the opening and closing of ion channels in the plasma membrane (see Stryer, 1986; Yau and Baylor, 1989). The first demonstration that cGMP may gate an outer-segment membrane conductance came from the experiments of Fesenko, Kolesnikov, and Lyubarsky (1985), who formed inside-out patches from frog rod outer segments and perfused the cytoplasmic surface of the patch with cyclic nucleotide. A typical result from their experiments is given in Fig. 16.5A. The inside-out patch was voltage-clamped and its conductance measured with 10 mV voltage pulses (lower trace). Perfusion of the cytosolic surface of the outer-segment plasma membrane with cGMP produced a large increase in the amplitude of the currents elicited by the voltage pulses (upper trace), indicative of an increase in membrane conductance. Other cyclic nucleotides (including cAMP) were much less effective. Since the recording in Fig. 16.5A was made in the absence of added ATP, the cGMP apparently activates the conductance of the outer segment directly, like a transmitter agonist but binding to the cytoplasmic side of the channel rather than to the extracellular side.

The recordings of Fesenko and collaborators were the first evidence for an important new family of channels gated by cyclic nucleotides (see Yau and Chen, 1995; Zimmerman, 1995; Finn, Grunwald, and Yau, 1996; Zagotta and Siegelbaum, 1996). When these channels were first isolated and their gene cloned (from rods—Cook, Hanke, and Kaupp, 1987; Kaupp et al., 1989), a surprising discovery was made. Cyclic-nucleotide-gated channels look a lot like *Shaker* K⁺ channels (Fig. 16.5B). All of the members of the cyclic-nucleotide-gated channel family appear to have six transmembrane domains, with both the N-terminal and C-terminal regions facing the cytoplasm. Figure 16.5C compares the sequence of the fourth transmembrane domain of the rod channel with *Shaker* S4. The similarity is remarkable: there are positively charged amino acids at some of the positions occupied by arginines and lysines in *Shaker*, though there are negatively charged and neutral amino acids at other positions, and the rod channel is only weakly voltage-dependent.

The cyclic-nucleotide-gated channels also have a recognizable P domain with significant sequence identity to the homologous region of the *Shaker* channel. There is excellent evidence that the P domain of cyclic-nucleotide-gated channels is responsible for ion permeation (Heginbotham, Abramson, and MacKinnon, 1992; Goulding et al., 1993), just as for *Shaker*. Furthermore, the amino-

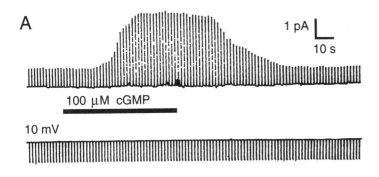

A

1 pA

10 s

100 μM cGMP

10 mV

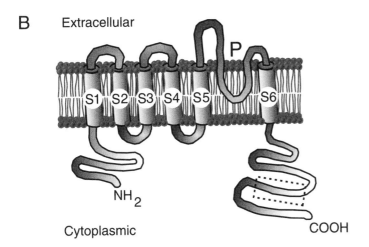

B Extracellular

P

S1 S2 S3 S4 S5 S6

NH₂

Cytoplasmic COOH

Fig. 16.5 Cyclic-nucleotide-gated channels in rods. **(A)** Activation of conductance in isolated patches from rod outer segments by cGMP. Inside-out patch pulled from outer segment of frog rod was perfused with 100 μM cGMP (indicated by horizontal bar). Lower trace shows timing of 10 mV voltage pulses, upper trace the resulting current. Increase in current indicates increase in conductance of patch, caused by opening of cyclic-nucleotide-gated channels. (Reprinted from Fesenko, Kolesnikov, and Lyubarsky, 1985, with permission of the authors and of Macmillan Magazines Limited.) **(B)** Hypothesized structure of cyclic-nucleotide-gated channels. Transmembrane domains are labeled S1–S6, and part of protein responsible at least in part for forming the ion channel is labeled as *P* (P domain). Dotted box on carboxyl-terminal tail indicates approximate position of cyclic-nucleotide-binding site. (After Finn, Grunwald, and Yau, 1996, and Zagotta and Siegelbaum, 1996.) **(C)** Comparison of S4 domain for the *Shaker* potassium channel and α subunit of bovine rod cyclic-nucleotide-gated channel (*bRCNC*). Identical amino acids in the two sequences are set in bold, and dots mark positions of positively charged amino acids in *Shaker,* which are characteristic of S4 domains in voltage-gated channels. (Reprinted from Finn, Grunwald, and Yau, 1996, with permission of the authors and of Annual Reviews, Inc.)

C · · · · · · ·
S4 region

Shaker L A I L**R**V I**RL**V**R**V F**R** I F K L S**R**H S K G

bRCNC Y P E I**R**L N**RL**L**R**I S**R** M F E F F Q R T E T

terminal 20 amino acids forming the "ball peptide" responsible for rapid inactivation of the *Shaker* channel (see Chapter 6) can block cyclic-nucleotide-gated channels (Kramer, Goulding, and Siegelbaum, 1994), probably by binding to residues in the P domain. This observation may have no physiological relevance, since cyclic-nucleotide-gated channels do not themselves contain a sequence homologous to the "ball peptide" and do not normally show voltage-dependent inactivation. Nevertheless, this surprising finding indicates cyclic-nucleotide-gated channels and voltage-gated channels are closely related and that one may have evolved from the other, or the two may have evolved from a common ancestor.

Like *Shaker* channels, the cyclic-nucleotide-gated channels are probably tetramers (Liu, Tibbs, and Siegelbaum, 1996). In rods the channels are heterotetramers, consisting of at least two different subunits. The first of the rod channels whose gene was cloned (by Kaupp et al., 1989) is now referred to as the α subunit. This channel can be expressed and will form homomultimeric channels with some but not all of the properties of native channels. Native channels also contain a second subunit, called β, which does not form channels by itself; however, when α and β are expressed together, channels are formed with properties similar to those recorded from rod outer segments (Chen et al., 1993; Körschen et al., 1995).

The sequences of both the α and β subunits of the rod channel (and of other cyclic-nucleotide-gated channels whose genes have been cloned) have a domain near the C terminus with considerable homology to cyclic-nucleotide-binding domains in protein kinases PKA and PKG (dotted box in Fig. 16.5B). This sequence appears to be largely responsible for determining the binding affinity of the channel for cyclic nucleotides (Goulding, Tibbs, and Siegelbaum, 1994). The rod channel has a much higher affinity for cGMP than for cAMP or for other cyclic nucleotides, but this is not true for all members of this family. As we shall see later in this chapter, olfactory receptor neurons also have cyclic-nucleotide-gated channels, but these channels have a much more nearly equal affinity for cGMP and cAMP.

Both rod and olfactory channels are permeable to monovalent and divalent cations, including Ca^{2+}. The Ca^{2+} permeation is of particular interest and has been extensively studied, since it resembles Ca^{2+} permeation through voltage-gated Ca^{2+} channels (see Chapter 7). There is considerable evidence, for example, that Ca^{2+} binds to an extracellular site in the mouth of both the rod and olfactory channels, and that the permeability of the channel to monovalent ions is considerably reduced in the presence of divalents. The block by divalents is voltage-dependent in rods (see Fig. 16.8B) and in olfactory neurons (Zufall and Firestein, 1993) and seems to be due to binding to a ring of glutamate residues at the mouth of the channel pore, in a position analogous to a similar ring of glutamate residues in voltage-gated calcium channels (Root and MacKinnon, 1993; Eismann et al., 1994). These observations reemphasize the close resemblance and probable evolutionary kinship of cyclic-nucleotide and voltage-gated channels.

The Photoreceptor Light Response

The activation of PDE and the decrease in cGMP concentration are directly responsible for the photoreceptor light response (see Yau and Baylor, 1989; McNaughton, 1990; Baylor, 1992; Pugh and Lamb, 1993; Yau, 1994). In a rod outer segment in darkness, the resting free cGMP concentration is of the order of 3–4 μM. The total cGMP concentration is much higher than this, but much of this cGMP is tightly bound, for example to noncatalytic sites on the PDE, and exchanges with free cGMP only rather slowly (see Bownds and Arshavsky, 1995). Light reduces the free cGMP concentration, and the channels close.

Before I describe in detail the properties of the photoreceptor light response, it may be helpful to begin with an overview (see Fig. 16.6). The cyclic-nucleotide-gated channels are cation-selective and permeable to both Na^+ and K^+, with a reversal potential under physiological conditions near zero. Since the photoreceptor resting membrane potential is about -35 mV, a negative or inward current flows through these channels in darkness, carried principally by Na^+. The Na^+ coming into the outer segment is pumped out of the rod by a Na^+/K^+ ATPase located principally on the plasma membrane of the inner segment (Bok, 1988; Schneider, Shyjan, and Levenson, 1991). This ATPase pumps Na^+ out in exchange for K^+ in, and the inward movement of K^+ is mostly compensated by K^+ flowing outward through the cyclic-nucleotide-gated channels and through K^+ channels located in the inner segment.

The cyclic-nucleotide-gated channels are permeable to divalent cations in addition to monovalent cations, and under physiological conditions approximately 15 percent of the current entering a rod outer segment (and an even higher percentage entering a cone— Perry and McNaughton, 1991) is carried by Ca^{2+}. This Ca^{2+} is pumped outward by a Ca^{2+} exchanger similar to the one described

Fig. 16.6 Channels and transporters in rod photoreceptors. Outer segment contains cyclic-nucleotide-gated channels, permeable to both monovalent and divalent cations. Most of the inward current through these channels is carried by Na^+ and Ca^{2+}. The outer segment also contains a Na^+/Ca^{2+}-K^+ transporter, which transports 1 Ca^{2+} and 1 K^+ out of the rod in exchange for 4 Na^+ inward. The inner segment contains a Na^+/K^+ ATPase, which transports 3 Na^+ out of the cell in exchange for 2 K^+, as well as K^+-selective channels and channels selective for both Na^+ and K^+ and activated by hyperpolarization (I_h). Finally, the synaptic terminal contains L-type Ca^{2+} channels that mediate Ca^{2+} influx and trigger synaptic transmitter release, as well as a Ca^{2+} ATPase that pumps out entering Ca^{2+}, probably in exchange for H^+.

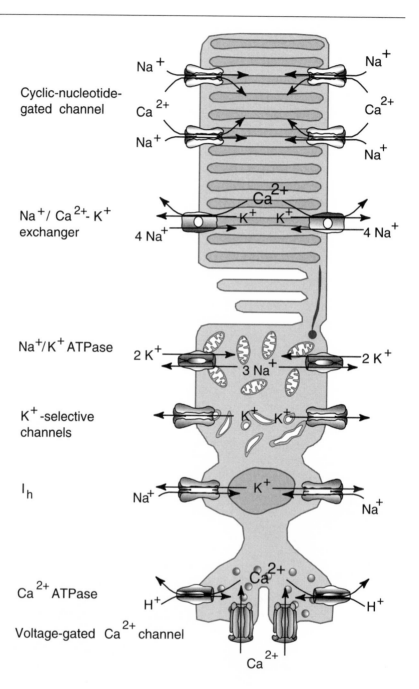

in Chapter 4 but with a different stoichiometry: it transports one Ca^{2+} and one K^+ outward, in exchange for 4 Na^+ inward (Cervetto et al., 1989). Since this exchanger uses the outward gradient of K^+ in addition to the inward Na^+ gradient, it is even more powerful than the 1 Ca^{2+}:3 Na^+ transporters found in most other cells. The rod transporter seems to be predominantly in the outer segment (see Kaupp and Koch, 1992; Kim et al., 1998). Ca^{2+} also enters the rod through L-type voltage-gated Ca^{2+} channels in the inner segment, which are responsible for regulating the release of synaptic transmitter. The Ca^{2+} entering the inner segment is apparently pumped out not by a transporter but rather by a Ca^{2+} ATPase located near the synaptic terminal (Krizaj and Copenhagen, 1997, 1998; Taylor, Morgans, Berntson, and Wässle, 1997).

The Polarity and Waveform of the Light Response

Light decreases the probability of opening of the cyclic-nucleotide-gated channels and reduces the flux of Na^+ (and Ca^{2+}) entering the outer segment. This causes the membrane potential of the rod to go negative, that is, to *hyperpolarize*. Fig. 16.7A shows the change in membrane potential produced by a series of brief light flashes of increasing intensity, recorded from a salamander rod with an intracellular microelectrode (from Baylor and Nunn, 1986). In darkness, the membrane potential is intermediate between the equilibrium potential for K^+ (-80 to -90 mV) and the reversal potential for the cyclic-nucleotide-gated channels (near zero mV). As the cyclic-nucleotide-gated channels close in the light, the membrane potential moves in a negative direction closer to the equilibrium potential for K^+ (E_K). The brighter the light, the larger the hyperpolarization. In very bright light there is in addition a rapid relaxation in the voltage response (at the arrow in Fig. 16.7A). This is not the result of any change in the cyclic-nucleotide-gated channels but is caused by a separate conductance in the inner segment, called i_h (see Fig. 16.6), which is gated by membrane hyperpolarization (see Pape, 1996). This conductance is specifically blocked by low concentrations of extracellular Cs^+ (see for example Hestrin, 1987), and Cs^+ eliminates the rapid relaxation of the voltage response (Fain et al., 1978).

Fig. 16.7 Electrical responses from rods. Three different ways of recording the light response of a salamander rod are illustrated here. All recordings in this figure were made from the same cell. For each part of the figure, the rod was stimulated at $t = 0$ with 11 ms flashes of increasing light intensity, from 1.5 to 430 photons per μm^2, and the responses to these flashes were superimposed. **(A)** Voltage responses, recorded with an intracellular microelectrode in the inner segment (V_m). Resting membrane potential was -34 mV, and light flashes produced a graded hyperpolarization. Bright flashes showed in addition a sudden relaxation of voltage *(arrow)*, produced by the voltage-dependent gating of the I_h current. **(B)** Suction-electrode recording. The outer segment of the rod was gently drawn up into the bore of a suction pipette, which was connected to a current-measuring amplifier (I_s). Current responses are to the same flashes as in **(A)** and were recorded simultaneously. **(C)** Voltage clamp. Two microelectrodes were inserted into the rod inner segment, one to record membrane potential (V_m) and the other to inject current. The membrane potential was clamped to -34 mV (lowermost trace), and suction-electrode (I_s) and total membrane currents (I_{vc}) were recorded simultaneously to the same series of flashes as in **(A)** and **(B)**. Total membrane current was initially zero, since cell in darkness was in steady state. Change in total current upon illumination, caused by closing of cyclic-nucleotide-gated channels, was larger than change in suction-electrode current because the suction electrode did not record current from the entire outer segment, and because some current was lost through the low-resistance seal between the suction pipette and the cell. (Data replotted, with cartoons added, from Baylor and Nunn, 1986.)

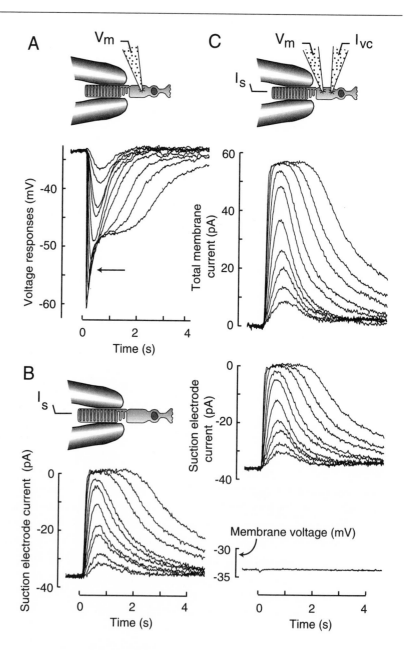

The current through the cyclic-nucleotide-gated channels can be measured in two ways. In the first, the outer segment is pulled up into a suction electrode, and the inside of this electrode is connected directly to a current-measuring amplifier. This method measures the current entering the outer segment, which is the current passing through the cyclic-nucleotide-gated channels, since the cyclic-nucleotide-gated channels are almost completely confined to the outer segment, and since few if any channels of any other type seem to be functional in this part of the rod. Typical results obtained by this method are shown in Fig. 16.7B, from the same cell whose voltage responses are presented in Fig. 16.7A. An inward current sustained in darkness (called the *dark current*) is transiently decreased when the rod is illuminated with a brief flash. The brightest flashes close all of the cyclic-nucleotide-gated channels and reduce the current entering the outer segment to zero.

One disadvantage of suction-electrode recording is that it does not voltage-clamp the cell. Since

$$\Delta i = \Delta g(V_m - E_{rev}) \qquad (1)$$

and E_{rev} is near zero, Δi is approximately $\Delta g(V_m)$, and changes in membrane voltage like those shown in Fig. 16.7A may influence the waveform of the currents. The influence of membrane voltage on the waveform of the currents was examined by Baylor and Nunn (1986), who recorded outer-segment currents with suction electrodes from rods that were simultaneously voltage-clamped. A representative example of their results is given in Fig. 16.7C—again for the same cell just described. The total membrane current measured with voltage clamp is initially zero, since in darkness the cell is at steady state and the current entering the outer segment through the cyclic-nucleotide-gated channels is exactly balanced by current leaving the inner segment. Since the inner-segment currents are unaffected by illumination, the time course of the total membrane current reflects the time course in the change of the outer-segment conductance, just as currents recorded from voltage-clamped squid axons reflect the time course of changes in Na^+ and K^+ conductance. The exposure to light closes channels whose reversal potential is near zero (see Eqn. 1), so the total membrane current is outward (positive) since Δg and $(V_m - E_{rev})$ are both negative.

Suction-electrode recordings were made simultaneously from this same rod under voltage clamp (Fig. 16.7C, lower current traces). The amplitude of the suction-electrode currents recorded under voltage clamp is smaller than that of the total membrane currents, in part because current was lost through the seal between the pipette and the cell, and in part because not all of the outer segment was sucked into the pipette. What is remarkable, however, is that the amplitude and time course of the suction-electrode currents in Fig. 16.7C are quite similar to those for the currents recorded in Fig. 16.7B, for which no voltage clamp was used. This means that changes in photoreceptor membrane voltage have only a small effect on the current through the cyclic-nucleotide-gated channels.

Voltage-clamp recordings from photoreceptors have provided useful information about the conductance responsible for the light response. Fig. 16.8A shows the effect of membrane potential on the polarity and amplitude of the outer-segment current, recorded with a suction electrode from a voltage-clamped rod. In this experiment, the holding potential was varied, and the change in current was measured in response to a bright (saturating) light flash (applied at arrows). When the holding potential was set to the resting potential (-31 mV for this cell), the dark current was about -11 pA, somewhat smaller than for the cell in Fig. 16.7. Light transiently decreased the current to zero. As the holding potential was made more negative (to -61 mV), the dark current also became more negative, as Eqn. (1) predicts, but the light flash again brought the current to zero. Fig. 16.8A shows, in fact, that a bright light flash brings the current to zero regardless of the holding potential, and the reason for this is quite simple. In bright light all of the cyclic-nucleotide-gated channels are closed, so Δg goes to zero. When Δg is zero, Δi is also zero, regardless of the value of V_m.

At positive holding potentials, the dark current for the cell in Fig. 16.8A became outward and increased dramatically as the holding potential was increased. This can be seen more clearly in Fig. 16.8B, which gives current-voltage relations for the same cell in darkness, in the presence of a steady light (which reduced the current by about a factor of two), and in bright light. In bright light, there was no current since the channels were all closed,

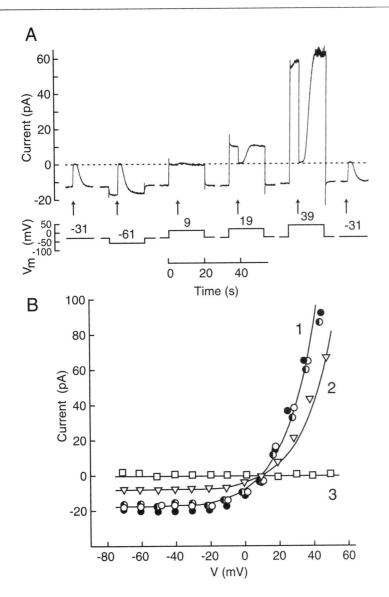

Fig. 16.8 Voltage dependence of light-activated current in rod photoreceptor. Rod was voltage clamped as in Fig. 16.7. **(A)** Membrane voltage is traced at bottom, with arrows indicating timing of bright, saturating light flashes. Upper traces show outer segment current recorded with a suction-electrode under voltage clamp (as for lower current traces in Fig. 16.7C). Note that bright light always brings the current to zero, since bright light closes all the cyclic-nucleotide-gated channels. In darkness on the other hand, the current is dramatically altered by membrane potential, since the cyclic-nucleotide-gated channels are open in darkness, and their conductance is voltage-dependent (largely as a result of a voltage-dependent block of the channels by divalent ions). **(B)** Current-voltage curve for rod in **(A)**. Current was measured in response to brief voltage pulses in darkness (curve 1), in steady light, which closed about half the cyclic-nucleotide-gated channels (curve 2), and in saturating light, which closed all of the channels (curve 3). Sequence of measurements was as follows: darkness *(open circles),* half-saturating light *(inverted triangles),* darkness *(filled circles),* saturating light *(open squares),* and darkness *(half-filled circles).* Each point is the average of several measurements. In saturating light, current is zero at all voltages because the channels are closed. In darkness, the current-voltage curve reflects the voltage-dependence of the cyclic-nucleotide-gated current. In half-saturating light, the curve is half-way between the curves in darkness and saturating light. (Reprinted from Baylor and Nunn, 1986, with permission of D. A. Baylor and of the Physiological Society.)

and the *i–V* curve was a straight line along the voltage axis. In the dark, the *i–V* curve reflects the voltage dependence of the cyclic-nucleotide-gated channels and is quite nonlinear, largely as the result of a voltage-dependent block of the channels by Ca^{2+} and Mg^{2+} (see Yau and Baylor, 1989; Yau, 1994).

Box 16.1

SINGLE-QUANTUM RESPONSES OF RODS

The behavioral experiments of Hecht, Shlaer, and Pirenne (1942) first indicated that rods are so sensitive that they are capable of detecting single photons of light. Early attempts to record the responses of rods to single photons with intracellular microelectrodes were unsuccessful, because the rods in many lower vertebrates are electrically coupled to one another by an extensive network of gap junctions. As a consequence, a photon absorbed by a rhodopsin molecule in one receptor can produce a voltage change in many other cells, and this effectively smooths out the Poisson variability expected from quantal responses (Fain, 1975). Intact rods in lower vertebrates show so little variability in the amplitude of responses to dim light that they give the impression of being able to respond to only a fraction of a photon.

Suction electrode recordings from isolated rods reveal a different story. The first measurements of this kind, made by Baylor, Lamb, and Yau (1979) from amphibian retina, offer clear evidence of responses to single photons. The recordings in the accompanying figure are from a similar study from primate retina (Baylor, Nunn, and Schnapf, 1984). Part A reproduces the responses to 51 flashes at 4 s intervals to a light so dim that many of the flashes failed to evoke a response. Some responses were a bit less than 1 pA in amplitude, and a few were twice as large. These records are reminiscent of the recordings of synaptic quantal responses described in Chapter 8 (see Fig. 8.14). The graphs in part B are amplitude histograms for responses from two cells to a similar series of flashes, fitted with the Poisson distribution (as in Fig. 8.15). This remarkable ability of the rods to detect single photons of light is a result both of the high gain of the transduction mechanism and of the very low rate of spontaneous noise.

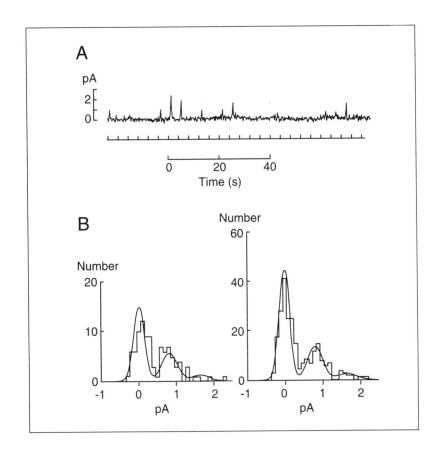

Calcium

The closing of the cyclic-nucleotide-gated channels in the outer segment not only decreases the entry of Na$^+$ into the rod, it also decreases the entry of Ca^{2+}. In darkness, approximately 10^7 Ca^{2+} ions enter an amphibian rod outer segment each second, and this Ca^{2+} is efficiently removed by the Na$^+$/Ca^{2+}-K$^+$ transporter. In the light, the probability of opening of the cyclic-nucleotide-gated channels is decreased and less Ca^{2+} enters the cell. The Na$^+$/Ca^{2+}-K$^+$ transporter will at least initially continue to remove Ca^{2+} at the same rate as in darkness, and the intracellular free-Ca^{2+} concentration will decrease. Provided the Na$^+$ and K$^+$ gradients are not greatly altered by light exposure, the rate of the transporter should be a function primarily of the intracellular Ca^{2+} concentration. As the Ca^{2+} concentration declines, the rate of Ca^{2+} transport will also decline, and Ca^{2+} influx and efflux will reach a new steady state at a lower free-Ca^{2+} concentration. The brighter the light, the smaller the Ca^{2+} influx, and the lower the free-Ca^{2+} concentration at steady state.

Evidence that light decreases the photoreceptor's intracellular Ca^{2+} concentration was first obtained from recordings of Na^+/Ca^{2+}-K^+ exchange currents (Yau and Nakatani, 1985) and then later by direct measurement, first with aequorin (McNaughton, Cervetto, and Nunn, 1986) and then with fura-2 (Ratto et al., 1988), indo (Gray-Keller and Detwiler, 1994), and fluo-3 (Sampath et al., 1998). The measurement in Fig. 16.9 is typical. In these experiments (from Sampath et al., 1998), an argon laser was focused on the outer segment of a salamander rod with spot confocal optics (Escobar et al., 1994). The rod was held in a suction electrode by its inner segment to permit a clear optical path for the laser spot (see Fig. 16.9A). Since the rod was not voltage-clamped, no current was injected into the cell externally, and any current entering the outer segment must be exactly compensated by current *leaving* the inner segment. Thus it does not matter which end of the cell was pulled into the suction electrode. The current recorded from the two ends of the cell must be equal in amplitude (though of course opposite in sign).

Figs. 16.9B and C show a simultaneous recording of the change in outer-segment current, measured as the negative of the current recorded from the inner segment, and the fluorescence from the fluo-3 Ca^{2+} indicator dye, measured with a photodiode. The laser used to excite the fluo-3 was sufficiently bright and of the appropriate wavelength to provide a bright-light stimulus to the rod. The channels all rapidly closed, leaving only a slowly declining inward current due to the Na^+/Ca^{2+}-K^+ transporter, which is electrogenic (arrow in Fig. 16.9B—see Yau and Nakatani, 1985; Hodgkin, McNaughton, and Nunn, 1987). The fluorescence signal from the fluo-3 also declined (Fig. 16.9C), indicating a decrease in Ca^{2+} concentration. The Ca^{2+} falls from 600–700 nM in darkness to about 30 nM in bright light (see also Gray-Keller and Detwiler, 1994).

A

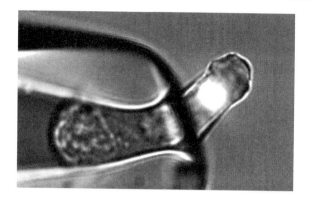

B

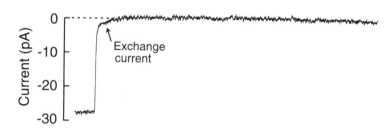

C

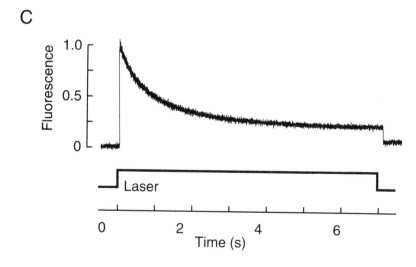

Fig. 16.9 Light-dependent change in Ca^{2+} concentration in a rod outer segment. **(A)** Experimental preparation. Inner segment of dissociated salamander rod is pulled up into a suction electrode to record current. A spot from an argon laser was focused onto the outer segment, and this spot was used both to provide a saturating light stimulus to the rod and to measure the Ca^{2+} concentration. Free-Ca^{2+} concentration was estimated from the fluorescence of the dye fluo-3, which was loaded into rods by incubating isolated photoreceptors with fluo-3-AM. **(B)** Outer-segment current measured as in **(A)** to 7-second exposure of argon laser. Arrow indicates inward current produced by Na^{+}/Ca^{2+}-K^{+} exchange transport. Current of exchanger is inward since stoichiometry of exchanger is 4 Na^{+} in for 1 Ca^{2+} out and 1 K^{+} out; in other words, a net movement of one charge into the cell accompanies each Ca^{2+} transported outward. **(C)** Fluo-3 fluorescence measured with a photodiode and plotted as a fraction of maximum fluorescence. Decline of fluorescence indicates decline of Ca^{2+} concentration, which other measurements show to be from a resting level of about 670 nM in darkness to about 30 nM in bright light. Note that the time course of Ca^{2+} is approximately the same as the time course of decline of the exchanger current in **(B)**. ((**A**), Unpublished data of A. P. Sampath, H. R. Matthews, M. C. Cornwall, and G. L. Fain; **(B)** and **(C)**, data replotted from Sampath et al., 1998.)

Light Adaptation

The fall in the Ca^{2+} concentration produced by the closing of the cyclic-nucleotide-gated channels is important, since Ca^{2+} appears to function as a second messenger in both rods and cones and is principally if not exclusively responsible for regulating the sensitivity of the transduction cascade in steady background light (see Fain and Matthews, 1990; Koutalos and Yau, 1996). This process is called *light adaptation:* the sensitivity of a photoreptor is altered in background light, much as hair cell sensitivity is altered by steady mechanical stimulation (see Fig. 15.10).

The effect of steady background light on a rod is shown in Fig. 16.10 (from Matthews, 1990). In part A, the rod in darkness was stimulated with brief flashes at intensities that increased by about a factor of 4. The peak amplitude of these responses can be imagined to trace out a *response-intensity curve,* giving the peak amplitude as a function of flash intensity. In parts B and C of this figure, these same flashes were repeated for this same rod but in the presence of two different steady background lights. The backgrounds produced a maintained decrease in the current entering the cyclic-nucleotide-gated channels, and a decrease in the amplitude of the response to flashes. They also shifted the response-intensity curve to higher flash intensities, so that brighter flashes were required to elicit even a minimal response from the cell.

The decrease in sensitivity produced by background light is perhaps clearer in Fig. 16.10D (from Fain and Cornwall, 1993). Here the responses of a rod to brief flashes in darkness and in the presence of several different background intensities have been superimposed. Since the intensities of the flashes in darkness and in the different backgrounds were not the same, the responses in each case have been divided by their flash intensities (in photons per μm^2) and plotted in units of sensitivity. As the background intensity was increased, the sensitivity declined. Notice also that the *waveform* of the response was altered. At each of the progressively brighter background intensities, the responses rose along approximately the same initial curve but began to decline at progressively earlier times. These recordings illustrate that one of the principal mechanisms for the sensitivity decrease is an acceleration in the time course of response decay (Baylor and Hodgkin, 1974).

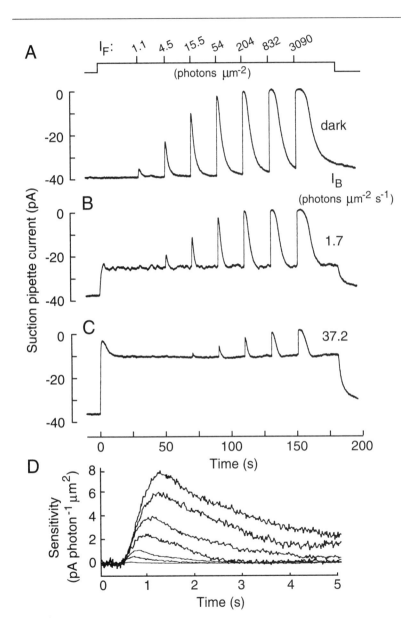

Fig. 16.10 Light adaptation in photoreceptors. For the top three recordings, a single rod was exposed to brief flashes of increasing light intensity (I_F) in darkness **(A)** or in the presence of steady background light (**B** and **C**). Uppermost trace shows timing of background exposures (for parts **B** and **C**), indicated by long-duration upward deflection beginning at $t = 0$; and timing of 20 ms, 500 nm light flashes, indicated by much briefer upward deflections. Intensities of flashes are given in units of photons per μm^2 (per flash) and are the same for **(A)**–**(C)**. **(A)** Salamander rod responses in darkness. Flash intensities increase progressively by about a factor of 4, so that increase in peak response amplitude can be imagined to trace out a response-intensity curve for the dark-adapted rod. **(B)** Same rod as in **(A)**, exposed to steady background light (I_B) of 1.7 photons $\mu m^{-2} s^{-1}$. **(C)** As in **(B)**, but for steady light of 37.2 photons $\mu m^{-2} s^{-1}$. Replotted from Matthews, 1990.) **(D)** Responses of salamander rod in darkness (largest response) and in the presence of background lights of progressively increasing intensity from 0.042 to 20 photons $\mu m^{-2} s^{-1}$. Responses were elicited by brief flashes superimposed on top of steady light (as in **B** and **C**). Since different flash intensities were used for different backgrounds, response amplitudes have been divided by the appropriate flash intensities to give units of sensitivity (pA photon^{-1} μm^2). Background lights produce a progressive decrease in sensitivity and speed up the decline of the response. (From Fain and Cornwall, 1993, reprinted with permission of the authors and of MIT Press.)

These changes in sensitivity and response waveform do not occur in the absence of a change in Ca^{2+}. One way to show this is to
prevent the Ca^{2+} inside the rod from changing, for example by
greatly reducing Ca^{2+} influx (by buffering the Ca^{2+} in the Ringer
solution to a low level with EGTA) and by blocking Ca^{2+} efflux
by removing Na^+ from the Ringer (and so blocking $Na^+/Ca^{2+}-K^+$
transport). When rods (and cones) are simultaneously exposed to
such a low-Ca^{2+}, zero-Na^+ solution, light adaptation does not occur (Matthews et al., 1988; Nakatani and Yau, 1988). These
and other experiments (Koutalos and Yau, 1996) provide considerable evidence that Ca^{2+} is primarily responsible for modulating the
transduction cascade in the presence of background light.

How does Ca^{2+} do this? The answer is still not entirely clear,
though there are a number of excellent suggestions (see Fig. 16.11).
On the one hand, there is good evidence that the Ca^{2+} concentration modulates the rate of the guanylyl cyclase (Koch and Stryer,
1988; Gorczyca et al., 1994). The predominant guanylyl cyclase
in rod outer segments is a membrane-bound protein, not the soluble guanylyl cyclases described in Chapter 13. The rod cyclase is
regulated not by NO but rather by Ca^{2+}: in high Ca^{2+}, the cyclase
is inactivated by small-molecular-weight Ca^{2+}-binding proteins,
called GCAPs, which bind to the cyclase (see Polans, Baehr, and
Palczewski, 1996). As the Ca^{2+} level falls in steady background
light, the Ca^{2+} comes off its binding site on the GCAPs, and these
proteins now stimulate the cyclase. The rate of cyclase turnover increases, generating more cGMP.

The guanylyl cyclase plays an important role in the adaptation
of the rod. A flash of light activates the PDE and decreases the
cGMP concentration, and the guanylyl cyclase then resynthesizes
new cGMP, so the cGMP concentration can return to its previous
level. In the presence of a steady background light, there is a steady
hydrolysis of cGMP by the PDE and a decrease in the intracellular
free-Ca^{2+} concentration. As the Ca^{2+} falls, the cyclase activity increases until the synthesis of cGMP equals its rate of hydrolysis.
Were this not to occur, the rod would remain saturated in background light with all of its cGMP-gated channels closed and with
no further responsiveness to changes in illumination.

In addition to regulation of the cyclase, several other Ca^{2+}-de-
pendent reactions have been proposed to modulate the sensi-

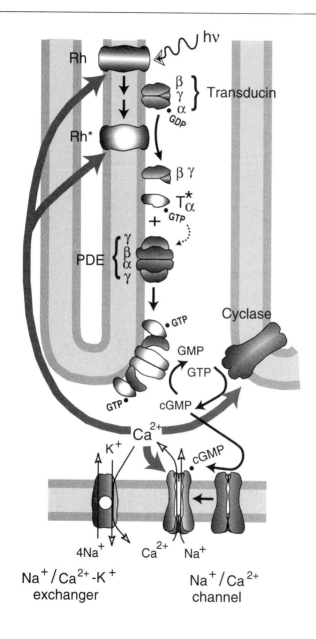

Fig. 16.11 Mechanism of adaptation in vertebrate photoreceptor. Excitation of rhodopsin *(Rh)* by light *(hν)* produces activated $T_\alpha \cdot GTP$, which binds to and activates the PDE. The PDE hydrolyzes cGMP to GMP, decreasing the cGMP concentration and closing the channels. This decreases the intracellular free-Ca^{2+} concentration. Ca^{2+} plays a key role in modulating the enzymes of transduction *(large arrows)* and is principally if not entirely responsible for light adaptation. Ca^{2+} regulates the cyclase *via* small-molecular-weight binding proteins called GCAPs (not shown). A decrease in Ca^{2+} concentration speeds up the cyclase and the synthesis of cGMP from GTP, preventing the saturation of the rod in background light. Ca^{2+} also regulates the cGMP-gated channel, so that a decline in free-Ca^{2+} concentration decreases the apparent affinity of the channel for cGMP. Finally, Ca^{2+} acts at some stage early in transduction, perhaps regulating the gain or lifetime of activated rhodopsin *(Rh*).* (After Fain, Matthews, and Cornwall, 1996, and Pugh and Lamb, 1993.)

tivity of the rod. There is good evidence that some early stage in the transduction cascade also contributes to light adaptation (Koutalos, Nakatani, and Yau, 1995; Matthews, 1996). Calcium may alter the gain of formation of Rh* (Lagnado and Baylor, 1994) or the lifetime of photoactivated rhodopsin (Torre, Matthews, and Lamb, 1986; Sagoo and Lagnado, 1997), perhaps by regulating the activity of the rhodopsin kinase (Kawamura, 1993). In addition, Ca^{2+} together with calmodulin (Hsu and Molday, 1993) and perhaps some other binding protein (Gordon, Downing-Park, and Zimmerman, 1995) has been shown to alter the apparent affinity of the cyclic-nucleotide-gated channels for cGMP (see Molday, 1996). All of these reactions are potentially important mechanisms that could affect the sensitivity of the transduction cascade.

Bleaching Adaptation

After light converts 11-*cis* retinal to all-*trans* retinal (Fig. 16.3A and C), the bond between the all-*trans* chromophore and the terminal amino group of lysine is hydrolyzed (in vertebrates) to form free all-*trans* retinal. In order to restore rhodopsin to its dark-adapted form, the all-*trans* retinal must be converted to all-*trans* retinol by the enzyme retinol dehydrogenase within the photoreceptor, and it must then leave the rod or cone and be transported by *interphotoreceptor retinoid binding protein* (or *IRBP*) within the extracellular space to a layer of cells called the *retinal pigment epithelium* (or *RPE*), adjacent to the photoreceptor's outer segments (see Fain, Matthews, and Cornwall, 1996). Within the RPE, the all-*trans* chromophore is converted back to 11-*cis* by the enzyme retinoid isomerase, and 11-*cis* retinal is then transported by IRBP back to the photoreceptors to regenerate the photopigment to its dark-adapted form.

When photoreceptors are exposed to light so bright that a large fraction of the photopigment is bleached, sensitivity is reduced and recovers only as the pigment is regenerated. This process is called *dark or bleaching adaptation* (see Fain and Cornwall, 1993; Fain, Matthews, and Cornwall, 1996). One of the most interesting features of bleaching adaptation is that the decrease in the sensitivity of the photoreceptor is larger than would be expected simply from the decrease in pigment concentration. That is, bleaching seems capable of decreasing the sensitivity of the photoreceptor to a greater extent than would be predicted from the loss in the number of rhodopsins available to absorb a photon.

Part of the decrease in sensitivity produced by large bleaches seems to be the result of a signal produced by bleached pigment. Bleached pigment stimulates the transduction cascade (Cornwall and Fain, 1994) by activating transducin (Matthews, Cornwall, and Fain, 1996), though with a much smaller gain than when Rh* activates transducin. The activation of the cascade closes cyclic-nucleotide-gated channels and decreases the Ca^{2+} concentration (Sampath et al., 1998), and the decrease in Ca^{2+} produces a modulation of the transduction cascade (Matthews, Fain, and Cornwall, 1996) much like that produced by background stimulation (Jones, Cornwall, and Fain, 1996). Regeneration of the pigment by the addition of 11-*cis* retinal and re-formation of the Schiff base between the chromophore and the opsin lysine then restores the Ca^{2+} concentration and sensitivity to their dark-adapted levels.

II: OLFACTORY RECEPTOR NEURONS

The mechanism of transduction in olfactory receptor neurons has many similarities to that in photoreceptors (see Reed, 1992; Zufall, Firestein, and Shepherd, 1994; Firestein, 1996; Buck, 1996; Hildebrand and Shepherd, 1997). Vertebrate olfactory receptor neurons are bipolar neurons that lie in an epithelial layer called the *olfactory mucosa* (see Fig. 16.12A). Instead of outer segments, olfactory neurons have numerous cilia (Fig. 16.12B), which emerge from a terminal swelling at the cell's epithelial surface called the *dendritic knob*. The cilia project up above the epithelial surface into a layer of mucous and appear to contain all of the elements of the transduction cascade: the receptors, G proteins, effectors, second messengers, and ion channels.

Odorant molecules bind to receptor proteins called *odorant receptors*, which appear to work much like rhodopsin or the β-adrenergic receptor. They couple to a specialized G protein, which in turn activates an adenylyl cyclase. The cyclase increases the cAMP concentration, and cAMP binds directly to cyclic-nucleotide-gated channels similar in structure to those in the outer

Fig. 16.12 Anatomy of olfactory receptors. **(A)** Olfactory mucosa of the nose is an epithelial layer consisting of receptor cells, supporting cells, and basal cells. Numerous cilia emerge from a terminal swelling of the receptor cell called the *dendritic knob.* These cilia contain all of the elements of the transduction cascade and function much like the outer segments of rods and cones. Receptors also have axons, which communicate sensory signals to the olfactory bulb in the CNS. (After Keverne, 1982.) **(B)** Single olfactory receptor cell dissociated from the nasal epithelium of salamander, shown in a phase contrast micrograph *(left)* and in silhouette *(right).* Note cilia emerging from dendritic knob. Scale bar, 10 μm. (Reprinted from Leinders-Zufall et al., 1997, with the permission of the authors and of the Society for Neuroscience.)

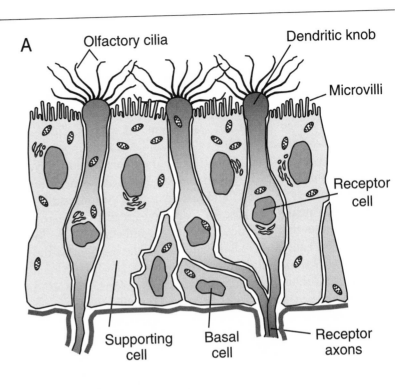

A

Olfactory cilia
Dendritic knob
Microvilli
Receptor cell
Supporting cell
Basal cell
Receptor axons

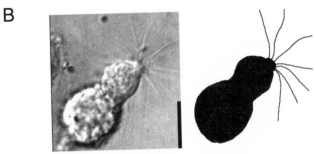

B

segments of photoreceptor cells. The opening of these channels produces an inward current that depolarizes the cell. In contrast to photoreceptors, however, olfactory receptor neurons produce action potentials and have axons that directly enter the central nervous system; they synapse onto specialized structures, called *glomeruli,* within the olfactory bulb of the brain.

Odorant Receptors

The discovery that odorant molecules activate an adenylyl cyclase in isolated receptor cell cilia (Pace et al., 1985; Sklar, Anholt, and Snyder, 1986) suggested that olfaction may be a specialized form of metabotropic transduction. Buck and Axel (1991) concluded that odorant receptors may therefore be members of the heptahelical receptor superfamily and used conserved sequences from proteins in this superfamily to clone the first genes of odorant receptor molecules. In so doing, they discovered a large family of perhaps 500–1,000 molecules, localized to the olfactory epithelium, that appear to be responsible for olfactory reception. Members of this family are quite variable in sequence, particularly for amino acids within the transmembrane domains, where the binding sites for odorant molecules are probably located.

When *in situ* hybridization was used to localize neurons expressing odorant receptors within the olfactory mucosa, several interesting discoveries were made (see Buck, 1996). Each odorant receptor is expressed by only a small proportion of the receptor cells, consistent with the possibility that each receptor cell expresses only a single odorant receptor protein. Cells expressing a given receptor protein are not grouped together but are widely distributed throughout the epithelium, though they are segregated into one of at least four broad zones (Ressler, Sullivan, and Buck, 1993; Vassar, Ngai, and Axel, 1993). The wide distribution of the cells may be necessary to provide a large surface of epithelium for odorant detection, for each of the different odorant receptor molecules. Remarkably, the axons of cells expressing the same odorant receptor molecules all converge within the olfactory bulb and synapse together onto a small number of glomeruli, providing specialized centers of integration for each of the different varieties of receptor protein (Vassar et al., 1994; Ressler, Sullivan, and Buck, 1994; Mombaerts et al., 1996).

Mechanism of Transduction

The primary mechanism for olfactory transduction is shown in Fig. 16.13. Olfactory receptor neurons contain a specialized G pro-

Fig. 16.13 Mechanism of olfactory transduction. Binding of odorant molecules to receptors facilitates the exchange of GTP for GDP on the α subunit of the G_{olf} protein. The $G_\alpha \cdot$GTP then binds to adenylyl cyclase, which synthesizes cAMP. Olfactory receptors, like photoreceptors, contain cyclic-nucleotide-gated channels, which are gated either by cGMP or cAMP. Synthesis of cAMP by the adenylyl cyclase opens the channels, producing an influx of both Na^+ and Ca^{2+} and depolarization of the cell. Ca^{2+} is known to bind to calmodulin *(CaM)*, which interacts with the channel, decreasing the apparent affinity of the channel for cAMP. This appears to be a major mechanism of adaptation in olfactory receptors. Ca^{2+}/calmodulin has also been hypothesized to regulate the activation rate of adenylyl cyclase and phosphodiesterase *(PDE)*, which hydrolyzes cAMP. Finally, Ca^{2+} can gate the opening of Ca^{2+}-dependent Cl^- channels in the receptor membrane (not shown), which can produce a considerable fraction of the electrical response of the cell to odorant. The response of the receptor is terminated by phosphorylation by a G-protein receptor kinase *(GRK)* and perhaps also by other kinases, such as protein kinase A *(PKA)*. Phosphorylation of the receptor facilitates the binding of arrestin and the termination of receptor activation. (After Buck, 1996.)

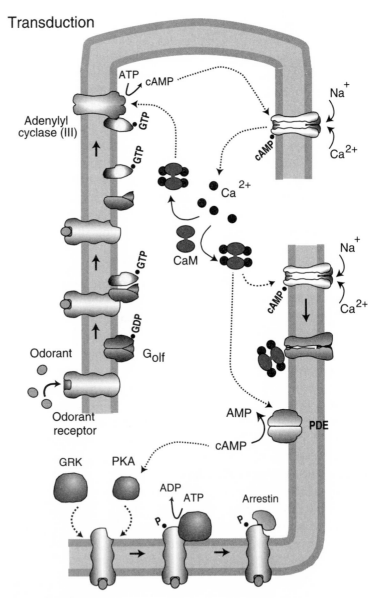

tein called G_{olf}, which is abundant in olfactory cell cilia (Jones and Reed, 1989). The α subunit of G_{olf} is a member of the α_s subfamily (see Table 11.1), with α_s and α_{olf} sharing 88 percent sequence identity. It would therefore not be too surprising if G_{olf} were coupled to an adenylyl cyclase. Olfactory cilia contain a high concentration of a Ca^{2+}/calmodulin-sensitive adenylyl cyclase (type III), which is again apparently localized to the cilia (Bakalyar and Reed, 1990); they also contain Ca^{2+}/calmodulin-sensitive phosphodiesterase, which may be responsible for hydrolyzing cAMP during the declining phase of the odorant response (Yan et al., 1995). Within the membrane of the cilia are cyclic-nucleotide-gated channels, and inside-out patches from the cilia respond to cyclic nucleotides much as inside-out patches from rods do (Nakamura and Gold, 1987). There is, however, one striking difference: patches from cilia are gated by cAMP as well as by cGMP, whereas rod patches are rather insensitive to cAMP.

When isolated olfactory receptor neurons are perfused with odorant molecules, they respond with inward currents (if they are voltage-clamped) or with depolarizations and action potentials (if they are not). Fig. 16.14 (from Firestein, Picco, and Menini, 1993) shows current responses from three olfactory receptor neurons recorded with a whole-cell voltage clamp. Each cell was perfused with three different odorants, for a duration indicated by the downward-going electrical artifacts (from the perfusion system). These recordings demonstrate that different cells, presumably each containing different odorant receptor proteins, are characterized by responses to many different odorants, with some cells responding widely to many odorants and others more narrowly to just a few. A single odorant molecule seems therefore to produce a spectrum of responses in many different receptor cells, and it is this spectrum of responses that is probably responsible for our sensation of particular smells.

Olfactory Cyclic-Nucleotide-Gated Channels

The electrical response of an olfactory receptor neuron is initiated by the binding of cAMP to cyclic-nucleotide-gated channels in the membrane of the cilia. These channels closely resemble those in rods. Two olfactory channel subunits have been described: an α,

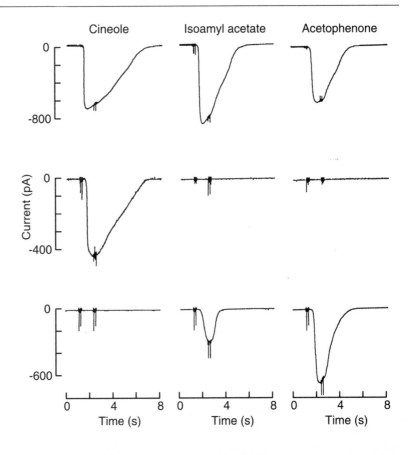

Fig. 16.14 Whole-cell patch recordings from dissociated salamander olfactory receptors, with $V_H = -55$ mV. Responses are to the odorants cineole, isoamyl acetate, and acetophenone, which were perfused onto the receptors at a concentration of 0.5 mM. The duration of the odorant exposure was 1.2 s, as indicated in several of the recordings by the downward-going electrical artifacts produced by the perfusion system at the beginning and end of the stimulus. Each row shows response from the same cell for each of the three odorants. Note the variety of responses to these odorants for the three cells illustrated. (Reprinted from Firestein, Picco, and Menini, 1993, with permission of the authors and of the Physiological Society.)

which can be expressed by itself to form homomultimeric channels (Dhallan et al., 1990; Ludwig et al., 1990); and a β, which cannot (Bradley et al., 1994; Liman and Buck, 1994). Co-expression of α and β cRNA produces channels with many of the properties of native channels, including an enhanced sensitivity to gating by cAMP (Bradley et al., 1994; Liman and Buck, 1994).

Olfactory cyclic-nucleotide-gated channels, like those in rods, are permeable to a variety of monovalent ions, including Na^+ and K^+ (see Zufall, Firestein, and Shepherd, 1994; Finn, Grunwald, and Yau, 1996; Zagotta and Siegelbaum, 1996), and to divalents, including Ca^{2+}. Because of the Ca^{2+} permeability of olfactory channels, Ca^{2+} carries a significant percentage of the current through the open channels (see for example Frings et al., 1995). This has several important consequences. The influx of Ca^{2+} causes an increase in intracellular Ca^{2+} concentration (see for example Leinders-Zufall et al., 1997), which may affect the activity of the adenylyl cyclase and PDE, which are both Ca^{2+}/calmodulin-sensitive (see Fig. 16.13). The increase in Ca^{2+} also gates a Ca^{2+}-dependent Cl^- current, which can generate a considerable portion of the actual response of olfactory neurons to perfused odorants (Kurahashi and Yau, 1993; Lowe and Gold, 1993a).

Adaptation

Ca^{2+} is also responsible for adaptation of olfactory cell responses. It is a common experience that the conscious sensation of smell fades with time. Olfactory cell responses also decrease in amplitude during maintained perfusion with an odorant, and this decrease is almost completely abolished in the absence of extracellular Ca^{2+} (Kurahashi and Shibuya, 1990; Zufall, Shepherd, and Firestein, 1991). The Ca^{2+} could be acting on one or more of the enzymes of transduction, as in photoreceptors, but the results in Fig. 16.15 indicate that the primary effect is on the channels. In these experiments (from Kurahashi and Menini, 1997), adapation was compared for odorant exposures and for photolysis of caged cAMP that had been dialyzed into the cell from a whole-cell patch pipette.

Figure 16.15A shows the current responses of an olfactory receptor neuron to odorant and caged cAMP. The response to the photolysis of caged cAMP has a shorter latency, since photolysis opens the channels directly, without prior activation of the enzymes of the cascade (see also Lowe and Gold, 1993b). The response to cAMP is comparable in amplitude to the response to the odorant, however, if the odorant concentration and photolysis light intensity are suitably adjusted. Part B of this figure shows that responses to odorants adapt both further responses to odorants and responses to cAMP uncaging. In other experiments, this adaptation was shown to be abolished when Ca^{2+} was removed from the extracellular solution or when the cell was held at a potential of +100 mV, which is near E_{Ca} (at which point little Ca^{2+} would flow into the cell). Kurahashi and Menini also found that if the responses to the odorant and uncaged cAMP are of equal amplitude, they produce an equal depression to subsequent responses (Fig. 16.15C).

The reason these results are so surprising is that they show that

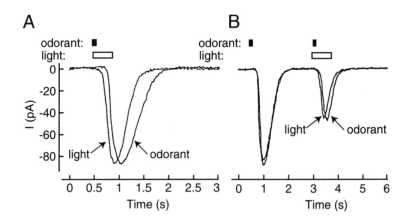

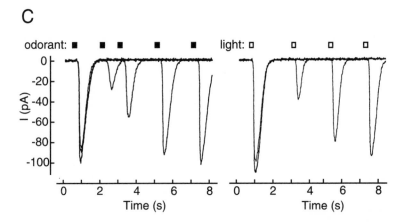

Fig. 16.15 Adaptation in olfactory receptors is produced by modulation of the cyclic-nucleotide-gated channels. Whole-cell patch recordings from receptors dissociated from the olfactory epithelium of the newt, with pipettes containing caged cAMP. The cAMP was uncaged by photolysis with flashes of ultraviolet light; $V_H = -50$ mV. **(A)** Comparison of time course of current response to the odorant amylacetate and to light exposure (which releases cAMP). Light intensity and odorant concentration were adjusted to produce responses of same peak amplitude. The approximately 200 ms delay of the odorant response was probably caused by the slow time course of transduction cascade. **(B)** Responses for the same cell as in **(A)** to same concentrations of odorant and same intensity of uncaging light (adjusted to produce equal responses in the absence of adaptation). Initial exposure to the odorant adapted the response to the second application of odorant, and a quantitatively similar adaptation was produced for the response to uncaged cAMP. **(C)** Comparison of time course of adaptation following stimulation by odorant (amylacetate) and by uncaging of cAMP. *Left:* Responses to the same odorant concentration given initially and then again after 1.5, 2.5, 4.5, and 6.5 s. *Right:* Responses to identical ultraviolet flashes given initially and then again after 3, 5, and 7 s. The time course of recovery from adaptation was similar for odorant and cAMP. (Reprinted with minor modification from Kurahashi and Menini, 1997, with permission of the authors and of Macmillan Magazines Limited.)

odorants and even cAMP can adapt further responses to cAMP. This would be unlikely if adaptation were caused by a modulation of the enzymes of transduction, since regulation at this level would simply alter the rate of synthesis or degradation of the cyclic nucleotide. If odorants can adapt responses to cAMP, the adaptation is most likely produced at the level of the channels.

Since adaptation depends upon the entry of Ca^{2+} into the cell, Ca^{2+} entry would appear to modulate the channels. The probable mechanism for this effect was discovered by Chen and Yau (1994), who showed that the effective affinity of the channel for cAMP is greatly reduced by Ca^{2+}/calmodulin. This effect is similar to the one previously demonstrated for rods (Hsu and Molday, 1993) but appears to be much stronger for the cyclic-nucleotide-gated channels of olfactory neurons. Whereas Ca^{2+}/calmodulin binds to the β subunit of the rod channel, it binds to the α subunit of the olfactory channel, near the amino terminus (Liu et al., 1994). Since calmodulin is abundant in olfactory receptor cilia, it is likely that a depression in the gating of the channel by cAMP produced by direct binding of Ca^{2+}/calmodulin causes much of the decrease in responsiveness of the cell to prolonged stimulation.

Alternative Mechanisms of Transduction

The G_{olf}-mediated activation of adenylyl cyclase and increase in cAMP outlined in Fig. 16.13 is probably the major mechanism of transduction in vertebrate olfactory receptor neurons, but there may also be other signaling cascades that may directly generate or modulate receptor cell responses. Some neurons in the primary olfactory epithelium or in a secondary structure called the *vomeronasal organ* do not appear to contain the molecules of the adenylyl cyclase cascade (such as G_{olf}, adenyly cyclase III, or the α subunit of the channel); these neurons may use other molecules in some alternative transduction mechanism (see for example Berghard, Buck, and Liman, 1996; Juilfs et al., 1997).

Olfactory neurons in some invertebrates appear to use IP_3 as a signaling molecule in olfactory transduction (Breer, Boekhoff, and Tareilus, 1990; see Ache and Zhainazarov, 1995), and an odorant-induced increase in IP_3 has also been reported in vertebrates (Boekhoff et al., 1990). Although an odorant-induced increase in IP_3 may modulate transduction in olfactory epithelium, it is unlikely to be the primary messenger. In transgenic mice for which the cyclic-nucleotide-gated channels have been eliminated, all responses to odorants appear to be abolished (Brunet, Gold, and Ngai, 1996). Since cyclic-nucleotide-gated channels seem to be essential for the production of an odorant response, it is likely that the primary second messenger in most olfactory neurons is a cyclic nucleotide.

The cyclic-nucleotide-gated channels in olfactory neurons respond to both cAMP and cGMP. Both particulate (Fülle et al., 1995) and soluble guanylyl cyclase (Ingi and Ronnett, 1995) have been localized to olfactory neurons and may serve as alternative signal-transducing proteins. Odorant-induced increases in cGMP have been observed both from isolated cilia (Breer, Klemm, and Boekhoff, 1992) and from cultures of olfactory neurons (Verma et al., 1993). This increase in cGMP may be produced at least in part by soluble guanylyl cyclase, stimulated by CO (see Chapter 13). Olfactory neurons contain a high concentration of heme oxygenase, an enzyme that generates CO (Verma et al., 1993). Increasing evidence indicates that a CO-mediated increase in cGMP (Ingi and Ronnett, 1995) may activate the cyclic-nucleotide-gated channels with a slow time course and produce a long-lasting form of olfactory adaptation (Leinders-Zufall, Shepherd, and Zufall, 1995, 1996; Zufall and Leinders-Zufall, 1997).

Summary

Sensory transduction in the vertebrate photoreceptor and the vertebrate olfactory receptor neuron is a metabotropic process. These two cells have much in common. In both there is a specific region specialized for sensory transduction: the outer segment for rods and cones, and the sensory cilia for olfactory receptor neurons. Within these regions, there is a high concentration of the primary detector of the sensory signal, which in each case is a heptahelical receptor protein. In olfactory cells these proteins seem similar to other metabotropic receptor proteins, but the receptor proteins in rods and cones (called rhodopsins) are somewhat unusual. They are covalently bound to a small-molecular-weight molecule (11-*cis* retinal) in a pocket resembling the binding pocket of the β-adrenergic receptor. The 11-*cis* retinal is bound to the protein when the receptor is in the unstimulated state—that is, in darkness. Light produces a photoisomerization of the retinal, which is responsible for triggering the light response.

Both photoreceptors and olfactory receptor neurons contain a variety of specialized proteins that mediate signal transduction. These include G proteins (G_{olf} and transducin), effector molecules (PDE and adenylyl cyclase), and cyclic-nucleotide-gated channels. In rods and cones, activation of PDE by light decreases the concentration of cGMP and decreases the probability that channels will open. As a result, the current through the outer segment membrane decreases, and the cell hyperpolarizes. In olfactory neurons, activation of adenylyl cyclase increases the cAMP concentration. This increases the probability that channels will open and depolarizes the cell. The channels of olfactory cells can also be activated by changes in cGMP concentration, and there is increasing evidence that odors may activate a soluble guanylyl cyclase, perhaps via a change in CO concentration, which may modulate the activity of the transduction cascade.

One of the most remarkable similarities between olfactory receptor neurons and photoreceptors (and hair cells—see Chapter 15) is that adaptation seems to be mostly if not entirely produced by a change in intracellular free-Ca^{2+} concentration. In photoreceptors, Ca^{2+} may modulate the guanylyl cyclase as well as other proteins in the transduction cascade, including rhodopsin. Ca^{2+}, in concert with calmodulin and perhaps other small-molecular-weight Ca^{2+}-binding proteins, may also modulate the probability of opening of the cyclic-nucleotide-gated channels. In olfactory neurons, the effect of Ca^{2+} on the channels is considerable, altering the effective affinity of the channels for cAMP by as much as 20-fold.

Transduction by metabotropic sensory receptors has attracted considerable interest, and much is known about receptors in other sensory systems and in other species. Some taste receptors (bitter, sweet) trigger metabotropic cascades, and molecular and cellular techniques are beginning to resolve many long-standing questions about the mechanism of transduction in these receptors (see Stewart, DeSimone, and Hill, 1997). Considerable attention has been given to the study of photoreception in arthropods, particularly *Drosophila*, for which powerful genetic techniques are available (see Pak, 1995; Zuker, 1996). It is of some interest that both photoreceptors and olfactory receptor neurons in arthropods respond to stimulation with a large and rapid activation of PLC and IP_3 turnover. The mechanism of transduction is still not entirely clear in these species but may eventually provide an interesting comparison to the mechanisms for vertebrates described in this chapter.

Appendix: Symbols Used

a	radius of cell or cable (cm)
A	ampere; unit of measure of current
A	cross-sectional area of cable $= \pi a^2$ (cm²)
β	partition coefficient
c	concentration (mol l⁻¹)
C	coulomb; unit of measure of charge
C	capacitance (F)
c_j^{in}	concentration of jth ion species just inside internal surface of membrane (mol l⁻¹)
c_j^{out}	concentration of jth ion species just inside external surface of membrane (mol l⁻¹)
cm	centimeter; unit of measure of length
c_m	capacitance of 1 cm of cable $= C_m 2\pi a$ (F cm⁻¹)
C_m	specific capacitance of cell membrane (F cm⁻²)
CV	coefficient of variation (standard deviation divided by mean)
δ	thickness of membrane (cm)
D	diameter of dendrite entering branch point (cm)
d_j	diameter of dendritic branch j leaving branch point (cm)
D_j	diffusion constant for jth ion
e	elementary charge (1.6021×10^{-19} C)
E	electric field across membrane (V cm⁻¹); also, constant value of electric field in derivation of Goldman equation (V cm⁻¹)
E_{eq}	equilibrium potential (V)

E_{Na}, E_K equilibrium potentials for Na$^+$ and K$^+$; in parallel conductance model, reversal potentials for Na$^+$ and K$^+$ channels (V)

E_{rev} reversal potential (V)

erf error function

$erfc$ complement of error function $= 1 - erf$

F   farad; unit of measure of capacitance

F Faraday (96,487 C mol^{-1}); also, mechanical force (N)

g conductance (S, ℧)

G Gibbs free energy (J)

g_j gap-junctional conductance (S)

$\overline{g}_K$, $\overline{g}_{Na}$ maximum value of K$^+$ and Na$^+$ conductances in Hodgkin-Huxley model (S cm^{-2})

g_m specific conductance of cell membrane (S cm^{-2})

h inactivation parameter for Na$^+$ conductance in Hodgkin-Huxley model; h_∞, value of h at steady state

i current (A)

I_0 amplitude of injected current for cable (A)

i_a current passing down cytoplasm of cable (A)

i_C displacement current (A)

i_j gap-junctional current (A)

I_j current density for jth ion species (A cm^{-2})

i_l, i_{Na}, i_K current densities of parallel conductance model, for leakage, Na$^+$, and K$^+$ (A cm^{-2})

i_m membrane current density of cell (A cm^{-2}) or cable (A cm^{-1})

$i\rho_{Na}$, $i\rho_K$ Na$^+$/K$^+$ ATPase pump currents for Na$^+$ and K$^+$ (A)

i_R current through resistor (A)

I_S steady-state current (A)

i_T total current (A)

J   joule; unit of measure of energy

K   degree Kelvin; unit of measure of temperature

k Boltzmann constant (1.3805 × 10^{-23} J K^{-1}); also, spring constant (J cm^{-1})

λ length constant of cable (cm)

l   liter; unit of measure of volume

μ chemical potential (J mol^{-1}); as prefix in unit of measure, *micro-* (= 1/10^6)

μ^0 standard chemical potential (J mol^{-1})

m	Mean quantal content; also, activation parameter for Na$^+$ conductance in Hodgkin-Huxley model; m_∞, value of m at steady state
M	molar; unit of measure of concentration
mm	millimeter; unit of measure of length
mM	millimolar; unit of measure of concentration
mol	mole; unit of measure of quantity
ms	millisecond; unit of measure of time
mV	millivolt; unit of measure of electrical potential
n	activation parameter for Hodgkin-Huxley model for K$^+$ conductance; n_∞, value of n at steady state
N	newton; unit of measure of force
N_A	Avogadro's number (6.023×10^{23} atoms, ions, or molecules)
p	probability
p_i	probability of observing i events in binomial or Poisson equation
p_0	in Poisson equation, probability of failure
P_j	permeability constant of jth ion species (cm s^{-1})
p_o	probability of a channel being open
Φ_j	flux of jth ion species (mol s^{-1} cm^{-2})
Φ_j^d	diffusive flux (mol s^{-1} cm^{-2})
Φ_j^e	electrophoretic flux (mol s^{-1} cm^{-2})
ψ	electrical potential of a solution (V)
q	charge (C)
r	electrogenicity of Na$^+$/K$^+$ ATPase (absolute value of ratio of Na$^+$ and K$^+$ pump currents = 1.5)
R	resistance (Ω); also gas constant (8.31 J K^{-1} mol^{-1})
r_a	specific resistance of cytoplasm per unit length of cable (1 cm) = R_a/A (Ω cm^{-1})
R_a	specific resistance of cytoplasm (Ω cm)
R_{in}	input resistance (Ω)
r_m	resistance of 1 cm of cable = $R_m/2\pi a$ (Ω cm)
r_o	resistance per unit length of extracellular space or solution (Ω cm^{-1})
R_m	specific resistance of cell membrane (Ω cm^2)
R_s	series resistance of voltage clamp (Ω)
σ^2	variance
s	second; unit of measure of time

S	siemens; unit of measure of conductance
τ	time constant (s)
t	time (s)
T	time normalized to time constant of cable $= t/\tau$
u	mobility of ion in solution (cm^2 s^{-1} V^{-1})
V	volt; unit of measure of electrical potential
V	voltage, electrical potential (V)
V_0	initial voltage; voltage at time zero (V)
V_c	command voltage of voltage clamp (V)
V_H	holding voltage (V); i.e., command potential before test pulse (V)
V_j	gap-junctional voltage (V)
V_m	membrane potential (V)
V_m'	approximate value of membrane potential in voltage-clamp circuit $= V_m + i_m R_S$ (V)
$V_m - E_{eq}$	driving force (V)
V_ρ	contribution of Na$^+$/K$^+$ ATPase pump to resting membrane potential (V)
x	distance (cm)
X	distance normalized to length constant of cable $= x/\lambda$
z	valence (charge) of an ion
Ω	ohm; unit of measure of resistance
$\mho$	"mho" $= 1/\Omega$; unit of measure of conductance

References

1. Introduction

Ascher, P., and Nowak, L. 1988. The role of divalent cations in the N-methyl-D-aspartate responses of mouse central neurones in culture. *Journal of Physiology* 399:247–266.

Baylor, D. A., Fuortes, M. G. F., and O'Bryan, P. M. 1971. Receptive fields of cones in the retina of the turtle. *Journal of Physiology* 214:265–294.

Baylor, D. A., and Hodgkin, A. L. 1974. Changes in time scale and sensitivity in turtle photoreceptors. *Journal of Physiology* 242:729–758.

Baylor, D. A., Lamb, T. D., and Yau, K.-W. 1979. Responses of retinal rods to single photons. *Journal of Physiology* 288:613–634.

Benzer, T. I., and Raftery, M. A. 1973. Solubilization and partial characterization of the tetrodotoxin binding component from nerve axons. *Biochemical and Biophysical Research Communications* 51:939–944.

Brown, K. T., and Flaming, D. G. 1977. New microelectrode techniques for intracellular work in small cells. *Neuroscience* 2:813–827.

Catterall, W. A. 1992. Cellular and molecular biology of voltage-gated sodium channels. *Physiological Reviews* 72:S15–S48.

Eccles, J. C. 1964. *The Physiology of Synapses*. Berlin: Springer-Verlag.

Edwards, F. A., Konnerth, A., Sakmann, B., and Takahashi, T. 1989. A thin slice preparation for patch clamp recordings from neurones of the mammalian central nervous system. *Pflügers Archiv* 414:600–612.

Fain, G. L. 1976. Sensitivity of toad rods: Dependence on wavelength and background. *Journal of Physiology* 261:71–101.

Fain, G. L., Matthews, H. R., and Cornwall, M. C. 1996. Dark adaptation in vertebrate photoreceptors. *Trends in Neurosciences* 19:502–507.

Goldin, A. L. 1992. Maintenance of *Xenopus laevis* and oocyte injection. *Methods in Enzymology* 207:266–279.

Grenningloh, G., Rienitz, A., Schmitt, B., Methfessel, C., Zensen, M., Beyreuther, K., Gundelfinger, E., and Betz, H. 1987. The strychnine-binding subunit of the glycine receptor shows homology with nicotinic acetylcholine receptors. *Nature* 328:215–220.

Hamill, O. P., Marty, A., Neher, E., Sakmann, B., and Sigworth, F. J. 1981. Improved patch-clamp techniques for high-resolution current recording from cells and cell-free membrane patches. *Pflügers Archiv* 391:85–100.

Henderson, R., and Wang, J. 1972. Solubilization of a specific tetrodotoxin-binding component from garfish olfactory nerve membrane. *Biochemistry* 11:4565–4569.

Hollman, M., O'Shea-Greenfield, A., Rogers, S. W., and Heinemann, S. 1989. Cloning by functional expression of a member of the glutamate receptor family. *Nature* 342:643–648.

Horn, R., and Marty, A. 1988. Muscarinic activation of ionic currents measured by a new whole-cell recording method. *Journal of General Physiology* 92:145–159.

Hubel, D. H., and Wiesel, T. N. 1977. Functional architecture of macaque monkey visual cortex: Ferrier lecture. *Proceedings of the Royal Society of London B* 198:1–59.

Javitt, D. C., and Zukin, S. R. 1991. Recent advances in the phencyclidine model of schizophrenia. *American Journal of Psychiatry* 148:1301–1308.

Johnson, J. W., and Ascher, P. 1987. Glycine potentiates the NMDA response in cultured mouse brain neurons. *Nature* 325:529–531.

Kamb, A., Iverson, L. E., and Tanouye, M. A. 1987. Molecular characterization of *Shaker*, a *Drosophila* gene that encodes a potassium channel. *Cell* 50:405–413.

Katz, B., and Miledi, R. 1972. The statistical nature of the acetylcholine potential and its molecular components. *Journal of Physiology* 224:665–699.

Kaupp, U. B., Niidome, T., Tanabe, T., Terada, S., Bönigk, W., Stühmer, W., Cook, N. J., Kangawa, K., Matsuo, H., Hirose, T., Miyata, T., and Numa, S. 1989. Primary structure and functional expression from complementary DNA of the rod photoreceptor cyclic GMP-gated channel. *Nature* 342:762–766.

Koutalos, Y., and Yau, K.-W. 1996. Regulation of sensitivity in vertebrate rod photoreceptors by calcium. *Trends in Neurosciences* 19:73–81.

Kubo, T., Fukuda, K., Mikami, A., Maeda, A., Takahashi, H., Mishina, M., Haga, T., Haga, K., Ichiyama, A., Kangawa, K., Kojima, M., Matsuo, H., Hirose, T., and Numa, S. 1986. Cloning, sequencing and expression of complementary DNA encoding the muscarinic acetylcholine receptor. *Nature* 323:411–416.

Ling, G., and Gerard, R. W. 1949. The normal membrane potential of frog sartorius fibers. *Journal of Cellular and Comparative Physiology* 34:383–396.

Magee, J. C., and Johnston, D. 1995. Characterization of single voltage-gated Na^+ and Ca^{2+} channels in apical dendrites of rat CA1 pyramidal neurons. *Journal of Physiology* 487:67–90.

Markram, H., Lübke, J., Frotscher, M., and Sakmann, B. 1997. Regulation of synaptic efficacy by coincidence of postsynaptic APs and EPSPs. *Science* 275:213–215.

Marty, A., and Neher, E. 1995. Tight-seal whole-cell recording. In *Single-Channel Recording,* ed. B. Sakmann and E. Neher, pp. 31–52. New York: Plenum Press.

Mayer, M. L., Westbrook, G. L., and Guthrie, P. B. 1984. Voltage-dependent block by Mg^{2+} of NMDA responses in spinal cord neurones. *Nature* 309:261–263.

McBain, C. J., and Mayer, M. L. 1994. N-methyl-D-aspartic acid receptor structure and function. *Physiological Reviews* 74:723–760.

Moriyoshi, K., Masu, M., Ishii, T., Shigemoto, R., Mizuno, N., and Nakanishi, S. 1991. Molecular cloning and characterization of the rat NMDA receptor. *Nature* 354:31–37.

Neher, E., and Sakmann, B. 1976. Single-channel currents recorded from membrane of denervated frog muscle fibers. *Nature* 260:799–802.

Noda, M., Shimizu, S., Tanabe, T., Takai, T., Kayano, T., Ikeda, T., Takahashi, H., Nakayama, H., Kanaoka, Y., Minamino, N., Kangawa, K., Matsuo, H., Raftery, M. A., Hirose, T., Inayama, S., Hayashida, H., Miyata, T., and Numa, S. 1984. Primary structure of *Electrophorus electricus* sodium channel deduced from cDNA sequence. *Nature* 312:121–127.

Nowak, L., Bregestovski, P., Ascher, P., Herbet, A., and Prochiantz, A. 1984. Magnesium gates glutamate-activated channels in mouse central neurones. *Nature* 307:462–465.

Papazian, D. M., Schwarz, T. L., Tempel, B. L., Jan, Y. N., and Jan, L. Y. 1987. Cloning of genomic and complementary DNA from *Shaker,* a putative potassium channel gene from *Drosophila. Science* 237:749–753.

Pongs, O., Kecskemethy, N., Muller, R., Krah-Jentgens, I., Baumann, A., Kiltz, H. H., Canal, I., Llamazares, S., and Ferrsu, A. 1988. *Shaker* encodes a family of putative potassium channel proteins in the nervous system of *Drosophila. EMBO Journal* 7:1087–1096.

Ramón y Cajal, S. 1909. *Histologie du Système Nerveux de l'Homme et des Vertebres,* vol. 1. Madrid: Instituto Ramón y Cajal.

Sakmann, B., and Neher, E. (eds.). 1995. *Single-Channel Recording.* New York: Plenum Press.

Sakmann, B., and Stuart, G. 1995. Patch-pipette recordings from the soma, dendrites, and axon of neurons in brain slices. In *Single-Channel Record-*

ing, ed. B. Sakmann and E. Neher, pp. 199–211. New York: Plenum Press.

Schofield, P. R., Darlison, M. G., Fujita, N., Burt, D. R., Stephenson, F. A., Rodriguez, H., Rhee, L. M., Ramachandran, J., Reale, V., Glencorse, T. A., Seeburg, P. H. and Barnard, E. A. 1987. Sequence and functional expression of the GABA$_A$ receptor shows a ligand-gated receptor super-family. *Nature* 328:221–227.

Sigworth, F. J., and Neher, E. 1980. Single Na$^+$ channel currents observed in cultured rat muscle cells. *Nature* 287:447–449.

Stuart, G. J., and Sakmann, B. 1994. Active propagation of somatic action potentials into neocortical pyramidal cell dendrites. *Nature* 367:69–72.

Stühmer, W. 1992. Electrophysiological recording from *Xenopus* oocytes. *Methods in Enzymology* 207:319–339.

Swanson, R., and Folander, K. 1992. *In vitro* synthesis of RNA for expression of ion channels in *Xenopus* oocytes. *Methods in Enzymology* 207:310–319.

Tanabe, T., Takeshima, H., Mikami, A., Flockerzi, V., Takahashi, H., Kangawa, K., Kojima, M., Matsuo, H., Hirose, T., and Numa, S. 1987. Primary structure of the receptor for calcium channel blockers from skeletal muscle. *Nature* 328:313–318.

Tempel, B. L., Papazian, D. M., Schwarz, T. L., Jan, Y. N., and Jan, L. Y. 1987. Sequence of a probable potassium channel component encoded at *Shaker* locus of *Drosophila*. *Science* 237:770–775.

Watson, J. D., Gilman, M., Witkowski, J., and Zoller, M. 1992. *Recombinant DNA,* 2d ed. New York: W. H. Freeman.

Zukin, R. S., and Bennett, M. V. L. 1995. Alternatively spliced isoforms of the NMDAR1 receptor subunit. *Trends in Neurosciences* 18:306–313.

2. Passive Electrical Properties of Neurons

Deisz, R. A., Fortin, G., and Zieglgänsberger, W. 1991. Voltage dependence of excitatory postsynaptic potentials of rat neocortical neurons. *Journal of Neurophysiology* 65:371–382.

De Schutter, E. 1989. Computer software for development and simulation of compartmental models of neurons. *Computers in Biology and Medicine* 19:71–81.

——— 1992. A consumer guide to neuronal modeling software. *Trends in Neurosciences* 15:462–464.

Famiglietti, E. V. 1991. Synaptic organization of starburst amacrine cells in rabbit retina: Analysis of serial thin sections by electron microscopy and graphic reconstruction. *Journal of Comparative Neurology* 309:40–70.

Fatt, P., and Katz, B. 1951. An analysis of the end-plate potential recorded with an intracellular electrode. *Journal of Physiology* 115:320–370.

Hodgkin, A. L., and Rushton, W. A. H. 1946. The electrical constants of a crustacean nerve fibre. *Proceedings of the Royal Society of London B* 133:444–479.

Jack, J. J. B., Noble, D., and Tsien, R. W. 1975. *Electric Current Flow in Excitable Cells.* Oxford: Clarendon Press.

Johnston, D., Magee, J. C., Colbert, C. M., and Christie, B. R. 1996. Active properties of neuronal dendrites. *Annual Review of Neuroscience* 19:165–186.

Koch, C., and Poggio, T. 1985. A simple algorithm for solving the cable equation in dendritic trees of arbitrary geometry. *Journal of Neuroscience Methods* 12:303–315.

Llinás, R. R. 1988. The intrinsic electrophysiological properties of mammalian neurons: Insights into central nervous system function. *Science* 242:1654–1664.

Major, G., Evans, J. D., and Jack, J. J. B. 1993. Solutions for transients in arbitrarily branching cables: I. Voltage recording with a somatic shunt. *Biophysical Journal* 65:423–449.

Major, G., Larkman, A. U., Jonas, P., Sakmann, B., and Jack, J. J. B. 1994. Detailed passive cable models of whole-cell recorded CA3 pyramidal neurons in rat hippocampal slices. *Journal of Neuroscience* 14:4613–4638.

Miller, R. F., and Bloomfield, S. A. 1983. Electroanatomy of a unique amacrine cell in the rabbit retina. *Proceedings of the National Academy of Sciences USA* 80:3069–3073.

Rall, W. 1959. Branching dendritic trees and motoneuron membrane resistivity. *Experimental Neurology* 1:491–527.

——— 1960. Membrane potential transients and membrane time constant of motoneurons. *Experimental Neurology* 2:503–532.

——— 1962. Electrophysiology of a dendritic neuron model. *Biophysical Journal* (Supplement) 2:145–167.

——— 1964. Theoretical significance of dendritic tree for neuronal input-output relations. In *Neural Theory and Modeling,* ed. R. F. Reiss, pp. 73–97. Stanford, CA: Stanford University Press.

——— 1969. Time constants and electrotonic length of membrane cylinders and neurons. *Biophysical Journal* 9:1483–1508.

——— 1977. Core conductor theory and cable properties of neurons. In *Handbook of Physiology, Section 1: The Nervous System, Volume 1: Cellular Biology of Neurons, Part 1,* ed. E. R. Kandel, pp. 39–97. Bethesda, MD: American Physiological Society.

——— 1989. Cable theory for dendritic neurons. In *Methods in Neuronal*

Modeling, ed. C. Koch and I. Segev, pp. 9–62. Cambridge, MA: MIT Press.

Sakmann, B. and Neher, E. 1995. Geometric parameters of pipettes and membrane patches. In *Single-Channel Recording,* 2d ed., ed. B. Sakmann and E. Neher, pp. 637–650. New York: Plenum Press.

Segev, I., Fleshman, J. W., and Burke, R. E. 1989. Compartmental models of complex neurons. In *Methods in Neuronal Modeling,* ed. C. Koch and I. Segev, pp. 63–96. Cambridge, MA: MIT Press.

Segev, I., Rinzel, J., and Shepherd, G. M. (eds.). 1995. *The Theoretical Foundation of Dendritic Function.* Collected Papers of Wilfred Rall. Cambridge, MA: MIT Press.

Spruston, N., and Johnston, D. 1992. Perforated patch-clamp analysis of the passive membrane properties of three classes of hippocampal neurons. *Journal of Neurophysiology* 67:508–529.

Stuart, G. J., and Sakmann, B. 1994. Active propagation of somatic action potentials into neocortical pyramidal cell dendrites. *Nature* 367:69–72.

——— 1995. Amplification of EPSPs by axosomatic sodium channels in neocortical pyramidal neurons. *Neuron* 15:1065–1076.

Tauchi, M., and Masland, R. H. 1984. The shape and arrangement of the cholinergic neurons in the rabbit retina. *Proceedings of the Royal Society of London B* 223:101–119.

Wong, R. O. L., and Collin, S. P. 1989. Dendritic maturation of displaced putative cholinergic amacrine cells in the rabbit retina. *Journal of Comparative Neurology* 287:164–178.

Yuste, R., and Tank, D. W. 1996. Dendritic integration in mammalian neurons, a century after Cajal. *Neuron* 16:701–716.

Zhou, Z. J., Cheney, M., and Fain, G. L. 1996. Starburst amacrine cells change from spiking to non-spiking neurons during visual development. *Investigative Ophthalmology and Visual Science* 37:S1153.

Zhou, Z. J., and Fain, G. L. 1996. Starburst amacrine cells change from spiking to nonspiking neurons during retinal development. *Proceedings of the National Academy of Sciences USA* 93:8057–8062.

3. Ion Permeability and Membrane Potentials

Bormann, J., Hamill, O. P., and Sakmann, B. 1987. Mechanism of anion permeation through channels gated by glycine and γ-aminobutyric acid in mouse cultured spinal neurones. *Journal of Physiology* 385:243–286.

Goldman, D. E. 1943. Potential, impedance, and rectification in membranes. *Journal of General Physiology* 27:37–60.

Hille, B. 1975. Ionic selectivity of Na and K channels of nerve membranes. In *Membranes—A Series of Advances,* Vol. 3: *Lipid Bilayers and Biological*

Membranes: Dynamic Properties, ed. G. Eisenman, pp. 255–323. New York: Marcel Dekker.

Hodgkin, A. L., and Horowicz, P. 1959. The influence of potassium and chloride ions on the membrane potential of single muscle fibres. *Journal of Physiology* 148:127–160.

Hodgkin, A. L., and Katz, B. 1949. The effect of sodium ions on the electrical activity of the giant axon of the squid. *Journal of Physiology* 108:37–77.

4. Ion Pumps and Homeostasis

Allbritton, N. L., Meyer, T., and Stryer, L. 1992. Range of messenger action of calcium ion and inositol 1,4,5-trisphosphate. *Science* 258:1812–1815.

Allen, T. J. A., Noble, D., and Reuter, H. 1989. *Sodium-Calcium Exchange: Proceedings of the First International Symposium.* Oxford: Oxford University Press.

Alper, S. L. 1991. The band 3-related anion exchanger (AE) gene family. *Annual Review of Physiology* 53:549–564.

Alvarez-Leefmans, F. J. 1990. Intracellular Cl⁻ regulation and synaptic inhibition in vertebrate and invertebrate neurons. In *Chloride Channels and Carriers in Nerve, Muscle, and Glial Cells,* ed. F. J. Alvarez-Leefmans and J. M. Russell, pp. 109–158. New York: Plenum Press.

Alvarez-Leefmans, F. J., Gamiño, S. M., Giraldez, F. and Noguerón, I. 1988. Intracellular chloride regulation in amphibian dorsal root ganglion neurones studied with ion-selective microelectrodes. *Journal of Physiology* 406:225–246.

Baker, P. F., Blaustein, M. P., Hodgkin, A. L., and Steinhardt, R. A. 1969. The influence of calcium on sodium efflux in squid axons. *Journal of Physiology* 200:431–458.

Baker, P. F., and DiPolo, R. 1984. Axonal calcium and magnesium homeostasis. *Current Topics in Membranes and Transport* 22:195–247.

Baylor, D. A., and Nicholls, J. G. 1969. After-effects of nerve impulses on signalling in the central nervous system of the leech. *Journal of Physiology* 203:571–589.

Bianchini, L., and Pouysségur, J. 1994. Molecular structure and regulation of vertebrate Na⁺/H⁺ exchangers. *Journal of Experimental Biology* 196:337–345.

Blaustein, M. P. 1988. Calcium transport and buffering in neurons. *Trends in Neurosciences* 11:438–443.

Blaustein, M. P., DiPolo, R., and Reeves, J. P. 1991. *Sodium-Calcium Exchange: Proceedings of the Second International Conference. Annals of New York Academy of Science* 639:1–671.

Blostein, R., and Polvani, C. 1991. Proton transport, charge transfer, and variable stoichiometry of the Na,K-ATPase. In *The Sodium Pump: Structure, Mechanism, and Regulation,* ed. J. H. Kaplan and P. De Weer, pp. 289–301. New York: Rockefeller University Press.

Bormann, J., Hamill, O. P., and Sakmann, B. 1987. Mechanism of anion permeation through channels gated by glycine and γ-aminobutyric acid in mouse cultured spinal neurones. *Journal of Physiology* 385:243–286.

Boron, W. F. 1984. Regulation of axonal pH. *Current Topics in Membranes and Transport* 22:249–269.

Boron, W. F., and Russell, J. M. 1983. Stoichiometry and ion dependencies of the intracellular-pH-regulating mechanism in squid giant axons. *Journal of General Physiology* 81:373–399.

Brindley, F. J., Jr. 1978. Calcium buffering in squid axons. *Annual Review of Biophysics and Bioengineering* 7:363–392.

Brown, J. E., and Lisman, J. E. 1972. An electrogenic sodium pump in *Limulus* ventral photoreceptor cells. *Journal of General Physiology* 59:720–733.

Gaillard, S., and Dupont, J.-L. 1990. Ionic control of intracellular pH in rat cerebellar Purkinje cells maintained in culture. *Journal of Physiology* 425:71–83.

Garrahan, P. J., and Glynn, I. M. 1967. The stoichiometry of the sodium pump. *Journal of Physiology* 192:217–235.

Glynn, I. M. 1993. "All hands to the sodium pump." *Journal of Physiology* 462:1–30.

Gorman, A. L. F., and Marmor, M. F. 1970. Contributions of the sodium pump and ionic gradients to the membrane potential of a molluscan neurone. *Journal of Physiology* 210:897–917.

Gunter, T. E., and Pfeiffer, D. R. 1990. Mechanisms by which mitochondria transport calcium. *American Journal of Physiology* 258:C755–C786.

Harvey, W. R., and Nelson, N. (eds.). 1994. Transporters. Volume 196 of *The Journal of Experimental Biology.* Cambridge, England: The Company of Biologists Limited.

Heizmann, C. W., and Hunziker, W. 1990. Intracellular calcium-binding molecules. In *Intracellular Calcium Regulation,* ed. F. Bronner, pp. 211–248. New York: Wiley-Liss.

Hilgemann, D. W., Nicoll, D. A., and Philipson, K. D. 1991. Charge movement during Na^+ translocation by native and cloned cardiac Na^+/Ca^{2+} exchanger. *Nature* 352:715–718.

Hodgkin, A. L. 1964. *The Conduction of the Nervous Impulse: The Sherrington Lectures, VII.* Liverpool: Liverpool University Press.

Hodgkin, A. L., and Horowicz, P. 1959. The influence of potassium and chloride ions on the membrane potential of single muscle fibers. *Journal of Physiology* 148:127–160.

Hodgkin, A. L., and Keynes, R. D. 1957. Movements of labelled calcium in squid giant axons. *Journal of Physiology* 138:253–281.

Horisberger, J.-D., Lemas, V., Kraehenbühl, J.-P., and Rossier, B. C. 1991. Structure-function relationship of Na,K-ATPase. *Annual Review of Physiology* 53:565–584.

Inesi, G., and Kirtley, M. R. 1992. Structural features of cation transport ATPases. *Journal of Bioenergetics and Biomembranes* 24:271–283.

Kaila, K., Saarikoski, J., and Voipio, J. 1990. Mechanism of action of GABA on intracellular pH and on surface pH in crayfish muscle fibers. *Journal of Physiology* 427:241–260.

Kawamura, M., and Noguchi, S. 1991. Possible role of the β-subunit in the expression of the sodium pump. In *The Sodium Pump: Structure, Mechanism, and Regulation*, ed. J. H. Kaplan and P. De Weer, pp. 46–61. New York: Rockefeller University Press.

Keynes, R. D. 1963. Chloride in the squid giant axon. *Journal of Physiology* 169:690–705.

Kirtley, M. E., Sumbilla, C., and Inesi, G. 1990. Mechanisms of calcium uptake and release by sarcoplasmic reticulum. In *Intracellular Calcium Regulation*, ed. F. Bronner, pp. 249–270. New York: Wiley-Liss.

Koike, H., Brown, H. M., and Hagiwara, S. 1971. Hyperpolarization of a barnacle photoreceptor membrane following illumination. *Journal of General Physiology* 57:723–737.

Läuger, P. 1991. *Electrogenic Ion Pumps*. Sunderland, MA: Sinauer.

Lingrel, J. B. 1992. Na,K-ATPase: Isoform structure, function, and expression. *Journal of Bioenergetics and Biomembranes* 24:263–270.

Lingrel, J. B., and Kuntzweiler, T. 1994. Minireview: Na$^+$,K$^+$-ATPase. *Journal of Biological Chemistry* 269:19659–19662.

Maunsbach, A. B., Skriver, E., and Hebert, H. 1991. Two-dimensional crystals and three-dimensional structure of Na,K-ATPase analyzed by electron microscopy. In *The Sodium Pump: Structure, Mechanism, and Regulation*, ed. J. H. Kaplan and P. De Weer, pp. 159–172. New York: Rockefeller University Press.

McGrail, K. M., Phillips, J. M., and Sweadner, K. J. 1991. Immunofluorescent localization of three Na,K-ATPase isozymes in the rat central nervous system: Both neurons and glia can express more than one Na,K-ATPase. *Journal of Neuroscience* 11:381–391.

McGrail, K. M., and Sweadner, K. J. 1989. Complex expression patterns for Na,K-ATPase isoforms in retina and optic nerve. *European Journal of Neuroscience* 2:170–176.

Mercer, R. W. 1993. Structure of the Na,K-ATPase. *International Review of Cytology* 137C:139–168.

Mohraz, M., Arystarkhova, E., and Sweadner, K. J. 1994. Immunoelectron microscopy of epitopes on Na,K-ATPase catalytic subunit. *Journal of Biological Chemistry* 269:2929–2936.

Moody, W. J., Jr. 1981. The ionic mechanism of intracellular pH regulation in crayfish neurones. *Journal of Physiology* 316:293–308.

——— 1984. Effects of intracellular H^+ on the electrical properties of excitable cells. *Annual Review of Neuroscience* 7:257–278.

Neher, E., and Augustine, G. J. 1992. Calcium gradients and buffers in bovine chromaffin cells. *Journal of Physiology* 450:273–301.

Nicoll, D. A., Longoni, S., and Philipson, K. D. 1990. Molecular cloning and functional expression of the cardiac sarcolemmal Na^+-Ca^{2+} exchanger. *Science* 250:562–565.

Petersen, O. H., Petersen, C. C. H., and Kasai, H. 1994. Calcium and hormone action. *Annual Review of Physiology* 56:297–319.

Philipson, K. D., and Nicoll, D. A. 1993. Molecular and kinetic aspects of sodium-calcium exchange. *International Review of Cytology* 137C:199–227.

Post, R. L., and Jolly, D. C. 1957. The linkage of sodium, potassium, and ammonium active transport across the human erythrocyte membrane. *Biochimica et Biophysica Acta* 25:118–128.

Pozzan, T., Rizzuto, R., Volpe, P., and Meldolesi, J. 1994. Molecular and cellular physiology of intracellular calcium stores. *Physiological Reviews* 74:595–636.

Rakowski, R. F. 1991. Stoichiometry and voltage dependence of the Na^+/K^+ pump in squid giant axons and *Xenopus* oocytes. In *The Sodium Pump: Structure, Mechanism, and Regulation,* ed. J. H. Kaplan and P. De Weer, pp. 339–353. New York: Rockefeller University Press.

Requena, J., Whittembury, J., Scarpa, A., Brinley, J. F., Jr., and Mullins, L. J. 1991. Intracellular ionized calcium changes in squid giant axons monitored by fura-2 and aequorin. *Annals of the New York Academy of Sciences* 639:112–125.

Reeves, J. P., Condrescu, M., Chernaya, G., and Gardner, J. P. 1994. Na^+/Ca^{2+} antiport in the mammalian heart. *Journal of Experimental Biology* 196:375–388.

Reuss, L., Russell, J. M., Jr., and Jennings, M. L. (eds.). 1993. *Molecular Biology and Function of Carrier Proteins.* Society of General Physiologists, 46th Annual Symposium. New York: Rockefeller University Press.

Russell, J. M. 1984. Chloride in the squid axon. *Current Topics in Membranes and Transport* 22:177–193.

Russell, J. M., and Boron, W. F. 1990. Chloride transport in squid giant axon.

In *Chloride Channels and Carriers in Nerve, Muscle, and Glial Cells,* ed. F. J. Alvarez-Leefmans and J. M. Russell, pp. 85–107. New York: Plenum Press.

Sachs, J. R. 1991. Successes and failures of the Albers-Post model in predicting ion flux kinetics. In *The Sodium Pump: Structure, Mechanism, and Regulation,* ed. J. H. Kaplan and P. De Weer, pp. 249–266. New York: Rockefeller University Press.

Schlue, W. R., and Thomas, R. C. 1985. A dual mechanism for intracellular pH regulation by leech neurons. *Journal of Physiology* 364:327–338.

Schwiening, C. J., and Boron, W. F. 1994. Regulation of intracellular pH in pyramidal neurons from the rat hippocampus by Na$^+$-dependent Cl$^-$-HCO$_3^-$ exchange. *Journal of Physiology* 475:59–67.

Schwiening, C. J., Kennedy, H. J., and Thomas, R. C. 1993. Calcium-hydrogen exchange by the plasma membrane Ca-ATPase of voltage-clamped snail neurons. *Proceedings of the Royal Society of London B* 253:285–289.

Sweadner, K. J. 1991. Overview: Subunit diversity in the Na,K-ATPase. In *The Sodium Pump: Structure, Mechanism, and Regulation,* ed. J. H. Kaplan and P. De Weer, pp. 63–76. New York: Rockefeller University Press.

——— 1995. Na,K-ATPase and its isoforms. In *Neuroglia,* ed. H. Kettenmann and B. R. Ransom, pp. 259–272. Oxford: Oxford University Press.

Thomas, R. C. 1969. Membrane current and intracellular sodium changes in a snail neurone during extrusion of injected sodium. *Journal of Physiology* 201:495–514.

——— 1972. Electrogenic sodium pump in nerve and muscle cells. *Physiological Reviews* 52:563–594.

——— 1977. The role of bicarbonate, chloride and sodium ions in the regulation of intracellular pH in snail neurons. *Journal of Physiology* 273:317–338.

——— 1982. Electrophysiology of the sodium pump in a snail neuron. *Current Topics in Membranes and Transport* 16:3–16.

Tse, M., Levine, S., Yun, C., Brant, S., Counillon, L. T., Pouysségur, J., and Donowitz, M. 1993. Structure/function studies of the epithelial isoforms of the mammalian Na$^+$/H$^+$ exchanger gene family. *Journal of Membrane Biology* 135:93–108.

Tse, A., Tse, F. W., and Hille, B. 1994. Calcium homeostasis in identified rat gonadotrophs. *Journal of Physiology* 477:511–525.

Weinman, E. J., and Shenolikar, S. 1993. Regulation of the renal brush border membrane Na$^+$-H$^+$ exchanger. *Annual Review of Physiology* 55:289–304.

Wright, E. M. 1978. Transport processes in the formation of the cerebrospinal fluid. *Reviews of Physiology, Biochemistry and Pharmacology* 83:1–34.

Wuytack, F., and Raeymaekers, L. 1992. The Ca^{2+}-transport ATPases from the plasma membrane. *Journal of Bioenergetics and Biomembranes* 3:285–300.

Zeuthen, T. 1994. Cotransport of K^+, Cl^- and H_2O by membrane proteins from choroid plexus epithelium of *Necturus maculosus*. *Journal of Physiology* 478:203–219.

5. Action Potentials: The Hodgkin-Huxley Experiments

Armstrong, C. M. 1975. Potassium pores of nerve and muscle membranes. In *Membranes—A Series of Advances,* Vol. 3: *Lipid Bilayers and Biological Membranes: Dynamic Properties,* ed. G. Eisenman, pp. 325–358. New York: Marcel Dekker.

Armstrong, C. M., and Binstock, L. 1965. Anomalous rectification in the squid giant axon injected with tetraethylammonium chloride. *Journal of General Physiology* 48:859–872.

Bernstein, J. 1902. Untersuchungen zur Thermodynamik der bioelektrischen Ströme. Erster Teil. *Pflügers Archiv* 92:521–562.

Bernstein, J. 1912. *Elektrobiologie.* Braunschweig: Viewig.

Chandler, W. K., and Meeves, H. 1965. Voltage clamp experiments on internally perfused giant axons. *Journal of Physiology* 180:788–820.

Cole, K. S. 1949. Dynamic electrical characteristics of the squid axon membrane. *Archives des Sciences Physiologiques* 3:253–258.

Curtis, H. J., and Cole, K. S. 1942. Membrane resting and action potentials from the squid giant axon. *Journal of Cellular and Comparative Physiology* 19:135–144.

Hille, B. 1967. The selective inhibition of delayed potassium currents in nerve by tetraethylammonium ion. *Journal of General Physiology* 50:1287–1302.

Hille, B. 1970. Ionic channels in nerve membranes. *Progress in Biophysical and Molecular Biology* 21:3–32.

Hille, B. 1975. Ionic selectivity of Na and K channels of nerve membranes. In *Membranes—A Series of Advances,* Vol. 3: *Lipid Bilayers and Biological Membranes: Dynamic Properties,* ed. G. Eisenman, pp. 255–323. New York: Marcel Dekker.

Hille, B. 1992. *Ionic Channels of Excitable Membranes.* Sunderland, MA: Sinauer Associates.

Hodgkin, A. L. 1964. *The Conduction of the Nervous Impulse: The Sherrington Lectures, VII.* Liverpool: Liverpool University Press.

Hodgkin, A. L. 1976. Chance and design in electrophysiology: An informal account of certain experiments on nerve carried out between 1934 and 1952. *Journal of Physiology* 263:1–21.

Hodgkin, A. L., and Huxley, A. F. 1939. Action potentials recorded from inside a nerve fibre. *Nature* 144:710–711.

—— 1945. Resting and action potentials in single nerve fibers. *Journal of Physiology* 104:176–195.

—— 1952a. Currents carried by sodium and potassium ions through the membrane of the giant axon of *Loligo*. *Journal of Physiology* 116:449–472.

—— 1952b. The components of membrane conductance in the giant axon of *Loligo*. *Journal of Physiology* 116:473–496.

—— 1952c. The dual effect of membrane potential on sodium conductance in the giant axon of *Loligo*. *Journal of Physiology* 116:497–506.

—— 1952d. A quantitative description of membrane current and its application to conduction and excitation in nerve. *Journal of Physiology* 117:500–544.

Hodgkin, A. L., Huxley, A. F., and Katz, B. 1952. Measurement of current-voltage relations in the membrane of the giant axon of *Loligo*. *Journal of Physiology* 116:424–448.

Hodgkin, A. L., and Katz, B. 1949. The effect of sodium ions on the electrical activity of the giant axon of the squid. *Journal of Physiology* 108:37–77.

Keynes, R. D. 1963. Chloride in the squid giant axon. *Journal of Physiology* 169:690–705.

Latorre, R., and Miller, C. 1983. Conduction and selectivity in potassium channels. *Journal of Membrane Biology* 71:11–30.

MacKinnon, R., and Yellen, G. 1990. Mutations affecting TEA blockade and ion permeation in voltage-activated K^+ channels. *Science* 250:276–279.

Marmont, G. 1949. Studies on the axon membrane. I. A new method. *Journal of Cellular and Comparative Physiology* 34:351–382.

Overton, E. 1902. Beiträge zur allgemeinen Muskel- und Nervenphysiologie. II. Über die Unentbehrlichkeit von Natrium- (oder Lithium-) Ionen für den Contractsionsact des Muskels. *Pflügers Archiv* 92:346–386.

Young, J. Z. 1936. Structure of nerve fibres and synapses in some invertebrates. *Cold Spring Harbor Symposium on Quantitative Biology* 4:1–6.

6. *The Structure and Function of Voltage-Gated Channels*

Adelman, J. P. 1995. Proteins that interact with the pore-forming subunits of voltage-gated ion channels. *Current Opinion in Neurobiology* 5:286–295.

Aggarwal, S. K., and MacKinnon, R. 1996. Contribution of the S4 segment to gating charge in the *Shaker* K^+ channel. *Neuron* 16:1169–1177.

Aldrich, R. W., Corey, D. P., and Stevens, C. F. 1983. A reinterpretation of mammalian sodium channel gating based on single channel recording. *Nature* 306:436–441.

Armstrong, C. M. 1975. Potassium pores of nerve and muscle membranes. In *Membranes—A Series of Advances,* Vol. 3: *Lipid Bilayers and Biological Membranes: Dynamic Properties,* ed. G. Eisenman, pp. 325–358. New York: Marcel Dekker.

Armstrong, C. M., and Bezanilla, F. 1973. Currents related to movement of the gating particles of the sodium channels. *Nature* 242:459–461.

——— 1974. Charge movement associated with the opening and closing of the activation gates of the Na channels. *Journal of General Physiology* 63:533–552.

——— 1977. Inactivation of the sodium channel. II. Gating current experiments. *Journal of General Physiology* 70:567–590.

Armstrong, C. M., Bezanilla, F., and Rojas, E. 1973. Destruction of sodium conductance inactivation in squid axons perfused with pronase. *Journal of General Physiology* 62:375–391.

Baker, P. F., Hodgkin, A. L., and Shaw, T. I. 1962. Replacement of the axoplasm of giant nerve fibres with artificial solutions. *Journal of Physiology* 164:330–354.

Bezanilla, F., and Armstrong, C. M. 1977. Inactivation of the sodium channel. I. Sodium current experiments. *Journal of General Physiology* 70:549–566.

Bezanilla, F., Perozo, E., Papazian, D. M., and Stefani, E. 1991. Molecular basis of gating charge immobilization in *Shaker* potassium channels. *Science* 254:679–683.

Bezanilla, F., and Stefani, E. 1994. Voltage-dependent gating of ionic channels. *Annual Review of Biophysics and Biomolecular Structure* 23:819–846.

Brown, A. M. 1993. Functional bases for interpreting amino acid sequences of voltage-dependent K^+ channels. *Annual Review of Biophysics and Biomolecular Structure* 22:173–198.

Catterall, W. A. 1992. Cellular and molecular biology of voltage-gated sodium channels. *Physiological Reviews* 72:S15–S48.

Chandy, K. G., and Gutman, G. A. 1995. Voltage-gated potassium channel genes. In *Ligand- and Voltage-Gated Ion Channels,* ed. R. A. North, pp. 1–71. Boca Raton, FL: CRC Press.

Choi, K. L., Mossman, C., Aubé, J., and Yellen, G. 1993. The internal quaternary ammonium receptor site of *Shaker* potassium channels. *Neuron* 10:533–541.

Cole, K. S., and Moore, J. W. 1960. Potassium ion current in the squid giant axon: Dynamic characteristic. *Biophysical Journal* 1:1–14.

Demo, S. D., and Yellen, G. 1991. The inactivation gate of the *Shaker* K^+ channel behaves like an open-channel blocker. *Neuron* 7:743–753.

Goldin, A. L. 1995. Voltage-gated sodium channels. In *Ligand- and Voltage-Gated Ion Channels,* ed. R. A. North, pp. 73–111. Boca Raton, FL: CRC Press.

Goldman, L. 1976. Kinetics of channel gating in excitable membranes. *Quarterly Reviews of Biophysics* 9:491–526.

Hartmann, H. A., Kirsch, G. E., Drewe, J. A., Taglialatela, M., Joho, R. H., and Brown, A. M. 1991. Exchange of conduction pathways between two related K^+ channels. *Science* 251:942–944.

Heinemann, S. H., and Conti, F. 1992. Nonstationary noise analysis and application to patch clamp recordings. *Methods in Enzymology* 207:131–148.

Hille, B. 1989. Ionic channels: Evolutionary origins and modern roles. *Quarterly Journal of Experimental Physiology* 74:785–804.

Hirschberg, B., Rovner, A., Lieberman, M., and Patlak, J. 1995. Transfer of twelve charges is needed to open skeletal muscle Na^+ channels. *Journal of General Physiology* 106:1053–1068.

Honig, B. H., Hubbell, W. L., and Flewelling, R. F. 1986. Electrical interactions in membranes and proteins. *Annual Review of Biophysics and Biophysical Chemistry* 15:163–193.

Horn, R., and Vandenberg, C. A. 1984. Statistical properties of single sodium channels. *Journal of General Physiology* 84:505–534.

Hoshi, T., and Zagotta, W. N. 1993. Recent advances in the understanding of potassium channel function. *Current Opinion in Neurobiology* 3:283–290.

Hoshi, T., Zagotta, W. N., and Aldrich, R. W. 1990. Biophysical and molecular mechanisms of *Shaker* potassium channel inactivation. *Science* 250:533–538.

Isom, L. L., DeJongh, K. S., and Catterall, W. A. 1994. Auxiliary subunits of voltage-gated ion channels. *Neuron* 12:1183–1194.

Jan, L. Y., and Jan, Y. N. 1990. A superfamily of ion channels. *Nature* 345:672.

——— 1992. Structural elements involved in specific K^+ channel functions. *Annual Review of Physiology* 54:537–555.

——— 1994. Potassium channels and their evolving gates. *Nature* 371:119–122.

——— 1997. Cloned potassium channels from eukaryotes and prokaryotes. *Annual Review of Neuroscience* 20:91–123.

Kallen, R. G., Cohen, S. A., and Barchi, R. L. 1994. Structure, function and expression of voltage-dependent sodium channels. *Molecular Neurobiology* 7:383–428.

Kavanaugh, M. P., Varnum, M. D., Osborne, P. B., Christie, M. J., Busch, A. E., Adelman, J. P., and North, R. A. 1991. Interaction between tetraethylammonium and amino acid residues in the pore of cloned voltage-dependent potassium channels. *Journal of Biological Chemistry* 266:7583–7587.

Kellenberger, S., West, J. W., Scheuer, T., and Catterall, W. A. 1997. Molecular analysis of the putative inactivation particle in the inactivation gate of brain type IIA Na⁺ channels. *Journal of General Physiology* 109:589–605.

Keynes, R. D., and Rojas, R. 1974. Kinetics and steady-state properties of the charged system controlling sodium conductance in the squid giant axon. *Journal of Physiology* 239:393–434.

Kontis, K. J., and Goldin, A. L. 1993. Site-directed mutagenesis of the putative pore region of the rat IIA sodium channel. *Molecular Pharmacology* 43:635–644.

Kukuljan, M., Labarca, P., and Latorre, R. 1995. Molecular determinants of ion conduction and inactivation in K⁺ channels. *American Journal of Physiology* 268:C535–556.

Larsson, H. P., Baker, O. S., Dhillon, D. S., and Isacoff, E. Y. 1996. Transmembrane movement of the *Shaker* K⁺ channel S4. *Neuron* 16:387–397.

Latorre, R., and Miller, C. 1983. Conduction and selectivity in potassium channels. *Journal of Membrane Biology* 71:11–30.

Lopez, G. A., Jan, Y. N., and Jan, L. Y. 1994. Evidence that the S6 segment of the *Shaker* voltage-gated K⁺ channel comprises part of the pore. *Nature* 367:179–182.

MacKinnon, R. 1991. Determination of the subunit stoichiometry of a voltage-activated potassium channel. *Nature* 350:232–235.

MacKinnon, R., Aldrich, R. W., and Lee, A. W. 1993. Functional stoichiometry of Shaker potassium channel inactivation. *Science* 262:757–759.

MacKinnon, R., and Yellen, G. 1990. Mutations affecting TEA blockade and ion permeation in voltage-activated K⁺ channels. *Science* 250:276–279.

Mannuzzu, L. M., Moronne, M. M., and Isacoff, E. Y. 1996. Direct physical measure of conformational rearrangement underlying potassium channel gating. *Science* 271:213–216.

Neher, E., and Stevens, C. F. 1977. Conductance fluctuations and ionic pores in membranes. *Annual Review of Biophysics and Bioengineering* 6:345–381.

Noda, M., Shimizu, S., Tanabe, T., Takai, T., Kayano, T., Ikeda, T., Takahashi, H., Nakayama, H., Kanaoka, Y., Minamino, N., Kangawa, K., Matsuo, H., Raftery, M. A., Hirose, T., Inayama, S., Hayashida, H., Miyata, T., and Numa, S. 1984. Primary structure of *Electrophorus electricus* sodium channel deduced from cDNA sequence. *Nature* 312:121–127.

Noda, M., Suzuki, H., Numa, S., and Stühmer, W. 1989. A single point mutation confers tetrodotoxin and saxitoxin insensitivity on the sodium channel II. *FEBS Letters* 259:213–216.

Papazian, D. M., and Bezanilla, F. 1997. How does an ion channel sense voltage? *News in Physiological Sciences* 12:203–210.

Papazian, D. M., Schwarz, T. L., Tempel, B. L., Jan, Y. N., and Jan, L. Y. 1987. Cloning of genomic and complementary DNA from *Shaker*, a putative potassium channel gene from *Drosophila*. *Science* 237:749–753.

Papazian, D. M., Timpe, L. C., Jan, Y. N., and Jan, L. Y. 1991. Alteration of voltage-dependence of *Shaker* potassium channel by mutations in the S4 sequence. *Nature* 349:305–310.

Perozo, E., MacKinnon, R., Bezanilla, F., and Stefani, E. 1993. Gating currents from a nonconducting mutant reveal open-closed conformations in *Shaker* K$^+$ channels. *Neuron* 11:353–358.

Pongs, O. 1992. Molecular biology of voltage-dependent potassium channels. *Physiological Review* 72:S69–S88.

———— 1993. Shaker-related K$^+$ channels. *Seminars in Neuroscience* 54:93–100.

Rettig, J., Heinemann, S. H., Wunder, F., Lorra, C., Parcej, D. N., Dolly, J. O., and Pongs, O. 1994. Inactivation properties of voltage-gated K+ channels altered by presence of beta-subunit. *Nature* 369:289–94.

Satin, J., Kyle, J. W., Chen, M., Bell, P., Cribbs, L. L., Fozzard, H. A., and Rogart, R. B. 1992. A mutant of TTX-resistant cardiac sodium channels with TTX-sensitive properties. *Science* 256:1202–1205.

Schoppa, N. E., McCormack, K., Tanouye, M. A., and Sigworth, F. J. 1992. The size of gating charge in wild-type and mutant *Shaker* potassium channels. *Science* 255:1712–1715.

Seoh, S.-A., Sigg, D., Papazian, D. M., and Bezanilla, F. 1996. Voltage-sensing residues in the S2 and S4 segments of the *Shaker* K$^+$ channel. *Neuron* 16:1159–1167.

Sigworth, F. J. 1980. The variance of sodium current fluctuations at the node of Ranvier. *Journal of Physiology* 307:97–129.

———— 1993. Voltage gating of ion channels. *Quarterly Review of Biophysics* 27:1–40.

———— 1995. Charge movement in the sodium channel. *Journal of General Physiology* 106:1047–1051.

Sigworth, F. J., and Neher, E. 1980. Single Na$^+$ channel currents observed in cultured rat muscle cells. *Nature* 287:447–449.

Slesinger, P. A., Jan, Y. N., and Jan, L. Y. 1993. The S4-S5 loop contributes to the ion-selective pore of potassium channels. *Neuron* 11:739–749.

Stryer, L. 1995. *Biochemistry,* 4th ed. New York: W. H. Freeman.

Stühmer, W. 1991. Structure-function studies of voltage-gated ion channels. *Annual Review of Biophysics and Biophysical Chemistry* 20:65–78.

Stühmer, W., Conti, F., Suzuki, H., Wang, X., Noda, M., Yahogi, N., Kubo, H., and Numa, S. 1989. Structural parts involved in activation and inactivation of the sodium channel. *Nature* 339:597–603.

Taglialatela, M., Toro, L., and Stefani, E. 1992. Novel voltage clamp to record small, fast currents from ion channels expressed in *Xenopus* oocytes. *Biophysical Journal* 61:78–82.

Tasaki, I., Watanabe, A., and Takenaka, T. 1962. Resting and action potential of intracellularly perfused squid giant axon. *Proceedings of the National Academy of Sciences USA* 57:1350–1354.

Tempel, B. L., Papazian, D. M., Schwarz, T. L., Jan, Y. N., and Jan, L. Y. 1987. Sequence of a probable potassium channel component encoded at *Shaker* locus of *Drosophila*. *Science* 237:770–775.

Terlau, H., Heinemann, S. H., Stühmer, W., Pusch, M., Conti, F., Imoto, K., and Numa, S. 1991. Mapping the site of block by tetrodotoxin and saxitoxin of sodium channel II. *FEBS Letters* 293:93–96.

Vandenberg, C. A., and Bezanilla, F. 1991. A sodium channel gating model based on single channel, macroscopic ionic, and gating currents in the squid giant axon. *Biophysical Journal* 60:1511–1533.

Vassilev, P. M., Scheuer, T., and Catterall, W. A. 1988. Identification of an intracellular peptide segment involved in sodium channel inactivation. *Science* 241:1658–1661.

Watson, J. D., Gilman, M., Witkowski, J., and Zoller, M. 1992. *Recombinant DNA*, 2d ed. New York: W. H. Freeman.

West, J. W., Patton, D. E., Scheuer, T., Wang, Y., Goldin, A. L., and Catterall, W. A. 1992. A cluster of hydrophobic amino acid residues required for fast Na^+-channel inactivation. *Proceedings of the National Academy of Sciences USA* 89:10910–10914.

Yang, N., George, A. L., Jr., and Horn, R. 1996. Molecular basis of charge movement in voltage-gated sodium channels. *Neuron* 16:113–122.

Yang, N., and Horn, R. 1995. Evidence for voltage-dependent S4 movement in sodium channels. *Neuron* 15:213–218.

Yau, K.-W., and Chen, T.-Y. 1995. Cyclic nucleotide-gated channels. In *Ligand- and Voltage-Gated Ion Channels*, ed. R. A. North, pp. 307–335. Boca Raton, FL: CRC Press.

Yellen, G., Jurman, M. E., Abramson, T., and MacKinnon, R. 1991. Mutations affecting internal TEA blockade identify the probable pore-forming region of a K^+ channel. *Science* 251:939–942.

Zagotta, W. N., and Aldrich, R. W. 1990. Voltage-dependent gating of *Shaker* A-type potassium channels in *Drosophila* muscle. *Journal of General Physiology* 95:29–60.

Zagotta, W. N., Hoshi, T., and Aldrich, R. W. 1989. Gating of single Shaker potassium channels in *Drosophila* muscle and in *Xenopus* oocytes injected with Shaker mRNA. *Proceedings of the National Academy of Sciences USA* 86:7243–7247.

——— 1990. Restoration of inactivation in mutants of *Shaker* potassium channels by a peptide derived from ShB. *Science* 250:568–571.

7. The Diversity of Voltage-Gated Channels

Adelman, J. P., Shen, K.-Z., Kavanaugh, M. P., Warren, R. A., Wu, Y.-N., Lagrutta, A., Bond, C. T., and North, R. A. 1992. Calcium-activated potassium channels expressed from cloned complementary DNAs. *Neuron* 9:209–216.

Adrian, R. H. 1969. Rectification in muscle membrane. *Progress in Biophysics and Molecular Biology* 19:341–369.

Akopian, A. N., Sivilotti, L., and Wood, J. N. 1996. A tetrodotoxin-resistant voltage-gated sodium channel expressed by sensory neurons. *Nature* 379:257–262.

Aldrich, R. W., Corey, D. P., and Stevens, C. F. 1983. A reinterpretation of mammalian sodium channel gating based on single channel recording. *Nature* 306:436–441.

Almers, W., and McCleskey, E. W. 1984. Non-selective conductance in calcium channels of frog muscle: Calcium selectivity in a single-file pore. *Journal of Physiology* 353:585–608.

Almers, W., McCleskey, E. W., and Palade, P. T. 1984. A non-selective cation conductance in frog muscle membrane blocked by micromolar external calcium ions. *Journal of Physiology* 353:565–583.

Armstrong, C. M. 1975. Potassium pores of nerve and muscle membranes. In *Membranes—A Series of Advances,* Vol. 3: *Lipid Bilayers and Biological Membranes: Dynamic Properties,* ed. G. Eisenman, pp. 325–358. New York: Marcel Dekker.

Ashcroft, F. M. 1988. Adenosine 5′-triphosphate-sensitive potassium channels. *Annual Review of Neurosience* 11:97–118.

Ashford, M. L. J., Bond, C. T., Blair, T. A., and Adelman, J. P. 1994. Cloning and functional expression of a rat heart K_{ATP} channel. *Nature* 370:456–459.

Atkinson, N. S., Robertson, G. A., and Ganetzky, B. 1991. A component of calcium-activated potassium channels encoded by the *Drosophila slo* locus. *Science* 253:551–555.

Babenko, A. P., Aguilar-Bryan, L., and Bryan, J. 1998. A view of SUR/K_{IR}6X, K_{ATP} channels. *Annual Review of Physiology* 60:667–687.

Bader, C. R., Bernheim, L., and Bertrand, D. 1985. Sodium-activated potassium current in cultured avian neurones. *Nature* 317:540–542.

Bader, C. R., Bertrand, D., and Schwartz, E. A. 1982. Voltage-activated and calcium-activated currents in solitary rod inner segments from the salamander retina. *Journal of Physiology* 331:253–284.

Barres, B. A., Chun, L. L. Y., and Corey, D. P. 1989. Glial and neuronal forms of the voltage-dependent sodium channel: Characteristics and cell-type distribution. *Neuron* 2:1375–1388.

Barrett, E. F., and Barrett, J. N. 1976. Separation of two voltage-sensitive potassium currents, and demonstration of a tetrodotoxin-resistant calcium current in frog motoneurones. *Journal of Physiology* 255:737–774.

Barrett, J. N., Magleby, K. L., and Pallotta, B. S. 1982. Properties of single calcium-activated potassium channels in cultured rat muscle. *Journal of Physiology* 331:211–230.

Bean, B. P. 1989. Classes of calcium channels in vertebrate cells. *Annual Review of Physiology* 51:367–384.

Bean, B. P., and Mintz, I. M. 1994. Pharmacology of different types of calcium channels in rat neurons. In *Handbook of Membrane Channels,* ed. C. Peracchia, pp. 199–210. San Diego, CA: Academic Press.

Bezanilla, F., and Correa, A. M. 1995. Single-channel properties and gating of Na^+ and K^+ channels in the squid giant axon. In *Cephalopod Neurobiology,* ed. N. J. Abbott, R. Williamson, and L. Maddock, pp. 131–151. New York: Oxford University Press.

Blatz, A. L. 1990. Chloride channels in skeletal muscle. In *Chloride Channels and Carriers in Nerve, Muscle, and Glial Cells,* ed. F. J. Alvarez-Leefmans and J. M. Russell, pp. 407–420. New York: Plenum.

——— 1994. Chloride channels in skeletal muscle and cerebral cortical neurons. *Current Topics in Membranes* 42:131–151.

Blatz, A. L., and Magleby, K. L. 1987. Calcium-activated potassium channels. *Trends in Neurosciences* 10:463–467.

Brehm, P., and Eckert, R. 1978. Calcium entry leads to inactivation of calcium channel in *Paramecium. Science* 202:1203–1206.

Brüggemann, A., Pardo, L. A., Stühmer, W., and Pongs, O. 1993. *Ether-à-gogo* encodes a voltage-gated channel permeable to K^+ and Ca^{2+} and modulated by cAMP. *Nature* 365:445–448.

Burgess, D. L., Jones, J. M., Meisler, M. H., and Noebels, J. L. 1997. Mutation of the Ca^{2+} channel β subunit gene *Cchb4* is associated with ataxia and seizures in the lethargic (*lh*) mouse. *Cell* 88:385–392.

Butler, A., Tsunoda, S., McCobb, D. P., Wei, A., and Salkoff, L. 1993. *mSlo,* a complex mouse gene encoding "Maxi" calcium-activated potassium channels. *Science* 261:221–224.

Catterall, W. A., Seagar, M. J., and Takahashi, M. 1988. Molecular properties of dihydropyridine-sensitive calcium channels in skeletal muscle: Minireview. *Journal of Biological Chemistry* 263:3535–3538.

Chabala, L. D. 1984. The kinetics of recovery and development of potassium channel inactivation in perfused squid *(Loligo pealei)* giant axons. *Journal of Physiology* 356:193–220.

Chandy, K. G., and Gutman, G. A. 1995. Voltage-gated potassium channel genes. In *Ligand- and Voltage-Gated Ion Channels,* ed. R. A. North, pp. 1–71. Boca Raton, FL: CRC Press.

Chesnoy-Marchais, D. 1990. Hyperpolarization-activated chloride channels in *Aplysia* neurons. In *Chloride Channels and Carriers in Nerve, Muscle, and Glial Cells,* ed. F. J. Alvarez-Leefmans and J. M. Russell, pp. 367–382. New York: Plenum.

Christie, M. J., North, R. A., Osborne, P. B., Douglass, J., and Adelman, J. P. 1990. Heteropolymeric potassium channels expressed in *Xenopus* oocytes from cloned subunits. *Neuron* 4:405–411.

Conner, J. A., and Stevens, C. F. 1971a. Inward and delayed outward membrane currents in isolated neural somata under voltage clamp. *Journal of Physiology* 213:1–19.

——— 1971b. Voltage clamp studies of a transient outward membrane current in gastropod neural somata. *Journal of Physiology* 213:21–30.

——— 1971c. Prediction of repetitive firing behaviour from voltage clamp data on an isolated neurone soma. *Journal of Physiology* 213:31–53.

Crill, W. E. 1996. Persistent sodium current in mammalian central neurons. *Annual Review of Physiology* 58:349–362.

Dascal, N., Schreibmayer, W., Lim, N. F., Wang, W., Chavkin, C., DiMagno, L., Labarca, C., Kieffer, B. L., Gaveriaux-Ruff, C., Trollinger, D., Lester, H. A., and Davidson, N. 1993. Atrial G protein-activated K^+ channel: Expression cloning and molecular properties. *Proceedings of the National Academy of Sciences USA* 90:10235–10239.

Debanne, D., Guérineau, N. C., Gähwiler, B. H., and Thompson, S. M. 1997. Action-potential propagation gated by an axonal I_A-like K^+ conductance in hippocampus. *Nature* 389:286–289.

DeCoursey, T. E., and Cherny, V. V. 1994. Voltage-activated hydrogen ion currents. *Journal of Membrane Biology* 141:203–223.

deLeon, M., Wang, Y., Jones, L., Perez-Reyes, E., Wei, X., Soong, T. W., Snutch, T. P., and Yue, D. T. 1995. Essential Ca^{2+}-binding motif for Ca^{2+}-sensitive inactivation of L-type Ca^{2+} channels. *Science* 270:1502–1506.

De Schutter, E. 1986. Alternative equations for the molluscan ion currents described by Conner and Stevens. *Brain Research* 382:134–138.

DiFrancesco, D. 1994. Hyperpolarization-activated *(i$_f$)* current in heart. In *Handbook of Membrane Channels,* ed. C. Peracchia, pp. 335–343. San Diego, CA: Academic Press.

Doupnik, C. A., Davidson, N., and Lester, H. A. 1995. The inward rectifier potassium channel family. *Current Opinion in Neurobiology* 5:268–277.

Doyle, D. A., Cabral, J. M., Pfuetzner, R. A., Kuo, A., Gulbis, J. M., Cohen, S. L., Chait, B. T., and MacKinnon, R. 1998. The structure of the potassium channel: Molecular basis of K^+ conduction and selectivity. *Science* 280:69–77.

Dunlap, K., Luebke, J. I., and Turner, T. J. 1995. Exocytotic Ca^{2+} channels in mammalian central neurons. *Trends in Neurosciences* 18:89–98.

Eckert, R., and Chad, J. E. 1984. The inactivation of Ca channels. *Progress in Biophysics and Molecular Biology* 44:215–267.

Eckert, R., and Tillotson, D. L. 1981. Calcium-mediated inactivation of the calcium conductance in caesium-loaded giant neurones of *Aplysia californica*. *Journal of Physiology* 314:265–280.

Eliasof, S. D., and Werblin, F. S. 1993. Characterization of the glutamate transporter in retinal cones of the tiger salamander. *Journal of Neuroscience* 13:402–411.

Ellinor, P. T., Zhang, J.-F., Randall, A. D., Zhou, M., Schwarz, T. L., Tsien, R. W., and Horne, W. A. 1993. Functional expression of a rapidly inactivating neuronal calcium channel. *Nature* 363:455–458.

Elliott, A. A., and Elliott, J. R. 1993. Characterization of TTX-sensitive and TTX-resistant sodium currents in small cells from adult rat dorsal root ganglia. *Journal of Physiology* 463:39–56.

Fain, G. L., Gerschenfeld, H. M., and Quandt, F. N. 1980. Calcium spikes in toad rods. *Journal of Physiology* 303:495–513.

Fairman, W. A., Vandenberg, R. J., Arriza, J. L., Kavanaugh, M. P., and Amara, S. G. 1995. An excitatory amino-acid transporter with properties of a ligand-gated chloride channel. *Nature* 375:599–603.

Fakler, B., Brändle, U., Bond, C., Glowatzki, E., Koenig, C., Adelman, J. P., Zenner, H.-P., and Ruppersberg, J. P. 1994. A structural determinant of differential sensitivity of cloned inward rectifier K^+ channels to intracellular spermine. *FEBS Letters* 356:199–203.

Fakler, B., Brändle, U., Glowatzki, E., Zenner, H.-P., and Ruppersberg, J. P. 1994. $K_{ir}2.1$ inward rectifier K^+ channels are regulated independently by protein kinases and ATP hydrolysis. *Neuron* 13:1413–1420.

Fatt, P., and Ginsborg, B. L. 1958. The ionic requirements for the production of action potentials in crustacean muscle fibres. *Journal of Physiology* 142:516–543.

Fatt, P., and Katz, B. 1953. The electrical properties of crustacean muscle fibres. *Journal of Physiology* 120:171–204.

Ficker, E., and Heinemann, U. 1992. Slow and fast transient potassium currents in cultured rat hippocampal cells. *Journal of Physiology* 445:431–455.

Ficker, E., Taglialatela, M., Wible, B. A., Henley, C. M., and Brown, A. M. 1994. Spermine and spermidine as gating molecules for inward rectifier K^+ channels. *Science* 266:1068–1072.

Foskett, J. K. 1998. ClC and CFTR chloride channel gating. *Annual Review of Physiology* 60:689–717.

Fox, A. P., Nowycky, M. C., and Tsien, R. W. 1987. Kinetic and pharmacological properties distinguishing three types of calcium currents in chick sensory neurones. *Journal of Physiology* 394:149–172.

Franciolini, F., and Adams, D. J. 1994. Functional properties of background chloride channels. In *Handbook of Membrane Channels,* ed. C. Peracchia, pp. 255–266. San Diego, CA: Academic Press.

Franciolini, F., and Petris, A. 1990. Chloride channels of biological membranes. *Biochimica et Biophysica Acta* 1031:247–259.

Galvez, A., Gimenez-Gallego, G., Reuben, J. P., Roy-Contancin, L., Feigenbaum, P., Kaczorowski, G. J., and Garcia, M. L. 1990. Purification and characterization of a unique, potent, petidyl probe for the high conductance calcium-activated potassium channel from venom of the scorpion *Buthus tamulus*. *Journal of Biological Chemistry* 265:11083–11090.

Ganetzky, B., Warmke, J. W., Robertson, G., and Pallanck, L. 1995. New potassium channel gene families in flies and mammals: From mutants to molecules. In *Ion Channels and Genetic Diseases*, ed. D. C. Dawson and R. A. Frizzell, pp. 29–39. New York: Rockefeller University Press.

Gautron, S., Dos Santos, G., Pinto-Henrique, D., Koulakoff, A., Gros, F., and Berwald-Netter, Y. 1992. The glial voltage-gated sodium channel: Cell- and tissue-specific mRNA expression. *Proceedings of the National Academy of Sciences USA* 89:7272–7276.

Goldin, A. L. 1995. Voltage-gated sodium channels. In *Ligand- and Voltage-Gated Ion Channels*, ed. R. A. North, pp. 73–111. Boca Raton, FL: CRC Press.

Gorman, A. L. F., and Hermann, A. 1979. Internal effects of divalent cations on potassium permeability in molluscan neurones. *Journal of Physiology* 296:393–410.

Gorman, A. L. F., and Thomas, M. V. 1980a. Intracellular calcium accumulation during depolarization in a molluscan neurone. *Journal of Physiology* 308:259–285.

——— 1980b. Potassium conductance and internal calcium accumulation in a molluscan neurone. *Journal of Physiology* 308:287–313.

Grant, G. B., and Dowling, J. E. 1995. A glutamate-activated chloride current in cone-driven ON bipolar cells of the white perch retina. *Journal of Neuroscience* 15:3852–3862.

Grant, G. B., and Werblin, F. S. 1996. A glutamate-elicited chloride current with transporter-like properties in rod photoreceptors of the tiger salamander. *Visual Neuroscience* 13:135–144.

Hagiwara, S. 1973. Ca spike. *Advances in Biophysics* 4:71–102.

——— 1975. Ca-dependent action potential. In *Membranes—A Series of Advances*, Vol. 3: *Lipid Bilayers and Biological Membranes: Dynamic Properties*, ed. G. Eisenman, pp. 359–381. New York: Marcel Dekker.

Hagiwara, S., and Byerly, L. 1981. Calcium channel. *Annual Review of Neuroscience* 4:69–125.

Hagiwara, S., and Jaffe, L. A. 1979. Electrical properties of egg cell membranes. *Annual Reviews of Biophysics and Bioengineering* 8:385–416.

Hagiwara, S., Kusano, K., and Saito, N. 1961. Membrane changes of

Onchidium nerve cell in potassium-rich media. *Journal of Physiology* 155:470–489.

Hagiwara, S., Miyazaki, S., and Rosenthal, N. P. 1976. Potassium current and the effect of cesium on this current during anomalous rectification of the egg cell membrane of a starfish. *Journal of General Physiology* 67:621–638.

Hagiwara, S., and Naka, K. I. 1964. The initiation of spike potential in barnacle muscle fibers under low intracellular Ca^{++}. *Journal of General Physiology* 48:141–162.

Hagiwara, S., Ozawa, S., and Sand, O. 1975. Voltage clamp analysis of two inward current mechanisms in the egg cell membrane of a starfish. *Journal of General Physiology* 65:617–644.

Hagiwara, S., and Takahashi, K. 1974. The anomalous rectification and cation selectivity of the membrane of a starfish egg cell. *Journal of Membrane Biology* 18:61–80.

Hagiwara, S., and Yoshii, M. 1979. Effects of internal potassium and sodium on the anomalous rectification of the starfish egg as examined by internal perfusion. *Journal of Physiology* 292:251–265.

Hanrahan, J. W., Tabcharani, J. A., Becq, F., Mathews, C. J., Augustinas, O., Jensen, T. J., Chang, X.-B., and Riordan, J. R. 1995. Function and dysfunction of the CFTR chloride channel. In *Ion Channels and Genetic Diseases,* ed. D. C. Dawson and R. A. Frizzell, pp. 125–137. New York: Rockefeller University Press.

Heinemann, S. H., Rettig, J., Graack, H.-R., and Pongs, O. 1996. Functional characterization of K_v channel β-subunits from rat brain. *Journal of Physiology* 493:625–633.

Heinemann, S. H., Terlau, H., Stühmer, W., Imoto, K., and Numa, S. 1992. Calcium channel characteristics conferred on the sodium channel by single mutations. *Nature* 356:441–443.

Hess, P. 1990. Calcium channels in vertebrate cells. *Annual Review of Neuroscience* 13:337–356.

Hille, B., and Schwarz, W. 1978. Potassium channels as multi-ion single-file pores. *Journal of General Physiology* 72:409–442.

Ho, K., Nichols, C. G., Lederer, W. J., Lytton, J., Vassilev, P. M., Kanazirska, M. V., and Hebert, S. C. 1993. Cloning and expression of an inwardly rectifying ATP-regulated potassium channel. *Nature* 362:31–38.

Hodgkin, A. L., and Horowicz, P. 1960. The effect of sudden changes in ionic concentrations on the muscle membrane potential of single muscle fibres. *Journal of Physiology* 153:370–385.

Hoffman, D. A., Magee, J. C., Colbert, C. M., and Johnston, D. 1997. K^+ channel regulation of signal propagation in dendrites of hippocampal pyramidal neurons. *Nature* 387:869–875.

Hofmann, F., Biel, M., and Flockerzi, V. 1994. Molecular basis for Ca^{2+} channel diversity. *Annual Review of Neuroscience* 17:399–418.

Hoth, M., and Penner, R. 1992. Depletion of intracellular calcium stores activates a calcium current in mast cells. *Nature* 355:353–356.

Huguenard, J. R. 1996. Low-threshold calcium currents in central nervous system neurons. *Annual Review of Physiology* 58:329–348.

Imredy, J. P., and Yue, D. T. 1994. Mechanism of Ca^{2+}-sensitive inactivation of L-type Ca^{2+} channels. *Neuron* 12:1301–1318.

Isacoff, E. Y., Jan, Y. N., and Jan, L. Y. 1990. Evidence for the formation of heteromultimeric potassium channels in *Xenopus* oocytes. *Nature* 345:530–534.

Isom, L. L., DeJongh, K. S., and Catterall, W. A. 1994. Auxiliary subunits of voltage-gated ion channels. *Neuron* 12:1183–1194.

Jan, L. Y., and Jan, Y. N. 1994. Potassium channels and their evolving gates. *Nature* 371:119–122.

———— 1997. Cloned potassium channels from eukaryotes and prokaryotes. *Annual Review of Neuroscience* 20:91–123.

Jentsch, T. J. 1994. Molecular biology of voltage-gated chloride channels. *Current Topics in Membranes* 42:35–57.

Jentsch, T. J., Lorenz, C., Pusch, M., and Steinmeyer, K. 1995. Myotonias due to ClC-1 chloride channel mutations. In *Ion Channels and Genetic Diseases,* ed. D. C. Dawson and R. A. Frizzell, pp. 149–159. New York: Rockefeller University Press.

Ji, S., George, A. L., Horn, R., and Barchi, R. L. 1995. Sodium channel mutations and disorders of excitation in human skeletal muscle. In *Ion Channels and Genetic Diseases,* ed. D. C. Dawson and R. A. Frizzell, pp. 61–76. New York: Rockefeller University Press.

Kallen, R. G., Cohen, S. A., and Barchi, R. L. 1994. Structure, function and expression of voltage-dependent sodium channels. *Molecular Neurobiology* 7:383–428.

Katz, B. 1949. Les constantes électriques de la membrane du muscle. *Archives des Sciences Physiologiques* 3:285–299.

Kerr, L. M., and Yoshikami, D. 1984. A venom peptide with a novel presynaptic blocking action. *Nature* 308:282–284.

Ketchum, K. A., Joiner, W. J., Sellers, A. J., Kaczmarek, L. K., and Goldstein, S. A. N. 1995. A new family of outwardly rectifying potassium channel proteins with two pore domains in tandem. *Nature* 376:690–695.

Kim, M.-S., Morii, T., Sun, L.-X., Imoto, K., and Mori, Y. 1993. Structural determinants of ion selectivity in brain calcium channel. *FEBS Letters* 318:145–148.

Knaus, H.-G., Folander, K., Garcia-Calvo, M., Garcia, M. L., Kaczorowski, G. J., Smith, M., and Swanson, R. 1994. Primary sequence and immunological characterization of the beta-subunit of the high-conductance Ca^{2+}-activated K^+ channel from smooth muscle. *Journal of Biological Chemistry* 269:17274–17278.

Kofuji, P., Davidson, N., and Lester, H. A. 1995. Evidence that neuronal G-protein-gated inwardly rectifying K^+ channels are activated by $G\beta\gamma$ subunits and function as heteromultimers. *Proceedings of the National Academy of Sciences USA* 92:6542–6546.

Köhler, M., Hirschberg, B., Bond, C. T., Kinzie, J. M., Marrion, N. V., Maylie, J., and Adelman, J. P. 1996. Small-conductance, calcium-activated potassium channels from mammalian brain. *Science* 273:1709–1713.

Krapivinsky, G., Gordon, E. A., Wickman, K., Velimirović, Krapivinsky, L., and Clapham, D. E. 1995. The G-protein-gated atrial K^+ channel I_{KACh} is a heteromultimer of two inwardly rectifying K^+-channel proteins. *Nature* 374:135–141.

Kubo, Y., Baldwin, T. J., Jan, Y. N., and Jan, L. Y. 1993. Primary structure and functional expression of a mouse inward rectifier potassium channel. *Nature* 362:127–133.

Kubo, Y., Reuveny, E., Slesinger, P. A., Jan, Y. N., and Jan, L. Y. 1993. Primary structure and functional expression of a rat G-protein-coupled muscarinic potassium channel. *Nature* 364:802–806.

Latorre, R., and Miller, C. 1983. Conduction and selectivity in potassium channels. *Journal of Membrane Biology* 71:11–30.

Latorre, R., Oberhauser, A., Labarca, P., and Alvarez, O. 1989. Varieties of calcium-activated potassium channels. *Annual Review of Physiology* 51:385–399.

Leech, C. A., and Stanfield, P. R. 1981. Inward rectification in frog skeletal muscle fibres and its dependence on membrane potential and external potassium. *Journal of Physiology* 319:295–309.

Llinás, R. R. 1988. The intrinsic electrophysiological properties of mammalian neurons: Insights into central nervous system function. *Science* 242:1654–1664.

Llinás, R. R., Sugimori, M., Hillman, D. E., and Cherksey, B. 1992. Distribution and functional significance of the P-type voltage-dependent Ca^{2+} channels in the mammalian central nervous system. *Trends in Neurosciences* 15:351–355.

Lopatin, A. N., Makhina, E. N., and Nichols, C. G. 1994. Potassium channel block by cytoplasmic polyamines as the mechanism of intrinsic rectification. *Nature* 372:366–369.

Lu, Z., and MacKinnon, R. 1994. Electrostatic tuning of Mg^{2+} affinity in an inward-rectifier K^+ channel. *Nature* 371:243–246.

Luneau, C. J., Williams, J. B., Marshall, J., Levitan, E. S., Oliva, C., Smith, J. S., Antanavage, J., Folander, K., Stein, R. B., Swanson, R., Kaczmarek,

L. K., and Buhrow, S. A. 1991. Alternative splicing contributes to K⁺ channel diversity in the mammalian central nervous system. *Proceedings of the National Academy of Sciences USA* 88:3932–3936.

Marty, A. 1981. Ca-dependent K channels with large unitary conductance in chromaffin cell membranes. *Nature* 291:497–500.

Matsuda, H., Saigusa, A., and Irisawa, H. 1987. Ohmic conductance through the inwardly rectifying K channel and blocking by internal Mg^{2+}. *Nature* 325:156–159.

Mayer, M. L., Owen, D. G., and Barker, J. L. 1990. Calcium-dependent chloride currents in vertebrate neurons. In *Chloride Channels and Carriers in Nerve, Muscle, and Glial Cells,* ed. F. J. Alvarez-Leefmans and J. M. Russell, pp. 355–364. New York: Plenum Press.

Mayer, M. L., and Westbrook, G. L. 1983. A voltage-clamp analysis of inward (anomalous) rectification in mouse spinal sensory ganglion neurones. *Journal of Physiology* 340:19–45.

McCormack, K., McCormack, T., Tanouye, M., Rudy, B., and Stühmer, W. 1995. Alternative splicing of the human *Shaker* K⁺ channel β1 gene and functional expression of the β2 gene product. *FEBS Letters* 370:32–36.

McManus, O. B., Helms, L. M. H., Pallanck, L., Ganetzky, B., Swanson, R., and Leonard, R. J. 1995. Functional role of the β subunit of high conductance calcium-activated potassium channels. *Neuron* 14:645–650.

Meech, R. W., and Standen, N. B. 1975. Potassium activation in *Helix aspera* neurones under voltage clamp: A component mediated by calcium influx. *Journal of Physiology* 249:211–259.

Meech, R. W., and Strumwasser, F. 1970. Intracellular calcium injection activates potassium conductance in *Aplysia* nerve cells. *Federation Proceedings* 29:834a.

Miller, C., Moczydlowski, E., Latorre, R., and Phillips, M. 1985. Charybdotoxin, a protein inhibitor of single Ca^{2+}-activated K⁺ channels from mammalian skeletal muscle. *Nature* 313:316–318.

Miller, C., and Richard, E. A. 1990. The voltage-dependent chloride channel of torpedo electroplax: Intimations of molecular structure from quirks of single-channel function. In *Chloride Channels and Carriers in Nerve, Muscle, and Glial Cells,* ed. F. J. Alvarez-Leefmans and J. M. Russell, pp. 383–405. New York: Plenum.

Mintz, I. M., Venema, V. J., Swiderek, K. M., Lee, T. D., Bean, B. P., and Adams, M. E. 1992. P-type calcium channels blocked by the spider toxin ω-Aga-IVA. *Nature* 355:827–829.

Neely, A., Olcese, R., Wei, X., Birnbaumer, L., and Stefani, E. 1994. Ca^{2+}-dependent inactivation of a cloned cardiac Ca^{2+} channel α_1 subunit (α_{1C}) expressed in *Xenopus* oocytes. *Biophysical Journal* 66:1895–1903.

Neely, A., Wei, X., Olcese, R., Birnbaumer, L., and Stefani, E. 1993. Potentiation by the β subunit of the ratio of the ionic current to the charge movement in the cardiac calcium channel. *Science* 262:575–578.

Neher, E. 1971. Two fast transient current components during voltage clamp on snail neurons. *Journal of General Physiology* 58:36–53.

Nichols, C. G., Ho, K., and Herbert, S. 1994. Mg^{2+}-dependent inward rectification of ROMK1 potassium channels expressed in *Xenopus* oocytes. *Journal of Physiology* 476:399–409.

Nichols, C. G., and Lopatin, A. N. 1997. Inward rectifier potassium channels. *Annual Review of Physiology* 59:171–191.

Noceti, F., Toro, L., and Stefani, E. 1996. Are all the measured charges per channel coupled to pore opening in voltage-dependent channels? *Biophysical Journal* 70:A184.

Olcese, R., Qin, N., Schneider, T., Neely, A., Wei, X., Stefani, E., and Birnbaumer, L. 1994. The amino terminus of a calcium channel β subunit sets rates of channel inactivation independently of the subunit's effect on activation. *Neuron* 13:1433–1438.

Pape, H.-C. 1996. Queer current and pacemaker: The hyperpolarization-activated cation current in neurons. *Annual Review of Physiology* 58:299–327.

Pappone, P. A. 1980. Voltage-clamp experiments in normal and denervated mammalian skeletal muscle fibres. *Journal of Physiology* 306:377–410.

Perez-Reyes, E., and Schneider, T. 1995. Molecular biology of calcium channels. *Kidney International* 48:1111–1124.

Pessia, M., Bond, C. T., Kavanaugh, M. P., and Adelman, J. P. 1995. Contributions of the C-terminal domain to gating properties of inward rectifier potassium channels. *Neuron* 14:1039–1045.

Petris, A., Trequattrini, C., and Franciolini, F. 1994. Structural information on background chloride channels obtained by molecular genetics. In *Handbook of Membrane Channels,* ed. C. Peracchia, pp. 245–254. San Diego, CA: Academic Press.

Pragnell, M., De Waard, M., Mori, Y., Tanabe, T., Snutch, T. P., and Campbell, K. P. 1994. Calcium channel β-subunit binds to a conserved motif in the I-II cytoplasmic linker of the α_1-subunit. *Nature* 368:67–70.

Randall, A., and Tsien, R. W. 1995. Pharmacological dissection of multiple types of Ca^{2+} channel currents in rat cerebellar granule neurons. *Journal of Neuroscience* 15:2995–3012.

Rettig, J., Heinemann, S. H., Wunder, F., Lorra, C., Parcei, D. N., Dolly, O., and Pongs, O. 1994. Inactivation properties of voltage-gated K^+ channels altered by the presence of β-subunit. *Nature* 369:289–294.

Rudy, B. 1988. Diversity and ubiquity of K channels. *Neuroscience* 25:729–749.

Sah, P. 1996. Ca^{2+}-activated K^+ currents in neurones: Types, physiological roles and modulation. *Trends in Neurosciences* 19:150–154.

Sarao, R., Gupta, S. K., Auld, V. J., and Dunn, R. J. 1991. Developmentally regulated alternative RNA splicing of rat brain sodium channel mRNAs. *Nucleic Acids Research* 19:5673–5679.

Sather, W. A., Tanabe, T., Zhang, J.-F., Mori, Y., Adams, M. E., and Tsien, R. W. 1993. Distinctive biophysical and pharmacological properties of class A (BI) calcium channel α_1 subunits. *Neuron* 11:291–303.

Schaller, K. L., Krzemien, D. M., Yarowsky, P. J., Krueger, B. K., and Caldwell, J. H. 1995. A novel abundant sodium channel expressed in neurons and glia. *Journal of Neuroscience* 15:3231–3242.

Schlichter, R., Bader, C. R., and Bernheim, L. 1991. Development of anomalous rectification (I_h) and of a tetrodotoxin-resistant sodium current in embryonic quail neurones. *Journal of Physiology* 442:127–145.

Schneider, T., Wei, X., Olcese, R., Costantin, J. L., Neely, A., Palade, P., Perez-Reyes, E., Qin, N., Zhou, J., Crawford, G. D., Smith, R. G., Appel, S. H., Stefani, E., and Birnbaumer, L. 1994. Molecular analysis and functional expression of the human type E neuronal Ca^{2+} channel α_1 subunit. *Receptors and Channels* 2:255–270.

Schrempf, H., Schmidt, O., Kümmerlen, R., Hinnah, S., Müller, D., Betzler, M., Steinkamp, T., and Wagner, R. 1995. A prokaryotic potassium ion channel with two predicted transmembrane segments from *Streptomyces lividans. The EMBO Journal* 14:5170–5178.

Sheng, M., Liao, Y. J., Jan, Y. N., and Jan, L. Y. 1993. Presynaptic A-current based on heteromultimeric K^+ channels detected in vivo. *Nature* 365:72–75.

Sheng, M., Tsaur, M. L., Jan, Y. N., and Jan, L. Y. 1994. Contrasting subcellular localization of the Kv1.2 K^+ channel subunit in different neurons of rat brain. *Journal of Neuroscience* 14:2408–2417.

Silver, M. R., and DeCoursey, T. E. 1990. Intrinsic gating of inward rectifier in bovine pulmonary artery endothelial cells in the presence or absence of internal Mg^{2+}. *Journal of General Physiology* 96:109–133.

Sontheimer, H., and Richie, J. M. 1995. Voltage-gated sodium and calcium channels. In *Neuroglia,* ed. H. Kettenmann and B. R. Ransom, pp. 202–220. Oxford: Oxford University Press.

Soong, T. W., Stea, A., Hodson, C. D., Dubel, S. J., Vincent, S. R., and Snutch, T. P. 1993. Structure and functional expression of a member of the low voltage-activated calcium channel family. *Science* 260:1133–1136.

Spauschus, A., Lentes, K. U., Wischmeyer, E., Dissmann, E., Karschin, C., and Karschin, A. 1996. A G-protein-activated inwardly rectifying K^+ channel (GIRK 4) from human hippocampus associates with other GIRK channels. *Journal of Neuroscience* 16:930–938.

Standen, N. B., and Stanfield, P. R. 1978. Inward rectification in skeletal muscle: A blocking particle model. *Pflügers Archiv* 378:173–176.

Stanfield, P. R., Davies, N. W., Shelton, P. A., Sutcliffe, M. J., Khan, I. A., Brammar, W. J., and Conley, E. C. 1994. A single aspartate residue is involved in both intrinsic gating and blockage by Mg^{2+} of the inward rectifier, IRK1. *Journal of Physiology* 478:1–6.

Stea, A., Soong, T. W., and Snutch, T. P. 1995. Voltage-gated calcium channels. In *Ligand- and Voltage-Gated Ion Channels,* ed. R. A. North, pp. 113–151. Boca Raton, FL: CRC Press.

Stea, A., Tomlinson, J., Soong, T. W., Borinet, E., Dubel, S. J., Vincent, S. R., and Snutch, T. P. 1994. Localization and functional properties of a rat brain α_{1A} calcium channel reflect similarities to neuronal Q- and P-type channels. *Proceedings of the National Academy of Sciences USA* 91:10576–10580.

Storm, J. F. 1987. Action potential repolarization and a fast afterhyperpolarization in rat hippocampal pyramidal cells. *Journal of Physiology* 385:733–759.

——— 1988. Temporal integration by a slowly inactivating K^+ current in hippocampal neurons. *Nature* 336:379–381.

Strange, K., Emma, E., and Jackson, P. S. 1996. Cellular and molecular physiology of volume-sensitive anion channels. *Americal Journal of Physiology* 270 (*Cellular Physiology* 39):C711–C730.

Stühmer, W., Ruppersberg, J. P., Schröter, K. H., Sakmann, B., Stocker, M., Giese, K. P., Perschke, A., Baumann, A., and Pong, O. 1989. Molecular basis of functional diversity of voltage-gated potassium channels in mammalian brain. *EMBO Journal* 8:3235–3244.

Taglialatela, M., Wible, B. A., Caporaso, R., and Brown, A. M. 1994. Specification of pore properties by the carboxyl terminus of inwardly rectifying K^+ channels. *Science* 264:844–847.

Tanabe, T., Takeshima, H., Mikami, A., Flockerzi, V., Takahashi, H., Kangawa, K., Kojima, M., Matsuo, H., Hirose, T., and Numa, S. 1987. Primary structure of the receptor for calcium channel blockers from skeletal muscle. *Nature* 328:313–318.

Thomas, R. C., and Meech, R. W. 1982. Hydrogen ion currents and intracellular pH in depolarized voltage-clamped snail neurones. *Nature* 299:826–828.

Toledo-Aral, J. J., Moss, B. L., He, Z.-J., Koszowski, A. G., Whisenand, T., Levinson, S. R., Wolf, J. J., Silos-Santiago, I., Halegoua, S., and Mandel, G. 1997. Identification of PN1, a predominant voltage-dependent sodium channel expressed principally in peripheral neurons. *Proceedings of the National Academy of Sciences USA* 94:1527–1532.

Tseng-Crank, J., Godinot, N., Johansen, T. E., Ahring, P. K., Strøbæk, D.,

Mertz, R., Foster, C. D., Olensen, S.-P., and Reinhart, P. H. 1996. Cloning, expression, and distribution of a Ca^{2+}-activated K^+ channel β-subunit from human brain. *Proceedings of the National Academy of Sciences USA* 93:9200–9205.

Vandenberg, C. A. 1987. Inward rectification of a potassium channel in cardiac ventricular cells depends on internal magnesium ions. *Proceedings of the National Academy of Sciences USA* 84:2560–2564.

Wadiche, J. I., Amara, S. G., and Kavanaugh, M. P. 1995. Ion fluxes associated with excitatory amino acid transport. *Neuron* 15:721–728.

Warmke, J., Drysdale, R., and Ganetzky, B. 1991. A distinct potassium channel polypeptide encoded by the *Drosophila eag* locus. *Science* 252:1560–1562.

Waxman, S. G., Kocsis, J. D., and Black, J. A. 1994. Type III sodium channel mRNA is expressed in embryonic but not adult spinal sensory neurons, and is reexpressed following axotomy. *Journal of Neurophysiology* 72:466–470.

Wei, A., Covarrubias, M., Butler, A., Baker, K., Pak, M., and Salkoff, L. 1990. K^+ current diversity is produced by an extended gene family conserved in *Drosophila* and mouse. *Science* 248:599–603.

Wei, A., Solaro, C., Lingle, C., and Salkoff, L. 1994. Calcium sensitivity of BK-type K_{Ca} channels determined by a separable domain. *Neuron* 13:671–681.

Weiser, M., de Miera, E. V.-S., Kentros, C., Moreno, H., Franzen, L., Hillman, D., Baker, H., and Rudy, B. 1994. Differential expression of *Shaw*-related K^+ channels in the rat central nervous system. *Journal of Neuroscience* 14:949–972.

Weiss, D. S. 1994. Voltage-dependent kinetics of the fast chloride channel. In *Handbook of Membrane Channels,* ed. C. Peracchia, pp. 213–227. San Diego, CA: Academic Press.

Welsh, M. J., Anderson, M. P., Rich, D. P., Berger, H. A., and Sheppard, D. N. 1994. The CFTR chloride channel. *Current Topics in Membranes* 42:153–171.

Westenbroek, R. E., Hell, J. W., Warner, C., Dubel, S. J., Snutch, T. P., and Catterall, W. A. 1992. Biochemical properties and subcellular distribution of an N-type calcium channel α1 subunit. *Neuron* 9:1099–1115.

Wible, B. A., Taglialatela, M., Ficker, E., and Brown, A. M. 1994. Gating of inwardly rectifying K^+ channels localized to a single negatively charged residue. *Nature* 371:246–249.

Williams, M. E., Brust, P. F., Feldman, D. H., Patthi, S., Simerson, S., Maroufi, A., McCue, A. F., Veliçelebi, G., Ellis, S. B., and Harpold, M. M. 1992. Structure and functional expression of an ω-conotoxin-sensitive human N-type calcium channel. *Science* 257:389–395.

Wu, R.-L., and Barish, M. E. 1992. Two pharmacologically and kinetically distinct transient potassium currents in cultured embryonic mouse hippocampal neurons. *Journal of Neuroscience* 12:2235–2246.

Yang, J., Ellinor, P. T., Sather, W. A., Zhang, J.-F., and Tsien, R. W. 1993. Molecular determinants of Ca^{2+} selectivity and ion permeation in L-type Ca^{2+} channels. *Nature* 366:158–161.

Yang, J., Jan, Y. N., and Jan, L. H. 1995a. Control of rectification and permeation by residues in two distinct domains in an inward rectifier K^+ channel. *Neuron* 14:1047–1054.

—— 1995b. Determination of the subunit stoichiometry of an inwardly rectifying potassium channel. *Neuron* 15:1441–1447.

Zhang, J.-F., Ellinor, P. T., Aldrich, R. W., and Tsien, R. W. 1994. Molecular determinants of voltage-dependent inactivation in calcium channels. *Nature* 372:97–100.

Zhang, J.-F., Randall, A. D., Ellinor, P. T., Horne, W. A., Sather, W. A., Tanabe, T., Schwarz, T. L., and Tsien, R. W. 1993. Distinctive pharmacology and kinetics of cloned neuronal Ca^{2+} channels and their possible counterparts in mammalian CNS neurons. *Neuropharmacology* 32:1075–1088.

8. Presynaptic Mechanisms of Synaptic Transmission

Adler, E. M., Augustine, G. J., Duffy, S. N., and Charlton, M. P. 1991. Alien intracellular calcium chelators attenuate neurotransmitter release at the squid giant synapse. *Journal of Neuroscience* 11:1496–1507.

Adrian, R. H., Chandler, W. K., and Hodgkin, A. L. 1970. Voltage clamp experiments in striated muscle fibres. *Journal of Physiology* 208:607–644.

Allbritton, N. L., Meyer, T., and Stryer, L. 1992. Range of messenger action of calcium ion and inositol 1,4,5-trisphosphate. *Science* 258:1812–1815.

Almers, W. 1990. Exocytosis. *Annual Review of Physiology* 52:607–624.

Alvarez de Toledo, G., Fernandez-Chacon, R., and Fernandez, J. M. 1993. Release of secretory products during transient vesicle fusion. *Nature* 363:554–558.

Augustine, G. J., Charlton, M. P., and Smith, S. J. 1985a. Calcium entry into voltage-clamped presynaptic terminals of squid. *Journal of Physiology* 367:143–162.

—— 1985b. Calcium entry and transmitter release at voltage-clamped nerve terminals of squid. *Journal of Physiology* 367:163–181.

Bajjalieh, S. M., and Scheller, R. H. 1995. The biochemistry of neurotransmitter secretion. *Journal of Biological Chemistry* 270:1971–1974.

Barrio, L. C., Suchyna, T., Bargiello, T., Xu, L. X., Roginski, R. S., Bennett, M. V. L., and Nicholson, B. J. 1991. Gap junctions formed by connexins

26 and 32 alone and in combination are differently affected by applied voltage. *Proceedings of the National Academy of Sciences USA* 88:8410–8414.

Bekkers, J. M. 1994. Quantal analysis of synaptic transmission in the central nervous system. *Current Opinion in Neurobiology* 4:360–365.

Bennett, M. V. L., Barrio, L. C., Bargiello, T. A., Spray, D. C., Hertzberg, E., and Sáez, J. C. 1991. Gap junctions: New tools, new answers, new questions. *Neuron* 6:305–320.

Bennett, M. V. L., and Spray, D. C. 1985. *Gap Junctions.* Cold Spring Harbor, NY: Cold Spring Harbor Laboratory.

Betz, W. J., and Angleson, J. K. 1998. The synaptic vesicle cycle. *Annual Review of Neuroscience* 60:347–363.

Betz, W. J., and Bewick, G. S. 1993. Optical monitoring of transmitter release and synaptic vesicle recycling at the frog neuromuscular junction. *Journal of Physiology* 460:287–309.

Betz, W. J., Mao, F., and Bewick, G. S. 1992. Activity-dependent fluorescent staining and destaining of living vertebrate motor nerve terminals. *Journal of Neuroscience* 12:363–375.

Beyer, E. C. 1993. Gap junctions. *International Review of Cytology* 137C:1–37.

Bezprozvanny, I., Scheller, R. H., and Tsien, R. W. 1995. Functional impact of syntaxin on gating of N-type and Q-type calcium channels. *Nature* 378:623–626.

Borst, J. G. G., and Sakmann, B. 1996. Calcium influx and transmitter release in a fast CNS synapse. *Nature* 383:431–434.

Boyd, I. A., and Martin, A. R. 1956. The end-plate potential in mammalian muscle. *Journal of Physiology* 132:74–91.

Breckenridge, L. J., and Almers, W. 1987. Currents through the fusion pore that forms during exocytosis of a secretory vesicle. *Nature* 328:814–817.

Buchner, E., and Gundersen, C. B. 1997. The DnaJ-like cysteine string protein and exocytotic neurotransmitter release. *Trends in Neurosciences* 20:223–227.

Bullock, T. H., and Hagiwara, S. 1957. Intracellular recording from the giant synapse of the squid. *Journal of General Physiology* 40:565–577.

Burgoyne, R. D., and Morgan, A. 1995. Ca^{2+} and secretory-vesicle dynamics. *Trends in Neurosciences* 18:191–196.

Ceccarelli, B., Hurlbut, W. P., and Mauro, A. 1972. Depletion of vesicles from frog neuromuscular junctions by prolonged tetanic stimulation. *Journal of Cell Biology* 54:30–38.

Chad, J. E., and Eckert, R. 1984. Calcium domains associated with individual channels can account for anomalous voltage relations of Ca-dependent responses. *Biophysical Journal* 45:993–999.

Chandler, D. E., and Heuser, J. E. 1980. Arrest of membrane fusion events in mast cells by quick-freezing. *Journal of Cell Biology* 86:666–674.

Clark, A. W., Hurlbut, W. P., and Mauro, A. 1972. Changes in the fine structure of the neuromuscular junction of the frog caused by black widow spider venom. *Journal of Cell Biology* 52:1–14.

Clements, J. D. 1996. Transmitter timecourse in the synaptic cleft: Its role in central synaptic function. *Trends in Neurosciences* 19:163–171.

Cohen, M. W., Jones, O. T., and Angelides, K. J. 1991. Distribution of Ca^{2+} channels on frog motor nerve terminals revealed by fluorescent ω-conotoxin. *Journal of Neuroscience* 11:1032–1039.

Couteaux, R., and Pecot-Déchavassine, M. 1970. Vésicules synaptiques et poches au niveau des zones actives de la jonction neuromuscularie. *Comptes Rendus de l'Académie de la Science, Série D* (Paris) 271:2346–2349.

Dahl, G., Miller, T., Paul, D., Voellmy, R., and Werner, R. 1987. Expression of functional cell-cell channels from cloned rat liver gap junction complementary DNA. *Science* 236:1290–1293.

De Camilli, P., and Takei, K. 1996. Molecular mechanisms in synaptic vesicle endocytosis and recycling. *Neuron* 16:481–486.

del Castillo, J., and Katz, B. 1954a. The effect of magnesium on the activity of motor nerve endings. *Journal of Physiology* 124:553–559.

———— 1954b. Quantal components of the end-plate potential. *Journal of Physiology* 124:560–573.

Dermietzel, R., and Spray, D. C. 1993. Gap junctions in the brain: Where, what type, how many and why? *Trends in Neurosciences* 16:186–192.

De Robertis, E. D. P., and Bennett, H. S. 1955. Some features of the submicroscopic morphology of synapses in frog and earthworm. *Journal of Biophysical and Biochemical Cytology* 1:47–58.

DeVries, S. H., and Schwartz, E. A. 1989. Modulation of an electrical synapse between solitary pairs of catfish horizontal cells by dopamine and second messengers. *Journal of Physiology* 414:351–375.

———— 1992. Hemi-gap-junction channels in solitary horizontal cells of the catfish retina. *Journal of Physiology* 445:201–230.

Dodge, F. A., Jr., and Rahamimoff, R. 1967. Co-operative action of calcium ions in transmitter release at the neuromuscular junction. *Journal of Physiology* 193:419–432.

Douglas, W. W., and Poisner, A. M. 1966. Evidence that the secreting adrenal chromaffin cell releases catecholamines directly from ATP-rich granules. *Journal of Physiology* 183:236–248.

Ebihara, L. 1992. Expression of gap junctional proteins in *Xenopus* oocyte pairs. *Methods in Enzymology* 207:376–380.

Elfgang, C., Eckert, R., Lichtenberg-Fraté, H., Butterweck, A., Traub, O., Klein, R. A., Hülser, D. F., and Willecke, K. 1995. Specific permeability and selective formation of gap junction channels in connexin-transfected HeLa cells. *Journal of Cell Biology* 129:805–817.

Faber, D. S., Young, W. S., Legendre, P., and Korn, H. 1992. Intrinsic quantal variability due to stochastic properties of receptor-transmitter interactions. *Science* 258:1494–1498.

Fatt, P., and Katz, B. 1951. An analysis of the end-plate potential recorded with an intra-cellular electrode. *Journal of Physiology* 115:320–370.

——— 1952. Spontaneous subthreshold activity at motor nerve endings. *Journal of Physiology* 117:109–128.

Forti, L., Bossi, M., Bergamaschi, A., Villa, A., and Malgaroli, A. 1997. Loose-patch recordings of single quanta at individual hippocampal synapses. *Nature* 388:874–878.

Frerking, M., Borges, S., and Wilson, M. 1995. Variation in GABA mini amplitude is the consequence of variation in transmitter concentration. *Neuron* 15:885–895.

Furshpan, E. J., and Potter, D. D. 1959. Transmission at the giant motor synapses of the crayfish. *Journal of Physiology* 145:289–325.

Geppert, M., Goda, Y., Hammer, R. E., Li, C., Rosahl, T. W., Stevens, C. F., and Südhof, T. C. 1994. Synaptotagmin I: A major Ca^{2+} sensor for transmitter release at a central synapse. *Cell* 79:717–727.

Geppert, M., and Südhof, T. C. 1998. RAB3 and synaptotagmin: The yin and yang of synaptic membrane fusion. *Annual Review of Neuroscience* 21:75–95.

Giaume, C., Kado, R. T., and Korn, H. 1987. Voltage-clamp analysis of a crayfish rectifying synapse. *Journal of Physiology* 386:91–112.

Goodenough, D. A., Goliger, J. A., and Paul, D. L. 1996. Connexins, connexons, and intercellular communication. *Annual Review of Biochemistry* 65:475–502.

Gray, E. G. 1987. Synapse, morphology. In *Encyclopedia of Neuroscience*, vol. 2, ed. G. Adelman, pp. 1158–1162. Boston: Birkhäuser.

Gundersen, C. B., Mastrogiacomo, A., and Umbach, J. A. 1995. Cysteine-string proteins as templates for membrane fusion: Models of synaptic vesicle exocytosis. *Journal of Theoretical Biology* 172:269–277.

Hampson, E. C. G. M., Vaney, D. I., and Weiler, R. 1992. Dopaminergic modulation of gap junction permeability between amacrine cells in mammalian retina. *Journal of Neuroscience* 12:4911–4922.

Hanson, P. I., Roth, R., Morisaki, H., Jahn, R., and Heuser, J. E. 1997. Structure and conformational changes in NSF and its membrane receptor complexes visualized by quick-freeze/deep-etch electron microscopy. *Cell* 90:523–535.

Haydon, P. G., Henderson, E., and Stanley, E. F. 1994. Localization of individual calcium channels at the release face of a presynaptic nerve terminal. *Neuron* 13:1275–1280.

Heidelberger, R., Heinemann, C., Neher, E., and Matthews, G. 1994. Calcium dependence of the rate of exocytosis in a synaptic terminal. *Nature* 371:513–515.

Henkel, A. W., and Betz, W. J. 1995. Staurosporine blocks evoked release of FM1–43 but not acetylcholine from frog motor nerve terminals. *Journal of Neuroscience* 15:8246–8258.

Hessler, N. A., Shirke, A. M., and Malinow, R. 1993. The probability of transmitter release at a mammalian central synapse. *Nature* 366:569–572.

Heuser, J. E., and Miledi, R. 1971. Effect of lanthanum ions on function and structure of frog neuromuscular junctions. *Proceedings of the Royal Society of London B* 179:247–260.

Heuser, J. E., and Reese, T. S. 1973. Evidence for recycling of synaptic vesicle membrane during transmitter release at the frog neuromuscular junction. *Journal of Cell Biology* 57:315–344.

——— 1977. Structure of the synapse. In *Handbook of Physiology, Section 1: The Nervous System, Volume 1: Cellular Biology of Neurons, Part 1*, ed. E. R. Kandel, pp. 261–294. Bethesda, MD: American Physiological Society.

——— 1981. Structural changes after transmitter release at the frog neuromuscular junction. *Journal of Cell Biology* 88:564–580.

Heuser, J. E., Reese, T. S., Dennis, M. J., Jan, Y., Jan, L., and Evans, L. 1979. Synaptic vesicle exocytosis captured by quick freezing and correlated with quantal transmitter release. *Journal of Cell Biology* 81:275–300.

Hochner, B., Parnas, H., and Parnas, I. 1989. Membrane depolarization evokes neurotransmitter release in the absence of calcium entry. *Nature* 342:433–435.

Isaac, J. T. R., Nicoll, R. A., and Malenka, R. C. 1995. Evidence for silent synapses: Implications for the expression of LTP. *Neuron* 15:427–434.

Isaacson, J. S., and Walmsley, B. 1995. Counting quanta: direct measurements of transmitter release at a central synapse. *Neuron* 15:875–884.

Issa, N. P., and Hudspeth, A. J. 1994. Clustering of Ca^{2+} channels and Ca^{2+}-activated K^+ channels at fluorescently labeled presynaptic active zones of hair cells. *Proceedings of the National Academy of Sciences USA* 91:7578–7582.

Katz, B. 1969. *The Release of Neural Transmitter Substances*. Liverpool: Liverpool University Press.

Katz, B., and Miledi, R. 1965a. The effect of calcium on acetylcholine release from motor nerve terminals. *Proceedings of the Royal Society of London B* 161:496–503.

——— 1965b. The effect of temperature on the synaptic delay at the neuromuscular junction. *Journal of Physiology* 181:656–670.

——— 1967. A study of synaptic transmission in the absence of nerve impulses. *Journal of Physiology* 192:407–436.

Kelly, R. B. 1993. Storage and release of neurotransmitters. *Neuron* 10 (Supplement):43–53.

Konig, N., and Zampighi, G. 1995. Purification of bovine lens cell-to-cell channels composed of connexin44 and connexin50. *Journal of Cell Science* 108:3091–3098.

Korn, H., and Faber, D. S. 1979. Electrical interactions between vertebrate neurons: Field effects and electronic coupling. In *The Neurosciences: Fourth Study Program,* ed. F. O. Schmitt, and F. G. Worden, pp. 333–358. Cambridge, MA: MIT Press.

———— 1991. Quantal analysis and synaptic efficacy in the CNS. *Trends in Neurosciences* 14:439–445.

Korn, H., Mallet, A., Triller, A., and Faber, D. S. 1982. Transmission at a central inhibitory synapse. II. Quantal description of release, with a physical correlate for binomial *n*. *Journal of Neurophysiology* 48:679–707.

Lando, L., and Zucker, R. S. 1994. Ca^{2+} cooperativity in neurosecretion measured using photolabile Ca^{2+} chelators. *Journal of Neurophysiology* 72:825–830.

Lasater, E. M., and Dowling, J. E. 1985. Dopamine decreases conductance of the electrical junctions between cultured retinal horizontal cells. *Proceedings of the National Academy of Sciences USA* 82:3025–3029.

Lindau, M., and Almers, W. 1995. Structure and function of fusion pores in exocytosis and ectoplasmic membrane fusion. *Current Opinion in Cell Biology* 7:509–517.

Lisman, J. E., and Harris, K. M. 1993. Quantal analysis and synaptic anatomy—integrating two views of hippocampal plasticity. *Trends in Neurosciences* 16:141–147.

Littleton, J. T., and Bellen, H. J. 1995. Synaptotagmin controls and modulates synaptic-vesicle fusion in a Ca^{2+}-dependent manner. *Trends in Neurosciences* 18:177–183.

Littleton, J. T., Stern, M., Perin, M., and Bellen, H. J. 1994. Calcium dependence of neurotransmitter release and rate of spontaneous vesicle fusions are altered in *Drosophila* synaptotagmin mutants. *Proceedings of the National Academy of Sciences USA* 91:10888–10892.

Liu, G., and Tsien, R. W. 1995. Properties of synaptic transmission at single hippocampal synaptic boutons. *Nature* 375:404–408.

Llinás, R., Steinberg, I. Z., and Walton, K. 1981a. Presynaptic calcium currents in squid giant synapse. *Biophysical Journal* 33:289–322.

———— 1981b. Relationship between presynaptic calcium current and postsynaptic potential in squid giant synapse. *Biophysical Journal* 33:323–352.

Llinás, R., Sugimori, M., and Silver, R. B. 1992. Microdomains of high calcium concentration in a presynaptic terminal. *Science* 256:677–679.

Makowski, L., Caspar, D. L. D., Phillips, W. C., and Goodenough, D. A. 1977.

Gap junction structures. II. Analysis of the X-ray diffraction data. *Journal of Cell Biology* 74:629–645.

Mastrogiacomo, A., Parsons, S. M., Zampighi, G. A., Jenden, D. J., Umbach, J. A., and Gundersen, C. B. 1994. Cysteine string proteins: A potential link between synaptic vesicles and presynaptic Ca^{2+} channels. *Science* 263:981–982.

Matthews, G. 1996. Neurotransmitter release. *Annual Review of Neuroscience* 19:219–233.

Milks, L. C., Kumar, N. M., Houghten, R., Unwin, N., and Gilula, N. B. 1988. Topology of the 32-kd liver gap junction protein determined by site-directed antibody localizations. *EMBO Journal* 7:2967–2975.

Mills, S. L., and Massey, S. C. 1995. Differential properties of two gap junctional pathways made by AII amacrine cells. *Nature* 377:734–737.

Monck, J. R., de Toledo, G. A., and Fernandez, J. M. 1990. Tension in secretory granule membranes causes extensive membrane transfer through the exocytotic fusion pore. *Proceedings of the National Academy of Sciences USA* 87:7804–7808.

Monck, J. R., and Fernandez, J. M. 1992. Mini-review: The exocytotic fusion pore. *Journal of Cell Biology* 119:1395–1404.

———— 1994. The exocytotic fusion pore and neurotransmitter release. *Neuron* 12:707–716.

Mulkey, R. M., and Zucker, R. S. 1991. Action potentials must admit calcium to evoke transmitter release. *Nature* 350:153–155.

Murthy, V. N, Sejnowski, T. J. and Stevens, C. F. 1997. Heterogeneous release properties of visualized individual hippocampal synapses. *Neuron* 18:599–612.

Negishi, K., Salas, R., Parthe, V. and Drujan, B. D. 1988. Morphological and functional correlates of horizontal cells in the retina of a teleost fish (*Eugerres plumieri*). *Biomedical Research* (Supplement 2) 9:109–117.

Palay, S. L. 1956. Synapses in the central nervous system. *Journal of Biochemical and Biophysical Cytology* 2:193–202.

Paul, D. L. 1995. New functions for gap junctions. *Current Opinion in Cell Biology* 7:665–672.

Ramón, F., Zampighi, G. A., and Rivera, A. 1985. Control of junctional permeability. In *Gap Junctions*, ed. M. V. L. Bennett and D. C. Spray, pp. 155–166. Cold Spring Harbor, NY: Cold Spring Harbor Laboratory.

Ransom, B. R. 1995. Gap junctions. In *Neuroglia*, ed. H. Kettenmann and B. R. Ransom, pp. 299–318. Oxford: Oxford University Press.

Rash, J. E., Dillman, R. K., Bilhartz, B. L., Duffy, H. S., Whalen, L. R., and Yasumura, T. 1996. Mixed synapses discovered and mapped throughout mammalian spinal cord. *Proceedings of the National Academy of Sciences USA*, 93:4235–4239.

Rettig, J., Sheng, Z.-H., Kim, D. K., Hodson, C. D., Snutch, T. P., and

Catterall, W. A. 1996. Isoform-specific interaction of the α_{1A} subunits of brain Ca^{2+} channels with the presynaptic proteins syntaxin and SNAP-25. *Proceedings of the National Academy of Sciences USA* 93:7363–7368.

Roberts, W. M. 1993. Spatial calcium buffering in saccular hair cells. *Nature* 363:74–76.

——— 1994. Localization of calcium signals by a mobile calcium buffer in frog saccular hair cells. *Journal of Neuroscience* 14:3246–3262.

Roberts, W. M., Jacobs, R. A., and Hudspeth, A. J. 1990. Colocalization of ion channels involved in frequency selectivity and synaptic transmission at presynaptic active zones of hair cells. *Journal of Neuroscience* 10:3664–3684.

Robitaille, R., Adler, E. M., and Charlton, M. P. 1990. Strategic location of calcium channels at transmitter release sites of frog neuromuscular synapses. *Neuron* 5:773–779.

Robitaille, R., Garcia, M. L., Kaczorowski, G. J., and Charlton, M. P. 1993. Functional colocalization of calcium and calcium-gated potassium channels in control of transmitter release. *Neuron* 11:645–655.

Rörig, B., Klausa, G., and Sutor, B. 1995. Dye coupling between pyramidal neurons in developing rat prefrontal and frontal cortex is reduced by protein kinase A activation and dopamine. *Journal of Neuroscience* 15:7386–7400.

Rose, B., and Loewenstein, W. 1976. Permeability of a cell junction and the local cytoplasmic free ionized calcium concentration: A study with aequorin. *Journal of Membrane Biology* 28:87–119.

Rosenmund, C., Clements, J. D., and Westbrook, G. L. 1993. Nonuniform probability of glutamate release at a hippocampal synapse. *Science* 262:754–757.

Rothman, J. E. 1994. Mechanisms of intracellular protein transport. *Nature* 372:55–63.

Rothman, J. E., and Wieland, F. T. 1996. Protein sorting by transport vesicles. *Science* 272:227–234.

Ryan, T. A., Reuter, H., Wendland, B., Schweizer, F. E., Tsien, R. W., and Smith, S. J. 1993. The kinetics of synaptic vesicle recycling measured at single presynaptic boutons. *Neuron* 11:713–724.

Ryan, T. A., and Smith, S. J. 1995. Vesicle pool mobilization during action potential firing at hippocampal synapses. *Neuron* 14:983–989.

Ryan, T. A., Smith, S. J., and Reuter, H. 1996. The timing of synaptic vesicle endocytosis. *Proceedings of the National Academy of Sciences USA* 93:5567–5571.

Scheller, R. H. 1995. Membrane trafficking in the presynaptic nerve terminal. *Neuron* 14:893–897.

Schneider, F. H., Smith, A. D., and Winkler, H. 1967. Secretion from the adrenal medulla: Biochemical evidence for exocytosis. *British Journal of Pharmacology and Chemotherapy* 31:94–104.

Schweizer, F. E., Betz, H., and Augustine, G. J. 1995. From vesicle docking to endocytosis: Intermediate reactions of exocytosis. *Neuron* 14:689–696.

Smith, C. B., and Betz, W. J. 1996. Simultaneous independent measurement of endocytosis and exocytosis. *Nature* 380:531–534.

Smith, S. J., Buchanan, J., Osses, L. R., Charlton, M. P., and Augustine, G. J. 1993. The spatial distribution of calcium signals in squid presynaptic terminals. *Journal of Physiology* 472:573–593.

Spray, D. C., Harris, A. L., and Bennett, M. V. L. 1981. Equilibrium properties of a voltage-dependent junctional conductance. *Journal of General Physiology* 77:77–93.

Spray, D. C., Stern, J. H., Harris, A. L., and Bennett, M. V. L. 1982. Gap junctional conductance: Comparison of sensitivities to H^+ and Ca^{2+} ions. *Proceedings of the National Academy of Sciences USA* 79:441–445.

Spruce, A. E., Breckenridge, L. J., Lee, A. K., and Almers, W. 1990. Properties of the fusion pore that forms during exocytosis of a mast cell secretory vesicle. *Neuron* 4:643–654.

Stjärne, L., Greengard, P., Grillner, S., Hökfelt, T., and Ottoson, D. (eds.). 1994. *Molecular and Cellular Mechanisms of Neurotransmitter Release.* New York: Raven.

Südhof, T. C. 1995. The synaptic vesicle cycle: A cascade of protein-protein interactions. *Nature* 375:645–653.

Südhof, T. C., and Rizo, J. 1996. Synaptotagmins: C_2-domain proteins that regulate membrane traffic. *Neuron* 17:379–388.

Tingley, D. W. 1995. Synaptic-vesicle release: New pieces of a puzzling process. *Journal of NIH Research* 7 (12):46–49.

Tong, G., and Jahr, C. E. 1994. Multivesicular release from excitatory synapses of cultured hippocampal neurons. *Neuron* 12:51–59.

Turin, L., and Warner, A. E. 1980. Intracellular pH in early *Xenopus* embryos: Its effect on current flow between blastomeres. *Journal of Physiology* 300:489–504.

Unwin, N. 1989. The structure of ion channels in membranes of excitable cells. *Neuron* 3:665–676.

Unwin, P. N. T., and Zampighi, G. 1980. Structure of the junction between communicating cells. *Nature* 283:545–549.

Vaney, D. I. 1994. Patterns of neuronal coupling in the retina. *Progress in Retinal and Eye Research* 13:301–355.

von Gersdorff, H., and Matthews, G. 1994a. Dynamics of synaptic vesicle fusion and membrane retrieval in synaptic terminals. *Nature* 367:735–739.

——— 1994b. Inhibition of endocytosis by elevated internal calcium in a synaptic terminal. *Nature* 370:652–655.

White, T. W., Bruzzone, R., and Paul, D. L. 1995. The connexin family of intercellular channel forming proteins. *Kidney International* 48:1148–1157.

Whittaker, V. P., Michaelson, I. A., and Kirkland, R. J. A. 1964. The separation of synaptic vesicles from nerve-ending particles ("synaptosomes"). *Biochemical Journal* 90:293–303.

Wolburg, H., and Rohlmann, A. 1995. Structure-function relationships in gap junctions. *International Review of Cytology* 157:315–373.

Wu, L.-G., and Betz, W. J. 1996. Nerve activity but not intracellular calcium determines the time course of endocytosis at the frog neuromuscular junction. *Neuron* 17:769–779.

Yazejian, B., DiGregorio, D., Vergara, J. L., Poage, R. E., Meriney, S. D., and Grinnell, A. D. 1997. Direct measurements of presynaptic calcium and calcium-activated potassium currents regulating neurotransmitter release at cultured *Xenopus* nerve-muscle synapses. *Journal of Neuroscience* 17:2990–3001.

Yeager, M., and Gilula, N. B. 1992. Membrane topology and quaternary structure of cardiac gap junction ion channels. *Journal of Molecular Biology* 223:929–948.

Zucker, R. S. 1996. Exocytosis: A molecular and physiological perspective. *Neuron* 17:1049–1055.

9. *Excitatory Transmission*

Adams, D. J., Dwyer, T. M., and Hille, B. 1980. The permeability of endplate channels to monovalent and divalent metal cations. *Journal of General Physiology* 75:493–510.

Akabas, M. H., Kaufmann, C., Archdeacon, P., and Karlin, P. 1994. Identification of acetylcholine receptor channel-lining residues in the entire M2 segment of the α subunit. *Neuron* 13:919–927.

Anderson, C. R., and Stevens, C. F. 1973. Voltage clamp analysis of acetylcholine produced end-plate current fluctuations at frog neuromuscular junction. *Journal of Physiology* 235:655–691.

Angulo, M. C., Lambolez, B., Audinat, E., Hestrin, S., and Rossier, J. 1997. Subunit composition, kinetic, and permeation properties of AMPA receptors in single neocortical nonpyramidal cells. *Journal of Neuroscience* 17:6685–6696.

Assaf, S. Y., and Chung, S.-H. 1984. Release of endogenous Zn^{2+} from brain tissue during activity. *Nature* 308:734–736.

Barbour, B., Keller, B. U., Llano, I., and Marty, A. 1994. Prolonged presence of glutamate during excitatory synaptic transmission to cerebellar Purkinje cells. *Neuron* 12:1331–1343.

Bennett, J. A., and Dingledine, R. 1995. Topology profile for a glutamate receptor: Three transmembrane domains and a channel-lining reentrant membrane loop. *Neuron* 14:373–384.

Bertrand, D., Galzi, J. L., Devillers-Thiéry, A., Bertrand, S., and Changeux, J. P. 1993. Mutations at two distinct sites within the channel domain M2 alter calcium permeability of neuronal alpha 7 nicotinic receptor. *Proceedings of the National Academy of Sciences USA* 90:6971–6975.

Borowsky, B., and Hoffman, B. J. 1995. Neurotransmitter transporters: Molecular biology, function, and regulation. *International Review of Neurobiology* 38:139–199.

Boulter, J., Evans, K., Goldman, D., Martin, G., Treco, D., Heinemann, S., and Patrick, J. 1986. Isolation of a cDNA clone coding for a possible neural nicotinic acetylcholine receptor alpha-subunit. *Nature* 319:368–374.

Bowie, D., and Mayer, M. L. 1995. Inward rectification of both AMPA and kainate subtype glutamate receptors generated by polyamine-mediated ion channel block. *Neuron* 15:453–462.

Burnashev, N., Monyer, H., Seeburg, P. H., and Sakmann, B. 1992. Divalent ion permeability of AMPA receptor channels is dominated by the edited form of a single subunit. *Neuron* 8:189–198.

Burnashev, N., Schoepfer, R., Monyer, H., Ruppersberg, J. P., Günther, W., Seeburg, P. H., and Sakmann, B. 1992. Control by asparagine residues of calcium permeability and magnesium blockade in the NMDA receptor. *Science* 257:1415–1419.

Burnashev, N., Zhou, Z., Neher, E., and Sakmann, B. 1995. Fractional calcium currents through recombinant GluR channels of the NMDA, AMPA and kainate receptor subtypes. *Journal of Physiology* 485:403–418.

Castillo, P. E., Malenka, R. C., and Nicoll, R. A. 1997. Kainate receptors mediate a slow postsynaptic current in hippocampal CA3 neurons. *Nature* 388:182–186.

Chittajallu, R., Vignes, M., Dev, K. K., Barnes, J. M., Collingridge, G. L., and Henley, J. M. 1996. Regulation of glutamate release by presynaptic kainate receptors in the hippocampus. *Nature* 379:78–81.

Clarke, P. B. S., Schwartz, R. D., Paul, S. M., Pert, C. B., and Pert, A. 1985. Nicotinic binding in rat brain: Autoradiographic comparison of [^{3}H]acetylcholine, [^{3}H]nicotine, and [^{125}I]-α-bungarotoxin. *Journal of Neuroscience* 5:1307–1315.

Clarke, V. R. J., Ballyk, B. A., Hoo, K. H., Mandelzys, A., Pellizzari, A., Bath, C. P., Thomas, J., Sharpe, E. F., Davies, C. H., Ornstein, P. L., Schoepp, D. D., Kamboj, R. K., Collingridge, G. L., Lodge, D., and Bleakman, D. 1997. A hippocampal GluR5 kainate receptor regulating inhibitory synaptic transmission. *Nature* 389:599–603.

Clements, J. D. 1996. Transmitter timecourse in the synaptic cleft: Its role in central synaptic function. *Trends in Neurosciences* 19:163–171.

Clements, J. D., Lester, R. A. J., Tong, G., Jahr, C. E., and Westbrook, G. L. 1992. The time course of glutamate in the synaptic cleft. *Science* 258:1498–1501.

Cohen, B. N., Labarca, C., Czyzyk, L., Davidson, N., and Lester, H. A. 1992. $Tris^+/Na^+$ permeability ratios of nicotinic acetylcholine receptors are reduced by mutations near the intracellular end of the M2 region. *Journal of General Physiology* 99:545–572.

Collo, G., North, R. A., Kawashima, E., Merlo-Pich, E., Neidhart, S., Surprenant, A., and Buell, G. 1996. Cloning of $P2X_5$ and $P2X_6$ receptors and the distribution and properties of an extended family of ATP-gated ion channels. *Journal of Neuroscience* 16:2495–2507.

Colquhoun, D., and Sakmann, B. 1985. Fast events in single-channel currents activated by acetylcholine and its analogues at the frog muscle end-plate. *Journal of Physiology* 369:501–557.

Connolly, J., Boulter, J., and Heinemann, S. F. 1992. $\alpha4$–$2\beta2$ and other nicotinic acetylcholine receptor subtypes as targets of psychoactive and addictive drugs. *British Journal of Pharmacology* 105:657–666.

Cooper, E., Couturier, S., and Ballivet, M. 1991. Pentameric structure and subunit stoichiometry of a neuronal nicotinic acetylcholine receptor. *Nature* 350:235–238.

Couturier, S., Bertrand, D., Matter, J.-M., Hernandez, M.-C., Bertrand, S., Millar, N., Valera, S., Barkas, T., and Ballivet, M. 1990. A neuronal nicotinic acetylcholine receptor subunit ($\alpha7$) is developmentally regulated and forms a homo-oligomeric channel blocked by α-BTX. *Neuron* 5:847–856.

Craig, A. M., Blackstone, C. D., Huganir, R. L., and Banker, G. 1993. The distribution of glutamate receptors in cultured rat hippocampal neurons: Postsynaptic clustering of AMPA-selective subunits. *Neuron* 10:1055–1068.

Czajkowski, C., and Karlin, A. 1991. Agonist binding site of *Torpedo* electric tissue nicotinic acetylcholine receptor: A negatively-charged region of the δ subunit within 0.9 nm of the α subunit binding site disulfide. *Journal of Biological Chemistry* 266:22603–22612.

Dale, H. H., Feldberg, W., and Vogt, M. 1936. Release of acetylcholine at voluntary motor nerve endings. *Journal of Physiology* 86:353–380.

Donevan, S. D., and Rogawski, M. A. 1993. GYKI 52466, a 2,3-benzodiazepine, is a highly selective, noncompetitive antagonist of AMPA/kainate receptor responses. *Neuron* 10:51–59.

——— 1995. Intracellular polyamines mediate inward rectification of Ca^{2+}-permeable α-amino-3-α-amino-3-hydroxy-5-methylisoxazole-4-proprionic acid receptors. *Proceedings of the National Academy of Sciences USA* 92:9298–9302.

Dwyer, T. M., Adams, D. J., and Hille, B. 1980. The permeability of the endplate channel to organic cations in frog muscle. *Journal of General Physiology* 75:469–492.

Dzubay, J. A., and Jahr, C. E. 1996. Kinetics of NMDA channel opening. *Journal of Neuroscience* 16:4129–4134.

Edmonds, B., and Colquhoun, D. 1992. Rapid decay of averaged single-channel NMDA receptor activations recorded at low agonist concentrations. *Proceedings of the Royal Society of London B* 250:279–286.

Edmonds, B., Gibb, A. J., and Colquhoun, D. 1995a. Mechanisms of activation of muscle nicotinic acetylcholine receptors and the time course of endplate currents. *Annual Review of Physiology* 57:469–493.

———— 1995b. Mechanisms of activation of glutamate receptors and the time course of excitatory synaptic currents. *Annual Review of Physiology* 57:495–519.

Ehlers, M. D., Tingley, W. G., and Huganir, R. L. 1995. Regulated subcellular distribution of the NR1 subunit of the NMDA receptor. *Science* 269:1734–1737.

Ferrer-Montiel, A. V., and Montal, M. 1996. Pentameric subunit stoichiometry of a neuronal glutamate receptor. *Proceedings of the National Academy of Sciences USA* 93:2741–2744.

Flores, C. M., Rogers, S. W., Pabreza, L. A., Wolfe, B. B., and Kellar, K. J. 1992. A subtype of nicotinic cholinergic receptor in rat brain is comprised of α-4 and β-2 subunits and is up-regulated by chronic nicotine treatment. *Molecular Pharmacology* 41:31–37.

Geiger, J. R. P., Melcher, T., Koh, D.-S., Sakmann, B., Seeburg, P. H., Jonas, P., and Monyer, H. 1995. Relative abundance of subunit mRNAs determines gating and Ca^{2+} permeability of AMPA receptors in principal neurons and interneurons in rat CNS. *Neuron* 15:193–204.

Gibb, A. J., and Colquhoun, D. 1992. Activation of N-methyl-D-aspartate receptors by L-glutamate in cells dissociated from adult rat hippocampus. *Journal of Physiology* 456:143–179.

Gray, R., Rajan, A. S., Radcliffe, K. A., Yakehiro, M., and Dani, J. A. 1996. Hippocampal synaptic transmission enhanced by low concentrations of nicotine. *Nature* 383:713–716.

Hamill, O. P., and Sakmann, B. 1981. Multiple conductance states of single acetylcholine receptor channels in embryonic muscle cells. *Nature* 294:462–466.

Herb, A., Burnashev, N., Werner, P., Sakmann, B., Wisden, W., and Seeburg, P. H. 1992. The KA-2 subunit of excitatory amino acid receptors shows widespread expression in brain and forms ion channels with distantly related subunits. *Neuron* 8:775–785.

Herlitze, S., Villarroel, A., Witzemann, V., Koenen, M., and Sakmann, B. 1996. Structural determinants of channel conductance in fetal and adult rat muscle acetylcholine receptors. *Journal of Physiology* 492:775–787.

Hestrin, S. 1993. Different glutamate receptor channels mediate fast excitatory synaptic currents in inhibitory and excitatory cortical neurons. *Neuron* 11:1083–1091.

Hille, B., and Campbell, D. T. 1976. An improved vaseline gap voltage clamp for skeletal muscle fibers. *Journal of General Physiology* 67:265–293.

Hirai, H., Kirsch, J., Laube, B., Betz, H., and Kuhse, J. 1996. The glycine binding site of the N-methyl-D-aspartate receptor subunit NR1: Identification of novel determinants of coagonist potentation in the extracellular M3-M4 loop region. *Proceedings of the National Academy of Sciences USA* 93:6031–6036.

Hollmann, M., Hartley, M., and Heinemann, S. 1991. Ca^{2+} permeability of KA-AMPA-gated glutamate receptor channels depends on subunit composition. *Science* 252:851–853.

Hollmann, M., and Heinemann, S. 1994. Cloned glutamate receptors. *Annual Review of Neuroscience* 17:31–108.

Hollmann, M., Maron, C., and Heinemann, S. 1994. N-glycosylation site tagging suggests a three transmembrane domain topology for the glutamate receptor GluR1. *Neuron* 13:1331–1343.

Hollmann, M., O'Shea-Greenfield, A., Rogers, S. W., and Heinemann, S. 1989. Cloning by functional expression of a member of the glutamate receptor family. *Nature* 342:643–648.

Honoré, T., Davies, S. N., Drejer, J., Fletcher, E. J., Jacobsen, P., Lodge, D., and Nielsen, F. E. 1988. Quinoxalinediones: Potent competitive non-NMDA glutamate receptor antagonists. *Science* 241:701–704.

Howell, G. A., Welch, M. G., and Frederickson, C. J. 1984. Stimulation-induced uptake and release of zinc in hippocampal slices. *Nature* 308:736–738.

Huettner, J. E. 1990. Glutamate receptor channels in rat DRG neurons: Activation by kainate and quisqualate and blockade of desensitization by ConA. *Neuron* 5:255–266.

Huettner, J. E., and Bean, B. P. 1988. Block of N-methyl-D-aspartate-activated current by the anticonvulsant MK-801: Selective binding to open channels. *Proceedings of the National Academy of Sciences USA* 85:1307–1311.

Imoto, K., Busch, C., Sakmann, B., Mishina, M., Konno, T., Nakai, J., Bujo, H., Mori, Y., Fukuda, K., and Numa, S. 1988. Rings of negatively charged amino acids determine the acetylcholine receptor channel conductance. *Nature* 335:645–648.

Jackson, M. B. 1984. Spontaneous openings of the acetylcholine receptor channel. *Proceedings of the National Academy of Sciences USA* 81:3901–3904.

——— 1988. Dependence of acetylcholine receptor channel kinetics on agonist concentration in cultured mouse muscle fibres. *Journal of Physiology* 397:555–583.

Jackson, M. B., and Yakel, J. L. 1995. The 5-HT$_3$ receptor channel. *Annual Review of Physiology* 57:447–468.

Jahr, C. E. 1992. High probability opening of NMDA receptor channels by L-glutamate. *Science* 255:470–472.

——— 1994. NMDA receptor kinetics and synaptic function. *Seminars in Neurosciences* 6:81–86.

Johnson, J. W., and Ascher, P. 1987. Glycine potentiates the NMDA response in cultured mouse brain neurons. *Nature* 325:529–531.

Jones, M. V., and Westbrook, G. L. 1996. The impact of receptor desensitization on fast synaptic transmission. *Trends in Neurosciences* 19:96–101.

Karlin, A. 1993. Structure of nicotinic acetylcholine receptors. *Current Opinion in Neurobiology* 3:299–309.

Karlin, A., and Akabas, M. H. 1995. Toward a structural basis for the function of nicotinic acetylcholine receptors and their cousins. *Neuron* 15:1231–1244.

Katz, B., and Miledi, R. 1972. The statistical nature of the acetylcholine potential and its molecular components. *Journal of Physiology* 224:665–699.

Katz, B., and Thesleff, S. 1957. A study of the "desensitization" produced by acetylcholine at the motor end-plate. *Journal of Physiology* 138:63–80.

Keinänen, K., Wisden, W., Sommer, B., Werner, P., Herb, A., Verdoorn, T. A., Sakmann, B., and Seeburg, P. H. 1990. A family of AMPA-selective glutamate receptors. *Science* 249:556–560.

Keller, B. U., Konnerth, A., and Yaari, Y. 1991. Patch clamp analysis of excitatory synaptic currents in granule cells of rat hippocampus. *Journal of Physiology* 435:275–293.

Köhler, M., Burnashev, N., Sakmann, B., and Seeburg, P. H. 1993. Determinants of Ca^{2+} permeability in both TM1 and TM2 of high affinity kainate receptor channels: Diversity by RNA editing. *Neuron* 10:491–500.

Kubalek, E., Ralston, S., Lindstrom, J., and Unwin, N. 1987. Location of subunits within the acetylcholine receptor by electron image analysis of tubular crystals from *Torpedo marmorata*. *Journal of Cell Biology* 105:9–18.

Kuner, T., and Schoepfer, R. 1996. Multiple structural elements determine subunit specificity of Mg^{2+} block in NMDA receptor channels. *Journal of Neuroscience* 16:3549–3558.

Kutsuwada, T., Kashiwabuchi, N., Mori, H., Sakimura, K., Kushiya, E., Araki, K., Meguro, H., Masaki, H., Kumanishi, T., Arakawa, M., and Mishina, M. 1992. Molecular diversity of the NMDA receptor channel. *Nature* 358:36–41.

Lambert, J. J., Peters, J. A., and Hope, A. G. 1995. 5-HT$_3$ receptors. In *Ligand- and Voltage-Gated Ion Channels,* ed. R. A. North, pp. 177–211. Boca Raton, FL: CRC Press.

Lambolez, B., Ropert, N., Perrais, D., Rossier, J., and Hestrin, S. 1996. Correlation between kinetics and RNA splicing of α-amino-3-hydroxy-5-methylisoxazole-4-proprionic acid receptors in neocortical neurons. *Proceedings of the National Academy of Sciences USA* 93:1797–1802.

Le Novère, N., and Changeux, J. P. 1995. Molecular evolution of the nicotinic acetylcholine receptor: An example of multigene family in excitable cells. *Journal of Molecular Evolution* 40:155–72.

Lerma, J., Paternain, A. V., Naranjo, J. R., and Mellström, B. 1993. Functional kainate-selective glutamate receptors in cultured hippocampal neurons. *Proceedings of the National Academy of Sciences USA* 90:11688–11692.

Lester, H. A. 1992. The permeation pathway of neurotransmitter-gated ion channels. *Annual Review of Biophysics and Biomolecular Structure* 21:267–292.

Lester, H. A., Mager, S., Quick, M. W., and Corey, J. L. 1994. The permeation properties of neurotransmitter transporters. *Annual Review of Pharmacology and Toxicology* 34:219–249.

Lester, R. A. J., Clements, J. D., Westbrook, G. L., and Jahr, C. E. 1990. Channel kinetics determine the time course of NMDA receptor-mediated synaptic currents. *Nature* 346:565–567.

Lester, R. A. J., and Dani, J. A. 1995. Acetylcholine receptor desensitization induced by nicotine in rat medial habenula neurons. *Journal of Neurophysiology* 74:195–206.

Lester, R. A. J., and Jahr, C. E. 1992. NMDA channel behavior depends on agonist affinity. *Journal of Neuroscience* 12:635–643.

Lindstrom, J. M. 1995. Nicotinic acetylcholine receptors. In *Ligand- and Voltage-Gated Ion Channels,* ed. R. A. North, pp. 153–175. Boca Raton, FL: CRC Press.

Lingle, C. J., Maconochie, D., and Steinbach, J. H. 1992. Activation of skeletal muscle nicotinic acetylcholine receptors. *Journal of Membrane Biology* 126:195–217.

Lingueglia, E., Champigny, G., Lazdunski, M., and Barbry, P. 1995. Cloning of the amiloride-sensitive FMRFamide peptide-gated sodium channel. *Nature* 378:730–733.

Lipton, S. A., Aizenman, E., and Loring, R. H. 1987. Neuronal nicotinic acetylcholine responses in solitary mammalian retinal ganglion cells. *Pflügers Archiv* 410:37–43.

Lomeli, H., Mosbacher, J., Melcher, T., Höger, T., Geiger, J. R. P., Kuner, T., Monyer, H., Higuchi, M., Bach, A., and Seeburg, P. H. 1994. Control of kinetic properties of AMPA receptor channels by nuclear RNA editing. *Science* 266:1709–1713.

Lukasiewicz, P. D., and Roeder, R. C. 1995. Evidence for glycine modulation of excitatory synaptic inputs to retinal ganglion cells. *Journal of Neuroscience* 15:4592–4601.

Magleby, K. L., and Stevens, C. F. 1972. The effect of voltage on the time course of end-plate currents. *Journal of Physiology* 223:151–171.

Masland, R. H. 1988. Amacrine cells. *Trends in Neurosciences* 11:405–10.

Mathie, A., Colquhoun, D., and Cull-Candy, S. G. 1990. Rectification of currents activated by nicotinic acetylcholine receptors in rat sympathetic ganglion neurones. *Journal of Physiology* 427:625–655.

McBain, C. J., and Mayer, M. L. 1994. N-methyl-D-aspartatic acid receptor structure and function. *Physiological Reviews* 74:723–760.

McGehee, D. S., and Role, L. W. 1995. Physiological diversity of nicotinic acetylcholine receptors expressed by vertebrate neurons. *Annual Review of Physiology* 57:521–546.

McGehee, D. S., Heath, M. J. S., Gelber, S., Devay, P., and Role, L. W. 1995. Nicotine enhancement of fast excitatory synaptic transmission in CNS by presynaptic receptors. *Science* 269:1692–1696.

Meguro, H., Mori, H., Araki, K., Kushiya, E., Kutsuwada, T., Yamazaki, M., Kumanishi, T., Arakawa, M., Sakimura, K., and Mishina, M. 1992. Functional characterization of a heteromeric NMDA receptor channel expressed from cloned cDNAs. *Nature* 357:70–74.

Melcher, T., Maas, S., Herb, A., Sprengel, R., Seeburg, P. H., and Higuchi, M. 1996. A mammalian RNA editing enzyme. *Nature* 379:460–464.

Melcher, T., Maas, S., Higuchi, M., Keller, W., and Seeburg, P. H. 1995. Editing of α-amino-3-hydroxy-5-methylisoxazole-4-propionic acid receptor GluR-B pre-mRNA *in vitro* reveals site-selective adenosine to inosine conversion. *Journal of Biological Chemistry* 270:8566–8570.

Mishina, M., Takai, T., Imoto, K., Noda, M., Takahashi, T., Numa, S., Methfessel, C., and Sakmann, B. 1986. Molecular distinction between fetal and adult forms of muscle acetylcholine receptor. *Nature* 321:406–411.

Monyer, H., Burnashev, N., Laurie, D. J., Sakmann, B., and Seeburg, P. H. 1994. Developmental and regional expression in the rat brain and functional properties of four NMDA receptors. *Neuron* 12:529–540.

Monyer, H., Sprengel, R., Schoepfer, R., Herb, A., Higuchi, M., Lomeli, H., Burnashev, N. Sakmann, B., and Seeburg, P. H. 1992. Heteromeric NMDA receptors: Molecular and functional distinction of subtypes. *Science* 256:1217–1221.

Moriyoshi, K., Masu, M., Ishii, T., Shigemoto, R., Mizuno, N., and

Nakanishi, S. 1991. Molecular cloning and characterization of the rat NMDA receptor. *Nature* 354:31–37.

Mosbacher, J., Schoepfer, R., Monyer, H., Burnashev, N., Seeburg, P. H., and Ruppersberg, J. P. 1994. A molecular determinant for submillisecond desensitization in glutamate receptors. *Science* 266:1059–1062.

Neher, E., and Sakmann, B. 1976. Single-channel currents recorded from membrane of denervated frog muscle fibers. *Nature* 260:799–802.

Neher, E., and Stevens, C. F. 1977. Conductance fluctuations and ionic pores in membranes. *Annual Review of Biophysics and Bioengineering* 6:345–381.

Ortells, M. O., and Lunt, G. G. 1995. Evolutionary history of the ligand-gated ion-channel superfamily of receptors. *Trends in Neurosciences* 18:121–127.

Otis, T. S., Wu, Y.-C., and Trussell, L. O. 1996. Delayed clearance of transmitter and the role of glutamate transporters at synapses with multiple release sites. *Journal of Neuroscience* 16:1634–1644.

Otis, T. S., Zhang, S., and Trussell, L. O. 1996. Direct measurement of AMPA receptor desensitization induced by glutamatergic synaptic transmission. *Journal of Neuroscience* 16:7496–7504.

Ozawa, S., and Rossier, J. 1996. Molecular basis for functional differences of AMPA-subtype glutamate receptors. *News in Physiological Science* 11:77–82.

Pan, Z. Z., Tong, G., and Jahr, C. E. 1993. A false transmitter at excitatory synapses. *Neuron* 11:85–91.

Partin, D. M., Patneau, D. K., Winters, C. A., Mayer, M. L., and Buonanno, A. 1993. Selective modulation of desensitization at AMPA versus kainate receptors by cyclothiazide and concanavalin A. *Neuron* 11:1069–1082.

Paternain, A. V., Morales, M., and Lerma, J. 1995. Selective antagonism of AMPA receptors unmasks kainate receptor-mediated responses in hippocampal neurons. *Neuron* 14:185–189.

Patneau, D. K., and Mayer, M. L. 1991. Kinetic analysis of interactions between kainate and AMPA: Evidence for activation of a single receptor in mouse hippocampal neurons. *Neuron* 6:785–798.

Patrick, J., Boulter, J., Goldman, D., Gardner, P., and Heinemann, S. 1987. Molecular biology of nicotinic acetylcholine receptors. *Annals of the New York Academy of Sciences* 505:194–207.

Peters, S., Koh, J., and Choi, D. W. 1987. Zinc selectively blocks the action of N-methyl-D-aspartate on cortical neurons. *Science* 236:589–593.

Picciotto, M. R., Zoli, M., Léna, C., Bessis, A., Lallemand, Y., LeNovèra, N., Vincent, P., Pich, E. M., Brûlet, P., and Changeux, J.-P. 1995. Abnormal avoidance learning in mice lacking functional high-affinity nicotine receptor in the brain. *Nature* 374:65–67.

Puchalski, R. B., Louis, J.-C., Brose, N., Traynelis, S. F., Egebjerg, J., Kukekov, V., Wenthold, R. J., Rogers, S. W., Lin, F., Moran, T., Morrison, J. H., and Heinemann, S. F. 1994. Selective RNA editing and subunit assembly of native glutamate receptors. *Neuron* 13:131–147.

Ramirez-Latorre, J., Yu, C. R., Qu, X., Perin, F., Karlin, A., and Role, L. 1996. Functional contributions of $\alpha5$ subunit to neuronal acetylcholine receptor channels. *Nature* 380:347–351.

Rodríguez-Moreno, A., Herreras, O., and Lerma, J. 1997. Kainate receptors presynaptically downregulate GABAergic inhibition in the rat hippocampus. *Neuron* 19:893–901.

Role, L. W., and Berg, D. K. 1996. Nicotinic receptors in the development and modulation of CNS synapses. *Neuron* 16:1077–1085.

Rueter, S. M., Burns, C. M., Coode, S. A., Mookherjee, P., and Emeson, R. B. 1995. Glutamate receptor RNA editing *in vitro* by enzymatic conversion of adenosine to inosine. *Science* 267:1491–1494.

Sachs, F. 1983. Is the acetylcholine receptor a unit-conductance channel? In *Single-Channel Recording,* ed. B. Sakmann and E. Neher, pp. 365–376. New York: Plenum Press.

Sands, S. B., and Barish, M. E. 1992. Neuronal nicotinic acetylcholine receptor currents in phaeochromocytoma (PC12) cells: Dual mechanisms of rectification. *Journal of Physiology* 447:467–487.

Sargent, P. B. 1993. The diversity of neuronal nicotinic acetylcholine receptors. *Annual Review of Neuroscience* 16:403–443.

Seeburg, P. H. 1996. The role of RNA editing in controlling glutamate receptor channel properties. *Journal of Neurochemistry* 66:1–5.

Séguéla, P., Haghighi, A., Soghomonian, J.-J., and Cooper, E. 1996. A novel neuronal P_{2X} ATP receptor ion channel with widespread distribution in the brain. *Journal of Neuroscience* 16:448–455.

Séguéla, P., Wadiche, J., Dineley-Miller, K., Dani, J. A., and Patrick, J. W. 1993. Molecular cloning, functional properties, and distribution of rat brain α_7: A nicotinic cation channel highly permeable to calcium. *Journal of Neuroscience* 13:596–604.

Silver, R. A., Colquhoun, D., Cull-Candy, S. G., and Edmonds, B. 1996. Deactivation and desensitization of non-NMDA receptors in patches and the time course of EPSCs in rat cerebellar granule cells. *Journal of Physiology* 493:167–173.

Simpson, L., and Emeson, R. B. 1996. RNA editing. *Annual Review of Neuroscience* 19:27–52.

Sivilotti, L., and Colquhoun, D. 1995. Acetylcholine receptors: Too many channels, too few functions. *Science* 269:1681–1682.

Sommer, B., Keinänen, K., Verdoorn, T. A., Wisden, W., Burnashev, N., Herb, A., Köhler, M., Takagi, T., Sakmann, B., and Seeburg, P. H. 1990. Flip and flop: A cell-specific functional switch in glutamate-operated channels of the CNS. *Science* 249:1580–1585.

Sommer, B., Köhler, M., Sprengel, R., and Seeburg, P. H. 1991. RNA editing in brain controls a determinant of ion flow in glutamate-gated channels. *Cell* 67:11–19.

Soto, F., Garcia-Guzman, M., Gomez-Hernandez, J. M., Hollmann, M., Karschin, C., and Stühmer, W. 1996. P2X$_4$: An ATP-activated ionotropic receptor cloned from rat brain. *Proceedings of the National Academy of Sciences USA* 93:3684–3688.

Sprengel, R., and Seeburg, P. H. 1995. Ionotropic glutamate receptors. In *Ligand- and Voltage-Gated Ion Channels,* ed. R. A. North, pp. 213–263. Boca Raton, FL: CRC Press.

Steinlein, O. K., Mulley, J. C., Propping, P., Wallace, R. H., Phillips, H. A., Sutherland, G. R., Scheffer, I. E., and Berkovic, S. F. 1995. A missense mutation in the neuronal nicotinic acetylcholine receptor α4 subunit is associated with autosomal dominant nocturnal frontal lobe epilepsy. *Nature Genetics* 11:201–203.

Stroud, R. M., McCarthy, M. P., and Shuster, M. 1990. Nicotinic acetylcholine receptor superfamily of ligand-gated ion channels. *Biochemistry* 29:11009–11023.

Sucher, N. J., and Deitcher, D. L. 1995. PCR and patch-clamp analysis of single neurons. *Neuron* 14:1095–1100.

Supplisson, S., and Bergman, C. 1997. Control of NMDA receptor activation by a glycine transporter co-expressed in *Xenopus* oocytes. *Journal of Neuroscience* 17:4580–4590.

Surprenant, A., Buell, G., and North, R. A. 1995. P$_{2X}$ receptors bring new structure to ligand-gated ion channels. *Trends in Neurosciences* 18:224–229.

Swanson, G. T., Feldmeyer, D., Kaneda, M., and Cull-Candy, S. G. 1996. Effect of RNA editing and subunit co-assembly on single-channel properties of recombinant kainate receptors. *Journal of Physiology* 492:129–142.

Takeuchi, N. 1963. Effects of calcium on the conductance change of the end-plate membrane during the action of transmitter. *Journal of Physiology* 167:141–155.

Takeuchi, A., and Takeuchi, N. 1959. Active phase of frog's end-plate potential. *Journal of Neurophysiology* 22:395–411.

——— 1960. On the permeability of end-plate membrane during the action of transmitter. *Journal of Physiology* 154:52–67.

Trussell, L. O., and Fischbach, G. D. 1989. Glutamate receptor desensitization and its role in synaptic transmission. *Neuron* 3:209–218.

Unwin, N. 1993a. Nicotinic acetylcholine receptor at 9 Å resolution. *Journal of Molecular Biology* 229:1101–1124.

——— 1993b. Neurotransmitter action: Opening of ligand-gated ion channels. *Neuron* 10 (supplement):31–41.

——— 1995. Acetylcholine receptor channel imaged in the open state. *Nature* 373:37–43.

Verdoorn, T. A., Burnashev, N., Monyer, H., Seeburg, P. H., and Sakmann, B. 1991. Structural determinants of ion flow through recombinant glutamate receptor channels. *Science* 252:1715–1718.

Vernallis, A. B., Conroy, W. G., and Berg, D. K. 1993. Neurons assemble acetylcholine receptors with as many as three kinds of subunits while maintaining subunit segregation among receptor subtypes. *Neuron* 10:451–464.

Vidal, C., and Changeux, J.-P. 1996. Neuronal nicotinic acetylcholine receptors in the brain. *News in Physiological Science* 11:202–208.

Vignes, M., and Collingridge, G. L. 1997. The synaptic activation of kainate receptors. *Nature* 388:179–182.

Villarroel, A., Herlitze, S., Witzemann, V., Könen, M., and Sakmann, B. 1992. Asymmetry of the rat acetylcholine receptor subunits in the narrow region of the pore. *Proceedings of the Royal Society of London B* 249:317–324.

Westbrook, G. L., and Mayer, M. L. 1987. Micromolar concentrations of Zn^{2+} antagonize NMDA and GABA responses of hippocampal neurons. *Nature* 328:640–643.

Whiting, P., and Lindstrom, J. 1987. Purification and characterization of nicotinic acetylcholine receptor from rat brain. *Proceedings of the National Academy of Sciences USA* 84:595–599.

Wilding, T. J., and Huettner, J. E. 1995. Differential antagonism of alpha-amino-3-hydroxy-5-methyl-4-isoxazolepropionic acid-preferring and kainate-preferring receptors by 2,3-benzodiazepines. *Molecular Pharmacology* 3:582–587.

——— 1997. Activation and desensitization of hippocampal kainate receptors. *Journal of Neuroscience* 17:2713–2721.

Wo, Z. G., and Oswald, R. E. 1994. Transmembrane topology of two kainate receptor subunits revealed by N-glycosylation. *Proceedings of the National Academy of Sciences USA* 91:7154–7158.

Wollmuth, L. P., Kuner, T., Seeburg, P. H., and Sakmann, B. 1996. Differential contribution of the NR1- and NR2A-subunits to the selectivity filter of recombinant NMDA receptor channels. *Journal of Physiology* 491:779–797.

Wonnacott, S. 1997. Presynaptic nicotinic ACh receptors. *Trends in Neurosciences* 20:92–98.

Wonnacott, S., Drasdo, A., Sanderson, E., and Rowell, P. 1990. Presynaptic nicotinic receptors and the modulation of transmitter release. In *The Biology of Nicotine Dependence: Ciba Foundation Symposium 152,* ed. G. Bock and J. Marsh, pp. 87–105. New York: Wiley.

Yang, J.-H., Sklar, P., Axel, R., and Maniatis, T. 1995. Editing of glutamate receptor subunit B pre-mRNA *in vitro* by site-specific deamination of adenosine. *Nature* 374:77–81.

Yazejian, B., and Fain, G. L. 1993. Whole-cell currents activated at nicotinic acetylcholine receptors on ganglion cells isolated from goldfish retina. *Visual Neuroscience* 10:353–361.

Zhang, Z.-W., Coggan, J. S., and Berg, D. K. 1996. Synaptic currents generated by neuronal acetylcholine receptors sensitive to α-bungarotoxin. *Neuron* 17:1231–1240.

Zhang, Z-W., Vijayaraghavan, S., and Berg, D. K. 1994. Neuronal acetylcholine receptors that bind α-bungarotoxin with high affinity function as ligand-gated ion channels. *Neuron* 12:167–177.

Zorumski, C. F., Yamada, K. A., Price, M. T., and Olney, J. W. 1993. A benzodiazepine recognition site associated with the non-NMDA glutamate receptor. *Neuron* 10:61–67.

Zukin, R. S., and Bennett, M. V. L. 1995. Alternatively spliced isoforms of the NMDAR1 receptor subunit. *Trends in Neurosciences* 18:306–313.

10. Inhibitory Transmission

Adams, P. R., and Brown, D. A. 1975. Actions of γ-aminobutyric acid on sympathetic ganglion cells. *Journal of Physiology* 250:85–120.

Akabas, M. H., Kaufmann, C., Archdeacon, P., and Karlin, P. 1994. Identification of acetylcholine receptor channel-lining residues in the entire M2 segment of the α subunit. *Neuron* 13:919–927.

Alger, B. E., and Nicoll, R. A. 1982. Pharmacological evidence for two kinds of GABA receptor on rat hippocampal pyramidal cells studied *in vitro.* *Journal of Physiology* 328:125–141.

Amin, J., and Weiss, D. S. 1993. $GABA_A$ receptor needs two homologous domains of the β-subunit for activation by GABA but not by pentobarbital. *Nature* 366:565–569.

Bormann, J., Hamill, O. P., and Sakmann, B. 1987. Mechanism of anion permeation through channels gated by glycine and γ-aminobutyric acid in mouse cultured spinal neurones. *Journal of Physiology* 385:243–286.

Bormann, J., Runström, N., Betz, H., and Langosch, D. 1993. Residues within transmembrane segment M2 determine chloride conductance of glycine receptor homo- and hetero-oligomers. *EMBO Journal* 12:3729–3737.

Borst, J. G. G., Lodder, J. C., and Kits, K. S. 1994. Large amplitude variability of GABAergic IPSCs in melanotropes from *Xenopus laevis:* Evidence that quantal size differs between synapses. *Journal of Neurophysiology* 71:639–655.

Chang, Y., Wang, R., Barot, S., and Weiss, D. S. 1996. Stoichiometry of a recombinant GABA$_A$ receptor. *Journal of Neuroscience* 16:5415–5424.

Clements, J. D. 1996. Transmitter timecourse in the synaptic cleft: Its role in central synaptic function. *Trends in Neurosciences* 19:163–171.

Cohen, B. N., Fain, G. L., and Fain, M. J. 1989. GABA and glycine channels in isolated ganglion cells from goldfish retina. *Journal of Physiology* 418:53–82.

Davies, P. A., Hanna, M. C., Hales, T. G., and Kirkness, E. F. 1997. Insensitivity to anaesthetic agents conferred by a class of GABA$_A$ receptor subunit. *Nature* 385:820–823.

DeKoninck, Y., and Mody, I. 1994. Noise analysis of miniature IPSCs in adult rat brain slices: Properties and modulation of synaptic GABA$_A$ receptor channels. *Journal of Neurophysiology* 71:1318–1335.

Dudel, J., and Kuffler, S. W. 1961. Presynaptic inhibition at the crayfish neuromuscular junction. *Journal of Physiology* 155:543–562.

Ebihara, S., Shirato, K., Harata, N., and Akaike, N. 1995. Gramicidin-perforated patch recording: GABA response in mammalian neurones with intact intracellular chloride. *Journal of Physiology* 484:77–86.

Eccles, J. C. 1964. *The Physiology of Synapses.* New York: Springer-Verlag.

Eghbali, M., Curmi, J. P., Birnir, B., and Gage, P. W. 1997. Hippocampal GABA$_A$ channel conductance increased by diazepam. *Nature* 388:71–75.

Feigenspan, A., Wässle, H., and Bormann, J. 1993. Pharmacology of GABA receptor Cl$^-$ channels in rat retinal bipolar cells. *Nature* 361:159–162.

ffrench-Constant, R. H., Rocheleau, T. A., Steichen, J. C., and Chalmers, A. E. 1993. A point mutation in a *Drosophila* GABA receptor confers insecticide resistance. *Nature* 363:449–451.

Franks, N. P., and Lieb, W. R. 1994. Molecular and cellular mechanisms of general anaesthesia. *Nature* 367:607–614.

Frerking, M., Borges, S., and Wilson, M. 1995. Variation in GABA mini amplitude is the consequence of variation in transmitter concentration. *Neuron* 15:885–895.

Galzi, J.-L., Devillers-Thiéry, A., Hussy, N., Bertrand, S., Changeux, J.-P., and Bertrand, D. 1992. Mutations in the channel domain of a neuronal nicotinic receptor convert ion selectivity from cationic to anionic. *Nature* 359:500–505.

Gingrich, K. J., Roberts, W. A., and Kass, R. S. 1995. Dependence of the GABA$_A$ receptor gating kinetics on the α-subunit isoform: Implications for structure-function relations and synaptic transmission. *Journal of Physiology* 489:529–543.

Grenningloh, G., Rienitz, A., Schmitt, B., Methfessel, C., Zensen, M., Beyreuther, K., Gundelfinger, E., and Betz, H. 1987. The strychnine-binding subunit of the glycine receptor shows homology with nicotinic acetylcholine receptors. *Nature* 328:215–220.

Hamill, O. P., and Sakmann, B. 1981. Multiple conductance states of single acetylcholine receptor channels in embryonic muscle cells. *Nature* 294:462–466.

Jackson, M. B., and Zhang, S. J. 1995. Action potential propagation and propagation block by GABA in rat posterior pituitary nerve terminals. *Journal of Physiology* 483:597–611.

Jones, M. V., and Westbrook, G. L. 1995. Desensitized states prolong $GABA_A$ channel responses to brief agonist pulses. *Neuron* 15:181–191.

Kaila, K., and Voipio, J. 1990. GABA-activated bicarbonate conductance: Influence on E_{GABA} and on postsynaptic pH regulation. In *Chloride Channels and Carriers in Nerve, Muscle, and Glial Cells,* ed. F. J. Alvarez-Leefmans and J. M. Russell, pp. 331–352. New York: Plenum.

Kirsch, J., Wolters, I., Triller, A., and Betz, H. 1993. Gephyrin antisense oligonucleotides prevent glycine receptor clustering in spinal neurons. *Nature* 366:745–748.

Kuhse, J., Betz, H., and Kirsch, J. 1995. The inhibitory glycine receptor: Architecture, synaptic localization, and molecular pathology of a postsynaptic ion-channel complex. *Current Opinion in Neurobiology* 5:318–323.

Kuhse, J., Laube, B., Magalei, D., and Betz, H. 1993. Assembly of the inhibitory glycine receptor: Identification of amino acid sequence motifs governing subunit stoichiometry. *Neuron* 11:1049–1056.

Langosch, D. 1995. Inhibitory glycine receptors. In *Ligand- and Voltage-Gated Ion Channels,* ed. R. A. North, pp. 291–305. Boca Raton, FL: CRC Press.

Langosch, D., Thomas, L., and Betz, H. 1988. Conserved quaternary structure of ligand-gated ion channels: The postsynaptic glycine receptor is a pentamer. *Proceedings of the National Academy of Sciences USA* 85:7394–7398.

Lester, R. A. J., and Jahr, C. E. 1992. NMDA channel behavior depends on agonist affinity. *Journal of Neuroscience* 12:635–643.

Lüddens, H., Korpi, E. R., and Seeburg, P. H. 1995. $GABA_A$/benzodiazepine receptor heterogeneity: Neurophysiological implications. *Neuropharmacology* 34:245–254.

Lukasiewicz, P. D., Maple, B. R., and Werblin, F. S. 1994. A novel GABA receptor on bipolar cell terminals in the tiger salamander retina. *Journal of Neuroscience* 14:1202–1212.

Macdonald, R. L., and Olsen, R. W. 1994. GABA$_A$ receptor channels. *Annual Review of Neuroscience* 17:569–602.

Macdonald, R. L., Rogers, C. J., and Twyman, R. E. 1989a. Barbiturate regulation of kinetic properties of the GABA$_A$ receptor channel of mouse spinal neurones in culture. *Journal of Physiology* 417:483–500.

———— 1989b. Kinetic properties of the GABA$_A$ receptor main conductance state of mouse spinal cord neurones in culture. *Journal of Physiology* 410:479–499.

MacInnes, D. A. 1961. *The Principles of Electrochemistry.* New York: Dover.

MacNeil, M. A., and Masland, R. H. 1998. Extreme diversity among amacrine cells: Implications for function. *Neuron* 20:971–982.

Maconochie, D. J., and Knight, D. E. 1989. A method for making solution changes in the sub-millisecond range at the tip of a patch pipette. *Pflügers Archiv* 414:589–596.

Maconochie, D. J., Zempel, J. M., and Steinbach, J. H. 1994. How quickly can GABA$_A$ receptors open? *Neuron* 12:61–71.

McKernan, R. M., and Whiting, P. J. 1996. Which GABA$_A$-receptor subtypes really occur in brain? *Trends in Neurosciences* 19:139–143.

Mody, I., DeKoninck, Y., Otis, T. S., and Soltesz, I. 1994. Bridging the cleft at GABA synapses in the brain. *Trends in Neurosciences* 17:517–525.

Newland, C. F., and Cull-Candy, S. G. 1992. On the mechanism of action of picrotoxin on GABA receptor channels in dissociated sympathetic neurones of the rat. *Journal of Physiology* 447:191–213.

Nicoll, R. A. 1988. The coupling of neurotransmitter receptors to ion channels in the brain. *Science* 241:545–551.

Ortells, M. O., and Lunt, G. G. 1995. Evolutionary history of the ligand-gated ion-channel superfamily of receptors. *Trends in Neurosciences* 18:121–127.

Pritchett, D. B., and Seeburg, P. H. 1991. γ-Aminobutyric acid type A receptor point mutation increases the affinity of compounds for the benzodiazepine site. *Proceedings of the National Academy of Sciences USA* 88:1421–1425.

Pritchett, D. B., Sontheimer, H., Shivers, B. D., Ymer, S., Kettenmann, H., Schofield, P. R., and Seeburg, P. H. 1989. Importance of a novel GABA$_A$ receptor subunit for benzodiazepine pharmacology. *Nature* 338:582–585.

Puia, G., Costa, E., and Vicini, S. 1994. Functional diversity of GABA-activated Cl$^-$ currents in Purkinje versus granule neurons in rat cerebellar slices. *Neuron* 12:117–126.

Qian, H., and Dowling, J. E. 1993. Novel GABA responses from rod-driven retinal horizontal cells. *Nature* 361:162–164.

——— 1994. Pharmacology of novel GABA receptors found on rod horizontal cells of the white perch retina. *Journal of Neuroscience* 14:4299–4307.

Rogers, C. J., Twyman, R. E., and Macdonald, R. L. 1994. Benzodiazepine and β-carboline regulation of single GABA_A receptor channels of mouse spinal neurones in culture. *Journal of Physiology* 475:69–82.

Saxena, N. C., and Macdonald, R. L. 1994. Assembly of GABA_A receptor subunits: Role of the δ subunit. *Journal of Neuroscience* 14:7077–7086.

Schmieden, V., Kuhse, J., and Betz, H. 1993. Mutation of glycine receptor subunit creates β-alanine receptor responsive to GABA. *Science* 262:256–258.

Schofield, P. R., Darlison, M. G., Fujita, N., Burt, D. R., Stephenson, F. A., Rodriguez, H., Rhee, L. M., Ramachandran, J., Reale, V., Glencorse, T. A., Seeburg, P. H., and Barnard, E. A. 1987. Sequence and functional expression of the GABA_A receptor shows a ligand-gated receptor super-family. *Nature* 328:221–227.

Shimada, S., Cutting, G. R., and Uhl, G. R. 1992. γ-Aminobutyric acid A or C receptor? γ-Aminobutyric acid rho 1 receptor RNA induces bicuculline-, barbiturate-, and benzodiazepine-insensitive γ-aminobutyric acid responses in *Xenopus* oocytes. *Molecular Pharmacology* 41:683–687.

Sieghart, W. 1995. Structure and pharmacology of γ-aminobutyric acid_A receptor subtypes. *Pharmacological Reviews* 47:181–234.

Smith, G. B., and Olsen, R. W. 1994. Identification of a [³H]muscimol photoaffinity substrate in the bovine γ-aminobutyric acid_A receptor α subunit. *Journal of Biological Chemistry* 269:20380–20387.

——— 1995. Functional domains of GABA_A receptors. *Trends in Pharmacological Sciences* 16:162–168.

Stryer, L. 1995. *Biochemistry,* 4th ed. New York: W. H. Freeman.

Tretter, V., Ehya, N., Fuchs, K., and Sieghart, W. 1997. Stoichiometry and assembly of a recombinant GABA_A receptor subtype. *Journal of Neuroscience* 17:2728–2737.

Twyman, R. E., Rogers, C. J., and Macdonald, R. L. 1990. Intraburst kinetic properties of the GABA_A receptor main conductance state of mouse spinal cord neurones in culture. *Journal of Physiology* 423:193–220.

Tyndale, R. F., Olsen, R. W., and Tobin, A. J. 1995. GABA_A receptors. In *Ligand- and Voltage-Gated Ion Channels,* ed. R. A. North, pp. 265–290. Boca Raton, FL: CRC Press.

Verdoorn, T. A. 1994. Formation of heteromeric γ-aminobutyric acid type A receptors containing two different α subunits. *Molecular Pharmacology* 45:475–480.

Wang, T.-L., Guggino, W. B., and Cutting, G. R. 1994. A novel γ-aminobutyric acid receptor subunit (ρ_2) cloned from human retina forms bicuculline-insensitive homooligomeric receptors in *Xenopus* oocytes. *Journal of Neuroscience* 14:6524–6531.

Weiss, D. S., and Magleby, K. L. 1989. Gating scheme for single GABA-activated Cl$^-$ channels determined from stability plots, dwell-time distributions, and adjacent-interval durations. *Journal of Neuroscience* 9:1314–1324.

Whiting, P. J., McKernan, R. M., and Wafford, K. A. 1995. Structure and pharmacology of vertebrate GABA$_A$ receptor subtypes. *International Review of Neurobiology* 38:95–138.

Xu, M., and Akabas, M. H. 1996. Identification of the channel-lining residues in the M2 membrane-spanning segment of the GABA$_A$ receptor α1 subunit. *Journal of General Physiology* 107:195–205.

Xu, M., Covey, D. F., and Akabas, M. H. 1995. Interaction of picrotoxin with GABA$_A$ receptor channel-lining residues probed in cysteine mutants. *Biophysical Journal* 69:1858–1867.

Yoon, K.-W., Covey, D. F., and Rothman, S. M. 1993. Multiple mechanisms of picrotoxin block of GABA-induced currents in rat hippocampal neurons. *Journal of Physiology* 464:423–439.

Zhang, H.-G., ffrench-Constant, R. H., and Jackson, M. B. 1994. A unique amino acid of the *Drosophila* GABA receptor with influence on drug sensitivity by two mechanisms. *Journal of Physiology* 479:65–75.

Zhang, S. J., and Jackson, M. B. 1993. GABA-activated chloride channels in secretory nerve endings. *Science* 259:531–534.

——— 1995. GABA$_A$ receptor activation and the excitability of nerve terminals in the rat posterior pituitary. *Journal of Physiology* 483:583–595.

11. Receptors and G Proteins

Baldwin, J. M. 1994. Structure and function of receptors coupled to G proteins. *Current Opinion in Cell Biology* 6:180–190.

Baude, A., Nusser, Z., Roberts, J. D. B., Mulvihill, E., McIlhinney, R. A. J., and Somogyi, P. 1993. The metabotropic glutamate receptor (mGluR1α) is concentrated at perisynaptic membrane of neuronal subpopulations as detected by immunogold reaction. *Neuron* 11:771–787.

Berman, D. M., Kozasa, T., and Gilman, A. G. 1996. The GTPase-activating protein RGS4 stabilizes the transition state for nucleotide hydrolysis. *Journal of Biological Chemistry* 271:27209–27212.

Berman, D. M., Wilkie, T. M., and Gilman, A. G. 1996. GAIP and RGS4 are GTPase-activating proteins for the Gi subfamily of G protein alpha subunits. *Cell* 86:445–452.

Biddlecome, G. H., Berstein, G., and Ross, E. M. 1996. Regulation of phospholipase C-β1 by G_q and m1 muscarinic cholinergic receptor. *Journal of Biological Chemistry* 271:7999–8007.

Birnbaumer, L., and Birnbaumer, M. 1994. G proteins in signal transduction. In *Handbook of Biomembranes,* vol. 3, ed. M. Shinitzky, pp. 153–252. Rehovoth, Israel: Balaban Publishers.

Bourne, H. R. 1995. GTPases: A family of molecular switches and clocks. *Philosophical Transactions of the Royal Society of London B* 349:283–289.

Braun, A. P., and Schulman, H. 1995. The multifunctional calcium/calmodulin-dependent protein kinase: From form to function. *Annual Review of Physiology* 57:417–445.

Brown, E. M., Gamba, G., Riccardi, D., Lombardi, M., Butters, R., Kifor, O., Sun, A., Hediger, M. A., Lytton, J., and Hebert, S. C. 1993. Cloning and characterization of an extracellular Ca^{2+}-sensing receptor from bovine parathyroid. *Nature* 366: 575–580.

Campbell, V., Berrow, N., and Dolphin, A. C. 1993. $GABA_B$ receptor modulation of Ca^{2+} currents in rat sensory neurones by the G protein G_o: Antisense oligonucleotide studies. *Journal of Physiology* 470:1–11.

Clapham, D. E. 1994. Direct G protein activation of ion channels? *Annual Review of Neuroscience* 17:441–464.

Clapham, D. E., and Neer, E. J. 1993. New roles for G-protein βγ-dimers in transmembrane signaling. *Nature* 365:403–406.

Conklin, B. R., and Bourne, H. R. 1993. Structural elements of $G_α$ subunits that interact with $G_{βγ}$, receptors, and effectors. *Cell* 73:631–641.

Conklin, B. R., Farfel, Z., Lustig, K. D., Julius, D., and Bourne, H. R. 1993. Substitution of three amino acids switches receptor specificity of $G_qα$ to that of $G_iα$. *Nature* 363:274–276

Conn, P. J., and Patel, J. (eds.). 1994. *The Metabotropic Glutamate Receptors.* Totowa, NJ: Humana Press.

Farahbakhsh, Z. T., Hideg, K., and Hubbell, W. L. 1993. Photoactivated conformational changes in rhodopsin: A time-resolved spin label study. *Science* 262:1416–1419.

Farrens, D. L., Altenbach, C., Yang, K., Hubbell, W. L., and Khorana, H. G. 1996. Requirement of rigid-body motion of transmembrane helices for light activation of rhodopsin. *Science* 274:768–770.

Finkbeiner, S., and Greenberg, M. E. 1996. Ca^{2+}-dependent routes to Ras: Mechanisms for neuronal survival, differentiation, and plasticity? *Neuron* 16:233–236.

Freedman, N. J., and Lefkowitz, R. J. 1996. Desensitization of G protein-coupled receptors. *Recent Progress in Hormone Research* 51:319–353.

Fung, B. K.-K., and Stryer, L. 1980. Photolyzed rhodopsin catalyzes the exchange of GTP for bound GDP in retinal rod outer segments. *Proceedings of the National Academy of Sciences USA* 77:2500–2504.

Gudermann, T., Schöneberg, T., and Schultz, G. 1997. Functional and structural complexity of signal transduction via G-protein-coupled receptors. *Annual Review of Neuroscience* 20:399–427.

Hamm, H. E., and Gilchrist, A. 1996. Heterotrimeric G proteins. *Current Opinion in Cell Biology* 8:189–196.

Holmes, T. C., Fadool, D. A., and Levitan, I. B. 1996. Tyrosine phosphorylation of the Kv1.3 potassium channel. *Journal of Neuroscience* 16:1581–1590.

Ito, H., Tung, R. T., Sugimoto, T., Kobayashi, I., Takahashi, K., Katada, T., Ui, M., and Kurachi, Y. 1992. On the mechanism of G protein $\beta\gamma$ subunit activation of the muscarinic K^+ channel in guinea pig atrial cell membrane: Comparison with the ATP-sensitive K^+ channel. *Journal of General Physiology* 99:961–983.

Jelsema, C. L., and Axelrod, J. 1987. Stimulation of phospholipase A_2 activity in bovine rod outer segments by the $\beta\gamma$ subunits of transducin and its inhibition by the α subunit. *Proceedings of the National Academy of Sciences USA* 84:3623–3627.

Jonas, E. A., Knox, R. J., Kaczmarek, L. K., Schwartz, J. H., and Solomon, D. H. 1996. Insulin receptor in *Aplysia* neurons: Characterization, molecular cloning, and modulation of ion currents. *Journal of Neuroscience* 16:1645–1658.

Kaupmann, K., Huggel, K., Heid, J., Flor, P. J., Bischoff, S., Mickel, S. J., McMaster, G., Angst, C., Bittiger, H., Fröstl, W., and Bettler, B. 1997. Expression cloning of $GABA_B$ receptors uncovers similarity to metabotropic glutamate receptors. *Nature* 386:239–246.

Kleuss, C., Hescheler, J., Ewel, C., Rosenthal, W., Schultz, G., and Wittig, B. 1991. Assignment of G-protein subtypes to specific receptors inducing inhibition of calcium currents. *Nature* 353:43–48.

Kleuss, C., Scherübl, H., Hescheler, J., Schultz, G., and Wittig, B. 1992. Different β-subunits determine G-protein interaction with transmembrane receptors. *Nature* 358:424–426.

—— 1993. Selectivity in signal transduction determined by γ subunits of heterotrimeric G proteins. *Science* 259:832–834.

Kobilka, B. 1992. Adrenergic receptors as models for G protein-coupled receptors. *Annual Review of Neuroscience* 15:87–114.

Liggett, S. B., and Lefkowitz, R. J. 1994. Adrenergic receptor-coupled adenylyl cyclase systems: Regulation of receptor function by phosphorylation, sequestration, and downregulation. In *Regulation of Cellular Signal Transduction Pathways by Desensitization and Amplification,* ed. D. R. Sibley and M. D. Houslay, pp. 71–97. New York: John Wiley.

Llinás, R., Moreno, H., Sugimori, M., Mohammadi, M., and Schlessinger, J. 1997. Differential pre- and postsynaptic modulation of chemical transmission in the squid giant synapse by tyrosine phosphorylation. *Proceedings of the National Academy of Sciences USA* 94:1990–1994.

Nakanishi, S. 1994. Metabotropic glutamate receptors: Synaptic transmission, modulation, and plasticity. *Neuron* 13:1031–1037.

Neer, E. J. 1995. Heterotrimeric G proteins: Organizers of transmembrane signals. *Cell* 80:249–257.

Nusser, Z., Mulvihill, E., Streit, P., and Somogyi, P. 1994. Subsynaptic segregation of metabotropic and ionotropic glutamate receptors as revealed by immunogold localization. *Neuroscience* 61:421–427.

O'Hara, P. J., Sheppard, P. O., Thøgersen, H., Venezia, D., Haldeman, B. A., McGrane, V., Houamed, K. M., Thomsen, C., Gilbert, T. L., and Mulvihill, E. R. 1993. The ligand-binding domain in metabotropic glutamate receptors is related to bacterial periplasmic binding proteins. *Neuron* 11:41–52.

Pepperl, D. J., and Regan, J. W. 1994. Adrenergic receptors. In *G Protein-Coupled Receptors,* ed. S. J. Peroutka, pp. 45–78. Boca Raton, FL: CRC Press.

Peroutka, S. J. (ed.). 1994. *G Protein-Coupled Receptors.* Boca Raton, FL: CRC Press.

Pin, J.-P., and Bockaert, 1995. Get receptive to metabotropic glutamate receptors. *Current Opinion in Neurobiology* 5:342–349.

Pin, J.-P., and Duvoisin, R. 1995. The metabotropic glutamate receptors: Structure and functions. *Neuropharmacology* 34:1–26.

Premont, R. T., Inglese, J., and Lefkowitz, R. J. 1995. Protein kinases that phosphorylate activated G protein-coupled receptors. *FASEB Journal* 9:175–182.

Sánchez-Prieto, J., Budd, D. C., Herrero, I., Vánquez, E., and Nicholls, D. G. 1996. Presynaptic receptors and the control of glutamate exocytosis. *Trends in Neurosciences* 19:235–239.

Schertler, G. F. X., Villa, C., and Henderson, R. 1993. Projection structure of rhodopsin. *Nature* 362:770–772.

Schreibmayer, W., Dessauer, C. W., Vorobiov, D., Gilman, A. G., Lester, H. A., Davidson, N., and Dascal, N. 1996. Inhibition of an inwardly rectifying K^+ channel by G-protein α-subunits. *Nature* 380:624–627.

Simon, M. I., Strathmann, M. P., and Gautam, N. 1991. Diversity of G proteins in signal transduction. *Science* 252:802–808.

Spiegel, A. M., Jones, T. L. Z., Simonds, W. F., and Weinstein, L. S. 1994. *G Proteins.* Austin, TX: R. G. Landes Company.

Sternweis, P. C. 1994. The active role of βγ in signal transduction. *Current Opinion in Cell Biology* 6:198–203.

Strader, C. D., Fong, T. M., Tota, M. R., and Underwood, D. 1994. Structure and function of G protein-coupled receptors. *Annual Review of Biochemistry* 63:101–132.

Streuli, M. 1996. Protein tyrosine phosphatases in signaling. *Current Opinion in Cell Biology* 8:182–188.

Takahashi, K., Tsuchida, K., Tanabe, Y., Masu, M., and Nakanishi, S. 1993. Role of the large extracellular domain of metabotropic glutamate receptors in agonist selectivity determination. *Journal of Biological Chemistry* 268:19341–19345.

Unger, V. M., Hargrave, P. A., Baldwin, J. M., and Schertler, G. F. X. 1997. Arrangement of rhodopsin and transmembrane α-helices. *Nature* 389:203–206.

Wang, Y. T., and Salter, M. W. 1994. Regulation of NMDA receptors by tyrosine kinases and phosphatases. *Nature* 369:233–235.

Watson, S., and Arkinstall, S. (eds.). 1994. *The G-Protein Linked Receptor Facts Book*. London: Academic Press.

Wedegaertner, P. B., Wilson, P. T., and Bourne, H. R. 1995. Lipid modification of trimeric G proteins. *Journal of Biological Chemistry* 270:503–506.

Wickman, K. D., and Clapham, D. E. 1995. G-protein regulation of ion channels. *Current Opinion in Neurobiology* 5:278–285.

Yuen, P. S. T., and Garbers, D. L. 1992. Guanylyl cyclase-linked receptors. *Annual Review of Neuroscience* 15:193–225.

12. Effector Molecules

Bean, B. P. 1989. Neurotransmitter inhibition of neuronal calcium currents by changes in channel voltage dependence. *Nature* 340:153–156.

Birnbaumer, L., and Birnbaumer, M. 1994. G proteins in signal transduction. In *Handbook of Biomembranes,* vol. 3, ed. M. Shinitzky, pp. 153–252. Rehovoth, Israel: Balaban Publishers.

Bourinet, E., Soong, T. W., Stea, A., and Snutch, T. P. 1996. Determinants of the G protein-dependent opioid modulation of neuronal calcium channels. *Proceedings of the National Academy of Sciences USA* 93:1486–1491.

Brown, A. M., Yatani, A., Imoto, Y., Kirsch, G., Hamm, H., Codina, J., Mattera, R., and Birnbaumer, L. 1988. Direct coupling of G proteins to ionic channels. *Cold Spring Harbor Symposia on Quantitative Biology* 53:365–373.

Browning, M. D., and Rogers, S. W. 1994. Ligand-gated ion channels: Molecular structure and functional regulation by phosphorylation. In *Regulation of Cellular Signal Transduction Pathways by Desensitization and*

Amplification, ed. D. R. Sibley and M. D. Houslay, pp. 307–339. New York: John Wiley.

Catterall, W. A. 1994. Modulation of sodium and calcium channels by protein phosphorylation. In *Regulation of Cellular Signal Transduction Pathways by Desensitization and Amplification,* ed. D. R. Sibley and M. D. Houslay, pp. 341–361. New York: John Wiley.

Clapham, D. E. 1994. Direct G protein activation of ion channels? *Annual Review of Neuroscience* 17:441–464.

Cooper, D. M. F., Mons, N., and Karpen, J. W. 1995. Adenylyl cyclases and the interaction between calcium and cAMP signalling. *Nature* 374:421–424.

Copenhagen, D. R., and Jahr, C. E. 1989. Release of endogenous excitatory amino acids from turtle photoreceptors. *Nature* 341:536–539.

Dascal, N., Schreibmayer, W., Lim, N. F., Wang, W., Chavkin, C., DiMagno, L., Labarca, C., Kieffer, B. L., Gaveriaux-Ruff, C., Trollinger, D., Lester, H. A., and Davidson, N. 1993. Atrial G protein-activated K^+ channel: Expression cloning and molecular properties. *Proceedings of the National Academy of Sciences USA* 90:10235–10239.

de la Villa, P., Kurahashi, T., and Kaneko, A. 1995. L-Glutamate-induced responses and cGMP-activated channels in three subtypes of retinal bipolar cells dissociated from the cat. *Journal of Neuroscience* 15:3571–3582.

Delcour, A. H., and Tsien, R. W. 1993. Altered prevalence of gating modes in neurotransmitter inhibition of N-type calcium channels. *Science* 259:980–984.

Divecha, N., and Irvine, R. F. 1995. Phospholipid signaling. *Cell* 80:269–278.

Dolphin, A. C. 1995. Voltage-dependent calcium channels and their modulation by neurotransmitters and G proteins. *Experimental Physiology* 80:1–36.

Doupnik, C. A., Davidson, N., and Lester, H. A. 1995. The inward rectifier potassium channel family. *Current Opinion in Neurobiology* 5:268–277.

Dowling, J. E. 1987. *The Retina: An Approachable Part of the Brain.* Cambridge, MA: Harvard University Press.

Dunwiddie, T. V., and Lovinger, D. M. (eds.). 1993. *Presynaptic Receptors in the Mammalian Brain.* Boston: Birkhäuser.

Exton, J. H. 1994a. Phosphatidylcholine breakdown and signal transduction. *Biochimica et Biophysica Acta* 1212:26–42.

———— 1994b. Phosphoinositide phospholipases and G proteins in hormone action. *Annual Review of Physiology* 56:349–369.

———— 1996. Regulation of phosphoinositide phospholipases by hormones, neurotransmitters, and other agonists linked to G proteins. *Annual Review of Pharmacology and Toxicology* 36:481–509.

Finn, J. T., Grunwald, M. W., and Yau, K.-W. 1996. Cyclic nucleotide-gated ion channels: An extended family with diverse functions. *Annual Review of Physiology* 58:395–426.

Francis, S. H., and Corbin, J. D. 1994. Structure and function of cyclic nucleotide-dependent protein kinases. *Annual Review of Physiology* 56:237–272.

Gershon, E., Weigl, L., Lotan, I., Schreibmayer, W., and Dascal, N. 1992. Protein kinase A reduces voltage-dependent Na$^+$ current in *Xenopus* oocytes. *Journal of Neuroscience* 12:3743–3752.

Gudermann, T., Schöneberg, T., and Schultz, G. 1997. Functional and structural complexity of signal transduction via G-protein-coupled receptors. *Annual Review of Neuroscience* 20:399–427.

Hannun, Y. A. 1994. The sphingomyelin cycle and the second messenger function of ceramide. *Journal of Biological Chemistry* 269:3125–3128.

———— 1996. Functions of ceramide in coordinating cellular responses to stress. *Science* 274:1855–1859.

Hargrave, P. A., and Hamm, H. E. 1994. Regulation of visual transduction. In *Regulation of Cellular Signal Transduction Pathways by Desensitization and Amplification*, ed. D. R. Sibley and M. D. Houslay, pp. 25–67. New York: John Wiley.

Herlitze, S., Garcia, D. E., Mackie, K., Hille, B., Scheuer, T., and Catterall, W. A. 1996. Modulation of Ca^{2+} channels by G-protein βγ subunits. *Nature* 380:258–262.

Herlitze, S., Hockerman, G. H., Scheuer, T., and Caterall, W. A. 1997. Molecular determinants of inactivation and G protein modulation in the intracellular loop connecting domains I and II of the calcium channel α_{1A} subunit. *Proceedings of the National Academy of Sciences USA* 94:1512–1516.

Hille, B. 1992. G protein-coupled mechanisms and nervous signaling. *Neuron* 9:187–195.

———— 1994. Modulation of ion-channel function by G-protein-coupled receptors. *Trends in Neurosciences* 17:531–536.

Hockberger, P., Toselli, M., Swandulla, D., and Lux, H. D. 1989. A diacylglycerol analogue reduces neuronal calcium currents independently of protein kinase C activation. *Nature* 338:340–342.

House, C., and Kemp, B. E. 1987. Protein kinase C contains a pseudosubstrate prototope in its regulatory domain. *Science* 238:1726–1728.

Huang, C.-L., Slesinger, P. A., Casey, P. J., Jan, Y. N., and Jan, L. Y. 1995. Evidence that direct binding of G$_{\beta\gamma}$ to the GIRK1 G protein-gated inwardly rectifying K$^+$ channel is important for channel activation. *Neuron* 15:1133–1143.

Hunter, T. 1995. Protein kinases and phosphatases: The yin and yang of protein phosphorylation and signaling. *Cell* 80:225–236.

Ikeda, S. R. 1996. Voltage-dependent modulation of N-type calcium channels by G-protein βγ subunits. *Nature* 380:255–258.

Inanobe, A., Morishige, K.-I., Takahashi, N., Ito, H., Yamada, M., Takumi, T., Nishina, H., Takahashi, K., Kanaho, Y., Katada, T., and Kurachi, Y. 1995. G$_{βγ}$ directly binds to the carboxyl terminus of the G protein-gated muscarinic K$^+$ channel, GIRK1. *Biochemical and Biophysical Research Communications* 212:1022–1028.

Ito, H., Tung, R. T., Sugimoto, T., Kobayashi, I., Takahashi, K., Katada, T., Ui, M., and Kurachi, Y. 1992. On the mechanism of G protein βγ subunit activation of the muscarinic K$^+$ channel in guinea pig atrial cell membrane: Comparison with the ATP-sensitive channel. *Journal of General Physiology* 99:961–983.

Jan, L. Y., and Jan, Y. N. 1997. Cloned potassium channels from eukaryotes and prokaryotes. *Annual Review of Neuroscience* 20:91–123.

Jelsema, C. L., and Axelrod, J. 1987. Stimulation of phospholipase A$_2$ activity in bovine rod outer segments by the βγ subunits of transducin and its inhibition by the α subunit. *Proceedings of the National Academy of Sciences USA* 84:3623–3627.

Jonas, E. A., and Kaczmarek, L. K. 1996. Regulation of potassium channels by protein kinases. *Current Opinion in Neurobiology* 6:318–323.

Karschin, C., Dißmann, E., Stühmer, W., and Karschin, A., 1996. IRK(1–3) and GIRK(1–4) inwardly rectifying K$^+$ channel mRNAs are differentially expressed in the adult rat brain. *Journal of Neuroscience* 16:3559–3570.

Kim, D., and Clapham, D. E. 1989. Potassium channels in cardiac cells activated by arachidonic acid and phospholipids. *Science* 244:1174–1176

Kleuss, C., Hescheler, J., Ewel, C., Rosenthal, W., Schultz, G., and Wittig, B. 1991. Assignment of G-protein subtypes to specific receptors inducing inhibition of calcium currents. *Nature* 353:43–48.

Kofuji, P., Davidson, N., and Lester, H. A. 1995. Evidence that neuronal G-protein-gated inwardly rectifying K$^+$ channels are activated by Gβγ subunits and function as heteromultimers. *Proceedings of the National Academy of Sciences USA* 92:6542–6546.

Krapivinsky, G., Krapivinsky, L., Wickman, K., and Clapham, D. E. 1995. Gβγ binds directly to the G protein-gated K$^+$ channel, I$_{KACh}$. *Journal of Biological Chemistry* 270:29059–29062.

Kubo, Y., Reuveny, E., Slesinger, P. A., Jan, Y. N., and Jan, L. Y. 1993. Primary structure and functional expression of a rat G-protein-coupled muscarinic potassium channel. *Nature* 364:802–806.

Kurachi, Y., Nakajima, T., and Sugimoto, T. 1986. On the mechanism of activation of muscarinic K⁺ channels by adenosine in isolated atrial cells: Involvement of GTP-binding proteins. *Pflügers Archiv* 407:264–274.

Levitan, I. B. 1994. Modulation of ion channels by protein phosphorylation and dephosphorylation. *Annual Review of Physiology* 56:193–212.

Li, M., West, J. W., Lai, Y., Scheuer, T., and Catterall, W. A. 1992. Functional modulation of brain sodium channels by cAMP-dependent phosphorylation. *Neuron* 8:1151–1159.

Liao, Y. J., Jan, Y. N., and Jan, L. Y. 1996. Heteromultimerization of G-protein-gated inwardly rectifying K⁺ channel proteins GIRK1 and GIRK2 and their altered expression in *weaver* brain. *Journal of Neuroscience* 16:7137–7150.

Lieberman, D. N., and Mody, I. 1994. Regulation of NMDA channel function by endogenous Ca²⁺-dependent phosphatase. *Nature* 369:235–239.

Liscovitch, M., and Cantley, L. C. 1994. Lipid second messengers. *Cell* 77:329–334.

Loewi, O. 1921. Über humorale Ubertragbarkeit der Herznervenwirkung. I. Mitteilung. *Pflügers Archiv* 189:239–242.

Logothetis, D. E., Kurachi, Y., Galper, J., Neer, E. J., and Clapham, D. E. 1987. The βγ subunits of GTP-binding proteins activate the muscarinic K⁺ channel in heart. *Nature* 325:321–326.

Masu, M., Iwakabe, H., Tagawa, Y., Miyoshi, T., Yamashita, M., Fukuda, Y., Sasaki, H., Hiroi, K., Nakamura, Y., Shigemoto, R., Takada, M., Nakamura, K., Nakao, K., Katsuki, M., and Nakanishi, S. 1995. Specific deficit of the ON response in visual transmission by targeted disruption of the mGluR6 gene. *Cell* 80:757–765.

Meldrum, E., Parker, P. J., and Carozzi, A. 1991. The PtdIns-PLC superfamily and signal transduction. *Biochimica et Biophysica Acta* 1092:49–71.

Miyake, M., Christie, M. J., and North, R. A. 1989. Single potassium channels opened by opioids in rat locus ceruleus neurons. *Proceedings of the National Academy of Sciences USA* 86:3419–3422.

Mochly-Rosen, D. 1995. Localization of protein kinase by anchoring proteins: A theme in signal transduction. *Science* 268:247–251.

Navarro, B., Kennedy, M. E., Velimirović, B., Bhat, D., Peterson, A. S., and Clapham, D. E. 1996. Nonselective and Gβγ-insensitive *weaver* K⁺ channels. *Science* 272:1950–1953.

Nawy, S., and Copenhagen, D. R. 1987. Multiple classes of glutamate receptor on depolarizing bipolar cells in retina. *Nature* 325:56–58.

Nawy, S., and Jahr, C. E. 1990. Suppression by glutamate of cGMP-activated conductance in retinal bipolar cells. *Nature* 346:269–271.

———— 1991. cGMP-gated conductance in retinal bipolar cells is suppressed by the photoreceptor transmitter. *Neuron* 7:677–683.

Negishi, K., Kato, S., and Teranishi, T. 1988. Dopamine cells and rod bipolar cells contain protein kinase C-like immunoreactivity in some vertebrate retinas. *Neuroscience Letters* 94:247–252.

Nishizuka, Y. 1995. Protein kinase C and lipid signaling for sustained cellular responses. *FASEB Journal* 9:484–496.

Nomura, A., Shigemoto, R., Nakamura, Y., Okamoto, N., Mizuno, N., and Nakanishi, S. 1994. Developmentally regulated postsynaptic localization of a metabotropic glutamate receptor in rat rod bipolar cells. *Cell* 77:361–369.

North, R. A. 1989. Drug receptors and the inhibition of nerve cells. *British Journal of Pharmacology* 98:13–28.

North, R. A., and Williams, J. T. 1985. On the potassium conductance increased by opioids in rat locus coeruleus neurones. *Journal of Physiology* 364:265–280.

Patil, P. G., de Leon, M., Reed, R. R., Dubel, S., Snutch, T. P., and Yue, D. T. 1996. Elementary events underlying voltage-dependent G-protein inhibition of N-type calcium channels. *Biophysical Journal* 71:2509–2521.

Piomelli, D. 1993. Arachidonic acid in cell signaling. *Current Opinion in Cell Biology* 5:274–280.

Ponce, A., Bueno, E., Kentros, C., Vega-Saenz de Miera, E., Chow, A., Hillman, D., Chen, S., Zhu, L., Wu, M. B., Wu, X., Rudy, B., and Thornhill, W. B. 1996. G-protein-gated inward rectifier K^+ channel proteins (GIRK1) are present in the soma and dendrites as well as in nerve terminals of specific neurons in the brain. *Journal of Neuroscience* 16:1990–2001.

Qin, N., Platano, D., Olcese, R., Stefani, E., and Birnbaumer, L. 1997. Direct interaction of $G_{\beta\gamma}$ with a C-terminal $G_{\beta\gamma}$-binding domain of the Ca^{2+} channel α_1 subunit is responsible for channel inhibition by G protein-coupled receptors. *Proceedings of the National Academy of Sciences USA* 94:8866–8871.

Raymond, L. A., Blackstone, C. D., and Huganir, R. L. 1993. Phosphorylation of amino acid neurotransmitter receptors in synaptic plasticity. *Trends in Neurosciences* 16:147–153.

Reuveny, E., Slesinger, P. A., Inglese, J., Morales, J. M., Iñiguez-Lluhl, J. A., Lefkowitz, R. J., Bourne, H. R., Jan, Y. N., and Jan, L. Y. 1994. Activation of the cloned muscarinic potassium channel by G protein $\beta\gamma$ subunits. *Nature* 370:143–146.

Rhee, S. G., and Choi, K. D. 1992. Regulation of inositol phospholipid-specific phospholipase C isozymes. *Journal of Biological Chemistry* 267:12393–12396.

Robison, G. A., Butcher, R. W., and Sutherland, E. W. 1968. Cyclic AMP. *Annual Review of Biochemistry* 37:149–174.

———— 1971. *Cyclic AMP and Cell Function.* New York: Academic Press.

Roche, K. W., Tingley, W. G., and Huganir, R. L. 1994. Glutamate receptor phosphorylation and synaptic plasticity. *Current Opinion in Neurobiology* 4:383–388.

Rosenmund, C., Carr, D. W., Bergeson, S. E., Nilaver, G., Scott, J. D., and Westbrook, G. L. 1994. Anchoring of protein kinase A is required for modulation of AMPA/kinase receptors on hippocampal neurons. *Nature* 368:853–856.

Schiller, P. H., Sandell, J. H., and Maunsell, J. H. R. 1986. Functions of the ON and OFF channels of the visual system. *Nature* 322:824–825.

Schreibmayer, W., Dessauer, C. W., Vorobiov, D., Gilman, A. G., Lester, H. A., Davidson, N., and Dascal, N. 1996. Inhibition of an inwardly rectifying K^+ channel by G-protein α-subunits. *Nature* 380:624–627.

Schreibmayer, W., Frohnwieser, B., Dascal, N., Platzer, D., Spreitzer, B., Zechner, R., Kallen, R. G., and Lester, H. A. 1994. β-Adrenergic modulation of currents produced by rat cardiac Na^+ channels expressed in *Xenopus laevis* oocytes. *Receptors and Channels* 2:339–350.

Shiells, R. A., and Falk, G. 1990. Glutamate receptors of rod bipolar cells are linked to a cyclic GMP cascade via a G-protein. *Proceedings of the Royal Society of London B* 242:91–94.

——— 1994. Responses of rod bipolar cells isolated from dogfish retinal slices to concentration-jumps of glutamate. *Visual Neuroscience* 11:1175–1183.

Slesinger, P. A., Reuveny, E., Jan, Y. N., and Jan, L. Y. 1995. Identification of structural elements involved in G protein gating of the GIRK1 potassium channel. *Neuron* 15:1145–1156.

Smith, R. D., and Goldin, A. L. 1996. Phosphorylation of brain sodium channels in the I-II linker modulates channel function in *Xenopus* oocytes. *Journal of Neuroscience* 16:1965–1974.

Soejima, M., and Noma, A. 1984. Mode of regulation of the ACh-sensitive K-channel by the muscarinic receptor in rabbit atrial cells. *Pflügers Archiv* 400:424–431.

Stea, A., Soong, T. W., and Snutch, T. P. 1995. Determinants of PKC-dependent modulation of a family of neuronal calcium channels. *Neuron* 15:929–940.

Stryer, L. 1995. *Biochemistry*, 4th ed. New York: W. H. Freeman.

Sunahara, R. K., Dessauer, C. W., and Gilman, A. G. 1996. Complexity and diversity of mammalian adenylyl cyclases. *Annual Review of Pharmacology and Toxicology* 36:461–480.

Sutherland, E. W. 1972. Studies on the mechanism of hormone action. *Science* 177:401–408.

Swartz, K. J. 1993. Modulation of Ca^{2+} channels by protein kinase C in rat central and peripheral neurons: Disruption of G protein-mediated inhibition. *Neuron* 11:305–320.

Swartz, K. J., and Bean, B. P. 1992. Inhibition of calcium channels in rat CA3 pyramidal neurons by a metabotropic glutamate receptor. *Journal of Neuroscience* 12:4358–4371.

Swartz, K. J., Merritt, A., Bean, B. P., and Lovinger, D. M. 1993. Protein kinase C modulates glutamate receptor inhibition of Ca^{2+} channels and synaptic transmission. *Nature* 361:165–168.

Takahashi, T., Forsythe, I. D., Tsujimoto, T., Barnes-Davies, M., and Onodera, K. 1996. Presynaptic calcium current modulation by a metabotropic glutamate receptor. *Science* 274:594–597.

Tanaka, C., and Nishizuka, Y. 1994. The protein kinase C family for neuronal signaling. *Annual Review of Neuroscience* 17:551–567.

Tang, W.-J., and Gilman, A. G. 1991. Type-specific regulation of adenylyl cyclase by G protein βγ subunits. *Science* 254:1500–1503.

——— 1992. Adenylyl cyclases. *Cell* 70:869–872.

Trudeau, L.-E., Emery, D. G., and Haydon, P. G. 1996. Direct modulation of the secretory machinery underlies PKA-dependent synaptic facilitation in hippocampal neurons. *Neuron* 17:789–797.

Tsien, R. W. 1973. Adrenaline-like effects of intracellular iontophoresis of cyclic AMP in cardiac Purkinje fibres. *Nature New Biology* 245:120–122.

Villafranca, J. E., Kissinger, C. R., and Parge, H. E. 1996. Protein serine/threonine phosphatases. *Current Opinion in Biotechnology* 7:397–402.

Waard, M. D., Liu, H., Walker, D., Scott, V. E. S., Gurnett, C. A., and Campbell, K. P. 1997. Direct binding of G-protein βγ complex to voltage-dependent calcium channels. *Nature* 385:446–450.

Walaas, S. I., and Greengard, P. 1991. Protein phosphorylation and neuronal function. *Pharmacological Reviews* 43:299–349.

Wang, L.-Y., Orser, B. A., Brautigan, D. L., and MacDonald, J. F. 1994. Regulation of NMDA receptors in cultured hippocampal neurons by protein phosphatases 1 and 2A. *Nature* 369:230–232.

Wera, S., and Hemmings, B. A. 1995. Serine/threonine protein phosphatases. *Biochemical Journal* 311:17–29.

Wickman, K. D., and Clapham, D. E. 1995. G-protein regulation of ion channels. *Current Opinion in Neurobiology* 5:278–285.

Wickman, K. D., Iñiguez-Lluhl, J. A., Davenport, P. A., Taussig, R., Krapivinsky, G. B., Linder, M. E., Gilman, A. G., and Clapham, D. E. 1994. Recombinant G-protein βγ-subunits activate the muscarinic-gated atrial potassium channel. *Nature* 368:255–257.

Yang, J., and Tsien, R. W. 1993. Enhancement of N- and L-type calcium channel currents by protein kinase C in frog sympathetic neurons. *Neuron* 10:127–136.

Zagotta, W. N., and Siegelbaum, S. A. 1996. Structure and function of cyclic nucleotide-gated channels. *Annual Review of Neuroscience* 19:235–263.

Zamponi, G. W., Bourinet, E., Nelson, D., Nargeot, J., and Snutch, T. P. 1997.

Crosstalk between G proteins and protein kinase C mediated by the calcium channel α_1 subunit. *Nature* 385:442–446.

13. Calcium and Nitric Oxide

Adams, S. R., Kao, J. P. Y., Grynkiewicz, G., Minta, A., and Tsien, R. Y. 1988. Biologically useful chelators that release Ca^{2+} upon illumination. *Journal of the Americal Chemical Society* 110:3212–3220.

Adams, S. R., and Tsien, R. Y. 1993. Controlling cell chemistry with caged compounds. *Annual Review of Physiology* 55:755–784.

Adler, E. M., Augustine, G. J., Duffy, S. N., and Charlton, M. P. 1991. Alien intracellular calcium chelators attenuate neurotransmitter release at the squid giant synapse. *Journal of Neuroscience* 11:1496–1507.

Barria, A., Muller, D., Derkach, V., Griffith, L. C., and Soderling, T. R. 1997. Regulatory phosphorylation of AMPA-type glutamate receptors by CaM-KII during long-term potentiation. *Science* 276:2042–2045.

Berridge, M. J. 1993. Inositol trisphosphate and calcium signalling. *Nature* 361:315–325.

——— 1995. Capacitative calcium entry. *Biochemical Journal* 312:1–11.

Berridge, M. J., Cheek, T. R., Bennett, D. L., and Bootman, M. D. 1996. Ryanodine receptors and intracellular calcium signaling. In *Ryanodine Receptors,* ed. V. Sorrentino, pp. 119–153. Boca Raton, FL: CRC Press.

Berridge, M. J., and Dupont, G. 1994. Spatial and temporal signalling by calcium. *Current Opinion in Cell Biology* 6:267–274.

Bezprozvanny, I. 1996. Inositol (1,4,5)-trisphosphate receptors: Functional properties, modulation, and role in calcium wave propagation. In *Organellar Ion Channels and Transporters,* ed. D. E. Clapham and B. E. Ehrlich, pp. 75–86. New York: Rockefeller University Press.

Bezprozvanny, I., and Ehrlich, B. E. 1995. The inositol 1,4,5-trisphosphate ($InsP_3$) receptor. *Journal of Membrane Biology* 145:205–216.

Bezprozvanny, I., Watras, J., and Ehrlich, B. E. 1991. Bell-shaped calcium-response curves of Ins(1,4,5)P3- and calcium-gated channels from endoplasmic reticulum of cerebellum. *Nature* 351:751–754.

Blackstone, C. D., Supattapone, S., and Snyder, S. H. 1989. Inositolphospholipid-linked glutamate receptors mediate cerebellar parallel-fiber—Purkinje-cell synaptic transmission. *Proceedings of the National Academy of Sciences USA* 86:4316–4320.

Bootman, M. D., and Berridge, M. J. 1995. The elemental principles of calcium signaling. *Cell* 83:675–678.

Braun, A. P., and Schulman, H. 1995. The multifunctional calcium/calmodulin-dependent protein kinase: From form to function. *Annual Review of Physiology* 57:417–445.

Bredt, D. S., and Snyder, S. H. 1989. Nitric oxide mediates glutamate-linked enhancement of cGMP levels in the cerebellum. *Proceedings of the National Academy of Sciences USA* 86:9030–9033.

——— 1990. Isolation of nitric oxide synthetase, a calmodulin-requiring enzyme. *Proceedings of the National Academy of Sciences USA* 87:682–685.

Burnett, A. L., Lowenstein, C. J., Bredt, D. S., Chang, T. S. K., and Snyder, S. H. 1992. Nitric oxide: A physiologic mediator of penile erection. *Science* 257:401–403.

Clapham, D. E. 1995. Calcium signaling. *Cell* 80:259–268.

——— 1996. TRP is cracked, but is CRAC TRP? *Neuron* 16:1069–1072.

Clapham, D. E., and Sneyd, J. 1995. Intracellular calcium waves. In *Advances in Second Messenger and Phosphoprotein Research,* vol. 30, ed. A. R. Means, pp. 1–24. New York: Raven.

Cobbold, P. H., and Lee, J. A. C. 1991. Aequorin measurements of cytoplasmic free calcium. In *Cellular Calcium: A Practical Approach,* ed. J. G. McCormack and P. H. Cobbold, pp. 55–81. Oxford: IRL Press at Oxford University Press.

Cohen, P., and Klee, C. B. (eds.). 1988. *Calmodulin.* Amsterdam: Elsevier.

Crane, B. R., Arvai, A. S., Gachhui, R., Wu, C., Ghosh, D. K., Getzoff, E. D., Stuehr, D. J., and Tainer, J. A. 1997. The structure of nitric oxide synthase oxygenase domain and inhibitor complexes. *Science* 278:425–431.

Dalva, M. B., and Katz, L. C. 1994. Rearrangements of synaptic connections in visual cortex revealed by laser photostimulation. *Science* 265:255–258.

Dawson, T. M., and Snyder, S. H. 1994. Gases as biological messengers: Nitric oxide and carbon monoxide in the brain. *Journal of Neuroscience* 14:5147–5159.

Dousa, T. P., Chini, E. N., and Beers, K. W. 1996. Adenine nucleotide diphosphates: Emerging second messengers acting via intracellular Ca^{2+} release. *Americal Journal of Physiology* 271 (*Cell Physiology* 40):C1007–C1024.

Ehrlich, B. E., Kaftan, E., Bezprozvannaya, S., and Bezprozvanny, I. 1994. The pharmacology of intracellular Ca^{2+}-release channels. *Trends in Pharmacological Sciences* 15:145–149.

Eilers, J., Augustine, G. J., and Konnerth, A. 1995. Subthreshold synaptic Ca^{2+} signalling in fine dendrites and spines of cerebellar Purkinje neurons. *Nature* 373:155–158.

Eilers, J., Schneggenburger, R., and Konnerth, A. 1995. Patch clamp and calcium imaging in brain slices. In *Single-Channel Recording,* 2d ed., ed. B. Sakmann and E. Neher, pp. 213–229. New York: Plenum Press.

Ellis-Davies, G. C. R., and Kaplan, J. H. 1994. Nitrophenyl-EGTA, a photolabile chelator that selectively binds Ca^{2+} with high affinity and releases it rapidly upon photolysis. *Proceedings of the National Academy of Sciences USA* 91:187–191.

Escobar, A. L., Cifuentes, F., and Vergara, J. L. 1995. Detection of Ca^{2+}-transients elicited by flash photolysis of DM-nitrophen with a fast calcium indicator. *FEBS Letters* 364:335–338.

Escobar, A. L., Velez, P., Kim, A. M., Cifuentes, F., Fill, M., and Vergara, J. L. 1997. Kinetic properties of DM-nitrophen and calcium indicators: Rapid transient response to flash photolysis. *European Journal of Physiology* 434:615–631.

Fasolato, C., Innocenti, B., and Pozzan, T. 1994. Receptor-activated Ca^{2+} influx: How many mechanisms for how many channels? *Trends in Pharmacological Sciences* 15:77–83.

Francis, S. H., and Corbin, J. D. 1994. Structure and function of cyclic nucleotide-dependent protein kinases. *Annual Review of Physiology* 56:237–272.

Furchgott, R. F. 1988. Studies on the relaxation of rabbit aorta by sodium nitrite: The basis for the proposal that the acid-activatable inhibitory factor from bovine retractor penis is organic nitrite and the endothelium-derived relaxing factor is nitric oxide. In *Mechanims of Vasodilation,* ed. P. M. Vanhoutte, pp. 31–36. New York: Raven.

Furchgott, R. F., and Zawadzki, J. V. 1980. The obligatory role of endothelial cells in the relaxation of arterial smooth muscle by acetylcholine. *Nature* 288:373–376.

Galione, A., and Summerhill, R. 1996. Regulation of ryanodine receptors by cyclic ADP-ribose. In *Ryanodine Receptors,* ed. V. Sorrentino, pp. 51–70. Boca Raton, FL: CRC Press.

Galione, A., White, A., Willmott, N., Turner, M., Potter, B. V. L., and Watson, S. P. 1993. cGMP mobilizes intracellular Ca^{2+} in sea urchin eggs by stimulating cyclic ADP-ribose synthesis. *Nature* 365:456–459.

Garthwaite, J. 1991. Glutamate, nitric oxide and cell-cell signalling in the nervous system. *Trends in Neurosciences* 14:60–67.

Garthwaite, J., and Boulton, C. L. 1995. Nitric oxide signaling in the central nervous system. *Annual Review of Physiology* 57:683–706.

Garthwaite, J., Charles, S. L., and Chess-Williams, R. 1988. Endothelium-derived relaxing factor release on activation of NMDA receptors suggests role as intercellular messenger in the brain. *Nature* 336:385–388.

Ghosh, A., and Greenberg, M. E. 1995. Calcium signaling in neurons: Molecular mechanisms and cellular consequences. *Science* 268:239–247.

Gillo, B., Chorna, I., Cohen, H., Cook, B., Manistersky, I., Chorev, M., Arnon, A., Pollock, J. A., Selinger, Z., and Minke, B. 1996. Coexpression of *Drosophila* TRP and TRP-like proteins in *Xenopus* oocytes reconstitutes capacitative Ca^{2+} entry. *Proceedings of the National Academy of Sciences USA* 93:14146–14151.

Gnegy, M. E. 1993. Calmodulin in neurotransmitter and hormone action. *Annual Review of Pharmacology and Toxicology* 33:45–70.

Griffith, O. W., and Stuehr, D. J. 1995. Nitric oxide synthases: Properties and catalytic mechanism. *Annual Review of Physiology* 57:707–736.

Grynkiewicz, G., Poenie, M., and Tsien, R. Y. 1985. A new generation of Ca^{2+} indicators with greatly improved fluorescence properties. *Journal of Biological Chemistry* 260:3440–3450.

Hanson, P. I., Meyer, T., Stryer, L., and Schulman, H. 1994. Dual role of calmodulin in autophosphorylation of multifunctional CaM kinase may underlie decoding of calcium signals. *Neuron* 12:943–956.

Hanson, P. I., and Schulman, H. 1992. Neuronal Ca^{2+}/calmodulin-dependent protein kinases. *Annual Review of Biochemistry* 61:559–601.

Harootunian, A. T., Kao, J. P. Y., Paranjape, S., and Tsien, R. Y. 1991. Generation of calcium oscillations in fibroblasts by positive feedback between calcium and IP$_3$. *Science* 251:75–78.

Hastings, J. W., Mitchell, G., Mattingly, P. H., Blinks, J. R., and Van Leeuwen, M. 1969. Response of aequorin bioluminescence to rapid changes in calcium concentration. *Nature* 222:1047–1050.

Haugland, R. P. 1996. *Handbook of Fluorescent Probes and Research Chemicals,* 6th ed., pp. 503–522. Eugene, OR: Molecular Probes.

Hobbs, A. J., and Ignarro, L. J. 1997. The nitric oxide-cyclic GMP signal transduction system. In *Nitric Oxide and the Lung,* ed. W. M. Zapol and K. D. Bloch, pp. 1–57. New York: Marcel Dekker.

Hoth, M., and Penner, R. 1992. Depletion of intracellular calcium stores activates a calcium current in mast cells. *Nature* 355:353–356.

———— 1993. Calcium release-activated calcium current in rat mast cells. *Journal of Physiology* 465:359–386.

Hua, S.-Y., Tokimasa, T., Takasawa, S., Furuya, Y., Nohmi, M., Okamoto, H., and Kuba, K. 1994. Cyclic ADP-ribose modulates Ca^{2+} release channels for activation by physiological Ca^{2+} entry in bullfrog sympathetic neurons. *Neuron* 12:1073–1079.

Iadecola, C. 1997. Bright and dark sides of nitric oxide in ischemic brain injury. *Trends in Neurosciences* 20:132–139.

Ignarro, L. J. 1990. Biosynthesis and metabolism of endothelium-derived nitric oxide. *Annual Review of Pharmacology and Toxicology* 30:535–560.

Ignarro, L. J., Buga, G. M., Wood, K. S., Byrns, R. E., and Chaudhuri, G. 1987. Endothelium-derived relaxing factor produced and released from artery and vein is nitric oxide. *Proceedings of the National Academy of Sciences USA* 84:9265–9269.

Kanaseki, T., Ikeuchi, Y., Sugiura, H., and Yamauchi, T. 1991. Structural features of Ca^{2+}/calmodulin-dependent protein kinase II revealed by electron microscopy. *Journal of Cell Biology* 115:1049–1060.

Kaplan, J. H., and Ellis-Davies, G. C. R. 1988. Photolabile chelators for the rapid photorelease of divalent cations. *Proceedings of the National Academy of Sciences USA* 85:6571–6575.

Kaplan, J. H., Forbush, B., III, and Hoffman, J. F. 1978. Rapid photolytic release of adenosine 5′-triphosphate from a protected analogue: Utilization by the Na:K pump of human red blood cell ghosts. *Biochemistry* 17:1929–1935.

Khodakhah, K., and Ogden, D. 1993. Functional heterogeneity of calcium release by inositol trisphosphate in single Purkinje neurones, cultured cerebellar astrocytes, and peripheral tissues. *Proceedings of the National Academy of Sciences USA* 90:4976–4980.

———— 1995. Fast activation and inactivation of inositol trisphosphate-evoked Ca^{2+} release in rat cerebellar Purkinje neurones. *Journal of Physiology* 487:343–358.

Knapp, A. G., and Dowling, J. E. 1987. Dopamine enhances excitatory amino acid-gated conductances in cultured retinal horizontal cells. *Nature* 325:437–439.

Kolaj, M., Cerne, R., Cheng, G., Brickey, D. A., and Randić, M. 1994. Alpha subunit of calcium/calmodulin-dependent protein kinase enhances excitatory amino acid and synaptic responses of rat spinal dorsal horn neurons. *Journal of Neurophysiology* 72:2525–2531.

Lai, Y., Nairn, A. C., and Greengard, P. 1986. Autophosphorylation reversibly regulates the Ca^{2+}/calmodulin-dependence of Ca^{2+}/calmodulin-dependent protein kinase II. *Proceedings of the National Academy of Sciences USA* 83:4253–4257.

Lechleiter, J., Girard, S., Peralta, E., and Clapham, D. 1991. Spiral calcium wave propagation and annihilation in *Xenopus laevis* oocytes. *Science* 252:123–126.

Lee, H. C. 1996. Cyclic ADP-ribose: A mediator of a calcium signaling pathway. In *Ryanodine Receptors,* ed. V. Sorrentino, pp. 31–50. Boca Raton, FL: CRC Press.

Levitan, I. B. 1994. Modulation of ion channels by protein phosphorylation and dephosphorylation. *Annual Review of Physiology* 56:193–212.

Lewis, R. S., Dolmetsch, R. E., and Zweifach, A. 1996. Positive and negative regulation of depletion-activated calcium channels by calcium. In *Organellar Ion Channels and Transporters,* ed. D. E. Clapham and B. E. Ehrlich, pp. 241–254. New York: Rockefeller University Press.

Linden, D. J., Smeyne, M., and Connor, J. A. 1994. *Trans*-ACPD, a metabotropic receptor agonist, produces calcium mobilization and an inward current in cultured cerebellar Purkinje neurons. *Journal of Neurophysiology* 71:1992–1998.

Llano, I., DiPolo, R., and Marty, A. 1994. Calcium-induced calcium release in cerebellar Purkinje cells. *Neuron* 12:663–673.

Llano, I., Dreessen, J., Kano, M., and Konnerth, A. 1991. Intradendritic release of calcium induced by glutamate in cerebellar Purkinje cells. *Neuron* 7:577–583.

Lledo, P.-M., Hjelmstad, G. O., Mukherji, S., Soderling, T. R., Malenka, R. C., and Nicoll, R. A. 1995. Calcium/calmodulin-dependent kinase II and long-term potentiation enhance synaptic transmission by the same mechanism. *Proceedings of the National Academy of Sciences USA* 92:11175–11179.

Makings, L. R., and Tsien, R. Y. 1994. Caged nitric oxide. *Journal of Biological Chemistry* 269:6282–6285.

Marietta, M. A. 1994. Nitric oxide synthase: Aspects concerning structure and catalysis. *Cell* 78:927–930.

Mathes, C., Fleig, A., and Penner, R. 1997. Calcium-release-activated-calcium current (ICRAC): A direct target for sphingosine. Submitted for publication.

Mathes, C., and Thompson, S. H. 1994. Calcium current activated by muscarinic receptors and thapsigargin in neuronal cells. *Journal of General Physiology* 104:107–121.

McCormack, J. G., and Cobbold, P. H. 1991. *Cellular Calcium: A Practical Approach*. Oxford: IRL Press at Oxford University Press.

McGlade-McCulloh, E., Yamamoto, H., Tan, S.-E., Brickey, D. A., and Soderling, T. R. 1993. Phosphorylation and regulation of glutamate receptors by calcium/calmodulin-dependent protein kinase II. *Nature* 362:640–642.

Meissner, G. 1994. Ryanodine receptor/Ca^{2+} release channels and their regulation by endogenous effectors. *Annual Review of Physiology* 56:485–508.

Meyer, T., Hanson, P. I., Stryer, L., and Schulman, H. 1992. Calmodulin trapping by calcium-calmodulin-dependent protein kinase. *Science* 256:1199–1202.

Meyer, T., and Stryer, L. 1991. Calcium spiking. *Annual Review of Biophysics and Biophysical Chemistry* 20:153–174.

Mikoshiba, K., Furuichi, T., Miyawaki, A., Yoshikawa, S., Nakade, S., Michikawa, T., Nakagawa, T., Okano, H., Kume, S., Muto, A., Aruga, J., Yamada, N., Hamanaka, Y., Fujino, I., and Kobayashi, M. 1993. Structure and function of inositol 1,4,5-trisphosphate receptor. *Annals of the New York Academy of Sciences* 707:178–197.

Miller, S. G., and Kennedy, M. B. 1986. Regulation of brain type II $Ca^{2+}/$

calmodulin-dependent protein kinase by autophosphorylation: A Ca^{2+}-triggered molecular switch. *Cell* 44:861–870.

Minke, B., and Selinger, Z. 1996. The roles of *trp* and calcium in regulating photoreceptor function in *Drosophila*. *Current Opinion in Neurobiology* 6:459–466.

Minta, A., Kao, J. P. Y., and Tsien, R. Y. 1989. Fluorescent indicators for cytosolic calcium based on rhodamine and fluorescein chromophores. *Journal of Biological Chemistry* 264:8171–8178.

Nakanishi, S., Maeda, N., and Mikoshiba, K. 1991. Immunohistochemical localization of an inositol 1,4,5-trisphosphate receptor, P_{400}, in neural tissue: Studies in developing and adult mouse brain. *Journal of Neuroscience* 11:2075–2086.

Neher, E. 1989. Combined fura-2 and patch clamp measurements in rat peritoneal mast cells. In *Neuromuscular Junction,* ed. L. C. Sellin, R. Libelius, and S. Thesleff, pp. 65–76. Amsterdam: Elsevier.

Neher, E., and Augustine, G. J. 1992. Calcium gradients and buffers in bovine chromaffin cells. *Journal of Physiology* 450:273–301.

Nelson, R. J., Demas, G. E., Huang, P. L., Fishman, M. C., Dawson, V. L., Dawson, T. M., and Snyder, S. H. 1995. Behavioural abnormalities in male mice lacking neuronal nitric oxide syntase. *Nature* 378:383–386.

Nerbonne, J. M. 1996. Caged compounds: Tools for illuminating neuronal responses and connections. *Current Opinion in Neurobiology* 6:379–386.

Nori, A., Gorza, L., and Volpe, P. 1996. Expression of ryanodine receptors. In *Ryanodine Receptors,* ed. V. Sorrentino, pp. 101–117. Boca Raton, FL: CRC Press.

Otis, T., Zhang, S., and Trussell, L. O. 1996. Direct measurement of AMPA receptor desensitization induced by glutamatergic synaptic transmission. *Journal of Neuroscience* 16:7496–7504.

Palmer, R. M. J., Ferrige, A. G., and Moncada, S. 1987. Nitric oxide release accounts for the biological activity of endothelium-derived relaxing factor. *Nature* 327:524–526.

Parekh, A. B., and Penner, R. 1996. Regulation of store-operated calcium currents in mast cells. In *Organellar Ion Channels and Transporters,* ed. D. E. Clapham and B. E. Ehrlich, pp. 231–239. New York: Rockefeller University Press.

Penner, R., Fasolato, C., and Hoth, M. 1993. Calcium influx and its control by calcium release. *Current Opinion in Neurobiology* 3:368–374.

Petersen, C. C. H., Berridge, M. J., Borgese, M. F., and Bennett, D. L. 1995. Putative capacitative calcium entry channels: Expression of a *Drosophila trp* and evidence for the existence of vertebrate homologues. *Biochemical Journal* 311:41–44.

Petersen, O. H., Petersen, C. C. H., and Kasai, H. 1994. Calcium and hormone action. *Annual Review of Physiology* 56:297–319.

Phillips, A. M., Bull, A., and Kelly, L. E. 1992. Identification of a *Drosophila* gene encoding a calmodulin-binding protein with homology to the *trp* phototransduction gene. *Neuron* 8:631–642.

Putney, J. W., Jr. 1986. A model for receptor-regulated calcium entry. *Cell Calcium* 7:1–12.

——— 1990. Capacitative calcium entry revisited. *Cell Calcium* 11:611–624.

Randriamampita, C., and Tsien, R. Y. 1993. Emptying of intracellular Ca^{2+} stores releases a novel small messenger that stimulates Ca^{2+} influx. *Nature* 364:809–814.

Roche, K. W., Tingley, W. G., and Huganir, R. L. 1994. Glutamate receptor phosphorylation and synaptic plasticity. *Current Opinion in Neurobiology* 4:383–388.

Schmidt, H. H. H. W., Lohmann, S. M., and Walter, U. 1993. The nitric oxide and cGMP signal transduction system: Regulation and mechanism of action. *Biochimica et Biophysica Acta* 1178:153–175.

Schmidt, H. H. H. W., and Walter, U. 1994. NO at work. *Cell* 78:919–925.

Schulman, H. 1995. Protein phosphorylation in neuronal plasticity and gene expression. *Current Opinion in Neurobiology* 5:375–381.

Schuman, E. M., and Madison, D. V. 1994. Nitric oxide and synaptic function. *Annual Review of Neuroscience* 17:153–183.

Sharp, A. H., McPherson, P. S., Dawson, T. M., Aoki, C., Campbell, K. P., and Snyder, S. H. 1993. Differential immunohistochemical localization of ionositol 1,4,5-trisphosphate- and ryanodine-sensitive Ca^{2+} release channels in rat brain. *Journal of Neuroscience* 13:3051–3063.

Shimomura, O., and Johnson, F. H. 1976. Calcium-triggered luminescence of the photoprotein aequorin. In *Calcium in Biological Systems,* ed. C. J. Duncan, pp. 41–54. Cambridge: Cambridge University Press.

Shmigol, A., Verkhratsky, A., and Isenberg, G. 1995. Calcium-induced calcium release in rat sensory neurons. *Journal of Physiology* 489:627–636.

Soderling, T. R. 1996. Structure and regulation of calcium/calmodulin-dependent protein kinases II and IV. *Biochimica et Biophysica Acta* 1297:131–138.

Sorrentino, V. 1996. Molecular biology of ryanodine receptors. In *Ryanodine Receptors,* ed. V. Sorrentino, pp. 85–100. Boca Raton, FL: CRC Press.

Svoboda, K., Denk, W., Kleinfeld, D., and Tank, D. W. 1997. *In vivo* dendritic calcium dynamics in neocortical pyramidal neurons. *Nature* 385:161–165.

Tan, S.-E., Wenthold, R. J., and Soderling, T. R. 1994. Phosphorylation of AMPA-type glutamate receptors by calcium/calmodulin-dependent protein kinase II and protein kinase C in cultured hippocampal neurons. *Journal of Neuroscience* 14:1123–1129.

Thomas, D., and Hanley, M. R. 1995. Evaluation of calcium influx factors from stimulated Jurkat T-lymphocytes by microinjection into *Xenopus* oocytes. *Journal of Biological Chemistry* 270:6429–6432.

Thomas, M. V. 1982. *Techniques in Calcium Research*. New York: Academic Press.

——— 1991. Metallochromic indicators. In *Cellular Calcium: A Practical Approach*, ed. J. G. McCormack and P. H. Cobbold, pp. 115–122. Oxford: IRL Press at Oxford University Press.

Tsien, R. Y. 1980. New calcium indicators and buffers with high selectivity against magnesium and protons: Design, synthesis, and properties of prototype structures. *Biochemistry* 19:2396–2404.

——— 1981. A non-disruptive technique for loading calcium buffers and indicators into cells. *Nature* 290:527–528.

Tsou, K., Snyder, G. L., and Greengard, P. 1993. Nitric oxide/cGMP pathway stimulates phosphorylation of DARPP-32, a dopamine- and cAMP-regulated phosphoprotein, in the substantia nigra. *Proceedings of the National Academy of Sciences USA* 90:3462–3465.

Umans, J. G., and Levi, R. 1995. Nitric oxide in the regulation of blood flow and arterial pressure. *Annual Review of Physiology* 57:771–790.

Vaca, L., Sinkins, W. G., Hu, Y., Kunze, D. L., and Schilling, W. P. 1994. Activation of recombinant *trp* by thapsigargin in Sf9 insect cells. *American Journal of Physiology* 267 (*Cell Physiology* 36):C1501–C1505.

Verkhratsky, A., and Shmigol, A. 1996. Calcium-induced calcium release in neurones. *Cell Calcium* 19:1–14.

Verma, A., Hirsch, D. J., Glatt, C. E., Ronnett, G. V., and Snyder, S. H. 1993. Carbon monoxide: A putative neural messenger. *Science* 259:381–384.

Wang, S. S.-H., and Augustine, G. J. 1995. Confocal imaging and local photolysis of caged compounds: Dual probes of synaptic function. *Neuron* 15:755–760.

Weinstein, H., and Mehler, E. L. 1994. Ca^{2+}-binding and structural dynamics in the functions of calmodulin. *Annual Review of Physiology* 56:213–236.

Wiebolt, R., Gee, K. R., Niu, L., Ramesh, D., Carpenter, B. K., and Hess, G. P. 1994. Photolabile precursors of glutamate: Synthesis, photochemical properties, and activation of glutamate receptors on a microsecond time scale. *Proceedings of the National Academy of Sciences USA* 91:8752–8756.

Wieboldt, R., Ramesh, D., Carpenter, B. K., and Hess, G. P. 1994. Synthesis and photochemistry of photolabile derivatives of γ-aminobutyric acid for chemical kinetic investigations of the γ-aminobutyric acid receptor in the millisecond time region. *Biochemistry* 33:1526–1533.

Yakel, J. L., Vissavajjhala, P., Derkach, V. A., Brickey, D. A., and Soderling, T. R. 1995. Identification of a Ca^{2+}/calmodulin-dependent protein kinase II regulatory phosphorylation site in non-*N*-methyl-D-aspartate glutamate receptors. *Proceedings of the National Academy of Sciences USA* 92:1376–1380.

Yuste, R., and Denk, W. 1995. Dendritic spines as basic functional units of neuronal integration. *Nature* 375:682–684.

Yuzaki, M., and Mikoshiba, K. 1992. Pharmacological and immunocytochemical characterization of metabotropic glutamate receptors in cultured Purkinje cells. *Journal of Neuroscience* 12:4253–4263.

Zhang, J., and Snyder, S. H. 1995. Nitric oxide in the nervous system. *Annual Review of Pharmacology and Toxicology* 35:213–233.

Zhu, X., Jiang, M., Peyton, M., Boulay, G., Hurst, R., Stefani, E., and Birnbaumer, L. 1996. *trp*, A novel mammalian gene family essential for agonist-activated capacitative Ca^{2+} entry. *Cell* 85:661–671.

Zitt, C., Zobel, A., Obukhov, G., Hartenneck, C., Kalkbrenner, F., Lückhoff, A., and Schultz, G. 1996. Cloning and functional expression of a human Ca^{2+}-permeable cation channel activated by calcium store depletion. *Neuron* 16:1189–1196.

Zweifach, A., and Lewis, R. S. 1993. Mitogen-regulated Ca^{2+} current of T lymphocytes is activated by depletion of intracellular Ca^{2+} stores. *Proceedings of the National Academy of Sciences USA* 90:6295–6299.

——— 1995. Rapid inactivation of depletion-activated calcium current (I_{CRAC}) due to local calcium feedback. *Journal of General Physiology* 105:209–226.

14. Long-Term Potentiation

Arai, A., and Lynch, G. 1992. Antagonists of the platelet-activating factor receptor block long-term potentiation in hippocampal slices. *European Journal of Neuroscience* 4:411–419.

Barria, A., Muller, D., Derkach, V., Griffith, L. C., and Soderling, T. R. 1997. Regulatory phosphorylation of AMPA-type glutamate receptors by CaM-KII during long-term potentiation. *Science* 276:2042–2045.

Barrionuevo, G., and Brown, T. H. 1983. Associative long-term potentiation in hippocampal slices. *Proceedings of the National Academy of Sciences USA* 80:7347–7351.

Bear, M. F., and Malenka, R. C. 1994. Synaptic plasticity: LTP and LTD. *Current Opinion in Neurobiology* 4:389–399.

Bekkers, J. M., and Stevens, C. F. 1990. Presynaptic mechanism for long-term potentiation in the hippocampus. *Nature* 346:724–729.

Bliss, T. V. P., and Collingridge, G. L. 1993. A synaptic model of memory: Long-term potentiation in the hippocampus. *Nature* 361:31–39.

Bliss, T. V. P., and Lømo, T. 1973. Long-lasting potentiation of synaptic transmission in the dentate area of the anaesthetized rabbit following stimulation of the perforant path. *Journal of Physiology* 232:331–356.

Blitzer, R. D., Wong, T., Nouranifar, R., Iyengar, R., and Landau, E. M. 1995. Postsynaptic cAMP pathway gates early LTP in the hippocampal CA1 region. *Neuron* 15:1403–1414.

Bolshakov, V. Y., and Siegelbaum, S. A. 1995. Regulation of hippocampal transmitter release during development and long-term potentiation. *Science* 269:1730–1734.

Braun, A. P., and Schulman, H. 1995. The multifunctional calcium/calmodulin-dependent protein kinase: From form to function. *Annual Review of Physiology* 57:417–445.

Castillo, P. E., Weisskopf, M. G., and Nicoll, R. A. 1994. The role of Ca^{2+} channels in hippocampal mossy fiber synaptic transmission and long-term potentiation. *Neuron* 12:261–269.

Collingridge, G. L., Kehl, S. J., and McLennan, H. 1983. Excitatory amino acids in synaptic transmission in the Schafffer collateral-commissural pathway of the rat hippocampus. *Journal of Physiology* 334:33–46.

Cummings, J. A., Mulkey, R. M., Nicoll, R. A., and Malenka, R. C. 1996. Ca^{2+} signaling requirements for long-term depression in the hippocampus. *Neuron* 16:825–833.

Dudek, S. M., and Bear, M. F. 1992 Homosynaptic long-term depression in area CA1 of hippocampus and effects of N-methyl-D-aspartate receptor blockade. *Proceedings of the National Academy of Sciences USA* 89:4363–4367.

Engert, F., and Bonhoeffer, T. 1997. Synapse specificity of long-term potentiation breaks down at short distances. *Nature* 388:279–284.

Frey, U., Huang, Y.-Y., and Kandel, E. R. 1993. Effects of cAMP simulate a late stage of LTP in hippocampal CA1 neurons. *Science* 260:1661–1664.

Fukunaga, K., Stoppini, L., Miyamoto, E., and Muller, D. 1993. Long-term potentiation is associated with an increased activity of Ca^{2+}/calmodulin-dependent protein kinase II. *Journal of Biological Chemistry* 268:7863–7867.

Gustafsson, B., Wigstrom, H., and Abraham, W. C. 1987. Long-term potentiation in the hippocampus using depolarizing current pulses as the conditioning stimulus to single volley synaptic potentials. *Journal of Neuroscience* 7:774–780.

Harris, E. W., and Cotman, C. W. 1986. Long-term potentiation of guinea pig mossy fiber responses is not blocked by N-methyl-D-aspartate antagonists. *Neuroscience Letters* 70:132–137.

Huang, Y.-Y., Li, X. C., and Kandel, E. R. 1994. cAMP contributes to mossy fiber LTP by initiating both a covalently mediated early phase and a macromolecular synthesis-dependent late phase. *Cell* 79:69–79.

Isaac, J. T. R., Nicoll, R. A., and Malenka, R. C. 1995. Evidence for silent synapses: Implications for the expression of LTP. *Neuron* 15:427–434.

Kato, K., Clark, G. D., Bazan, N. G., and Zorumski, C. F. 1994. Platelet-activating factor as a potential retrograde messenger in CA1 hippocampal long-term potentiation. *Nature* 367:175–179.

Kelso, S. R., Ganong, A. H., and Brown, T. H. 1986. Hebbian synapses in hippocampus. *Proceedings of the National Academy of Sciences USA* 83:5326–5330.

Klee, C. B. 1991. Concerted regulation of protein phosphorylation and dephosphorylation by calmodulin. *Neurochemical Research* 16:1059–1065.

Kullmann, D. M. 1994. Amplitude fluctuations of dual-component EPSCs in hippocampal pyramidal cells: Implications for long-term potentiation. *Neuron* 12:1111–1120.

Kullmann, D. M., and Nicoll, R. A. 1992. Long-term potentiation is associated with increases in quantal content and quantal amplitude. *Nature* 357:240–244.

Levy, W. B., and Steward, O. 1979. Synapses as associative memory elements in the hippocampal formation. *Brain Research* 175:233–245.

Liao, D., Hessler, N. A., and Malinow, R. 1995. Activation of postsynaptically silent synapses during pairing-induced LTP in CA1 region of hippocampal slice. *Nature* 375:400–404.

Lisman, J. 1989. A mechanism for the Hebb and the anti-Hebb processes underlying learning and memory. *Proceedings of the National Academy of Sciences USA* 86:9574–9578.

——— 1994. The CaM kinase II hypothesis for the storage of synaptic memory. *Trends in Neurosciences* 17:406–412.

Lisman, J. E., and Harris, K. M. 1993. Quantal analysis and synaptic anatomy—integrating two views of hippocampal plasticity. *Trends in Neurosciences* 16:141–147.

Lledo, P.-M., Hjelmstad, G. O., Mukherji, S., Soderling, T. R., Malenka, R. C., and Nicoll, R. A. 1995. Calcium/calmodulin-dependent kinase II and long-term potentiation enhance synaptic transmission by the same mechanism. *Proceedings of the National Academy of Sciences USA* 92:11175–11179.

Lynch, G., Larson, J., Kelso, S., Barrionuevo, G., and Schottler, F. 1983. Intracellular injections of EGTA block induction of hippocampal long-term potentiation. *Nature* 305:719–721.

Malenka, R. C., Kauer, J. A., Zucker, R., and Nicoll, R. A. 1988. Postsynaptic calcium is sufficient for potentiation of the hippocampal synaptic transmission. *Sciences* 242:81–84.

Malenka, R. C., Kauer, J. A., Perkel, B. J., and Nicoll, R. A. 1989. The impact of postsynaptic calcium on synaptic transmission—Its role in long-term potentiation. *Trends in Neurosciences* 12:444–450.

Malenka, R. C., Kauer, J. A., Perkel, D. J., Mauk, M. D., Kelly, P. T., Nicoll, R. A., and Waxham, M. N. 1989. An essential role for postsynaptic calmodulin and protein kinase activity in long-term potentiation. *Nature* 340:554–557.

Malgaroli, A., and Tsien, R. W. 1992. Glutamate-induced long-term potentiation of the frequency of miniature synaptic currents in cultured hippocampal neurons. *Nature* 357:134–139.

Malinow, R., and Miller, J. P. 1986. Postsynaptic hyperpolarization during conditioning reversibly blocks induction of long-term potentiation. *Nature* 320:529–530.

Malinow, R., Schulman, H., and Tsien, R. W. 1989. Inhibition of postsynaptic PKC or CaM KII blocks induction but not expression of LTP. *Science* 245:862–866.

Malinow, R., and Tsien, R. W. 1990. Presynaptic enhancement shown by whole-cell recordings of long-term potentiation in hippocampal slices. *Nature* 346:177–180.

Manabe, T., and Nicoll, R. A. 1994. Long-term potentiation: Evidence against an increase in transmitter release probability in the CA1 region of the hippocampus. *Science* 265:1888–1892.

Manabe, T., Renner, P., and Nicoll, R. A. 1992. Postsynaptic contribution to long-term potentiation revealed by the analysis of miniature synaptic currents. *Nature* 355:50–55.

Matthies, H. 1989. In search of cellular mechanisms of memory. *Progress in Neurobiology* 32:277–349.

McGlade-McCulloh, E., Yamamoto, H., Tan, S.-E., Brickey, D. A., and Soderling, T. R. 1993. Phosphorylation and regulation of glutamate receptors by calcium/calmodulin-dependent protein kinase II. *Nature* 362:640–642.

McNaughton, B. L., Douglas, R. M., and Goddard, G. V. 1978. Synaptic enhancement in fascia dentata: Cooperativity among coactive afferents. *Brain Research* 157:277–293.

Miller, S. G., and Kennedy, M. G. 1986. Regulation of brain type II $Ca^{2+}/$

calmodulin-dependent protein kinase by autophosphorylation: A Ca^{2+}-triggered molecular switch. *Cell* 44:861–870.

Mulkey, R. M., Endo, S., Shenolikar, S., and Malenka, R. C. 1994. Involvement of a calcineurin/inhibitor-1 phosphatase cascade in hippocampal long-term depression. *Nature* 369:486–488.

Mulkey, R. M., Herron, C. E., and Malenka, R. C. 1993. An essential role for protein phosphatases in hippocampal long-term depression. *Science* 261:1051–1055.

Mulkey, R. M., and Malenka, R. C. 1992. Mechanisms underlying induction of homosynaptic long-term depression in area CA1 of the hippocampus. *Neuron* 9:967–975.

Nicoll, R. A., Kauer, J. A., and Malenka, R. C. 1988. The current excitement in long-term potentiation. *Neuron* 1:97–103.

Nicoll, R. A., and Malenka, R. C. 1995. Contrasting properties of two forms of long-term potentiation in the hippocampus. *Nature* 377:115–118.

Nguyen, P. V., Abel, T., and Kandel, E. R. 1994. Requirement of a critical period of transcription for induction of a late phase of LTP. *Science* 265:1104–1107.

O'Dell, T. J., Grant, S. G. N., and Kandel, E. R. 1991. Long-term potentiation in the hippocampus is blocked by tyrosine kinase inhibitors. *Nature* 353:558–560.

O'Dell, T. J., Hawkins, R. D., Kandel, E. R., and Hawkins, R. D. 1991. Tests of the roles of two diffusible substances in long-term potentiation: Evidence for nitric oxide as a possible early retrograde messenger. *Proceedings of the National Academy of Sciences USA* 86:11285–11289.

Oliet, S. H. R., Malenka, R. C., and Nicoll, R. A. 1996. Bidirectional control of quantal size by synaptic activity in the hippocampus. *Science* 271:1294–1297.

Regehr, W. G., and Tank, D. W. 1990. Postsynaptic NMDA receptor-mediated calcium accumulation in hippocampal CA1 pyramidal cell dendrites. *Nature* 345:807–810.

Reymann, K. G., Brodemann, R., Kase, H., and Matthies, H. 1988. Inhibitors of calmodulin and protein kinase C block different phases of hippocampal long-term potentiation. *Brain Research* 461:388–392.

Sastry, B. R., Goh, J. W., and Auyeung, A. 1986. Associative induction of posttetanic and long-term potentiation in CA1 neurons of rat hippocampus. *Science* 232:988–990.

Schuman, E. M., and Madison, D. V. 1991. A requirement for the intercellular messenger nitric oxide in long-term potentiation. *Science* 254:1503–1506.

Shields, S. M., Ingebritsen, T. S., and Kelly, P. T. 1985. Identification of protein phosphatase 1 in synaptic junction: Dephosphorylation of endogenous calmodulin-dependent kinase II and synapse-enriched phosphoproteins. *Journal of Neuroscience* 5:3414–3422.

Silva, A. J., Stevens, C. F., Tonegawa, S., and Wang, Y. 1992. Deficient hippocampal long-term potentiation in α-calcium-calmodulin kinase II mutant mice. *Science* 257:201–206.

Squire, L. R., and Zola-Morgan, S. 1991. The medial temporal lobe memory system. *Science* 253:1380–1386.

Stevens, C. F., and Wang, Y. 1993. Reversal of long-term potentiation by inhibitors of haem oxygenase. *Nature* 364:147–149.

——— 1994. Changes in reliability of synaptic function as a mechanism for plasticity. *Nature* 371:704–707.

Thomas, M. J., Moody, T. D., Makhinson, M., and O'Dell, T. J. 1996. Activity-dependent β-adrenergic modulation of low frequency stimulation induced LTP in the hippocampal CA1 region. *Neuron* 17:475–482.

Weisskopf, M. G., Castillo, P. E., Zalutsky, R. A., and Nicoll, R. A. 1994. Mediation of hippocampal mossy fiber long-term potentiation by cyclic AMP. *Science* 265:1878–1882.

Williams, J. H., Errington, M. L., Li, Y.-G., Lynch, M. A., and Bliss, T. V. P. 1993. The search for retrograde messengers in long-term potentiation. *Seminars in the Neurosciences* 5:149–158.

Williams, J. H., Errington, M. L., Lynch, M. A., and Bliss, T. P. 1989. Arachidonic acid induces a long-term activity-dependent enhancement of synaptic transmission in the hippocampus. *Nature* 341:739–742.

Zalutsky, R., and Nicoll, R. A. 1990. Comparison of two forms of long-term potentiation in single hippocampal neurons. *Science* 248:1619–1624.

Zhuo, M., Hu, Y., Schultz, C., Kandel, E. R., and Hawkins, R. D. 1994. Role of guanylyl cyclase and cGMP-dependent protein kinase in long-term potentiation. *Nature* 368:635–639.

15. Mechanoreceptors

Art, J. J., and Fettiplace, R. 1987. Variation of membrane properties in hair cells isolated from the turtle cochlea. *Journal of Physiology* 385:207–242.

Art, J. J., Wu, Y.-C., and Fettiplace, R. 1995. The calcium-activated potassium channels of turtle hair cells. *Journal of General Physiology* 105:49–72.

Ashmore, J. F. 1987. A fast motile response in guinea-pig outer hair cells: The cellular basis of the cochlear amplifier. *Journal of Physiology* 388:323–347.

——— 1994. The cellular machinery of the cochlea. *Experimental Physiology* 79:113–134.

Ashmore, J. F., and Kolston, P. J. 1994. Hair cell based amplification in the cochlea. *Current Opinion in Neurobiology* 4:503–508.

Assad, J. A., and Corey, D. P. 1992. An active motor model for adaptation by vertebrate hair cells. *Journal of Neuroscience* 12:3291–3309.

Assad, J. A., Hacohen, N., and Corey, D. P. 1989. Voltage dependence of adaptation and active bundle movement in bullfrog saccular hair cells. *Proceedings of the National Academy of Sciences USA* 86:2918–2922.

Assad, J. A., Shepherd, G. M. G., and Corey, D. P. 1991. Tip-link integrity and mechanical transduction in vertebrate hair cells. *Neuron* 7:985–994.

Brehm, P., Kullberg, R., and Moody-Corbett, F. 1984. Properties of non-junctional acetylcholine receptor channels on innervated muscle of *Xenopus laevis*. *Journal of Physiology* 350:631–648.

Brown, H. M., Ottoson, D., and Rydqvist, B. 1978. Crayfish stretch receptor: An investigation with voltage-clamp and ion-sensitive electrodes. *Journal of Physiology* 284:155–179.

Brownell, W. E., Bader, C. R., Bertrand, D., and de Ribaupierre, Y. 1985. Evoked mechanical responses of isolated cochlear outer hair cells. *Science* 227:194–196.

Cody, A. R., and Russell, I. J. 1987. The responses of hair cells in the basal turn of the guinea-pig cochlea to tones. *Journal of Physiology* 383:551–569.

Corey, D. P., and Assad, J. A. 1992. Transduction and adaptation in vertebrate hair cells: Correlating structure with function. In *Sensory Transduction,* ed. D. P. Corey and S. D. Roper, pp. 325–342. New York: Rockefeller University Press.

Corey, D. P., and García-Añoveros, J. 1996. Mechanosensation and the DEG/ENaC ion channels. *Science* 273:323–324.

Corey, D. P., and Hudspeth, A. J. 1979. Ionic basis of the receptor potential in a vertebrate hair cell. *Nature* 281:675–678.

———— 1983. Kinetics of the receptor current in bullfrog saccular hair cells. *Journal of Neuroscience* 3:962–976.

Crawford, A. C., Evans, M. G., and Fettiplace, R. 1989. Activation and adaptation of transducer currents in turtle hair cells. *Journal of Physiology* 419:405–434.

———— 1991. The actions of calcium on the mechano-electrical transducer current of turtle hair cells. *Journal of Physiology* 434:369–398.

Crawford, A. C., and Fettiplace, R. 1981. An electrical tuning mechanism in turtle cochlear hair cells. *Journal of Physiology* 312:377–412.

Dallos, P. 1985. Response characteristics of mammalian cochlear hair cells. *Journal of Neuroscience* 5:1591–1608.

Dallos, P., and Cheatham, M. A. 1992. Cochlear hair cell function reflected in intracellular recordings *in vivo*. In *Sensory Transduction* (Society for

General Physiology Series, vol. 47), ed. D. P. Corey, and S. D. Roper, pp. 371–393. New York: Rockefeller University Press.

Denk, W., Holt, J. R., Shepherd, G. M. G., and Corey, D. P. 1995. Calcium imaging of single stereocilia in hair cells: Localization of transduction channels at both ends of tip links. *Neuron* 15:1311–1321.

Denk, W., and Svoboda, K. 1997. Photon upmanship: Why multiphoton imaging is more than a gimmick. *Neuron* 18:351–357.

Eatock, R. A., Corey, D. P., and Hudspeth, A. J. 1987. Adaptation of mechanoelectrical transduction in hair cells of the bullfrog's sacculus. *Journal of Neuroscience* 7:2821–2836.

Edwards, C., Ottoson, D., Rydqvist, B., and Swerup, C. 1981. The permeability of the transducer membrane of the crayfish stretch receptor to calcium and other divalent cations. *Neuroscience* 6:1455–1460.

Erxleben, C. 1989. Stretch-activated current through single ion channels in the abdominal stretch receptor organ of the crayfish. *Journal of General Physiology* 94:1071–1083.

Evans, B. N., and Dallos, P. 1993. Stereocilia displacement induced somatic motility of cochlear outer hair cells. *Proceedings of the National Academy of Sciences USA* 90:8347–8351.

Eyzaguirre, C., and Kuffler, S. W. 1955. Processes of excitation in the dendrites and in the soma of single isolated sensory nerve cells of the lobster and crayfish. *Journal of General Physiology* 39:87–119.

Fettiplace, R. 1992. The role of calcium in hair cell transduction. In *Sensory Transduction,* ed. D. P. Corey and S. D. Roper, pp. 343–356. New York: Rockefeller University Press.

Flock, Å. 1965. Transducing mechanisms in the lateral line canal organ receptors. *Cold Spring Harbor Symposia on Quantitative Biology* 30:133–145.

García-Añoveros, J., and Corey, D. P. 1997. The molecules of mechanosensation. *Annual Review of Neuroscience* 20:567–594.

Gillespie, P. G. 1995. Molecular machinery of auditory and vestibular transduction. *Current Opinion in Neurobiology* 5:449–455.

Gillespie, P. G., and Hudspeth, A. J. 1993. Adenine nucleoside diphosphates block adaptation of mechanoelectrical transduction in hair cells. *Proceedings of the National Academy of Sciences USA* 90:2710–2714.

Gillespie, P. G., Wagner, M. C., and Hudspeth, A. J. 1993. Identification of a 120 kd hair-bundle myosin located near stereociliary tips. *Neuron* 11:581–594.

Guharay, F., and Sachs, F. 1984. Stretch-activated single ion channel currents in tissue-cultured embryonic chick skeletal muscle. *Journal of Physiology* 352:685–701.

Hackney, C. M., and Furness, D. N. 1995. Mechanotransduction in vertebrate hair cells: Structure and function of the stereociliary bundle. *American Journal of Physiology* 268 (*Cell Physiology* 37):C1–C13.

Hacohen, N., Assad, J. A., Smith, W. J., and Corey, D. P. 1989. Regulation of tension on hair-cell transduction channels: Displacement and calcium dependence. *Journal of Neuroscience* 9:3988–3997.

Hamill, O. P., and McBride, D. W., Jr. 1996. A supramolecular complex underlying touch sensitivity. *Trends in Neurosciences* 19:258–261.

Hasson, T., Gillespie, P. G., Garcia, J. A., MacDonald, R. B., Zhao, Y., Yee A. G., Mooseker, M. S., and Corey, D. P. 1997. Unconventional myosins in inner-ear sensory epithelia. *Journal of Cell Biology* 137:1287–1307.

Holton, T., and Hudspeth, J. D. 1986. The transduction channel of hair cells from the bull-frog characterized by noise analysis. *Journal of Physiology* 375:195–227.

Howard, J., and Hudspeth, A. J. 1987. Mechanical relaxation of the hair bundle mediates adaptation in mechanoelectrical transduction by the bull-frog's saccular hair cell. *Proceedings of the National Academy of Sciences USA* 84:3064–3068.

Hudspeth, A. J. 1982. Extracellular current flow and the site of transduction by vertebrate hair cells. *Journal of Neuroscience* 2:1–10.

—— 1985. The cellular basis of hearing: The biophysics of hair cells. *Science* 230:745–752.

—— 1989. How the ear's works work. *Nature* 341:397–404.

Hudspeth, A. J., and Corey, D. P. 1977. Sensitivity, polarity, and conductance change in the response of vertebrate hair cells to controlled mechanical stimuli. *Proceedings of the National Academy of Sciences USA* 74:2407–2411.

Hudspeth, A. J., and Gillespie, P. G. 1994. Pulling springs to tune transduction: Adaptation by hair cells. *Neuron* 12:1–9.

Jaramillo, F., and Hudspeth, A. J. 1991. Localization of the hair cell's transduction channels at the hair bundle's top by iontophoretic application of a channel blocker. *Neuron* 7:409–420.

—— 1993. Displacement-clamp measurement of the forces exerted by gating springs in the hair bundle. *Proceedings of the National Academy of Sciences USA* 90:1330–1334.

Kachar, B., Brownell, W. E., Altschuler, R., and Fex, J. 1986. Electrokinetic shape changes of cochlear outer hair cells. *Nature* 322:365–368.

Kataoka, Y., and Ohmori, H. 1994. Activation of glutamate receptors in response to membrane depolarization of hair cells isolated from chick cochlea. *Journal of Physiology* 477:403–414.

Kimitsuki, T., and Ohmori, H. 1992. The effect of caged calcium release on the adaptation of the transduction current in chick hair cells. *Journal of Physiology* 458:27–40.

Lumpkin, E. A., and Hudspeth, A. J. 1995. Detection of Ca^{2+} entry through mechanosensitive channels localizes the site of mechanoelectrical transduction in hair cells. *Proceedings of the National Academy of Sciences USA* 92:10297–10301.

Mammano, F., and Ashmore, J. F. 1993. Reverse transduction measured in the isolated cochlea by laser Michelson interferometry. *Nature* 365:838–841.

Markin, V. S., and Hudspeth, A. J. 1995. Gating-spring models of mechanoelectrical transduction by hair cells of the internal ear. *Annual Review of Biophysics and Biomolecular Structure* 24:59–83.

Morris, C. E., and Horn, R. 1991. Failure to elicit neuronal macroscopic mechanosensitive currents anticipated by single-channel studies. *Science* 251:1246–1249.

Nakajima, S., and Onodera, K. 1969. Adaptation of the generator potential in the crayfish stretch receptors under constant length and constant tension. *Journal of Physiology* 200:187–204.

Ohmori, H. 1985. Mechano-electrical transduction currents in isolated vestibular hair cells of the chick. *Journal of Physiology* 359:189–217.

———— 1988. Mechanical stimulation and fura-2 fluorescence in the hair bundle of dissociated hair cells of the chick. *Journal of Physiology* 399:115–137.

Pickles, J. O. 1988. *An Introduction to the Physiology of Hearing,* 2d ed. New York: Academic.

Pickles, J. O., Comis, S. D., and Osborne, M. P. 1984. Cross-links between stereocilia in the guinea pig organ of Corti, and their possible relation to sensory transduction. *Hearing Research* 15:103–112.

Ricci, A. J., and Fettiplace, R. 1997. The effects of calcium buffering and cyclic AMP on mechanoelectrical transduction in turtle auditory hair cells. *Journal of Physiology* 501:111–124.

Russell, I. J., and Sellick, P. M. 1983. Low-frequency characteristics of intracellularly recorded receptor potentials in guinea-pig cochlear hair cells. *Journal of Physiology* 338:179–206.

Ryan, A. F., and Dallos, P. 1984. Physiology of the cochlea. In *Hearing Disorders,* 2d ed., ed. J. L. Northern, pp. 253–266. Boston: Little Brown and Company.

Sachs, F. 1992. Stretch-sensitive ion channels: An update. In *Sensory Transduction,* ed. D. P. Corey and S. D. Roper, pp. 241–260. New York: Rockefeller University Press.

Sackin, H. 1995. Mechanosensitive channels. *Annual Review of Physiology* 57:333–353.

Sand, O. 1975. Effects of different ionic environments on the mechanosensitivity of lateral line organs in the mudpuppy. *Journal of Comparative Physiology* 102:27–42.

Shepherd, G. M. G., and Corey, D. P. 1994. The extent of adaptation in bull-frog saccular hair cells. *Journal of Neuroscience* 14:6217–6229.

Solc, C. K., Derfler, B. H., Duyk, G. M., and Corey, D. P. 1994. Molecular cloning of myosins from the bullfrog saccular macula: A candidate for the hair cell adaptation motor. *Auditory Neuroscience* 1:63–75.

Sukharev, S. I., Blount, P., Martinac, B., Blattner, F. R., and Kung, C. 1994. A large-conductance mechanosensitive channel in *E. coli* encolded by *mscL* alone. *Nature* 368:265–268.

von Békésy, G. 1960. *Experiments in Hearing.* New York: McGraw-Hill.

Walker, R. G., and Hudspeth, A. J. 1996. Calmodulin controls adaptation of mechanoelectrical transduction by hair cells of the bullfrog's sacculus. *Proceedings of the National Academy of Sciences USA* 93:2203–2207.

Wiersma, C. A. 1967. *Invertebrate Nervous Systems.* Chicago: University of Chicago Press.

Yamoah, E. N., and Gillespie, P. G. 1996. Phosphate analogs block adaptation in hair cells by inhibiting adaptation-motor force production. *Neuron* 17:523–533.

Zhao, Y.-D., Yamoah, E. N., and Gillespie, P. G. 1996. Regeneration of broken tip links and restoration of mechanical transduction in hair cells. *Proceedings of the National Academy of Sciences USA* 93:15469–15474.

16. *Photoreceptors and Olfactory Receptors*

Ache, B. W., and Zhainazarov, A. 1995. Dual second-messenger pathways in olfactory transduction. *Current Opinion in Neurobiology* 5:461–466.

Arshavsky, V. Y., and Bownds, M. D. 1992. Regulation of deactivation of photoreceptor G protein by its target enzyme and cGMP. *Nature* 357:416–417.

Bakalyar, H. A., and Reed, R. R. 1990. Identification of a specialized adenylyl cyclase that may mediate odorant detection. *Science* 250:1403–1406.

Baylor, D. 1992. Transduction in retinal photoreceptor cells. In *Sensory Transduction,* ed. D. P. Corey and S. D. Roper, pp. 151–174. New York: Rockefeller University Press.

Baylor, D. A., and Hodgkin, A. L. 1974. Changes in time scale and sensitivity in turtle photoreceptors. *Journal of Physiology* 242:729–758.

Baylor, D. A., Lamb, T. D., and Yau, K.-W. 1979. Responses of retinal rods to single photons. *Journal of Physiology* 288:613–634.

Baylor, D. A., Matthews, G., and Yau, K.-W. 1980. Two components of electrical dark noise in toad retinal rod outer segments. *Journal of Physiology* 309:591–621.

Baylor, D. A., and Nunn, B. J. 1986. Electrical properties of the light-sensitive conductance of rods of the salamander *Ambystoma tigrinum. Journal of Physiology* 371:115–145.

Baylor, D. A., Nunn, B. J., and Schnapf, J. L. 1984. The photocurrent, noise, and spectral sensitivity of rods of the monkey *Macaca fascicularis. Journal of Physiology* 357:575–607.

Berghard, A., Buck, L. B., and Liman, E. R. 1996. Evidence for distinct signaling mechanisms in two mammalian olfactory sense organs. *Proceedings of the National Academy of Sciences USA* 93:2365–2369.

Boekhoff, I., Tareilus, E., Strotmann, J., and Breer, H. 1990. Rapid activation of alternative second messenger pathways in olfactory cilia from rats by different odorants. *EMBO Journal* 9:2453–2458.

Bok, D. 1988. Structure and function of the retinal pigment epithelium-photoreceptor complex. In *Retinal Diseases: Biomedical Foundations and Clinical Management,* ed. M. O. M. Tso, pp. 3–48. Philadephia: J. B. Lippincott.

Bowmaker, J. K., Dartnall, H. J. A., and Mollon, J. D. 1980. Microspectro-photometric demonstration of four classes of photoreceptor in an Old World primate, *Macaca fascicularis. Journal of Physiology* 298:131–143.

Bownds, M. D., and Arshavsky, V. Y. 1995. What are the mechanisms of photoreceptor adaptation? *Behavioral and Brain Sciences* 18:415–424.

Bradley, J., Li, J., Davidson, N., Lester, H. A., and Zinn, K. 1994. Heteromeric olfactory cyclic nucleotide-gated channels: A subunit that confers increased sensitivity to cAMP. *Proceedings of the National Academy of Sciences USA* 91:8890–8894.

Breer, H., Boekhoff, I., and Tareilus, E. 1990. Rapid kinetics of second messenger formation in olfactory transduction. *Nature* 345:65–68.

Breer, H., Klemm, T., and Boekhoff, I. 1992. Nitric oxide mediated formation of cyclic GMP in the olfactory system. *NeuroReport* 3:1030–1032.

Brunet, L. J., Gold, G. H., and Ngai, J. 1996. General anosmia caused by a targeted disruption of the mouse olfactory cyclic nucleotide-gated cation channel. *Neuron* 17:681–693.

Buck, L. B. 1996. Information coding in the vertebrate olfactory system. *Annual Review of Neuroscience* 19:517–544.

Buck, L., and Axel, R. 1991. A novel multigene family may encode odorant receptors: A molecular basis for odor recognition. *Cell* 65:175–187.

Cervetto, L., Lagnado, L., Perry, R. J., Robinson, D. W., and McNaughton, P. A. 1989. Extrusion of calcium from rod outer segments is driven by both sodium and potassium gradients. *Nature* 337:740–743.

Chen, J., Makino, C. L., Peachey, N. S., Baylor, D. A., and Simon, M. I. 1995. Mechanisms of rhodopsin inactivation in vivo as revealed by a COOH-terminal truncation mutant. *Science* 267:374–377.

Chen, T.-Y., Peng, Y.-W., Dhallan, R. S., Ahamed, B., Reed, R. R., and Yau, K.-W. 1993. A new subunit of the cyclic nucleotide-gated cation channel in retinal rods. *Nature* 362:764–767.

Chen, T.-Y., and Yau, K.-W. 1994. Direct modulation by Ca^{2+}-calmodulin of cyclic nucleotide-activated channel of rat olfactory receptor neurons. *Nature* 368:545–548.

Cobbs, W. H., and Pugh, E. N., Jr. 1987. Kinetics and components of the flash photocurrent of isolated retinal rods of the larval salamander, *Ambystoma tigrinum*. *Journal of Physiology* 394:529–572.

Cook, N. J., Hanke, W., and Kaupp, U. B. 1987. Identification, purification, and functional reconstitution of the cyclic GMP-dependent channel from rod photoreceptors. *Proceedings of the National Academy of Sciences USA* 84:585–589.

Cornwall, M. C., and Fain, G. L. 1994. Bleached pigment activates transduction in isolated rods of the salamander retina. *Journal of Physiology* 480:261–279.

Dhallan, R. S., Yau, K.-W., Schrader, K. A., and Reed, R. R. 1990. Primary structure and functional expression of a cyclic nucleotide-activated channel from olfactory neurons. *Nature* 347:184–187.

Eismann, E., Müller, F., Heinemann, S. H., and Kaupp, U. B. 1994. A single negative charge within the pore region of a cGMP-gated channel controls rectification, Ca^{2+} blockage, and ionic selectivity. *Proceedings of the National Academy of Sciences USA* 91:1109–1113.

Escobar, A. L., Monck, J. R., Fernandez, J. M., and Vergara, J. L. 1994. Localization of the site of Ca^{2+} release at the level of a single sarcomere in skeletal muscle fibres. *Nature* 367:739–741.

Fain, G. L. 1975. Quantum sensitivity of rods in the toad retina. *Science* 187:838–841.

Fain, G. L., and Cornwall, M. C. 1993. Light and dark adaptation in vertebrate photoreceptors. In *Contrast Sensitivity,* ed. R. Shapley and D. M.-K. Lam, pp. 3–32. Cambridge, MA: MIT Press.

Fain, G. L., and Matthews, H. R. 1990. Calcium and the mechanism of light adaptation in vertebrate photoreceptors. *Trends in Neurosciences* 13:378–384.

Fain, G. L., Matthews, H. R., and Cornwall, M. C. 1996. Dark adaptation in vertebrate photoreceptors. *Trends in Neurosciences* 19:502–507.

Fain, G. L., Quandt, F. N., Bastian, B. L., and Gerschenfeld, H. M. 1978. Contribution of a caesium-sensitive conductance increase to the rod photoresponse. *Nature* 272:467–469.

Farahbakhsh, Z. T., Hideg, K., and Hubbell, W. L. 1993. Photoactivated conformational changes in rhodopsin: A time-resolved spin label study. *Science* 262:1416–1419.

Farrens, D. L., Altenbach, C., Yang, K., Hubbell, W. L., and Khorana, H. G. 1996. Requirement of rigid-body motion of transmembrane helices for light activation of rhodopsin. *Science* 274:768–770.

Fesenko, E. E., Kolesnikov, S. S., and Lyubarsky, A. L. 1985. Induction by cyclic GMP of cationic conductance in plasma membrane of retinal rod outer segment. *Nature* 313:310–313.

Finn, J. T., Grunwald, M. E., and Yau, K.-W. 1996. Cyclic nucleotide-gated ion channels: An extended family with diverse functions. *Annual Review of Physiology* 58:395–426.

Firestein, S. 1996. Scentsational ion channels. *Neuron* 17:803–806.

Firestein, S., Picco, C., and Menini, A. 1993. The relation between stimulus and response in olfactory receptor cells of the tiger salamander. *Journal of Physiology* 468:1–10.

Frings, S., Seifert, R., Godde, M., and Kaupp, U. B. 1995. Profoundly different calcium permeation and blockage determine the specific function of distinct cyclic nucleotide-gated channels. *Neuron* 15:169–179.

Fülle, H.-J., Vassar, R., Foster, D. C., Yang, R.-B., Axel, R., and Garbers, D. L. 1995. A receptor guanylyl cyclase expressed specifically in olfactory sensory neurons. *Proceedings of the National Academy of Sciences USA* 92:3571–3575.

Fung, B. K.-K., and Stryer, L. 1980. Photolyzed rhodopsin catalyzes the exchange of GTP for bound GDP in retinal rod outer segments. *Proceedings of the National Academy of Sciences USA* 77:2500–2504.

Gorczyca, W. A., Gray-Keller, M. P., Detwiler, P. B., and Palczewski, K. 1994. Purification and physiological evaluation of a guanylate cyclase activating protein from retinal rods. *Proceedings of the National Academy of Sciences USA* 91:4014–4018.

Gordon, S. E., Downing-Park, J., and Zimmerman, A. L. 1995. Modulation of the cGMP-gated ion channel in frog rods by calmodulin and an endogenous inhibitory factor. *Journal of Physiology* 486:533–546.

Goulding, E. H., Tibbs, G. R., Liu, D., and Siegelbaum, S. A. 1993. Role of H5 domain in determining pore diameter and ion permeation through cyclic nucleotide-gated channels. *Nature* 364:61–64.

Goulding, E. H., Tibbs, G. R., and Siegelbaum, S. A. 1994. Molecular mechanism of cyclic-nucleotide-gated channel activation. *Nature* 372:369–374.

Gray-Keller, M. P., and Detwiler, P. B. 1994. The calcium feedback signal in the phototransduction cascade of vertebrate rods. *Neuron* 13:849–861.

Hargrave, P. A. 1995. Future directions for rhodopsin structure and function studies. *Behavioral and Brain Sciences* 18:403–414.

Hargrave, P. A., and Hamm, H. E. 1994. Regulation of visual transduction. In *Regulation of Cellular Signal Transduction Pathways by Desensitization and Amplification*, ed. D. R. Sibley and M. D. Houslay, pp. 25–67. New York: Wiley.

Hecht, S., Schlaer, S., and Pirenne, M. 1942. Energy, quanta and vision. *Journal of General Physiology* 25:819–840.

Heginbotham, L., Abramson, T., and MacKinnon, R. 1992. A functional connection between the pores of distantly related ion channels as revealed by mutant K^+ channels. *Science* 258:1152–1155.

Hestrin, S. 1987. The properties and function of inward rectification in rod photoreceptors of the tiger salamander. *Journal of Physiology* 390:319–333.

Hildebrand, J. G., and Shepherd, G. M. 1997. Mechanisms of olfactory discrimination: Converging evidence for common principles across phyla. *Annual Review of Neuroscience* 20:595–631.

Hodgkin, A. L., McNaughton, P. A., and Nunn, B. J. 1987. Measurement of sodium-calcium exchange in salamander rods. *Journal of Physiology* 391:347–370.

Hsu, Y.-T., and Molday, R. S. 1993. Modulation of the cGMP-gated channel of rod photoreceptor cells by calmodulin. *Nature* 361:76–79.

Ingi, T., and Ronnett, G. V. 1995. Direct demonstration of a physiological role for carbon monoxide in olfactory receptor neurons. *Journal of Neuroscience* 15:8214–8222.

Jelsema, C. L., and Axelrod, J. 1987. Stimulation of phospholipase A_2 activity in bovine rod outer segments by the βγ subunits of transducin and its inhibition by the α subunit. *Proceedings of the National Academy of Sciences USA* 84:3623–3627.

Jones, D. T., and Reed, R. R. 1989. G_{olf}: An olfactory neuron-specific G protein involved in odorant signal transduction. *Science* 244:790–795.

Jones, G. J., Cornwall, M. C., and Fain, G. L. 1996. Equivalence of background and bleaching desensitization in isolated rod photoreceptors of the larval tiger salamander. *Journal of General Physiology* 108:333–340.

Juilfs, D. M., Fülle, H.-J., Zhao, A. Z., Houslay, M. D., Garbers, D. L., and Beavo, J. A. 1997. A subset of olfactory neurons that selectively express cGMP-stimulated phosphodiesterase (PDE2) and guanylyl cyclase-D define a unique olfactory signal transduction pathway. *Proceedings of the National Academy of Sciences USA* 94:3388–3395.

Kaupp, U. B., and Koch, K.-W. 1992. Role of cGMP and Ca^{2+} in vertebrate photoreceptor excitation and adaptation. *Annual Review of Physiology* 54:153–175.

Kaupp, U. B., Niidome, T., Tanabe, T., Terada, S., Bönigk, W., Stühmer, W., Cook, N. J., Kangawa, K., Matsuo, H., Hirose, T., Miyata, T., and Numa, S. 1989. Primary structure and functional expression from complementary DNA of the rod photoreceptor cyclic GMP-gated channel. *Nature* 342:762–766.

Kawamura, S. 1993. Rhodopsin phosphorylation as a mechanism of cyclic GMP phosphodiesterase regulation by S-modulin. *Nature* 362:855–857.

Keverne, E. B. 1982. Chemical senses: Smell. In *The Senses,* ed. H. B. Barlow and J. D. Mollon, pp. 409–427. Cambridge: Cambridge University Press.

Koch, K.-W., and Stryer, L. 1988. Highly cooperative feedback control of retinal rod guanylate cyclase by calcium ions. *Nature* 334:64–66.

Körschen, H. G., Illing, M., Seifert, R., Sesti, F., Williams, A., Gotzes, S., Colville, C., Müller, F., Dosé, A., Godde, M., Molday, L., Kaupp, U. B., and Molday, R. S. 1995. A 240 kDa protein represents the complete β subunit of the cyclic nucleotide-gated channel from rod photoreceptor. *Neuron* 15:627–636.

Koutalos, Y., Nakatani, K., and Yau, K.-W. 1995. The cGMP-phosphodiesterase and its contribution to sensitivity regulation in retinal rods. *Journal of General Physiology* 106:891–921.

Koutalos, Y., and Yau, K.-W. 1996. Regulation of sensitivity in vertebrate rod photoreceptors by calcium. *Trends in Neurosciences* 19:73–81.

Kramer, R. H., Goulding, E., and Siegelbaum, S. A. 1994. Potassium channel inactivation peptide blocks cyclic nucleotide-gated channels by binding to the conserved pore domain. *Neuron* 12:655–662.

Krizaj, D., and Copenhagen, D. R. 1997. Calcium ATP-ase and not Na^+/Ca^{2+} exchange controls intracellular calcium in salamader photoreceptor inner segments. *Investigative Ophthalmology* 38 (*ARVO abstracts*):S615.

Kurahashi, T., and Menini, A. 1997. Mechanism of odorant adaptation in the olfactory receptor cell. *Nature* 385:725–729.

Kurahashi, T., and Shibuya, T. 1990. Ca^{2+}-dependent adaptive properties in the solitary olfactory receptor cell of the newt. *Brain Research* 515:261–268.

Kurahashi, T., and Yau, K.-W. 1993. Co-existence of cationic and chloride components in odorant-induced current of vertebrate olfactory receptor cells. *Nature* 363:71–74.

Lagnado, L., and Baylor, D. A. 1994. Calcium controls light-triggered formation of catalytically active rhodopsin. *Nature* 367:273–277.

Leinders-Zufall, T., Rand, M. N., Shepherd, G. M., Greer, C. A., and Zufall, F. 1997. Calcium entry through cyclic nucleotide-gated channels in individual cilia of olfactory receptor cells: Spatiotemporal dynamics. *Journal of Neuroscience* 17:4136–4148.

Leinders-Zufall, T., Shepherd, G. M., and Zufall, F. 1995. Regulation of cyclic nucleotide-gated channels and membrane excitability in olfactory receptor cells by carbon monoxide. *Journal of Neurophysiology* 74:1498–1508.

——— 1996. Modulation by cyclic GMP of the odour sensitivity of vertebrate olfactory receptor cells. *Proceedings of the Royal Society of London B* 263:803–811.

Liman, E. R., and Buck, L. B. 1994. A second subunit of the olfactory cyclic nucleotide-gated channel confers high sensitivity to cAMP. *Neuron* 13:611–621.

Liu, D. T., Tibbs, G. R., and Siegelbaum, S. A. 1996. Subunit stoichiometry of cyclic nucleotide-gated channels and effects of subunit order on channel function. *Neuron* 16:983–990.

Liu, M., Chen, T.-Y., Ahamed, B., Li, J., and Yau, K.-W. 1994. Calcium-calmodulin modulation of the olfactory cyclic nucleotide-gated cation channel. *Science* 266:1348–1354.

Lowe, G., and Gold, G. H. 1993a. Nonlinear amplification by calcium-dependent chloride channels in olfactory receptor cells. *Nature* 366:283–286.

——— 1993b. Contribution of the ciliary cyclic nucleotide-gated conductance to olfactory transduction in the salamander. *Journal of Physiology* 462:175–196.

Ludwig, J., Margalit, T., Eismann, E., Lancet, D., and Kaupp, U. B. 1990. Primary structure of cAMP-gated channel from bovine olfactory epithelium. *FEBS Letters* 270:24–29.

Matthews, H. R. 1990. Messengers of transduction and adaptation in vertebrate photoreceptors. In *Light and Life in the Sea,* ed. P. J. Herring, A. K. Campbell, M. Whitfield, and L. Maddock, pp. 185–198. Cambridge: Cambridge University Press.

——— 1996. Static and dynamic actions of cytoplasmic Ca^{2+} in the adaptation of responses to saturating flashes in salamander rods. *Journal of Physiology* 490:1–15.

Matthews, H. R., Cornwall, H. R., and Fain, G. L. 1996. Persistent activation of transducin by bleached rhodopsin in salamander rods. *Journal of General Physiology* 108:557–563.

Matthews, H. R., Fain, G. L., and Cornwall, M. C. 1996. Role of cytoplasmic calcium concentration in the bleaching adaptation of salamander cone photoreceptors. *Journal of Physiology* 490:293–303.

Matthews, H. R., Murphy, R. L. W., Fain, G. L., and Lamb, T. D. 1988. Photoreceptor light adaptation is mediated by cytoplasmic calcium concentration. *Nature* 334:67–69.

McNaughton, P. A. 1990. Light response of vertebrate photoreceptors. *Physiological Reviews* 70:847–883.

McNaughton, P. A., Cervetto, L., and Nunn, B. J. 1986. Measurement of the intracellular free calcium concentration in salamander rods. *Nature* 322:261–263.

Molday, R. S. 1996. Calmodulin regulation of cyclic-nucleotide-gated channels. *Current Opinion in Neurobiology* 6:445–452.

Mombaerts, P., Wang, F., Dulac, C., Chao, S. K., Nemes, A., Mendelsohn, M., Edmondson, J., and Axel, R. 1996. Visualizing an olfactory sensory map. *Cell* 87:675–686.

Nakamura, T., and Gold, G. H. 1987. A cyclic nucleotide-gated conductance in olfactory receptor cilia. *Nature* 325:442–444.

Nakatani, K., and Yau, X.-W. 1988. Calcium and light adaptation in retinal rods and cones. *Nature* 334:69–71.

Nunn, B. J., Schnapf, J. L., and Baylor, D. A. 1984. Spectral sensitivity of single cones in the retina of *Macaca fascicularis*. *Nature* 309:264–266.

Pace, U., Hanski, E., Salomon, Y., and Lancet, D. 1985. Odorant-sensitive adenylate cyclase may mediate olfactory reception. *Nature* 316:255–258.

Pak, W. L. 1995. *Drosophila* in vision research. *Investigative Ophthalmology and Vision Research* 36:2340–2357.

Palczewski, K., and Saari, J. C. 1997. Activation and inactivation steps in the visual transduction pathway. *Current Opinion in Neurobiology* 7:500–504.

Pape, H.-C. 1996. Queer current and pacemaker: The hyperpolarization-activated cation current in neurons. *Annual Review of Physiology* 58:299–327.

Perry, R. J., and McNaughton, P. A. 1991. Response properties of cones from the retina of the tiger salamander. *Journal of Physiology* 433:561–587.

Polans, A., Baehr, W., and Palczewski, K. 1996. Turned on by Ca^{2+}! The physiology and pathology of Ca^{2+}-binding proteins in the retina. *Trends in Neurosciences* 19:547–554.

Poo, M.-M., and Cone, R. A. 1974. Lateral diffusion of rhodopsin in the photoreceptor membrane. *Nature* 247:438–441.

Pugh, E. N., Jr., and Lamb, T. D. 1993. Amplification and kinetics of the activation steps in phototransduction. *Biochimica et Biophysica Acta* 1141:111–149.

Rao, V. R., and Oprian, D. D. 1996. Activating mutations of rhodopsin and other G protein-coupled receptors. *Annual Review of Biophysics and Biomolecular Structure* 25:287–314.

Ratto, G. M., Payne, R., Owen, W. G., and Tsien, R. Y. 1988. The concentration of cytosolic free calcium in vertebrate rod outer segments measured with Fura-2. *Journal of Neuroscience* 8:3240–3246.

Reed, R. R. 1992. Signaling pathways in odorant detection. *Neuron* 8:205–209.

Ressler, K. J., Sullivan, S. L., and Buck, L. B. 1993. A zonal organization of odorant receptor gene expression in the olfactory epithelium. *Cell* 73:597–609.

——— 1994. Information coding in the olfactory system: Evidence for a stereotyped and highly organized epitope map in the olfactory bulb. *Cell* 79:1245–1255.

Root, M. J., and MacKinnon, R. 1993. Identification of an external divalent cation-binding site in the pore of a cGMP-activated channel. *Neuron* 11:459–466.

Sagoo, M. S., and Lagnado, L. 1997. G-protein deactivation is rate-limiting for shut-off of the phototransduction cascade. *Nature* 389:392–395.

Sampath, A. P., Matthews, H. R., Cornwall, M. C., and Fain, G. L. 1998. Bleached pigment produces a maintained decrease in outer segment Ca^{2+} in salamander rods. *Journal of General Physiology* 111:1–12.

Schertler, G. F. X., and Hargrave, P. A. 1995. Projection structure of frog rhodopsin in two crystal forms. *Proceedings of the National Academy of Sciences USA* 92:11578–11582.

Schneider, B. G., Shyjan, A. W., and Levenson, R. 1991. Co-localization and polarized distribution of Na,K ATPase α3 and β2 subunits in photoreceptors cells. *Journal of Histochemistry and Cytochemistry* 39:507–517.

Sheikh, S. P., Zvyaga, T. A., Lichtarge, O., Sakmar, T. P., and Bourne, H. R. 1996. Rhodopsin activation blocked by metal-ion-binding sites linking transmembrane helices C and F. *Nature* 383:347–350.

Sklar, P. B., Anholt, R. R. H., and Snyder, S. H. 1986. The odorant-sensitive adenylate cyclase of olfactory receptor cells: Differential stimulation by distinct classes of odorants. *Journal of Biological Chemistry* 261:15538–15543.

Stewart, R. E., DeSimone, J. A., and Hill, D. L. 1997. New perspectives in gustatory physiology: Transduction, development, and plasticity. *American Journal of Physiology* 272 (*Cell Physiology* 41):C1–C26.

Stryer, L. 1986. Cyclic GMP cascade of vision. *Annual Review of Neuroscience* 9:87–119.

Tanford, C. 1961. *Physical Chemistry of Macromolecules*. New York: Wiley.

Taylor, W. R., Morgans, C. W., Berntson, A. K., and Wässle, H. 1997. A plasma-membrane calcium-ATPase is responsible for calcium extrusion from mammalian photoreceptor terminals. *Investigative Ophthalmology* 38 (*ARVO abstracts*): S723.

Torre, V., Matthews, H. R., and Lamb, T. D. 1986. Role of calcium in regulating the cyclic GMP cascade of phototransduction in retinal rods. *Proceedings of the National Academy of Sciences USA* 83:7109–7113.

Unger, V. M., Hargrave, P. A., Baldwin, J. M., and Schertler, G. F. X. 1997. Arrangement of rhodopsin transmembrane α-helices. *Nature* 389:203–206.

Vassar, R., Chao, S. K., Sitcheran, R., Nuñez, J. M., Vosshall, L. B., and Axel, R. 1994. Topographic organization of sensory projections to the olfactory bulb. *Cell* 79:981–991.

Vassar, R., Ngai, J., and Axel, R. 1993. Spatial segregation of odorant receptor expression in the mammalian olfactory epithelium. *Cell* 74:309–318.

Verma, A., Hirsch, D. J., Glatt, C. E., Ronnett, G. V., and Snyder, S. H. 1993. Carbon monoxide: A putative neural messenger. *Science* 259:381–384.

Vuong, T. M., Chabre, M., and Stryer, L. 1984. Millisecond activation of transducin in the cyclic nucleotide cascade of vision. *Nature* 311:659–661.

Yan, C., Zhao, A. Z., Bentley, J. K., Loughney, K., Ferguson, K., and Beavo, J. A. 1995. Molecular cloning and characterization of a calmodulin-dependent phosphodiesterase enriched in olfactory sensory neurons. *Proceedings of the National Academy of Sciences USA* 92:9677–9681.

Yau, K.-W. 1994. Phototransduction mechanism in retinal rods and cones. *Investigative Ophthalmology and Visual Science* 35:9–32.

Yau, K.-W., and Baylor, D. A. 1989. Cyclic GMP-activated conductance of retinal photoreceptor cells. *Annual Review of Neuroscience* 12:289–327.

Yau, K.-W., and Chen, T.-Y. 1995. Cyclic nucleotide-gated channels. In *Ligand- and Voltage-Gated Ion Channels,* ed. R. A. North, pp. 307–335. Boca Raton, FL: CRC Press.

Yau, K.-W., Matthews, G., and Baylor, D. A. 1979. Thermal activation of the visual transduction mechanism in retinal rods. *Nature* 279:806–807.

Yau, K. W., and Nakatani, K. 1985. Light-induced reduction of cytoplasmic free calcium in retinal rod outer segment. *Nature* 313:579–582.

Zagotta, W. N., and Siegelbaum, S. A. 1996. Structure and function of cyclic nucleotide-gated channels. *Annual Review of Neuroscience* 19:235–263.

Zimmerman, A. L. 1995. Cyclic nucleotide gated channels. *Current Opinion in Neurobiology* 5:296–303.

Zufall, F., and Firestein, S. 1993. Divalent cations block the cyclic nucleotide-gated channel of olfactory receptor neurons. *Journal of Neurophysiology* 69:1758–1768.

Zufall, F., Firestein, S., and Shepherd, G. M. 1994. Cyclic nucleotide-gated ion channels and sensory transduction in olfactory receptor neurons. *Annual Review of Biophysics and Biomolecular Structure* 23:577–607.

Zufall, F., and Leinders-Zufall, T. 1997. Identification of a long-lasting form of odor adaptation that depends on the carbon monoxide/cGMP second-messenger system. *Journal of Neuroscience* 17:2703–2712.

Zufall, F., Shepherd, G. M., and Firestein, S. 1991. Inhibition of the olfactory cyclic nucleotide gated ion channel by intracellular calcium. *Proceedings of the Royal Society of London B* 246:225–230.

Zuker, C. S. 1996. The biology of vision in *Drosophila. Proceedings of the National Academy of Sciences USA* 93:571–576.

References Added in Proof

DeVries, S. H., and Schwartz, E. A. 1999. Kainate receptors mediate synaptic transmission between cones and 'Off' bipolar cells in a mammalian retina. *Nature* 397:157–160.

Garbers, D. L., and Lowe, D. G. 1994. Guanylyl cylase receptors. *Journal of Biological Chemistry* 269:30741–30744.

Hayashi, T., Umemori, H., Mishina, M., and Yamamoto, T. 1999. The AMPA receptor interacts with and signals through the protein tyrosine kinase Lyn. *Nature* 397:72–76.

Kim, T. S., Reid, D. M., and Molday, R. S. 1998. Structure-function relationships and localization of the Na/Ca-K exchanger in rod photoreceptors. *Journal of Biological Chemistry* 273:16561–16567.

Krizaj, D., and Copenhagen, D. R. 1998. Compartmentalization of calcium extrusion mechanisms in the outer and inner segments of photoreceptors. *Neuron* 21:249–256.

Laube, B., Kuhse, J., and Betz, H. 1998. Evidence for a tetrameric structure of recombinant NMDA receptors. *Journal of Neuroscience* 18:2954–2961.

Li, P., Wilding, T. J., Kim, S. J., Calejesan, A. A., Huettner, J. E., and Zhuo, M. 1999. Kainate-receptor-mediated sensory synaptic transmission in mammalian spinal cord. *Nature* 397:161–164.

O'Brien, J., Bruzzone, R., White, T. W., Al-Ubaidi, M. R., and Ripps, H. 1998. Cloning and expression of two related connexins from the perch retina define a distinct subgroup of the connexin family. *Journal of Neuroscience* 18:7625–7637.

Perez-Reyes, E., Cribbs, L. L., Daud, A., Lacerda, A. E., Barclay, J., Williamson, M. P., Fox, M., Rees, M., and Lee, J. H. 1998. Molecular characterization of a neuronal low-voltage-activated T-type calcium channel. *Nature* 391:896–900.

Ramanathan, K., Michael, T. H., Jiang, G. J., Hiel, H., and Fuchs, P. A. 1999. A molecular mechanism for electrical tuning of cochlear hair cells. *Science* 283:215–217.

Rivera, C., Viopio, J., Payne, J. A., Ruusuvuori, E., Lahtinen, H., Lamsa, K., Pirvola, U., Saarma, M., and Kaila, K. 1999. The K^+/Cl^- co-transporter KCC2 renders GABA hyperpolarizing during neuronal maturation. *Nature* 397:251–255.

Rosenmund, C., Stern-Bach, Y., and Stevens, C. F. 1998. The tetrameric structure of a glutamate receptor channel. *Science* 280:1596–1599.

Segev, I., and Rall, W. 1998. Excitable dendrites and spines: Earlier theoretical insights elucidate recent direct observations. *Trends in Neurosciences* 21:453–60.

Sutton, R. B., Fasshauer, D., Jahn, R., and Brunger, A. T. 1998. Crystal structure of a SNARE complex involved in synaptic exocytosis at 2.4 Å resolution. *Nature* 395:347–353.

Unger, V. M., Kumar, N. M., Gilula, N. B., and Yeager, M. 1999. Three-dimensional structure of a recombinant gap junction membrane channel. *Science* 283:1176–1180.

Velte, T. J., and Miller, R. F. 1997. Spiking and nonspiking models of starburst amacrine cells in the rabbit retina. *Visual Neuroscience* 14:1073–1088.

Wang, Y., Small, D. L., Stanimirovic, D. B., Morley, P., and Durkin, J. P. 1997. AMPA receptor-mediated regulation of a G_i-protein in cortical neurons. *Nature* 389:502–504.

Index